BATES' GUIDE TO *Physical Examination and History Taking*

BATES' GUIDE TO

Chapter 1: Interviewing and the Health History
revised and expanded by

Elizabeth H. Naumburg, MD

Associate Professor of Family Medicine
University of Rochester School of Medicine and Dentistry
Rochester, New York

Chapter 14: The Pregnant Woman

Joyce Beebe Thompson
CNM, DrPH, FAAN, FACNM

Professor and Director
Graduate Program in Nurse Midwifery
School of Nursing
University of Pennsylvania
Philadelphia, Pennsylvania

Physical Examination and History Taking

Seventh Edition

Lynn S. Bickley, MD

Associate Professor of Medicine
University of Rochester School of Medicine and Dentistry
Rochester, New York

Robert A. Hoekelman, MD

Professor Emeritus of Pediatrics
University of Rochester School of Medicine and Dentistry
Rochester, New York

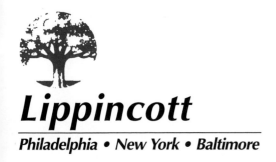

Lippincott

Philadelphia • New York • Baltimore

Acquisitions Editor: Ilze Rader
Associate Managing Editor: Barbara Ryalls
Senior Production Manager: Helen Ewan
Production Coordinator: Mike Carcel
Assistant Art Director: Kathy Kelley-Luedtke
Indexer: Katherine Pitcoff

Edition 7

8 7 6 5 4 3

Library of Congress Cataloging in Publication Data

Bickley, Lynn S.
    Bates' guide to physical examination and history taking / Lynn S.
Bickley, Robert A. Hoekelman. — 7th ed.
        p.   cm.
    Rev. ed. of: A guide to physical examination and history taking /
Barbara Bates, Lynn S. Bickley, Robert A. Hoekelman. 6th ed. c1995.
    Includes bibliographical references and index.
    ISBN 0-7817-1655-1 (alk. paper)
    1. Physical diagnosis.   2. Medical history taking.   I. Hoekelman,
Robert A.   II. Bates, Barbara, 1928–   Guide to physical examination
and history taking.   III. Title.
    [DNLM: 1. Physical Examination—methods.   2. Medical History
Taking—methods.   WB 205B583b   1999]
RC76.B37   1999
616.07'54—dc21
DNLM/DLC
for Library of Congress   98-21795
                                                            CIP

Care has been taken to confirm the accuracy of the information presented and to describe generally accepted practices. However, the authors, editors, and publisher are not responsible for errors or omissions or for any consequences from application of the information in this book and make no warranty, express or implied, with respect to the contents of the publication.

The authors, editors and publisher have exerted every effort to ensure that drug selection and dosage set forth in this text are in accordance with current recommendations and practice at the time of publication. However, in view of ongoing research, changes in government regulations, and the constant flow of information relating to drug therapy and drug reactions, the reader is urged to check the package insert for each drug for any change in indications and dosage and for added warnings and precautions. This is particularly important when the recommended agent is a new or infrequently employed drug.

Some drugs and medical devices presented in this publication have Food and Drug Administration (FDA) clearance for limited use in restricted research settings. It is the responsibility of the health care provider to ascertain the FDA status of each drug or device planned for use in their clinical practice.

To Barbara Bates,

whose clarity of thought and dialogue with readers and colleagues have illuminated the techniques of physical examination and interviewing and guided students to mastery for more than two decades.

Acknowledgments

To Barbara Bates, we extend appreciation for her detailed review of the 6th edition and for her insightful suggestions to improve the organization and text of the 7th edition.

For his extensive contributions to seven editions, we gratefully acknowledge Robert Hoekelman, MD, author of Chapter 19, The Physical Examination of Infants and Children, and the pediatric segments of Chapters 1 and 2, as well a continuing source of inspiration and advice. We extend thanks to Joyce Thompson, CNM, as author of Chapter 14, The Pregnant Woman, and welcome a new contributor, Elizabeth Naumburg, MD, who revised and expanded Chapter 1, Interviewing and the Health History. For their expertise and helpful suggestions, we thank Alexis Abernethy, MD, PhD, Denice Bellinger, PhD, Mel Callan, RNP, James Eichelberger, MD, Erdal Ertuck, MD, Jeffery Harp, MD, Trish Harren, Carl Hoffman, PhD, Suzanne Lee, MD, Joseph Modrak, MD, Eric Naumburg, MD, Randolph Schiffer, MD, David Siegel, MD, Peter Szilagyi, MD, and colleagues at the University of Rochester School of Nursing.

It has been a pleasure to work with a talented team at Lippincott Williams & Wilkins. Ilze Rader, senior editor of the project, has provided gentle guidance and literate critiques, promoting consistency in tone and approach. Susan Blaker has coordinated the art program, a special challenge with this edition, now enriched by color illustrations throughout the text. Mary Norris, as manuscript editor, has improved the style and substance of the text, and Barbara Ryalls, project editor, has orchestrated new additions and color changes with aplomb. Donna Hilton, Vice President and Publisher, has provided oversight from her long experience editing the Guide. We remain grateful to these editors as well as other members of Lippincott Williams & Wilkins who have contributed so much to this edition.

For the color photography illustrating techniques of examination and physical findings, we are grateful to the patience and skill of Royal Chamberlain, medical photographer at the University of Rochester School of Medicine and Dentistry. Able assistance was provided by Diego Cahn-Hidalgo, MD, who recruited many models for examiner and patient and helped to update the bibliography, and by Jeffrey Kaczorowski, MD, who worked on Chapter 19. We are grateful to Claretha Williams, Catherine Farrell, and Patricia Webb for preparation of the manuscript.

Contents

List of Tables

(C) denotes 4-color Tables

Introduction

Bates' Guide to Physical Examination and History Taking is designed for students in health care who are learning to talk with patients, to examine them, and to understand and assess their problems. The first three chapters deal with interviewing and the health history, common and important symptoms, and the assessment of mental status. Subsequent chapters devoted to body regions or body systems review the relevant anatomy and physiology, describe the sequence and techniques of physical examination, identify health promotion issues for screening and counseling, and help the student to recognize selected abnormalities. Two final chapters deal with clinical thinking and organizing the patient's record.

We assume that the students have had basic courses in human anatomy and physiology. Our sections on these subjects are intended to help students apply their knowledge in interpreting symptoms, examining the human body, and understanding physical signs.

Throughout the book, we have emphasized common or important problems rather than the rare and esoteric. Occasionally, a physical sign of a rare disorder has been included when it occupies a solid niche in classic physical diagnosis, or when recognizing the disorder is especially important for the health or even the life of the patient.

Most students will learn their examination skills by practicing first on each other. Most of the anatomy and physiology, some of the techniques, and many of the abnormal findings are common to both adults and children. Dr. Hoekelman's chapter on the examination of infants and children describes variations that occur in the younger age groups together with signs or conditions that are unique to them.

The Seventh Edition

The Seventh Edition marks a milestone for the *Guide to Physical Examination and History Taking*, as it passes from Barbara Bates, MD, to a new editor and author, Lynn Bickley, MD. A keen observer and meticulous editor, Dr. Bates has created a landmark text in the field of physical diagnosis and interviewing, used by healthcare professionals throughout the world. Ever responsive to the probing questions of students, Dr. Bates has brought the highest standards of accuracy and clarity to both content and illustration. Dr. Bickley, contributor to the sixth edition and a recognized teacher and clinician, continues the traditions of excellence that distinguish both layout and text.

As in previous editions, a number of changes make the book easier and more efficient to use. Readers will notice a new look to the *Guide*. Color now demarcates chapter sections more clearly and highlights topic headings and key tables, as well as the narrative of the comprehensive history in Chapter 1, the overview of a comprehensive examination in Chapter 4, and the sample patient write-up in Chapter 21. Four hundred new color photographs and drawings add extra clarity and dimension to techniques of examination and to physical findings, replacing the majority of black-and-white illustrations in previous editions.

Readers will note several changes in the text. Chapter 1, Interviewing and the Health History, now begins with a review of the structure and purposes of the health history, then describes setting the stage before the interview begins, and details the stages of the interview as the patient relates *the medical history*. Chapter 1 has been expanded to include new material pertaining to interviewing, bias and cultural differences, ethical considerations, aging, and language barriers and working with interpreters.

In recognition of the growing importance of evaluating musculoskeletal problems arising from sports-related injuries and aging, Chapter 17, The Musculoskeletal System, has been rewritten to provide more detail on soft tissue and bony structures for each joint in the Anatomy and Physiology sections. In Techniques of Examination readers will find added detail and illustrations on diagnostic maneuvers for assessing each joint and its structures, with relatively less emphasis on range-of-motion. These changes are designed to help students assess musculoskeletal problems of varying origin—soft tissue or bony, mechanical or traumatic.

Finally, in this edition we introduce a new section on Health Promotion and Counseling which follows Techniques of Examination. These sections draw attention to the importance of counseling our patients on key issues of health promotion—risk reduction for skin cancer, detection of deficits in vision and hearing, smoking cessation, control of hypertension and reduction of cardiac risk factors, patient self-examination of the breasts and testicles, and guidelines for mammography and testing for occult blood in the stool. The Health Promotion and Counseling sections also address concerns of growing importance to the health of our population: screening for infections from HIV and sexually transmitted diseases, prevention of osteoporosis, and detection of depression and dementia. Readers are encouraged to peruse three excellent sources for additional information on these topics: *The Guide to Clinical Preventive Services* by the US Preventive Services Task Force (1996), *Health Promotion and Disease Prevention in Clinical Practice* by Woolf et al (1996) and *The Clinician's Handbook on Preventive Services: Put Prevention Into Practice* by the American Nurses Association (1994). The Bibliography of the 7th edition provides additional references to new literature on interviewing, techniques of physical examination and physical diagnosis, and related issues in preventive health care.

Readers of previous editions will again note some changes in techniques and standards. The age-specific adult height-weight tables from Metropolitan have been reintroduced due to weight ranges reflecting size of frame. Transillumination of the sinuses has been discontinued as a routine technique due to its highly variable sensitivity and specificity for underlying sinus conditions. Categories of normal and high blood pressures have again been updated. Routine compression of a woman's nipple for discharge is now found under Special Techniques. In Chapter 18, The Nervous System, the Anatomy and Physiology section has been revised to achieve greater clarity.

Despite these changes, we have retained our basic organization. Students may study or review the Anatomy and Physiology sections according to their individual needs. From the sections on techniques, they can study how to do the examination, then practice it under faculty guidance, and review it again afterward. Techniques indicated for special situations are placed at the end of these sections so that they do not interfere with the flow of the usual examination. Faculty may choose which of these Special Techniques to include in their expectations of students.

Abnormalities appear in two places. The right-hand column of the technique sections introduces students to some common abnormal findings that might be present. Awareness of these findings, compared to the normal, improves the learners' observations. Tables that follow these sections give further information. They display or describe various conditions, enabling students to review, compare, and contrast them in a convenient format. These tables also serve as subsequent references.

Suggestions for Using the Book

Although a health history and a physical examination have somewhat similar goals in patient care, students often learn them separately, even from different faculty members. Nevertheless, interconnections should be made between them. We suggest that, as students learn successive parts of the physical examination, they also read the relevant sections in Chapter 2, "An Approach to Symptoms." In a few areas, the history and the examination do not quite match. Symptoms described under "The Chest" pertain to the chapters on both the thorax and lungs and the cardiovascular system. The symptoms of the urinary tract, moreover, relate to chapters on the abdomen, the prostate, and both male and female genitalia.

As students proceed through the body systems and regions, they should refer periodically to Chapter 4, "Physical Examination: Approach and Overview," and to Chapter 21, "The Patient's Record." They can thereby place their newly learned techniques in the sequence of both doing a comprehensive examination and describing it. A review of Chapter 20, "Clinical Thinking: From Data to Plan," will help them to select and analyze the data that they are learning to collect.

Skimming the tables of abnormalities serves to familiarize students with what they should be looking for and why they are asking certain questions. They should not, however, try to memorize the details that are presented there. The best time to learn about abnormalities and diseases is when a patient (real or described) appears with a problem. The student should then try to analyze the problem with this book, and pursue the subject in as much depth as necessary in other clinical texts or journals.

For relevant sources, see the Bibliography.

Related Learning Material

Bates Pocket Guide to Physical Examination and History Taking, 3rd edition, 1998 by Lynn Bickley and Robert A. Hoekelman is an abbreviated version of this text, designed for portability, review, and convenience. This pocket guide does not stand alone; reference to the text and illustrations of *Bates' Guide to Physical Examination and History Taking* is required for a more comprehensive study and understanding of these subjects. *A Visual Guide to Physical Examination*, 3rd edition, is a series of 12 video tapes available from Lippincott-Raven Publishers.

Equipment

Equipment necessary for a physical examination includes the following:

An ophthalmoscope and an otoscope. If the otoscope is to be used to examine children, it should allow for pneumatic otoscopy.

A flashlight or penlight

Tongue depressors

A ruler and flexible tape measure, preferably marked in centimeters

A thermometer

A watch with a second hand

A sphygmomanometer

A stethoscope with the following characteristics:
- Ear tips that fit snugly and painlessly. To get this fit, choose ear tips of the proper size, align the ear pieces with the angle of your ear canals, and adjust the spring of the connecting metal band to a comfortable tightness.
- Thick-walled tubing as short as feasible to maximize the transmission of sound: about 30 cm (12 inches) if possible and no longer than 38 cm (15 inches)
- A bell and a diaphragm with a good changeover mechanism

Gloves
Lubricant } For vaginal, rectal, and possibly oral examinations

Vaginal specula and equipment for cytological and perhaps bacteriological study

A reflex hammer

Tuning forks, ideally one of 128 Hz and one of 512 Hz

Safety pins or other disposable objects for testing two-point discrimination

Cotton for testing the sense of light touch

Two test tubes (optional) for testing temperature sensation

Paper and pen or pencil

BATES' GUIDE TO Physical Examination and History Taking

Interviewing and the Health History

The health history is a conversation with a purpose. As a clinician you will draw on many of the interpersonal skills that you use every day. But talk with patients has unique and important differences. Unlike other conversations in which you have responsibility largely for yourself, the interview has as its primary goal to improve the well-being of the patient. In the most basic sense, the purpose of the interview is to gather information from the patient, to establish a trusting and supportive relationship with the patient, and to offer information and counselling. Your relationship with the patient is a primary tool in your care of the patient's health. As a beginning clinician your energies will be focused on gathering information. Using the skills that support the relationship, you will allow the patient's story to unfold in its most full and detailed form. Providing emotional support not only enhances the gathering of information but in itself is part of the therapeutic process of patient care.

While listening to the patient's story, the clinician generates a series of hypotheses about the nature of the patient's concerns. The clinician tests these various hypotheses by asking for more detailed information. Eventually, as you gain more health information, you will offer this to the patient in language that the patient can understand. Even if you discover that little can be done for the patient's disease, your discussion with the person about the experience of being ill can be therapeutic. In the example that follows, a research protocol made the patient ineligible for treatment of her long-standing and severe arthritis.

> She had never talked about what the symptoms meant to her. She had never said: "This means that I can't go to the bathroom by myself, put my clothes on, even get out of bed without calling for help."
>
> When we finished (the physical assessment) I said something like: "Rheumatoid arthritis really has not been nice to you." She burst into tears, and her daughter did also, and I sat there, very close to losing it myself.
>
> She said: "You know, no one has ever talked about it as a personal thing before, no one's ever talked to me as if this were a thing that mattered, a personal event."
>
> That was the significant thing about the encounter. I didn't really have much else to offer ... Something really significant had happened between us, something that she valued and would carry away with her.*

* Hastings C: The lived experience of the illness: Making contact with the patient. In Benne P, Wrubel J: The Primacy of Caring: Stress and Coping in Health and Illness. Menlo Park, CA, Addison-Wesley, 1989.

Interviewing patients is much more than gathering pieces of information. Good interviewing requires both the knowledge of what information you need to obtain from the patient and skill in eliciting and responding to the patient's story. This chapter outlines the structure and purposes of the health history and describes a basic approach to interviewing. It explains useful interviewing techniques, suggests ways to address difficult issues, and explores how to talk with patients of different ages and needs. At the end of the chapter, a standard format for recording a comprehensive history for adults and for children covers the range of content you might include.

The Structure and Purposes of the Health History

The scope and focus of the health history vary according to the patient's agenda and problem, the clinician's goals for the visit, and the clinical setting (inpatient or outpatient, amount of time available, specialty or primary care). Often the clinician targets a specific complaint, such as a cough or painful urination; a limited approach tailored to that specific problem may then be indicated. In a primary care setting, the clinician is likely to address specific preventive or health maintenance issues such as smoking or high-risk sexual behaviors. A subspecialist may do an in-depth history to evaluate a specific problem that incorporates several areas of inquiry. In other settings, you will do a comprehensive health history. Knowing the content and relevance of all the components of a comprehensive health history enables you to pick the elements that will help most in evaluating the patient's concern in a context.

The Comprehensive Health History. The comprehensive health history has several parts, each with a specific purpose (see pp. 35–42). Together they give structure to your data collection and to your final record, but their order shown here should not dictate the sequence of the interview.

Selected introductory information in the health history typically precedes the account of the patient's story. *Identifying data,* such as age, birthplace, family members, and occupation, serve not only to establish who the patient is but also to give you basic information about the person you are talking to and what the likely problems might be. When patients do not initiate their own visits, the *source of referral* becomes important. It indicates that a written report may be necessary, and it helps you to understand the patient's possible motivations. Persons seen at the request of school authorities or an insurance company may have different goals than those who come on their own initiative. Under some circumstances, you may also wish to comment on the probable *reliability* of the source of your data. Reliability varies with knowledge, memory, trust, and motivation, among other factors, and is a judgment made at the end of the interaction, not at the beginning. (Note that in the written record, p. 35, introductory information also includes the *date* and, in rapidly changing circumstances, the *time.* The *source of the history,* whether it be the patient, family, friends, a letter of referral, or the past medical record, also deserves comment. It helps you to assess the value and possible biases of the information.)

The main part of the history starts with the patient's *chief complaints.* These are the one or more symptoms or other concerns for which the patient is seeking care or advice. The *present illness* section is the clinician's statement about the scope of the patient's presenting concerns. It amplifies the chief complaints and, in its written form, gives a full, clear, chronologic account of how each of the symptoms developed, their attributes, and their context. The present illness section pulls in relevant aspects of the patient's perspectives and pertinent parts of the *review of systems* (see below). The present illness section also includes how the patient thinks and feels about the illness, what concerns have led to seeking attention, and how the illness has affected the patient's daily life and functions. The *past history* explores childhood illnesses and any history of adult medical illnesses, surgery, obstetric or gynecologic events, and psychiatric conditions. Accidents and injuries, as well as transfusions, may also be included. It is wise to include issues relevant to *health maintenance,* including immunizations and screening examinations, lifestyle issues, and safety practices.

The *family history* helps you to assess the patient's risks of developing certain diseases and may also suggest family experiences relevant to the patient's concerns. The *personal and social history* includes information about the patient's education, family of origin, current household, and personal interests. It helps you in getting to know your patient as a person. It often suggests contributory factors in the patient's illness and helps you to evaluate the patient's sources of support, likely reactions to illness, coping mechanisms, strengths, and fears. Questions relating to the personal and social history should be woven throughout the interview.

In the *review of systems* you ask about common symptoms in each major body system, and thus try to identify problems that the patient has not mentioned. The main purpose of the review of systems is to make sure that you have not missed any important symptoms, particularly in areas that you have not already thoroughly explored while discussing the present illness. A fairly general question that introduces each system, or subset of a system, is helpful. It focuses the patient's attention, allows you to move from the general to the more specific in each system, and on occasion may be all you need to ask. For example:

How are your ears and hearing?
How about your lungs and breathing?
Any trouble with your heart?
How is your digestion? How about your bowels?

As you ask additional questions, the detail needed within each area depends on the patient's age, complaints, general state of health, and the purpose of the visit, among other variables. An older patient, who is at greater risk of heart disease, cancer, and hearing loss, for example, needs more detailed questioning in certain areas than does an apparently healthy 20-year-old.

Some clinicians like to combine the review of systems with the physical examination, asking about the ears, for example, while looking at them. When a patient has few symptoms, this combination can be efficient. When a patient has multiple symptoms, however, the flow of both the history and the examination is disrupted and necessary note taking becomes awkward. If you want to try the combination, it is probably wise to wait until you master the flow of the examination.

While the present illness is usually the single most important part of a history, important data are also discovered in subsequent parts of the interview. The review of systems may uncover material that requires as full an exploration as the present illness. You may learn of a parent's death or a prior illness. Here is a good opportunity to find out what it meant to the patient. "How was it for you then?" or "What were your feelings at the time?" *Keep your technique flexible.* Remember that interviewing the patient is a loosely structured process that you will organize into a written format only after the interview and examination are completed.

Setting the Stage for the Interview

Obtaining a health history requires planning. You are undoubtedly eager to establish contact with the patient, but there are several things to be considered before beginning the interview that are crucial to success.

Reviewing the Chart. Before seeing the patient, review the chart. The medical chart may give you valuable information about past diagnoses and treatments, but it should not prevent you from developing new approaches or ideas. The purpose of reviewing the chart is partly to gather information and partly to develop ideas about what might be explored with the patient. You should look at the identifying data (age, gender, address, health insurance), the problem list, the medication list, and other specific details, such as the documentation of allergies. Remember that the information contained in the chart is shaped by individual observers or by the institution that created the chart format and forms. What you learn from the chart may be incomplete or inconsistent with what you learn from the patient. The chart may not capture the essence of the person whom you are going to meet. If information from the patient and the chart differ, exploring such differences may give you new insights.

Clinician's Tasks. Before seeing a patient the clinician must clarify the goals for the interview. As a student, your goal may be to obtain a complete health history so that you can submit a write-up to your teacher. As a clinician, your goals for the interview may include completing forms needed for the hospital or testing hypotheses you have about the problem based on your review of the chart. A clinician must balance these clinician-centered goals with the goals of the patient. There can be a tension between the needs of the clinician, the needs of the institution, and the needs of the patient and their family. Part of the clinician's task is to keep these multiple agendas in mind. If you think through your goals prior to the interview, it will be easier during the interview to establish a healthy balance between your needs and the patient's.

Clinician's Mindset. As clinicians, we encounter a wide variety of people, each one unique. Establishing relationships with individuals representing a broad spectrum of age, social class, ethnicity, and health to illness is an uncommon opportunity. Being consistently open and respectful of human differences is one of the clinician's challenges. Because we bring our own values and assumptions to every encounter, we must work to clarify for ourselves how our expectations and reactions may affect what we hear and how we behave. *Self-reflection is a continual part of professional development in clinical practice.* The deepening personal awareness that emerges from our work with patients is one of the most rewarding aspects of patient care.

Clinician's Behaviors. Just as you observe the patient throughout the interview, the patient will be watching you. Consciously or not, you send messages through both your words and your behavior. You should be sensitive to those messages and manage them as well as you can. Posture, gestures, eye contact, and words can all express interest, attention, acceptance, and understanding. The skilled interviewer seems calm and unhurried, even when time is limited. Reactions that betray disapproval, embarrassment, impatience, or boredom block communication, as do behaviors that condescend, stereotype, or make fun of the patient. Although negative reactions such as these are normal and understandable, they should not be expressed. Guard against them, not only when talking with patients but also when discussing the patient with your colleagues in the hall or other public places.

Clinician's Appearance. Your personal appearance may also affect the ease with which you establish a relationship. Cleanliness, neatness, conservative dress, and a name tag are reassuring to the patient. Keep the patient's perspective about your appearance in mind. Remember that you want the patient to trust you.

Note Taking. As a novice, you will need to write down much of what you learn in a health history. While an experienced clinician can conduct an interview focused on a few problems without needing to take notes, no one can remember all the details of a comprehensive history. However, note taking should not divert your attention from the patient, nor should a written form prevent you from following your patient's lead. When the patient is talking about sensitive or disturbing material, put your pen down and be especially aware of maintaining eye contact. While eliciting a comprehensive health history, jot down short phrases, specific dates, or words rather than trying to put it into a final format. Most patients are accustomed to note taking, but some may seem uncomfortable with it. If so, explore their concerns and explain your desire to make an accurate record.

The Environment. Make the setting as private and comfortable as possible. Although you may have to talk with the patient under difficult circumstances, such as in a four-bed room or the corridor of a busy emergency department, a proper environment will improve communication. If there are privacy curtains, ask permission to pull them shut. Suggest moving to an empty room rather than having a conversation in a waiting area. *As the clinician, you should make the adjustments in location and seating that are necessary to make the patient and you comfortable.* It is always worth the time.

Learning About the Patient's Illness

Because you have invested time and energy into planning your approach to the patient, you are now fully ready to learn about the present illness and the patient's concerns. In general, an interview moves through stages. *Throughout this sequence you, the clinician, must be attuned to the patient's feelings, support their expression, respond to their content, and validate their significance.* The following stages are typical:

The Stages of the Interview

1. Greeting the patient and establishing rapport
2. Inviting the patient's story
3. Establishing the agenda for the interview
4. Generating and testing hypotheses about the nature of the problem(s) by expanding and clarifying the patient's story
5. Creating a shared understanding of the problem(s)
6. Negotiating a plan (includes further diagnostic evaluation, treatment, and patient education)
7. Planning for follow-up and closing the interview

As a student clinician, you will focus your interview on obtaining the patient's story and creating a shared understanding of the problem. As you become more experienced, the components of negotiating a plan will become more important. Even in a comprehensive health history, the interview should include the elements listed above.

Greeting the Patient and Establishing Rapport. Greet the patient by name and introduce yourself by name. Shake hands with the patient if you feel comfortable doing so. If this is the first contact, clarify your role, such as stating your status as a student and explaining your relation to the patient's care. It is always most appropriate to address the patient with a title, for example, Mr. O'Neil or Ms. Washington. Use of first names should be limited to conversation with a child or adolescent unless you know the patient well or the patient has specifically given you permission. Addressing unfamiliar adults as "granny" or "dear" tends to depersonalize and demean. Often other individuals are present in the room when you are going to conduct an interview. You need to find out the identity and the relationship to the patient of each of these individuals. Be sure to acknowledge and greet each person in turn. *When other individuals are present, ask the permission of the patient to con-*

duct the interview in front of them. State that you welcome the other individuals, but allow the patient to decide. For example, "I am comfortable with having your sister, Mrs. Jones, stay for the interview, but I want to make sure that this is also what you want," or "Would you prefer that I spoke to you alone or with your sister present?"

Arranging the Room. Position yourself at a distance from the patient that enhances comfortable conversation and good eye contact. You should be within several feet, close enough to be intimate but not awkward. Pull up a chair, if possible, and sit so that you are at eye level with the patient. Remember that interpersonal distance varies by culture and personal style. In an outpatient setting, sitting on a rolling stool can help you respond to patient cues. Avoid having physical barriers (e.g., desks, bedside tables) between you and the patient. Arrangements that indicate inequality of power or even disrespect, such as greeting and interviewing a woman while she is lying supine, positioned for a pelvic examination, are unacceptable. Lighting also makes a difference. Avoid sitting between a patient and a bright light or window. Although your view may be fine, the patient must squint uncomfortably toward your silhouette. You unwittingly conduct an interrogation, not a helping interview.

The Patient's Comfort. Be alert to the patient's comfort. In the office or clinic, there should be a suitable place for coats and belongings other than the patient's own lap. In the hospital, inquire how the patient is feeling and whether your visit now is convenient. Watch for indications of discomfort such as poor positioning or evidence of pain or anxiety. An improved position in bed or a brief delay so that the patient can say goodbye to visitors or finish using the bedpan may be the shortest route to a good history.

Establishing Rapport. The initial contact with the patient sets the foundation for the relationship. Be prepared to give your undivided attention. Spend enough time and energy on your greeting and the patient's response to achieve a level of comfort on the part of the patient. Use eye contact and attend to the relative physical position of you, the patient, and any other individuals in the room. As you begin the interview, do not read the chart or take notes.

Inviting the Patient's Story. Once rapport has been established, you need to determine the patient's reason for seeking health care, or the *chief complaint.* Begin your interview with a question that allows full freedom of response, often called an **open-ended question.** "What concerns bring you here today?" or "How can I help you?" After the patient answers, inquire again or even several times, "Anything else?" Note that these questions do not express your point of view or require a simple yes or no answer. When the patient has finished listing all his or her concerns, the next step is to encourage further description of each concern by saying, for example, "Tell me about your headaches."

Patients can seek health care for a routine visit for follow-up for hypertension, a complete physical examination, or a desire to discuss a health-related matter without actually having a specific complaint or problem.

At other times, patients may request a routine examination yet still have specific concerns that they are uncomfortable bringing to the forefront. In all these situations, *it is still important to start with the patient's story.* Additional examples of open-ended questions are, "Are there specific concerns that prompted you to schedule this appointment?" "What made you decide to come for health care now?"

Following the Patient's Leads. Good interviewing technique allows patients to recount their own stories spontaneously. If you intervene too early by asking specific questions prematurely, you risk trampling on the very information you are seeking. Your role, however, is not passive. You should listen actively and watch for clues to important symptoms, emotions, events, and relationships. At the initial part of the interview, using responses called **continuers** works best. They include nonverbal cues such as head nodding and verbal phrases such as "go on" or "I see." Continuing with open-ended questions and facilitative techniques (see p. 12), you will usually be able to obtain a general idea of the patient's principal problems and most of the necessary specifics.

You can then guide the patient into telling you more about the areas that seem most significant. This is done by using **direct questioning.** The process of direct questioning follows several guiding principles. *Questions should proceed from the general to the specific.* A possible sequence, for example, might be, "What was your chest pain like? Tell me more. Where did you feel it? Show me. Anywhere else? Did it travel anywhere? . . . to which fingers?"

Direct questions should not be leading questions. If a patient says yes to "Did your stools look like tar?" you must wonder if the description is the patient's or yours. A better wording is, "What color were your stools?" When possible, *ask questions that require a graded response* rather than a yes or no answer. "How many steps can you climb before getting short of breath?" is better than "Do you get short of breath climbing stairs?"

Sometimes patients seem quite unable to describe their symptoms without help. To minimize bias here, *offer multiple-choice answers.* "Is your pain aching, sharp, pressing, burning, shooting, or what?" Almost any direct question can allow at least two possible answers. "Do you bring up any phlegm with your cough, or is it dry?" *Ask one question at a time.* "Any tuberculosis, pleurisy, asthma, bronchitis, pneumonia?" may lead to a negative answer out of sheer confusion. Try, "Do you have any of the following problems?" and be sure to pause and establish eye contact with each problem listed.

Finally, *use language that is understandable and appropriate* to the patient. Although you might ask a trained health professional about dyspnea, the customary term is shortness of breath. As you learn and increasingly use medical language, it is easy to slip into using it with patients. This blocks communication. Appropriate words for symptoms are suggested in Chapter 2. Whenever possible, however, use the patient's words, *making sure you clarify their meaning.*

Establishing the sequence and time course of the patient's symptoms is important. You can encourage a chronologic account by such questions as "What then?" or "What happened next?" However, you will usually need further specific information to help you in testing the different hypotheses you have about the problem. Fill in the details with more direct questions that ask for specific information not already offered by the patient. *In general, an interview moves back and forth from open-ended questions to directed questions and then on to another open-ended question.*

Establishing an Agenda for the Interview. The clinician often approaches the interview with specific questions in mind. The patient will also have questions and concerns. It is important to identify all of the patient's concerns at the beginning of the encounter. This will help to ensure that everything is addressed, then or in the future. As a student, you may have enough time available to cover the breadth of both your concerns and the patient's concerns in one visit. However, for a clinician, time is almost always an issue. It may be necessary to focus the encounter by asking the patient to identify the one problem that is of most concern. An example of this might be, "You have told me about several different problems that are important for us to discuss. We need to decide which one or two problems to address today. Can you tell me which one is of greatest concern to you?" Stating that the other problems are also important and should be addressed in a future visit helps to establish the expectation of an ongoing collaboration. Then you can proceed with questions such as, "Tell me about that problem."

Generating and Testing Diagnostic Hypotheses. As you learn about the patient's story and the symptoms, you should be generating hypotheses about what body systems might be involved by a pathologic process. You test these theories by asking for specific information. Leg pain, for example, suggests a problem in the peripheral vascular, musculoskeletal, or nervous system. An associated swollen ankle may favor a vascular problem or a musculoskeletal problem when associated with aching joints. A severe pain that shoots down the back of one leg to below the knee indicates pressure on a nerve root.

If the present illness involves pain, for example, it is important to clarify the following elements:

The Seven Attributes of a Symptom
1. Its location. Where is it? Does it radiate?
2. Its quality. What is it like?
3. Its quantity or severity. How bad is it?
4. Its timing. When did (does) it start? How long does it last? How often does it come?
5. The setting in which it occurs, including environmental factors, personal activities, emotional reactions, or other circumstances that may have contributed to the illness
6. Factors that make it better or worse
7. Associated manifestations

Other symptoms should be described in similar terms. These attributes are fundamental in recognizing patterns of disease and differentiating one disease from another. As you learn more about diagnostic patterns, listening for and asking about these attributes will become more automatic. For additional data that will contribute to your analysis, use items from relevant sections of the review of systems. You can thus develop arguments for and against the various diagnostic possibilities. This kind of clinical thinking is illustrated by the tables in Chapter 2 and discussed further in Chapter 20.

Creating a Shared Understanding of the Problem. While the focus of this chapter is on the practical how-to's of patient interviewing, it is useful to have a working understanding of the difference between *illness* and *disease.* This distinction highlights the two different perspectives that should be examined in every good interview, and the need for the patient and the clinician to find common ground. *Illness* can be defined as the patient's experience of symptoms. The patient's perspective may be shaped by many factors, including prior personal or family health experiences, how the symptoms are affecting daily life, concerns about the severity of symptoms, and expectations about medical care. *Disease* is the explanation that the clinician brings to the symptoms. It is the way the clinician organizes what is learned from the patient into a coherent picture that leads to a medical diagnosis. *The health interview needs to take into account both of these views of reality.*

Even a chief complaint as straightforward as a sore throat can illustrate these divergent views. The patient may be most concerned about pain and difficulty in swallowing, a cousin who once was hospitalized with epiglottitis, or missing time from work. The clinician, however, may focus on specific points that differentiate strep pharyngitis from other etiologies and the most cost-effective treatment for a patient with a history of allergy to penicillin.

To satisfy both the patient's expectations and the clinician's agenda, and to provide good health care, the clinician continues beyond the attributes of the symptoms. To learn about the patient's illness, you ask *patient-centered questions* in the six domains listed below.

Eliciting the Patient's Perspective
1. The patient's thoughts about the nature and the cause of the problem
2. The patient's feelings about the problem, especially fears
3. The patient's expectations of the clinician and health care
4. The effect of the problem on the patient's life
5. Similar experiences in the patient's personal or family history
6. Any steps that the patient has taken to address the problem

Ask for the patient's ideas about the cause of the problem ("Why do you think you have this stomach ache?") and for the patient's feelings about the problem ("What worries you most about the pain?"). It may be helpful to ask the patient about prior experiences—"Has anything like this happened to you or your family before?" ("I think I might have an appendicitis. My uncle Charlie died of a ruptured appendix."). Ask what the patient has done so far to take care of the problem (most patients will have tried either over-the-counter medications or traditional remedies or sought advice of others). Inquire as to how the illness has affected the patient's lifestyle and functioning. This question is especially pertinent for a patient with chronic illness. "What can't you do now that you could do before? How has the backache, (shortness of breath, etc.), affected your ability to work? . . . your life at home? . . . your social activities? . . . your role as a parent? . . . your role as a husband or wife? . . . the way you feel about yourself as a person?"

Negotiating a Plan. Learning about the disease *and* conceptualizing the illness provide the opportunity for you and the patient to create a complete picture of the problem. This multifaceted picture then forms the basis for planning further evaluation (e.g., physical examination, laboratory tests, consultations) and negotiating a treatment plan.

Planning for Follow-up and Closing the Interview. You may find that ending the interview is difficult. Patients often have many questions and, if you have done your job well, they are enjoying talking with you. Giving a few minutes' notice before you are out of time can be helpful. Before gathering your papers or standing to leave the room, warn the patient, "We need to stop now. Do you have any questions about what we've covered?" Make sure the patient understands the shared treatment plan you have developed. Reviewing plans for evaluation and follow-up are helpful. "So, you will take the medicine as we discussed, get the blood test before you leave today, and make a follow-up appointment for 4 weeks." Address any fears or concerns that the patient expresses.

Allowing the patient to ask final clarifying questions is important. It is not, however, a time to bring up new topics. If that happens (and the problem is not life threatening), simple reassurance about your interest and plans for a future time to address the problem are appropriate. "That headache sounds concerning. Why don't you make an appointment for next week so we can discuss it." Reaffirming that you will continue to work with the patient to improve his or her health is always important.

The Skills of Good Interviewing

Skillful interviewing relies on the use of learnable techniques. You need to practice these techniques and find ways to be observed or recorded so that you can receive feedback on your progress. The following list describes some of the fundamental skills for enriching the interview as you follow the patient's leads.

Nonverbal Communication. Each of us sends and receives messages all the time that do not involve the use of speech. Becoming more aware of nonverbal communication allows you to use those cues effectively, both to "read" the patient and to send your own messages. Be alert to such attributes as eye contact, body posture, head position and movement (e.g., shaking or nodding), distance from the patient, and placement of arms or legs, such as crossed, neutral, or open. Matching body positions between you and the patient is a sign of increasing rapport. Moving closer to the patient or physical contact can be used to enhance communication of empathy or to help a patient gain control. Bringing nonverbal communication to the conscious level is the first step toward using this crucial form of communication.

Closely related to nonverbal communication is *paralanguage,* the qualities of speech. The pacing, tone, and volume of the patient's speech are all useful to observe, and can be mirrored to increase connection. Paralanguage and the patient's nonverbal communication also provide information about the patient's emotional state.

Facilitation. You use facilitation when by posture, actions, or words you encourage the patient to say more but do not specify the topic. Remaining silent yet attentive and relaxed is a cue for the patient to continue. Leaning forward, making eye contact, saying "Mm-hmm" or "Go on" or "I'm listening" all help the patient to continue.

Reflection. A simple repetition of the patient's words encourages the patient to give you more details. This is useful in eliciting both facts and feelings, as in the following example:

Patient:	The pain got worse and began to spread. (Pause)
Response:	Spread?
Patient:	Yes, it went to my shoulder and down my left arm to the fingers. It was so bad that I thought I was going to die. (Pause)
Response:	Going to die?
Patient:	Yes, It was just like the pain my father had when he had his heart attack, and I was afraid the same thing was happening to me.

This reflective technique has helped to reveal not only the location and severity of the pain but also its meaning to the patient. It did not bias the story or interrupt the patient's train of thought.

Clarification. Sometimes the patient's words are ambiguous or the associations are unclear. If you are to understand their meaning you must request clarification, as in "Tell me exactly what you meant by 'a cold' " or "You said you were behaving just like your mother. What did you mean?"

Summarization. Giving a capsule summary of the patient's story at some point in the interview is a very useful technique. It both indicates to the patient that you have been listening carefully and clarifies what you know and what you don't know. "Now, you said you've been coughing for 3 days, that it's especially bad at night, you are also now bringing up yellow phlegm. You have not had a fever or felt short of breath, but feel congested, with difficulty breathing through your nose. Anything else?" This also allows you, the clinician, to organize your thoughts in the process of diagnostic reasoning.

Validation. Another important way to make a patient feel safe is to legitimize or validate the patient's experience. If a patient who has been in a car accident has no significant physical injury but still is experiencing distress, you may reassure the patient that the experience is normal by stating something like "I can understand that the accident must have been very scary for you, and that may be why you continue to feel unsettled."

Empathic Responses. Expressing empathy is part of establishing a relationship with a patient and is also therapeutic. As patients talk with you they may express—with or without words—feelings they have not consciously acknowledged. These feelings are crucial to understanding their illness and to establishing a trusting relationship. *To empathize with your patient you must first identify the patient's feelings.* When you sense important but unexpressed feelings from the patient's face, voice, words, or behavior, inquire about them rather than assuming how the patient feels. You may simply ask, "How did you feel about that?"

When feelings are expressed, respond with understanding and acceptance. Responses may be as simple as "I understand," "That sounds upsetting," or "You seem sad." Empathy may also be nonverbal—for example, offering a tissue to a crying patient or gently placing your hand on an arm to convey understanding. In using an empathic response, be sure that you are responding correctly to what the patient has expressed. If you have acknowledged how upset a patient must have been at the death of a parent, when in fact the death relieved the patient from a long-standing financial and emotional burden, you have misunderstood the situation.

Reassurance. When you are talking with anxious patients, it is normal to want to reassure them. "Don't worry. Everything is going to be all right." While this may be appropriate in non-professional relationships, in your role as a clinician this approach is usually counterproductive. Unless you and the patient have had a chance to explore the nature of the anxiety, you may well be giving reassurance about the wrong thing. Moreover, premature reassurance blocks further communication. *The first step to effective reassurance involves identifying and accepting the patient's feelings.* This promotes a feeling of security. The final steps come much later in the health-care encounter, after you have completed the interview, the physical examination, and perhaps some laboratory studies. At that point you can interpret for the patient what is happening and deal openly with the real concerns.

Transitions. Patients often feel anxious and vulnerable. One way to make them more at ease is to keep them aware of how you are organizing the flow of the interview, examination, and closing discussion. Sharing this information gives the patient a greater sense of control. As you move from one part of the history to another and through the physical exam, you may orient the patient with brief transitional phrases. "Now I'd like to ask some questions about your past health." Be clear about what the patient should do or expect next. "Now I would like to examine you. I will step out for a few minutes. Please get completely undressed and put on this gown." By specifying whether the gown should open in the front or the back, you may earn the patient's gratitude and save yourself time.

Challenges to the Clinician

Taking a History on Sensitive Topics

Clinicians must ask patients about a variety of subjects that are emotionally laden or culturally sensitive. Initially, these discussions will be particularly difficult, but even experienced clinicians have some discomfort with specific topics. The list of these topics may include use or abuse of alcohol and drugs, sexual orientation or activities, death and dying, financial concerns, racial and ethnic experiences, family interactions, domestic violence, psychiatric illnesses, physical deformities, functioning of the urinary tract and bowel, and others. These areas are difficult to explore, partially because of societal taboos. We all know, for example, that talking about bowel function is not "polite table talk." In addition, there are strongly held cultural, societal, and personal beliefs about many of these topics. Bias about race, drug use, and homosexual practices are three obvious examples of areas that can prompt strong reactions and pose barriers during the interview. The following sections explore these and other important and sometimes sensitive areas, such as domestic violence, the dying patient, and mental illness.

Several basic principles can guide you in approaching any sensitive subject. The single most important rule is to *maintain a nonjudgmental approach*. The clinician's role is to learn about the patient and help the patient achieve better health. Disapproval of behaviors or elements in the health history will only interfere with this goal. Explaining to a patient why you need to know the information and putting it into context helps to orient the patient and allows you to collect your thoughts. For example, explain that "Because sexual practices put people at risk for certain diseases, I ask all of my patients the following questions." You should *use specific language*. Refer to genitalia with explicit words such as penis or vagina and avoid talking about "private parts." Make sure that the patient understands the words you may use. "By intercourse, I mean when a man inserts his penis into a woman's vagina." Familiarize yourself with some opening questions on sensitive topics and learn the additional kinds of data you need to make the desired assessments.

Other ways to become more comfortable with sensitive areas include: general reading about these topics in the medical and lay literature; talking to selected colleagues and teachers openly about your concerns; special courses that assist you in exploring your own feelings and reactions to these sensitive topics; and ultimately, your own life experience. Take advantage of all of these resources. Whenever possible, listen to experienced clinicians as they discuss such subjects with patients, and then try exploring some of these areas yourself. It is particularly important for you to actually practice talking about sensitive areas with patients. The range of topics that you can explore with comfort will widen progressively.

Bias and Cultural Differences. Developing the ability to interact with patients of many backgrounds is a lifelong professional goal. Review the examples below, which illustrate how unconscious bias and cultural differences can influence patient care.

> A 28-year-old cab driver from Ghana who had recently moved to the United States complained to a friend from home about U.S. medical care. He had gone to the clinic because of fever and fatigue. He described being weighed, having his temperature taken, and having a cloth wrapped tightly, to the point of pain, around his arm. The clinician, a 36-year-old African American from Washington, D.C., had asked him many questions, examined him, and wanted to take blood—which the patient had refused. His final comment was ". . . and she didn't even give me chloroquine!"—his primary reason for seeking care. The man from Ghana was expecting few questions, no exam, and treatment for malaria, which is what fever usually means in Ghana.

This example of how different expectations based on different countries of origin can lead to ineffective health care is a readily understandable and nonthreatening illustration of cross-cultural miscommunication. However, cross-cultural communication occurs in many clinical interactions and is usually more subtle.

> A 16-year-old African American high school student from a lower socioeconomic urban community came to the local teen health center because of painful menstrual cramps that were interfering with school. The clinician, a 30-year-old European American from a middle-class suburb, asked many questions that reflected incorrect assumptions. "So are you planning to finish high school? . . . What kind of job do you want then? . . . What kind of birth control do you want?" The teenager felt pressured to accept birth control despite stating clearly that she had not had intercourse, and didn't plan to until she was older, and married. She was an honor student and athlete planning to go to college and graduate school, but these goals were not uncovered. The issue of cramps was given little attention by the clinician— "Oh, you can just take some ibuprofen. They usually get better as you get older." The patient will not take the birth control pills that were prescribed nor will she seek health care soon again. She has experienced ineffective health care due to cross-cultural misunderstanding and clinician bias.

The failure in both of the cases above is due to the clinician's assumptions or biases. In the first case, the clinician did not take into account the many variables that can shape a patient's beliefs about health and attitudes toward medical care. In the second case, the clinician allowed stereotypes to dictate the agenda instead of listening to and respecting the patient as an individual. As individuals we each have our own cultural background and biases. These do not simply slip away as we become clinicians. As you encounter an expanding array of patient concerns, behaviors, and backgrounds, it is important to understand how culture shapes not just the patient's beliefs and behaviors but our own.

Culture is a system of shared ideas, rules, and meanings which individuals inherit or acquire that tells them how to view the world, how to experience it emotionally, and how to behave in relation to other people and to the environment. It can be understood as the "lens" through which individuals perceive and make sense out of the world they inhabit. While learning about specific cultural groups is important, without a framework it may lead to developing a series of stereotypes. Work on an appropriate and informed clinical approach to all patients *by becoming aware of your own biases and values, developing communication skills that transcend cultural differences, and building therapeutic partnerships based on respect for the patient's life experiences.* This framework will allow you to approach each patient as unique and distinct.[†]

Self-Awareness. Start by exploring your own cultural identity. How do you define yourself by ethnicity, class, region, religion, political affiliation . . .? Don't forget the characteristics that we often take for granted—gender, life roles, sexual orientation, physical ability, race—especially if we are in majority groups. What aspects of your family of origin do you identify with and how are you different from your family of origin?

Another, more challenging, part of learning about yourself is the task of bringing your own values and biases to a conscious level. *Values* are the standards we use to measure beliefs and behaviors, which may appear to be absolutes. *Biases* are the attitudes or feelings that we attach to the awareness of difference. Being attuned to difference is a normal, and in the distant past, life-preserving ability. Intuitively knowing members of one's own tribe is a survival skill that societally we have outgrown but is still actively at work. We often feel so guilty about our biases that it is hard to recognize and acknowledge them. Start with less threatening constructs, like the way an individual relates to time. This can be a culturally determined phenomenon. Are you always on time?—a positive value in the dominant Western culture. Or do you tend to run a little late? How do you feel about people who have the opposite habit from you? Next time you attend a meeting or class, notice who is early, on time, or late. Is it predictable? Think about the role of physical appearance. Do you consider yourself thin, medium, or heavy? How do you feel about your weight? What does prevailing U.S. culture teach us to value in body habitus? How do you feel about people who have different weights?

Learning About Others. Given the complexity of culture, no one can possibly know the health beliefs and practices of every culture and subculture. Therefore, remember that the patients you are working with are

---

[†] This approach reflects the conceptual framework of the Cross-Cultural Education Committee at the University of Rochester School of Medicine and Dentistry.

experts on their own unique cultural perspectives. Patients may not be able to identify or define their values or beliefs in the abstract, but should be able to respond to specific questions. Find out about the patient's cultural background. Use some of the same questions discussed in "eliciting the patient's perspective" (see p. 10). Maintain an open, respectful, and inquiring stance. "What did you hope to get from this visit?" If you have established rapport and trust, patients will be willing to teach you. Be ready to acknowledge your ignorance or bias. "I know very little about Ghana. What would have happened at a clinic there if you had these concerns?" Or, with the second patient and with much more difficulty, "I mistakenly made assumptions about you that are not right. I apologize. I must have some biases about teenage girls of color that I need to work on. Would you be willing to tell me more about yourself and your future goals?"

Learning about specific cultures is still valuable because it helps to expand what you, as a clinician, identify as areas you need to explore. Do some reading about the life experiences of ethnic or racial groups that live in your region. Go to movies that are made in different countries or explicitly present the perspective of different groups. Learn about the perspectives and concerns of different consumer groups with visible health agendas. Seek out healers of different disciplines and establish collegial relationships with them. Most importantly, be open to learning from your patients.

Building a Partnership. Through continual work on self-awareness and an active attempt to learn about the "lens" of others, the clinician lays the foundation for the collaborative relationship that will best support the health of the patient. Creating communication that is based on trust, respect, and a willingness to reexamine assumptions will allow patients to express aspects of their concerns that may run counter to the dominant culture. These concerns may be associated with strong feelings such as anger or shame. You, the clinician, must be willing to listen to and validate these feelings, and not let your own feelings prevent you from exploring painful areas. You must also be willing to reexamine your beliefs about what is the right approach to clinical care in a given situation. A willingness to be flexible and creative in your plans, a respect for patients' knowledge about their own best interests, and a conscious effort to clarify the truly acute or life-threatening risks to the patient's health are helpful approaches. Remember that if the patient stops listening, doesn't follow your advice, or doesn't return, your partnership has not been successful.

Alcohol and Drugs. One difficult area for many clinicians is asking patients about their use of alcohol and drugs, illegal or prescription. Yet alcohol and drugs are often directly related to a patient's symptoms, and the use of or dependence on a substance may affect future care. Remember that it is not your role to disapprove of the use of substances. It is your job to gather data, assess the impact on the patient's health, and plan a response.

Questions about alcohol and other drugs follow naturally after questions about coffee and cigarettes. "How much alcohol do you drink?" or "Tell me about your use of alcohol" are good opening questions that avoid the easy yes or no response. Learning about alcohol consumption is always relevant to complaints of abdominal pain. Asking about alcohol use may not be very helpful in detecting an alcohol problem. For this purpose, try two additional questions: "Have you ever had a drinking problem?" and "When was your last drink?" An affirmative answer to the first question, along with a drink within 24 hours, has been shown in at least one study to suggest a drinking problem. (Cyr MG, Wartman SA: The effectiveness of routine screening questions in the detection of alcoholism. JAMA 259:51–54, 1988)

Four other questions, known as the CAGE questions, are also helpful in detecting alcoholism. Their name comes from their themes of **C**utting down, **A**nnoyance by criticism, **G**uilty feelings, and **E**ye-openers.

The CAGE Questionnaire

Have you ever felt the need to Cut down on drinking?
Have you ever felt Annoyed by criticism of drinking?
Have you ever had Guilty feelings about drinking?
Have you ever taken a drink first thing in the morning (Eye-opener) to steady your nerves or get rid of a hangover?

Adapted from Mayfield D, McLeod G, Hall P: The CAGE questionnaire: Validation of a new alcoholism screening instrument. Am J Psychiatry 131:1121–1123, 1974.

Two or more affirmative answers suggest alcoholism. They also suggest further lines of inquiry. If indicated, ask about blackouts (loss of memory for events during drinking), seizures, accidents or injuries while drinking, and job losses, marital problems, or arrests. Mixing alcohol use and driving or operating machinery should be addressed specifically.

Questions about drugs take a similar pattern. "How much marijuana do you use? cocaine? heroin? other illegal drugs? How about prescription drugs such as sleeping pills? diet pills? pain-killers?" And further:

How do you feel when you take it?
Have you had any bad reactions? What happened?
Any drug-related accidents, injuries, or arrest? Job or family problems?
Have you ever tried to quit?

Addressing this area with adolescents can be even more challenging. It may be helpful to ask first about the use of such substances by friends or family members. "A lot of young people are using drugs these days. How about at your school? your friends?" After patients have found your response nonjudgmental and concerned, they may feel more comfortable telling you about their own patterns of use.

Remember that alcohol and drug use can start at young ages. These topics should be introduced, along with tobacco use, in front of the parent at age 6 or 7. Also, remember that drug use, in particular IV drug use, relates to the risk for a variety of other diseases, including HIV disease and hepatitis.

The Sexual History. Asking questions about sexual function and practices serves at least four purposes. (1) Sexual practices determine the risk of unwanted pregnancy and sexually transmitted diseases, including AIDS. Discussion may lead to preventing disease. (2) Sexual practices may be directly related to specific symptoms, and they need to be understood for diagnostic, therapeutic, and preventive reasons. (3) Many patients have questions or problems about sexuality that they would like to discuss with a professional if given the opportunity. Even if they choose not to discuss these questions on the first visit, they may feel free to do so at a later time if you have introduced the topic. (4) Sexual dysfunction is sometimes the consequence of medication which, if recognized, may be readily addressed.

Questions about sexual functions or practices may be relevant at multiple points in a patient's history. Sexual practices may be part of the lifestyle issues covered in the Personal and Social History, or for women may be covered in the Obstetric/Gynecologic history. If a patient's chief complaint involves genitourinary symptoms, a sexual history is included in the Present Illness section. Questions about sexuality can be an expansion of asking about the important relationships in the person's life, or specifically introduced as part of the Health Maintenance questions similar to those about drug use, diet, and exercise. Whenever a person has a chronic illness or serious symptoms such as pain or shortness of breath, sexual function may be affected. Asking about it in the context of other effects on the patient's life is a natural sequence of inquiry.

An *orienting sentence* or two is often helpful. "Now, to figure out why you have this discharge and what we should do about it, I need to ask you some questions about your sexual activity." If there have been no apparent sex-related complaints, a different introduction is indicated. "I'd like to ask you some questions about your sexual health and practices."

Questions about the patient's specific sexual behaviors and satisfaction with sexual function can both be addressed. Specific questions that should be addressed include:

1. "When was the last time you had intimate physical contact with anyone?" "Did that contact include sexual intercourse?" Using the term "sexually active" can be ambiguous. Patients have been known to reply, "No, I just lie there."
2. "Do you have sex with men, women, or both?" The health implications of heterosexual, homosexual, or bisexual relationships are significant.
3. "How many sexual partners have you had in the last 6 months?" Again, this question assumes that the patient may have had more than one partner. It is not meant to insult patients but to provide them with the easy opportunity to acknowledge multiple partners.

4. If the patient is engaged in heterosexual activity, it is important to ask both men and women about the use of birth control, and specifically the use of condoms. "What birth control are you currently using?" If the patient responds that he or she is not using any birth control, follow up with "Are you currently trying to become a parent?"
5. "Are you satisfied with your sexual function?"
6. "Are you concerned about HIV disease or AIDS?" This question, then, gives you an opportunity to ask about the specific behaviors that put a patient at risk for HIV disease, and to review those behaviors.

Note that these questions make no assumptions about marital status, sexual preference, or attitudes toward pregnancy or contraception. Listen to each of the patient's responses, and ask additional questions as indicated.

Remember that sexual behavior, too, can start at a young age. Introducing sexuality and encouraging parents to talk to their children about sexual behaviors at an early age are appropriate. It is often easier to discuss these normal physiologic functions with children before they have been heavily socialized outside the home. Because sexual behaviors of adolescents are often kept secret from parents, clinicians must be sensitive to the need for patient confidentiality, as discussed in the section about talking with adolescents (see p. 26).

Domestic and Physical Violence. Because of the high incidence of physical, sexual, and emotional abuse in our society, routine screening of all female patients for domestic violence is currently recommended. While not all victims of physical and sexual abuse are female, women are at a much greater risk. Initiating this part of the interview by indicating that the problem is common creates a context to normalize the questions. "Because violence is common in many women's lives, I've begun to ask about it routinely." "Are there times in your relationships that you feel unsafe or afraid?" "Many women tell me that someone at home is abusing or hurting them. Is this true for you?" "Are you currently in a relationship in which you have been physically hurt or threatened?"

Physical abuse—often not mentioned by the victim or the perpetrator—should be considered (1) when injuries are unexplained, seem inconsistent with the patient's story, are concealed by the patient, or cause embarrassment; (2) when the patient has delayed getting treatment for trauma; (3) when there is a past history of repeated injuries or "accidents"; and (4) when the patient or person close to the patient has a history of alcohol or drug abuse. At times, the behavior of the abuser raises suspicion: he (she) tries to dominate the interview, will not leave the room, or seems unusually anxious or solicitous. It is important in such situations to spend part of the interview alone with the patient.

Child abuse is also common in our culture. Asking parents about their approach to discipline is a normal part of well-child care. Another approach to consider is talking about how parents cope with the normal experience of babies who won't stop crying or children who have been misbehaving. "Most parents get very upset when their baby cries (or their child has been naughty). How do you feel when your baby cries?" "What do you do when your baby won't stop crying?" "Do you have any fears that you might hurt your child?" You should also inquire about other caretakers or people the child spends time with to explore possibilities of both physical and sexual abuse.

Mental Illness. Our society and many cultures have ingrained beliefs about mental illness that separate it and treat it differently than physical illness. Think about how easily people talk about diabetes and taking insulin compared to discussions of schizophrenia and the use of chlorpromazine. Asking specific questions about a history of mental illness in the individual patient and the family should include both open-ended questions—"Have you ever had any problem with emotional or mental illnesses?"—and specific questions about treatments—"Have you ever visited a counselor or psychotherapist?" "Have you or anyone in your family ever been hospitalized for an emotional or mental health problem?"

Many patients with schizophrenia or other psychotic disorders are able to function in the community. Such patients are frequently capable of telling you freely about their diagnoses, their symptoms, their hospitalizations, and their current medications. You should feel comfortable inquiring about these without embarrassment or circumlocution. You should always assess the degree to which symptoms are causing distress.

While *depression* is known to be a common problem with effective treatments, it is still underdiagnosed and undertreated, even among patients who are receiving health care. Some clinicians advocate screening all patients for depression. While this had not been accepted universally, it is important to be alert to the possibility of depression. Mood change might not be the presenting symptom; you should always ask about the specific symptoms of depression in patients who have fatigue, vague symptoms, weight loss, insomnia, or other clues to poor functioning. Two open-ended questions to use are, "How have your mood or spirits been over the past month?" and "What about your level of interest or pleasure in each day's activities?" To diagnose depression you must actively consider it as a possibility, identify it by knowing the typical symptoms, and explore its manifestations. Be sure you know how severe the depression is by asking for thoughts of suicide. "Have you ever thought about hurting yourself or ending your life?" Just as you would evaluate the severity of chest pain, you must evaluate the severity of depression. Both are potentially lethal.

Death and the Dying Patient. In communicating with fatally ill or dying patients, clinicians are at risk of avoiding the subject of death because of their own discomforts and anxieties. With the help of reading and discussion, you will need to work through your own feelings. As in any clinical situation, it is helpful to know what reactions the patient is likely to have.

Kübler-Ross has described five stages in a patient's response to impending death: denial and isolation, anger, bargaining, depression or preparatory grief, and acceptance. These stages may come sequentially or in different times and combinations. At each stage, your approach is basically the same. Be alert to the feelings of such patients and to cues that they want to talk about their feelings. Help them to bring out their concerns with nondirective techniques. Make openings for them to ask questions: "I wonder if you have any concerns about the operation? . . . your illness? . . . how it will be when you go home?" Explore these concerns and provide whatever information the patients request. Be wary of inappropriate reassurance. If you can explore and accept the patients' feelings, if you can answer the patients' questions, if you can assure and demonstrate your ability to stay with the patients throughout the illness, reassurance will grow where it really matters—within the patients themselves.

Fatally ill or dying patients rarely want to talk about their illnesses all the time, nor do they wish to confide in everyone they meet. Give such patients opportunities to talk, and listen receptively, but if the patient prefers to keep the conversation on a lighter plane you need not feel like a failure. *Remember that illness—even a terminal one—is only one small part of personhood.* A smile, a touch, an inquiry after a family member, a comment on the day's ball game, or even some gentle humor all recognize and reinforce other parts of the patient's individuality and help sustain the living person. To communicate appropriately, you have to get to know the patient; that is part of the helping process.

Understanding how a patient wishes to be treated at the end of life is an important part of a clinician's role. In general, however, our society avoids death and, in health care, it is usually seen as a failure. These factors, in addition to your own discomfort, may make it difficult for you, but this should not prevent you from asking specific questions. The health of the patient and the context of care will partially determine what needs to be discussed. With an ill patient in an acute hospital setting, the need to find out what a patient wants done in the event of a cardiac or respiratory arrest is usually mandatory. Asking about "DNR status" (Do Not Resuscitate) is often made more difficult by the lack of an established relationship with the patient and little knowledge of the patient's personal values or life experience. Patients may also have unrealistic beliefs about the effectiveness of resuscitation based on programming in the media. Find out about the patient's frame of reference. "What experiences have you had with the death of a close friend or relative?" "What do you know about cardiopulmonary resuscitation?" Educate patients about the likely success of cardiopulmonary resuscitation, especially in chronically ill or older patients. Assure them that attending to physical needs such as pain will be a priority.

In general, encouraging any adult, but more specifically the elderly or those with chronic illness, to complete health proxies or living wills is an important task. You can do this as part of a *values history*. A values history is a part of the interview aimed at finding out what is important to patients, what makes their life worth living, and at what point their life would no longer be worth living. Asking questions about how they spend their time on a daily basis, what brings them joy, and what they look forward to are useful. Make sure to clarify the specific meaning of any statements. "You said that you don't want to be a burden to your family. What exactly do you mean by that?" In addition, exploring any religious or spiritual framework the patient may believe in or practice is important in understanding how you and the patient can make the most appropriate decisions about health care.

Sexuality in the Clinician–Patient Relationship

Clinicians of both sexes will occasionally find themselves attracted to their patients. The emotional and physical intimacy of the clinician–patient relationship may make sexual feelings more likely to occur. If you become aware of such feelings, accept them as normal human responses, and think about them consciously to prevent them from affecting your behavior. If you deny these feelings, you are more likely to act inappropriately. Any sexual contact or romantic relationship with patients is entirely unethical; keep your relationship with the patient within professional bounds.

Occasionally, clinicians may meet patients who are frankly seductive or make sexual advances. Calmly but firmly, you should make clear that your relationship is professional, not personal. You may also wish to review your image. Have you been overly warm with the patient? Expressed your affection physically? Sought his or her emotional support? Has your clothing or demeanor been unconsciously seductive? It is your responsibility to avoid these problems.

Ethical Considerations

The area of medical ethics is broad, complex, and usually considered in the context of treatment decisions and research. But if you remember the importance of the clinician–patient relationship as a therapeutic alliance and the central role of the patient interview in creating that alliance, you will more readily understand the need to be guided by three fundamental principles: Nonmaleficence, Beneficence, and Autonomy.

Nonmaleficence or *primum non nocere* is commonly stated as "First, do no harm." In the context of an interview, harm can be done by giving information that is incorrect or not really related to the patient's problem. Harm can also be done by avoiding relevant topics or creating barriers to open communication. The degree to which a patient can communicate most fully his or her experiences, thoughts, and feelings helps to determine the accuracy of your assessment. **Beneficence** is the dictum that the clinician needs to "do good" for the patient. As clinicians, our actions need to be motivated by what is in the patient's best interest. This principle must be linked to *autonomy*, which is the patients' right to determine what is best for themselves.

As you can readily see, these principles can create challenges when deciding on the best course of action. A patient's ability to understand the medical thinking about a given situation and the ability of a clinician to understand the patient's perspective are integrally related.

Patients at Different Ages

As people develop, have families, and age, they provide you with special opportunities and require certain adaptations in your interviewing style.

Caring for Children

Unlike adults who frequently receive health care as individuals, children usually appear with a parent or caregiver. Even if adolescents come in alone, they are often seeking health care at the request of their parents—indeed, the parent is often sitting in the waiting room. This aspect of caring for children calls for some specific clinician approaches. You need to consider the needs and perspectives of both the child and the caregivers. In addition, because so much of the care of children is in the context of "well child care," the clinician may also have a set agenda such as immunizations, anticipatory guidance, or developmental assessment. The specific approaches related to caring for children expand on themes covered earlier in this chapter.

Establishing Rapport. With children, as with adults, begin the interview by greeting and establishing rapport with each person present. Refer to the infant or child by name rather than by "him," "her," or "the baby." Clarify the role or relationship of all of the adults and children. "Now, are you Jimmy's grandmother?" When the family structure is not immediately clear, you may avoid embarrassment by asking directly about other members. "Who else lives in the home?" "Who is Jimmy's father?" "Do you live together?" Address the parents as "Mr. Smith" and "Ms. Smith" rather than by their first names or "Mom" or "Dad." First names may be used with permission when you have established a reasonably long-standing relationship.

Establishing rapport with a 2-year-old is obviously different from establishing rapport with a 25-year-old. *The key here is to meet children on their level.* Use your personal experiences with interacting with children in other settings as a guide for how to engage children in the health-care context. Eye contact on their level (for example, sit on the floor if needed), playful engagement, and talking about what interests them are always helpful guides. Ask children about their clothes, a toy they have, what book or TV show they like, or their adult companion in an enthusiastic but gentle style. Spending time at the beginning of the interview to calm down and connect with an anxious child or crying infant can put both the child and the caregiver at ease.

Working With Families. One of the biggest challenges in working with more than one person is being conscious of where you direct your questions. While eventually you need to get information from both the child and the parent(s), it is useful to start with the child, if he or she is verbal. Even at the age of 3, some children can tell you the specific problem. Asking simple, open-ended questions—"Are you sick? . . . Tell me about it."—followed by more specific questions can often give you much of the history of the present illness. The parents can then verify the information, tell you additional details that give you the larger context, and identify other specific issues you need to address. Sometimes children are embarrassed to begin, but once the parent has started the conversation you can direct the questions back to the child.

> Your mother tells me that you get a lot of stomach aches. Tell me about them.
> Show me where you get the pain. What does it feel like?
> Is it a pin prick, or does it ache?
> Does it stay in the same spot, or does it move around?
> Anything else about feeling sick?
> What helps make it go away?
> What do you think causes it?
> How about missing school a lot?

In addition to the specific communication between clinician, patient, and family, the presence of multiple family members provides a rich opportunity to observe the interactions. While you talk with the parent, see how a young child relates to a new environment. It is normal for a toddler to open drawers, pull at paper, and wander around the room. An older child may be able to sit still or may get restless and start fidgeting. You may see specific examples of how the parents set limits on the child's actions or fail to when they should.

Multiple Agendas. As discussed earlier, each individual in the room, including the clinician, may have a different idea of the nature of the problem and what needs to be done about it. It is your job to discover as many of these perspectives and agendas as possible. In addition, family members who are not present (the absent parent or grandparent) may also have concerns. It is a good idea to ask specifically about those concerns. "If Suzie's father were here today, what questions or concerns would he have?" "Have you, Mrs. Jones, discussed this with your mother or anyone else?" "What does she think?" Mrs. Jones brings Suzie in for abdominal pain because she is worried that Suzie may have an ulcer. She is also worried about Suzie's eating habits. Suzie is not worried about the belly pain. It rarely interferes with what she wants to do. She is, however, worried about the changes in her body, especially her belief that she is getting fat. Mr. Jones thinks that Suzie's school work is not getting enough attention. You, as the clinician, need to balance these concerns with what you see as a healthy, 12-year-old girl in early puberty with some mild functional abdominal pain. Your goals need to include your agenda of helping the family to develop a realistic attitude toward the range of normal. You also need, however, to specifically address the concerns of Mr. and Mrs. Jones and Suzie.

The Family as Resource. Much of the information you obtain about a child will come from the family. In addition, most of the care provided to the child, both explicitly health related and in general, is provided by the family. *They are your major allies in caring for this child.* Recognizing the range of what is normal in parenting behavior will help you establish this alliance. Raising a child is not a medically defined task. It is determined by cultural, socioeconomic, and family practices. As clinicians, we know some specific approaches that enhance a child's healthy growth and development, and some specific approaches that are harmful. Beyond that, there is huge variation. Your ability to develop an alliance with the parents or caretakers will be most successful if you respect those limits. In addition, taking the stance that the parents are the experts in the care of their child and that you are there as a consultant will minimize the potential for parents to discount or ignore advice that they are given. There is a lot at stake for most parents as they try to cope with the problems of their children, so health practitioners who are supportive rather than judgmental are needed. Comments like, "Why didn't you bring him in sooner?" or "What did you do that for!" will not improve your rapport with a parent. Statements acknowledging the hard work of parenting and praising successes are always appreciated.

Hidden Agendas. Finally, as with adults, the chief complaint may not relate to the real reason the parent has brought the child to see you. The complaint may serve as a "ticket to care" or bridge to concerns that may not seem legitimate reasons for seeking care. Try to create an open and trusting atmosphere that allows parents to express all their concerns. If necessary, ask questions that will facilitate the process.

> Are there any other concerns with Johnny that you would like to tell me about?
> What did you hope I would be able to do for you today?
> Was there anything else that you wanted to tell/ask me today?

Talking with Adolescents

Adolescents, like most other people, will usually respond positively to anyone who demonstrates a genuine interest in them. It is important to show interest early and then sustain the connection if communication is to be effective. Adolescents are more likely to open up when the focus of the interview is on themselves and not on their problems. In contrast to most interviews, start with specific direct questions to build trust and rapport and get the flow of conversation going. You may have to do more talking than usual. A good way to begin the interview with adolescents is to chat informally about their friends, school, hobbies, and family. Using silence in an attempt to get adolescents to talk or asking about feelings directly is usually not a good idea. It is particularly important to use orienting (see p. 19) and transitional statements (see p. 13) and explain what you are going to do during the physical exam. The physical can be an opportunity to get the young person talking. Once rapport has been established, return to more open-ended questions. Make sure at that point to ask what concerns or questions the adolescent may have.

Remember also that adolescents' behavior is related to their developmental stage, not necessarily chronologic age or physical development. Their age and appearance may fool you into, assuming that they are functioning on a more future-oriented and realistic level. The reverse can also be true, especially in teens with delayed puberty or chronic illness.

Issues of *confidentiality* become important as children enter adolescence. Explain to both parents and adolescents that the best health care allows adolescents some degree of independence and confidentiality. It helps if the clinician starts asking the parent to leave the room for part of the interview when the child is 10 or 11. This prepares both caregivers and young people for future visits when the patient spends time alone with the clinician.

Speaking alone with an adolescent or a child should be done only after you have taken certain steps. Before the parent leaves the room, get relevant medical history from the parent (the patient may not know certain elements of past history) and clarify the parent's agenda for the visit. Also discuss confidentiality. *You should explain to both parents and children that confidentiality is to improve health care, not to keep secrets.* Adolescents need to know that what they discuss with you will be held in confidence. However, never offer unlimited confidentiality. Always be explicit that you may need to act on information that makes you concerned about the safety of the adolescent. "I will not tell your parents what we talk about, unless you give me permission or I am concerned about your safety—for example, if you talk to me about killing yourself and I think that there is a risk that you would actually try it."

Your goal as clinician is to help adolescents bring their concerns or questions to their parents whenever that is safe and realistic. Encourage adolescents to discuss sensitive issues with their parents, and offer to be present or help. While young people may believe that their parents would "kill them if they only knew," you may be able to promote more open dialogue. This takes a careful assessment of the parents' perspective and the full and explicit consent of the young person.

Aging Patients
At the other end of life's cycle, aging patients also have special needs and concerns. Their hearing and vision may be impaired, their responses may be slow, and they often have chronic illnesses with associated disabilities. For several reasons, elderly people may not report their symptoms. Some may be afraid or embarrassed to do so. Others may be trying to avoid the medical expenses or the discomforts of diagnosis and treatment. They may think their symptoms are merely a form of the aging process, or may simply have forgotten about them. Aging patients also may tell their histories more slowly than younger patients.

Give an elderly person extra time to respond to your questions if needed. Speak slowly and clearly but do not shout or raise your voice. A comfortable room, free of distractions and noise, is helpful. Ask to turn off the radio or television. Remember that visual cues may be more important, so make sure that your face is well lit. Do not try to accomplish everything in one visit. Multiple visits may be less fatiguing and more productive.

From middle age on, people become increasingly aware of their personal aging and may begin to measure their lives in terms of the years left rather than the years lived. It is normal for older people to reminisce about the past and to reflect upon previous experience, including joys, regrets, and conflicts. Listening to this process of life review can give you important insights and provide opportunities for you to support patients in working through painful feelings or recapturing experiences of joy or accomplishment.

While generalizations about elderly people are useful, you must recognize and avoid stereotypes that can block your understanding and enjoyment of each individual patient. Work to determine the unique priorities and goals of each patient. Learn how patients have handled problems in the past. Because they may pursue similar adaptive patterns in the present situation, this knowledge will help you plan with them. Find out how they perceive themselves and their situation. "Can you tell me how you feel about getting older? What kinds of things do you find most satisfying? What kinds of things worry you? What would you change if you could?"

Learning how elderly people (and others with chronic illness) function in their daily lives is essential to your understanding of and care for them. Establishing their level of function also provides a baseline for future comparisons. There are two standard categories of assessment, *physical activities of daily living* (ADLs) and *instrumental activities of daily living* (IADLs).

Activities of Daily Living (ADL)	
Physical ADLs	**Instrumental ADLs**
Bathing	Using the telephone
Dressing	Shopping
Toileting	Food preparation
Transfers	Housekeeping
Continence	Laundry
Feeding	Transportation
Taking medicine	Managing money

Can the patients perform the activities of daily living independently, do they need some help, or are they entirely dependent? Instead of asking about each area separately, have the patient go through a typical day, *in detail*. Start with an open-ended request—"Tell me about your day yesterday"—and then guide the story to a greater level of detail. "You got up at 8? How is it getting out of bed?" "What did you do next?" Ask how things have changed, who is available for help, and who actually does what to help. Keep safety as an important priority. Remember that increasing dependence on others is difficult for most people to accept.

Situations That Call for Specific Responses

Regardless of patient age, certain behaviors and special situations may particularly vex or perplex the practitioner. Your skills in handling these problems will evolve over a lifetime. *Always remember the importance of listening to the patient and clarifying the patient's agenda.*

Silence. Novice interviewers may grow uncomfortable during periods of silence, feeling somehow obligated to keep the conversation going. They need not feel so. Silences have many meanings and many uses. When recounting a present illness a patient frequently falls silent for short periods to collect thoughts, remember details, or decide whether or not to trust you enough to report something. An attentive posture on the interviewer's part is usually the best response here, sometimes followed by brief encouragement to continue. During periods of silence, be particularly alert to nonverbal cues, such as evidence that the patient is having difficulty controlling emotions. Depressed patients or those with dementia may have lost their usual spontaneity of expression, give short answers to questions, and fall silent quickly after each one. If you sense one of these problems, shift your inquiry to asking about the symptoms of depression or begin an exploratory mental status examination (see Ch. 3).

At times, a patient's silence results from interviewer error or insensitivity. Are you asking too many direct questions in rapid sequence? The patient may simply have yielded the initiative to you and taken the passive role you seem to expect. Have you offended the patient in any way?—for example, by signs of disapproval or criticism? Have you failed to recognize an overwhelming symptom such as pain, nausea, or dyspnea? If so, you may need to ask the patient directly, "You seem very quiet. Is there something I have done to upset you?"

Patients Who Like to Talk. The garrulous, rambling patient may be just as difficult as the silent one, possibly more so. Faced with limited time and a perceived need to "get the whole story," the interviewer may grow impatient, even exasperated. Although there are no perfect solutions for this problem, several techniques are helpful. First, you may need to shift your agenda and accept less than a comprehensive history. Second, give the patient free rein for the first 5 or 10 minutes of the interview. You will then have the chance to observe the patient's pattern of speech. Perhaps the patient has simply lacked a good listener for a long time and is expressing pent-up concerns. Maybe the patient's style is to tell detailed stories. Does the patient seem obsessively detailed or unduly anxious? Is there a flight of ideas or a disorganization of thought processes that suggests a psychotic disorder? Could it be confabulation? Third, try to focus the discussion on what seems to be most important to the patient. Show interest and ask questions in those areas. Interrupt if you must, but courteously. It is acceptable to be directive. A brief summary may help you change the topic while letting the patient know that you have both heard and understood. "As I understand it, your chest pains come frequently, last a long time, and do not necessarily stay in any one place. Now tell me about your breathing." Finally, do not let your impatience show. If you have used up the allotted time or, more likely, gone over it, explain that to the patient and arrange for a second meeting. Setting a time limit for the next appointment may be helpful. "I know we have much more to talk about. Can you come again next week? We will have a full hour then."

Patients with Multiple Symptoms. Some patients seem to have every symptom that you mention. They have an "essentially positive review of systems." Although it is conceivable that such a patient has multiple organic illnesses, a somatization disorder is much more likely. In such cases it will profit little to explore each symptom in detail. Focus on the meaning or function of the symptom and guide the interview into a psychosocial assessment.

Anxious Patients. Anxiety is a frequent and normal reaction to sickness, to treatment, and to the health-care system itself. For some patients anxiety is a filter for all their perceptions and reactions, and for others it may be part of their illness. Be sensitive to nonverbal and verbal clues. For example, anxious patients may sit tensely, fidgeting with their fingers or clothes. They may sigh frequently, lick their dry lips, sweat more than average, or actually tremble. Carotid pulsations may betray a rapid heart rate. Some anxious patients fall silent, unable to speak freely or confide. Others try to cover their feelings with words, busily avoiding their own basic problems. When you sense an underlying anxiety, encourage such patients to talk about their feelings.

Anger and Hostility. Patients have reasons to be angry: they are ill, they have suffered a loss, they lack their accustomed control over their own lives, they feel relatively powerless in the health-care system. They may direct this anger toward you. It is possible that you have justly earned their hostility. Were you late for your appointment, inconsiderate, insensitive, or angry yourself? If so, recognize the fact and try to make amends. More often, however, some of the response is a displacement of the patients' anger onto the clinician as a symbol of their pain.

Allow patients to get angry feelings off their chests. Accept their feelings without getting angry in return. Beware of joining such patients in their hostility toward another part of the clinic or hospital, even when you privately harbor similar feelings. *You can validate patients' feelings without agreeing with their reasons.* After a patient has calmed down, you may be able to help him or her to identify specific steps that will be useful in the future. Rational solutions to emotional problems are not always possible, however, and people need time to express their angry feelings and have them validated.

The Obstreperous Inebriate. Few patients can disrupt the clinic or emergency room more quickly than an acutely intoxicated person who is angry, belligerent, and uncontrolled. Before interviewing such a patient, it is wise to alert the security force of the hospital. As a clinician you have a right to feel and be safe. It is especially important to stay calm and appear accepting, not challenging. To do this, approach the patient as you would normally, but keep your posture relaxed and nonthreatening and your hands loosely open. Do not try to make inebriated patients lower their voices or stop cursing you or the staff, but listen carefully and try to understand what they are saying. Since some such persons feel trapped in small rooms, it is usually best to talk with them in an open area. You too are likely to feel more comfortable there.

Crying. Crying is an important clue to emotions. While it is often an expression of sadness, it can be due to anger or frustration. If the patient seems on the verge of tears, gentle probing or an empathic response may allow the patient to cry. It is usually therapeutic for the patient to allow this expression of feeling. Quiet acceptance is then appropriate. Offer a tissue, wait for recovery, perhaps make a facilitating or supportive remark: "It's good to get it out." In that kind of accepting context, most patients will soon compose themselves and will feel better and capable of continuing the discussion. Many people in our culture find that crying makes them uncomfortable. If that is true for you, as a clinician you will need to work to support patients in this important expression.

Confusing Behaviors or Histories. At times you may find yourself baffled, frustrated, and confused in your interaction with the patient. The history is vague and difficult to understand, ideas are poorly related to one another, and language is hard to follow. Even though you word your questions carefully, you seem unable to get clear answers. The patient's manner of relating to you may also seem peculiar: distant, aloof, inappropriate, or bizarre. Symptoms may be described in bizarre terms: "My fingernails feel too heavy" or "My stomach knots up like a snake." With the usual nondirective techniques, you may be able to get more information about the unusual qualities of the symptoms. These characteristics should alert you to possible alterations in mental status, such as psychosis or delirium that may be due to mental illnesses such as schizophrenia or some other cognitive dysfunction (see Ch. 3). Be particularly alert for delirium when dealing with an acutely ill or intoxicated patient, and for dementia when dealing with an elderly patient.

Patients with these problems may be unable to give clear histories. They may be vague and inconsistent about symptoms or events and unable to report when and how things happened. They may be inattentive to your questions and hesitant in their answers. Occasionally such patients may confabulate to fill in the gaps in their memories. When you suspect a cognitive disorder, such as dementia, do not spend too much time trying to get a detailed history. You will only tire and frustrate the patient as well as yourself. Shift your inquiry instead to an evaluation of mental status, checking particularly on level of consciousness, orientation, and memory (see Ch. 3). You can work the initial questions smoothly into the interview. "When was your last appointment at the clinic? Let's see, then, that was about how long ago?" "Your address now is?... and your phone number?" Responses can all be checked against the chart (presuming, of course, the chart is accurate).

Patients with Limited Intelligence. Patients of moderately limited intelligence can usually give adequate histories. You may, in fact, overlook their limitations and thereby make mistakes, such as omitting their dysfunction from a disability evaluation or giving instructions they cannot understand. If you suspect such problems, pay special attention to the patient's schooling and independent function. How far did they go in school? If they didn't finish, why not? What kinds of courses are (were) they taking? How did they do in those courses? Did they have any testing done? Are they living alone? Do they get help with any activities (e.g., transportation, shopping)? If you are unsure, you can make a smooth transition into a mental status examination, including simple calculations, vocabulary, information, and tests of abstract thinking (see Ch. 3). The sexual history is equally important and often overlooked in the care of these patients. When patients suffer from severe mental retardation, you will have to obtain their history from family or friends. Always first show interest in the patients themselves. Establish rapport and eye contact and engage in simple conversation. As with children, avoid "talking down" to mentally retarded patients and using affectations of speech or condescending behaviors. The patient, family members, caretakers, or friends will notice and appreciate respectful behavior.

Limited or No Ability to Read. Before giving written instructions, it may be advisable to assess a patient's reading ability. Literacy levels vary significantly, and marginal reading skills are more prevalent than commonly believed. People cannot read for many reasons: language barriers, learning disorders, poor vision, or lack of education. Illiterate people may try to hide their inability to read. Asking about educational level may be helpful, but can be misleading. Respond sensitively, and remember that illiteracy and lack of intelligence are not synonymous. When you give written instructions, check to see if the patient can read what you have written.

Language Barriers. Nothing will more surely convince you that a history is essential than having to do without one. When you cannot communicate with your patient because you speak different languages, take every possible step to find an interpreter. A few broken words and gestures are no substitute. The ideal interpreter is a neutral, objective person who is familiar with both languages. When family members or friends try to help, they are more likely to distort meanings and may also present confidentiality conflicts for both the patient and the interviewer. Many interpreters try to speed the process by telescoping a long communication into a few words. Try to make clear at the beginning that you need the interpreter to explain everything, not to interpret or summarize. Make your questions clear and short. You can also help the interpreter by outlining the goals for each segment of your history.

When available, written bilingual questionnaires are invaluable, especially for the review of systems. Before using one, however, be sure patients can read in their own language or can get help with the questionnaire. Some clinical settings have access to speaker-phone translators; use them if there are no better options.

Guidelines for Working With an Interpreter

1. Choose a trained interpreter when possible, in preference to a volunteer or family member.
2. Orient the interpreter to how you want the interview to proceed. Include reminders to translate 2 literal meanings and avoid interpretations or advice to the patient.
3. Arrange the room so that you and the patient have eye contact and you can read nonverbal cues. Seating the interpreter next to you works well.
4. Allow the interpreter and patient to establish rapport.
5. Address the patient directly ("How long have you been sick?" rather than "How long has he been sick?"). Use your body position to reinforce your rapport with the patient.
6. Keep statements short and simple. Think about the most important concepts to communicate.
7. Use the interpreter as a resource for cultural information.
8. Verify mutual understanding by asking the patient to report back what has been communicated.
9. Be patient. The interview will take more time and may provide less information.

Deaf and Hard-of-Hearing Patients. Communicating with people who are deaf presents many of the same problems as communicating with patients who speak a different language. Deaf people may preferentially use sign language, which is a unique language with its own syntax. In addition, the deaf often identify themselves as being part of a separate cultural group. Thus, this is often a truly cross-cultural communication. Find out the patient's preferred form of communication. If the patient knows sign language, make every effort to find an interpreter, using the principles identified above. Although very time consuming, handwritten questions and answers may be the only solution. When patients have partial hearing impairment or can read lips, face them directly, in good light. Speak slowly and in a relatively low-pitched voice. Do not let your voice trail off at the ends of sentences, avoid covering your mouth, and use gestures to reinforce your words. If the patient has unilateral hearing loss, arrange the seating for access to the hearing side. A person who has a hearing aid should, of course, wear it, and you should check to be sure that it is working. Patients who use glasses should use them, too; visual cues may help them to understand you better. Supplement any oral instructions with written ones. Written questionnaires are a great help.

Blind Patients. When meeting with a blind patient, shake the person's hand to establish contact and explain who you are and why you are there. If the room is unfamiliar, orient the patient to it and explain what is there and whether anyone else is present. Remember to respond vocally to such patients when they speak, since facilitative postures and gestures will not work. At the same time, guard against raising your voice unnecessarily.

Talking With Families or Friends. Some patients are totally unable to give their own histories due to age, dementia, or other limitations. Others may be unable to describe parts of the history, such as their behavior during a convulsion. Under these circumstances, you must try to find a third person from whom you can get the story. At times, although you may think you have a reasonably comprehensive knowledge of the patient, other sources may offer surprising and important information. A spouse, for example, may report significant family strains, depressive symptoms, or drinking habits that the person has denied.

The basic principles of interviewing apply to your conversations with relatives or friends. Find a private place to talk. Introduce yourself, state your purpose, inquire how they are feeling under the circumstances, and recognize and acknowledge their concerns. As you listen to their versions of the history, be alert for clues to the quality of their relationships with the patient. These may color their credibility or give you helpful ideas in planning the patient's care. It is also important to find out the basis for their knowledge. For example, when a child is brought in for health care, the adult may not be the primary or even frequent caregiver, just the most available ride. Always try to find the best informed source.

When seeking data from a third person, it is necessary to have the patient's approval. Assure such patients that you will keep confidential what they have already told you, or get their permission to share certain information. Data from other persons must also be held in confidence. Occasionally a relative or friend insists on accompanying the patient during the history or even the physical examination. If you can, ascertain his or her reasons as well as the patient's wishes. When patients can communicate at all, even just by facial expressions or gestures, it is important that they be given the chance to do so with complete confidentiality. It is usually possible to divide the interview into two parts—one with the patient alone and the other with both the patient and the second person. Each part has its own value.

Responding to Patients' Questions. Patients' questions may seek simple factual information. More often, however, they express feelings or concerns. Try to elicit these feelings or delve further, lest you offer a misguided answer.

Patient:	What are the effects of this blood pressure medicine?
Response:	There are several effects. Why do you ask?
Patient:	(Pause) Well, I was reading up on it in a friend's book. I read it could make me impotent.

Similar caution is indicated when patients seek advice for personal problems. Should the patient quit a stressful job, for example, or move to Arizona, or have an abortion? Before responding, find out what approaches the patient has considered, what pros and cons there might be to the possible solutions. A chance to talk through the problem with you is usually much more valuable and therapeutic than any answer you could give.

Finally, when the patient is asking for specific information about the diagnosis, progress, or treatment plan, answer when you can but be careful that your responses do not conflict with those provided by others. When you are unsure of the answer, offer to find out if you can. Alternatively, you can suggest that the patient ask Dr. X because Dr. X knows more about the case or is making that decision. Beware, however, of using this approach simply to avoid a difficult issue. If you carry the primary patient responsibility yourself, share your opinions, your plans, and the patient's prognosis with other members of the health-care team so that each in turn can communicate with the patient effectively.

The Content of a Comprehensive History

The items in a history vary with the patient's age, gender, and illness, with the clinician's specialty and available time, and with the goals of the visit. By learning and understanding all of the items in such a history you can select the ones you need. Two patterns of a comprehensive history are detailed in the next few pages: one for adults, the other for children. Technical terms for symptoms appear in these histories. Definitions of these terms, together with ways to ask about the symptoms, are included in Chapter 2. These patterns are the structure of the documentation or write-up. They do not determine the sequence of the information gathering or how the information is obtained.

COMPREHENSIVE HISTORY: ADULT PATIENT

Date and Time of History. The date is always important, and in rapidly changing circumstances it is always wise to document the time. (This is increasingly important to regulatory agencies.)

Identifying Data, including age, gender, marital status, and occupation

Source of History or Referral, such as patient, family, friend, officer, consultant, medical record. It helps the reader to assess the purpose of the history or referral.

Reliability, if relevant. For example, "The patient is consistent about the description of her symptoms but vague about when they began."

Chief Complaints, when possible in the patient's own words. "My stomach hurts and I feel awful." Sometimes patients have no overt complaints; ascertain their goals instead. "I have come for my regular checkup" or "I've been admitted for a thorough evaluation of my heart."

Present Illness

This section is a clear, chronologic account of the problems for which the patient is seeking care. *The data come from the patient, but the organization is yours.* The narrative should include the onset of the problem, the setting in which it developed, its manifestations, and any treatments. The principal symptoms should be described in terms of (1) location, (2) quality, (3) quantity or severity, (4) timing (i.e., onset, duration, and frequency), (5) the setting in which they occur, (6) factors that have aggravated or relieved them, and (7) associated manifestations. Also note significant negatives (the absence of certain symptoms that will aid in differential diagnosis). Other relevant information should be brought into the present illness section, such as risk factors for coronary artery disease if the chief complaint is chest pain, and current medications in a patient with syncope. A present illness description should also include patient's responses to his or her own symptoms and what effect the illness has had on the patient's life.

Current Medications, including dose and frequency of use. Also include home remedies, nonprescription drugs, vitamin/mineral or herbal supplements, birth control, and medicines borrowed from family members or friends. It is a good idea to ask patients to bring in all their medications and show you exactly what they take.

Allergies, including the specific reaction

Past History

Childhood Illnesses, such as measles, rubella, mumps, whooping cough, chickenpox, rheumatic fever, scarlet fever, polio

Adult Illnesses, including *Medical* (such as diabetes, hypertension, hepatitis, asthma, HIV disease, and information about hospitalizations); *Surgical* (include dates, indication, and outcome); *Obstetric/Gynecologic* (include obstetric history and menstrual history, birth control, number and gender of partners, at-risk practices); and *Psychiatric* (include dates, diagnoses, hospitalizations, treatments). Also includes *Accidents and Injuries* and *Transfusions*.

Current Health Status

Tobacco, including the type used (e.g., cigarettes, chewing tobacco) and amount and duration of use. Cigarette smoking is often reported in pack-years (a person who has smoked 1½ packs a day for 12 years has an 18 pack-year history). If someone has quit, note for how long.

Alcohol, Drugs, and Related Substances. See p. 17 for suggested methods of inquiry.

Exercise and Diet, including frequency of exercise, usual daily food intake, and any dietary supplements or restrictions. Ask about coffee, tea, and other caffeine-containing beverages.

Immunizations, such as tetanus, pertussis, diphtheria, polio, measles, rubella, mumps, influenza, hepatitis B, *Haemophilus influenzae* type b, and pneumococcal vaccine. Usually obtainable from medical records.

Screening Tests appropriate to the patient, such as tuberculin tests, Pap smears, mammograms, stools for occult blood, and cholesterol tests, together with the results and the dates they were last performed. The patient may not know this information. You may need to refer to the chart or get the patient's permission to obtain old medical records.

Safety Measures, such as use or nonuse of seat belts, bicycle helmets, sunblock, smoke detectors, and other devices related to specific hazards

Family History

Note the age and health, or age and cause of death, of each immediate family member (i.e., parents, siblings, spouse, and children). Data on grandparents or grandchildren may also be useful.

Note the occurrence within the family of any of the following conditions: diabetes, heart disease, hypercholesterolemia, high blood pressure, stroke, kidney disease, tuberculosis, cancer, arthritis, anemia, allergies, asthma, headaches, epilepsy, mental illness, alcoholism, drug addiction, and symptoms like those of the patient.

It may be useful to record this information in a diagram called a pedigree or genogram.

Personal and Social History

This is an outline or narrative-description that captures the important and relevant information about the patient as a person, lifestyle issues that create risk or promote health, and health maintenance measures.

Occupation and Education

Home Situation and Significant Others

Daily Life, particularly important in elderly patients or patients with disabilities to establish their baseline level of function. Can include *sleep patterns,* including times that the person goes to bed and awakens, daytime naps, and any difficulties in falling asleep or staying asleep

Important Experiences, including upbringing, schooling, military service, job history, financial situation, marriage, recreation, retirement

Leisure Activities/Hobbies (may be a clue to environmental exposures)

Religious Affiliation and Beliefs, relevant to perceptions of health, illness, and treatment

Review of Systems

General. Usual weight, recent weight change, any clothes that fit tighter or looser than before. Weakness, fatigue, fever

Skin. Rashes, lumps, sores, itching, dryness, color change, changes in hair or nails

Head. Headache, head injury, dizziness, lightheadedness

Eyes. Vision, glasses or contact lenses, last examination, pain, redness, excessive tearing, double vision, blurred vision, spots, specks, flashing lights, glaucoma, cataracts

Ears. Hearing, tinnitus, vertigo, earaches, infection, discharge. If hearing is decreased, use or nonuse of hearing aids

Nose and Sinuses. Frequent colds, nasal stuffiness, discharge, or itching, hay fever, nosebleeds, sinus trouble

Mouth and Throat. Condition of teeth, gums, bleeding gums, dentures, if any, and how they fit, last dental examination, sore tongue, dry mouth, frequent sore throats, hoarseness

Neck. Lumps, "swollen glands," goiter, pain, or stiffness in the neck

Breasts. Lumps, pain or discomfort, nipple discharge, self-examination practices

Respiratory. Cough, sputum (color, quantity), hemoptysis, dyspnea, wheezing, asthma, bronchitis, emphysema, pneumonia, tuberculosis, pleurisy, last chest x-ray

Cardiac. Heart trouble, high blood pressure, rheumatic fever, heart murmurs, chest pain or discomfort, palpitations, dyspnea, orthopnea, paroxysmal nocturnal dyspnea, edema, past electrocardiogram or other heart test results

Gastrointestinal. Trouble swallowing, heartburn, appetite, nausea, vomiting, regurgitation, vomiting of blood, indigestion. Frequency of bowel movements, color and size of stools, change in bowel habits, rectal bleeding or black tarry stools, hemorrhoids, constipation, diarrhea. Abdominal pain, food intolerance, excessive belching or passing of gas. Jaundice, liver or gallbladder trouble, hepatitis

Urinary. Frequency of urination, polyuria, nocturia, burning or pain on urination, hematuria, urgency, reduced caliber or force of the urinary stream, hesitancy, dribbling, incontinence, urinary infections, stones

Genital

Male. Hernias, discharge from or sores on the penis, testicular pain or masses, history of sexually transmitted diseases and their treatments. Sexual preference, interest, function, satisfaction, birth control methods, condom use, and problems. Exposure to HIV infection.

Female. Age at menarche; regularity, frequency, and duration of periods; amount of bleeding, bleeding between periods or after intercourse, last menstrual period; dysmenorrhea, premenstrual tension; age at menopause, menopausal symptoms, postmenopausal bleeding. If the patient was born before 1971, exposure to DES (diethylstilbestrol) from maternal use during pregnancy. Discharge, itching, sores, lumps, sexually transmitted diseases and treatments. Number of pregnancies, number and type of deliveries, number of abortions (spontaneous and induced); complications of pregnancy; birth control methods. Sexual preference, interest, function, satisfaction, any problems, including dyspareunia. Exposure to HIV infection.

Peripheral Vascular. Intermittent claudication, leg cramps, varicose veins, past clots in the veins

Musculoskeletal. Muscle or joint pains, stiffness, arthritis, gout, backache. If present, describe location and symptoms (e.g., swelling, redness, pain, tenderness, stiffness, weakness, limitation of motion or activity).

Neurologic. Fainting, blackouts, seizures, weakness, paralysis, numbness or loss of sensation, tingling of "pins and needles," tremors or other involuntary movements

Hematologic. Anemia, easy bruising or bleeding, past transfusions and any reactions to them

Endocrine. Thyroid trouble, heat or cold intolerance, excessive sweating, diabetes, excessive thirst or hunger, polyuria

Psychiatric. Nervousness, tension, mood including depression, memory

COMPREHENSIVE HISTORY: CHILD PATIENT

In addition to obvious age-related differences between the histories of children and those of adults, there are present and past historical data specifically pertinent to the assessment of infants, children, and adolescents. These relate particularly to the patient's chronologic age and stage of development. The child's history, then, follows an outline similar to that of the adult's history. When the topics are the same, information covered in the adult section has not been repeated here.

Identifying Data. Date and place of birth. Nickname. First names of parents (and last name of each, if different), their occupations, and where they may be reached during work hours

Chief Complaints. Make clear whether these are concerns of the patient, the parent(s), or both. In some instances, a third party such as a schoolteacher may have expressed concerns about the child.

Present Illness. Should include how other members of the family think about the patient's symptoms

Past History

Birth History. Particularly important during the first 2 years of life and for neurologic and developmental problems. Hospital records should be reviewed if preliminary information from the parent(s) indicates significant difficulties before, during, or after delivery.

Prenatal. Maternal health during pregnancy, including specific complications related to the pregnancy; tobacco, alcohol, and drugs (prescription and illegal) taken during pregnancy; duration of pregnancy; parental attitudes concerning the pregnancy

Natal. Nature of labor and type of delivery, including duration, analgesia used, and complications encountered; birth order if a multiple birth; birth weight

Neonatal. Onset of respirations; resuscitation efforts; Apgar scores (see Ch. 19) and estimation of gestational age (see Ch. 19). Specific problems with feeding, respiratory distress, cyanosis, jaundice, anemia, convulsions, congenital anomalies, infection. Early bonding and caregiving. Patterns of crying, sleeping, urination, and defecation

Childhood Illnesses. In addition to specific illnesses experienced, mention of any recent exposures to childhood illnesses should be made here.

Operations and Hospitalizations. The reactions of the child and parents to these events should be ascertained.

Accidents or Injuries

Allergies. Particular attention should be given to the allergies that are more prevalent during infancy and childhood—eczema, urticaria, allergic rhinitis, asthma, food intolerance, and insect hypersensitivity.

Feeding History. Particularly important during the first 2 years of life

Infancy. Method of feeding (breast, bottle, or a combination), type of formula used, introduction of solid foods, vitamin or iron supplements, water source (fluoride?), any parental concerns. If the chief complaint involves problems with growth, weight gain, or the gastrointestinal system, a much more detailed history is needed.

Childhood. Eating habits—likes and dislikes, typical types and amounts of food eaten, parental ideas about eating in general and specifically in relation to this child. Eating habits and body perceptions are particularly important for adolescents.

Growth and Development History. Particularly important during infancy and childhood and at any age when problems of delayed physical growth, psychomotor or intellectual retardation, or behavioral disturbances are present.

Physical Growth. Actual (or approximate) weight and height at birth and at 1, 2, 5, and 10 years; history of any slow or rapid gains or losses; tooth eruption or loss pattern.

Developmental Milestones. Ages at which patient held up head while in a prone position; rolled over from front to back and back to front, sat with support and alone, stood with support and alone, walked with support and alone, said first word, combinations of words, and sentences, tied own shoes, dressed without help, tooth eruption and loss pattern, percentile on growth chart at different ages if known

Social Development. *Sleep*—amount and patterns during day and at night, bedtime routines, type of bed and its location, nightmares, terrors, and somnambulation. *Toileting*—methods of training used, when bladder and bowel control attained, occurrence of enuresis or encopresis, parental attitudes, terms used within the family for urination and defecation. *Speech*—ability to communicate, estimate number of words in vocabulary, any speech abnormalities (hesitation, stuttering, lisping). *Personality*—ask the parent to describe the child; relationship with parents, siblings, and peers; group and independent activities and interests, congeniality, special friends (real or imaginary), major assets and skills, self-image. *Discipline*—methods used and satisfaction with the process, specific problems such as temper tantrums, aggressive behavior. *Schooling*—experience with day care, nursery school, kindergarten; age and adjustment upon entry; current parental and child satisfaction; academic achievement; school's concerns. *Sexuality*—parental teaching and responses to child's questions regarding sexuality, intercourse, masturbation, menstruation, nocturnal emissions, development of secondary sexual characteristics, AIDS and other sexually transmitted diseases

Health Maintenance

Immunizations. Specific dates of administration of each vaccine should be recorded so that an ongoing booster program can be maintained throughout childhood and adolescence. Parents should have their own written record of their child's immunizations. Any untoward reactions to specific vaccines should also be recorded. *This information should be obtained from a written record if possible.*

Screening Procedures. The dates and results of any screening tests performed should be recorded. These include blood pressure readings, vision, hearing, and tuberculin tests, blood lead levels, urinalysis, hematocrits, tests for phenylketonuria, galactosemia, and other genetic metabolic disorders (these may be mandated at birth by your state), and, for certain high-risk populations, sickle cell anemia, cholesterol, $alpha_1$-antitrypsin deficiency, and other tests that may be indicated.

Safety and Injury Prevention. Age-appropriate questions should be asked of the child and caregivers. Some topics include supervision in general, car seats, seat belts, bicycle helmets and habits; presence and storage of firearms; proximity to water (pools, ponds); ingestion; smoke detectors and fire safety.

Family History

The Family History includes individuals who live in the home and their relationship to the child, and relationships to first-degree relatives not living in the home. Note the occupational and health history of individuals in the home, caretakers, and first-degree relatives. Parental work schedules (who provides supervision after school); support available from relatives, friends, and neighbors; description of neighborhood in which the family lives. The ethnic and cultural milieu in which the family lives. Parental expectations and attitudes toward the patient in relation to siblings. (All or portions of this information may be recorded in the Present Illness section, if pertinent to it, or under Personal and Social History.) Consanguinity of the parents should be ascertained (by inquiring if they are "related by blood").

An Approach to Symptoms

While Chapter 1 deals with the general methods of interviewing, this chapter tailors those methods to common or important symptoms. It (1) defines the technical terms for the symptoms, (2) suggests ways of asking about them, and (3) outlines some of their most common mechanisms and causes.

Technical terms, of course, are not intended for use with most patients. As a clinician, however, you must learn to translate the patient's observations into words such as tinnitus, hemoptysis, or nocturia. You can then understand the professional literature and communicate clearly with your colleagues.

Data to gather about symptoms appear here in bold-faced type. Specific questions are suggested, especially in difficult or sensitive areas. When no suggestions are made, identify the *seven attributes of the symptom*, as described on p. 9, and use the general principles of interviewing that you have already learned.

The order used in this chapter resembles the review of systems in a comprehensive history. Interpretive comments on the meaning of certain symptoms appear in the right-hand columns, together with examples of specific abnormalities that may cause them. Tables at the end of the chapter compare various disorders and diseases according to their symptoms. When assessment of symptoms depends heavily on physical examination, reference is made to later chapters.

Obviously no table exhausts all the possible explanations for symptoms, nor can any table, which is necessarily oversimplified, capture the infinite variety of human perceptions and experience. Real patients seldom match a textbook in every detail.

One of the qualities that is difficult for a patient to communicate is color. A chart that includes the various colors of sputum, urine, and feces is often helpful in getting an accurate history. You can easily make such a chart by cutting rectangles out of the colored pages of a magazine and taping them to a small card. Colors should range from white to yellowish and light green for sputum; from pale to deep yellow, orange, pink, reddish, and brown for urine; and from gray and light tan to brown and black for feces. The bright and dark red colors of blood should also be included. These colors can be arranged into one scheme from which the patient can select the closest match.

Symptoms and Approaches to Them

General Symptoms

Changes in *body weight* result from quantitative changes in either the body tissues or the body fluids. *Weight gain* occurs when caloric intake exceeds caloric expenditure over a period of time, and typically appears as increased body fat. Weight gain may also result from an abnormal accumulation of body fluids. When the retention of fluid is relatively mild it may not be visible, but if several pounds of it accumulate it usually appears as edema.

Weight loss is an important symptom that has many causes. Mechanisms include one or more of the following: decreased intake of food for reasons that include anorexia, dysphagia, vomiting, and insufficient supplies of food; defective absorption of nutrients through the gastrointestinal tract; increased metabolic requirements; and loss of nutrients through the urine, feces, or injured skin.

A person may also lose weight when a fluid-retaining state improves or responds to treatment. Moreover, the greater part of the weight lost when a person starts on a low-calorie diet is fluid.

Good opening questions include "How often do you check your weight? Has it changed in the past year? . . . in what manner? Why has it changed, do you think? What would you like to weigh?" If weight change in either direction appears to be a problem, try to ascertain the amount of change, its timing, the setting in which it occurred, and any associated symptoms.

In the *overweight patient,* for example, when did the weight gain begin? Was the patient heavy as an infant or a child? Using milestones appropriate to the patient's age, inquire about the weight at the time of birth, on entrance to kindergarten, on graduation from high school or college, on discharge from the service, at marriage, following each pregnancy, at menopause, and on retirement. What was going on in the patient's life during the periods of weight gain? Has the patient tried to lose weight? How? With what results?

When the problem is *weight loss,* try to determine whether the intake of food has diminished proportionately or whether it has remained normal or even increased.

Symptoms associated with the weight loss often suggest its likely cause. So does a good psychosocial history. **Who cooks and shops for the patient? Where and with whom does the patient eat? Are there any difficulties in getting, storing, preparing, or chewing the food?**

Rapid changes in weight (over a few days) suggest changes in body fluids, not tissues.

See Table 16-3, Mechanisms and Patterns of Edema, pp. 480–481.

Causes of weight loss include gastrointestinal diseases; endocrine disorders (diabetes mellitus, hyperthyroidism, adrenal insufficiency); chronic infections; malignancies; chronic cardiac, pulmonary, or renal failure; depression; and anorexia nervosa.

Weight loss with a relatively high food intake suggests diabetes mellitus, hyperthyroidism, or malabsorption. Consider also binge eating (*bulimia*) with clandestine vomiting.

Poverty, old age, social isolation, physical disability, emotional or mental impairment, lack of teeth, ill-fitting den-

Does the patient restrict certain foods for medical, religious, or other reasons?

Throughout the history, be alert for manifestations of malnutrition. Symptoms here are often subtle and nonspecific: weakness, easy fatigability, cold intolerance, flaky dermatitis, and ankle swelling, among other examples. A good dietary history is mandatory.

Like weight loss, *fatigue* is a relatively nonspecific symptom with many causes. It refers to a sense of weariness or loss of energy that patients describe in various ways. "I've lost my pep. . . . I just feel blah. . . . I'm all in. . . . I can hardly get through the day. . . . By the time I get to the office I feel as though I've done a day's work." Because fatigue is a normal response to hard work, sustained stress, or grief, you must consider the context in which it occurs, but fatigue that is unrelated to such factors needs an explanation.

In infants and children, fatigue is not expressed verbally but is manifested by withdrawal from normal activities, irritability, loss of interest in the surroundings, and excessive sleeping.

Use open-ended questions to explore the attributes of the patient's fatigue, and get as clear an idea as possible of what the patient is experiencing. Important clues to the cause of the problem often lie in a good psychosocial history, review of systems, and exploration of sleep patterns.

Weakness is different from fatigue. It denotes a demonstrable loss of muscular power, and will be discussed later with other neurologic symptoms (see pp. 70–71).

Fever refers to an abnormal elevation in body temperature (see p. 000). **Ask about it when the patient has an acute or a chronic illness. Find out whether the patient has measured the temperature with a thermometer. Has the patient felt feverish or unusually hot, noted excessive sweating, or felt chilly and cold? Try to distinguish between subjective *chilliness* and a *shaking chill* in which the body shivers and the teeth chatter.**

Feelings of coldness, gooseflesh, and shivering accompany a rising temperature, while hot feelings and sweats accompany defervescence. The normal temperature rises during the day and falls during the night. When fever exaggerates this swing, *night sweats* occur. Malaise, headache, and pain in the muscles and joints often accompany fever.

Fever has many causes. **Focus your questions on the timing of the illness and its associated symptoms. Become familiar with patterns of infectious diseases to which your patient may have been subject, and inquire about travel, contacts with sick persons, or other un-**

tures, alcoholism, and drug abuse increase the likelihood of malnutrition.

Fatigue is a common symptom of depression and anxiety states, but consider also infections (such as hepatitis, infectious mononucleosis, and tuberculosis); endocrine disorders (hypothyroidism, adrenal insufficiency, diabetes mellitus, and panhypopituitarism); heart failure; chronic disease of the lungs, kidneys, or liver; electrolyte imbalance; moderate to severe anemia; malignancies; nutritional deficits; medications; and drug withdrawal.

Weakness, especially if localized in a neuroanatomic pattern, suggests a disorder of the nervous system or muscles.

Recurrent shaking chills suggest more extreme swings in temperature.

Feelings of heat and sweating also accompany menopause.

usual exposures. **Inquire about medications.** They may cause fever, while aspirin, acetaminophen, corticosteroids, and nonsteroidal anti-inflammatory drugs (NSAIDs) may mask it.

The Skin

Start your inquiry about the patient's skin with a few open-ended questions: "Have you noticed any changes in your skin? . . . your hair? . . . your nails? Have you had any rashes? . . . sores? . . . lumps? . . . itching? . . . any moles that have changed in appearance? Where? When?" Further questions are usually best deferred until the physical examination, when you can see what the patient is talking about.

See Chapter 6, The Skin.

Causes of generalized itching without obvious reason include dry skin, aging, pregnancy, uremia, obstructive jaundice, lymphomas and leukemia, drug reactions, and body lice.

The Head

Headache is an extremely common symptom. Although only a very small fraction of people with headaches harbor life-threatening problems as the cause, the symptom requires careful evaluation. Get as full a description as possible. After your usual open-ended approach, ask the patient to show you where the discomfort is. **Is it one-sided or bilateral? steady or throbbing? The single most important attribute of headache is its chronologic pattern. Are you dealing with a new and acute problem, a chronic and recurring one that has not changed very much in its pattern, or a chronic, recurring one that has recently changed its characteristics or become progressively severe? Does the pain recur at the same time every day? Associated symptoms and a family history may also give you important clues.**

See Table 2-1, Headaches, pp. 74–77. Tension and migraine headaches are the most common kinds of recurring headache. Changing or progressively severe headaches increase the likelihood of tumor or other demonstrable structural cause. Extremely severe headaches suggest subarachnoid hemorrhage or meningitis.

Inquire specifically about associated nausea and vomiting and about neurologic symptoms. Explore the physical and emotional settings in which the headaches occur.

Nausea and vomiting are common with migraine but also occur with brain tumors and subarachnoid hemorrhage.

Ask whether coughing, sneezing, or changing the position of the head affects the headache.

Such maneuvers may increase pain from brain tumor and acute sinusitis.

The Eyes

"How is your vision?" and **"Have you had any trouble with your eyes?"** conveniently start your inquiry about ocular problems. If the patient has noted a visual disturbance,

Refractive errors most commonly explain gradual blurring. High blood sugar levels may cause blurring.

• **Has it started suddenly or gradually?**

Sudden visual loss suggests retinal detachment, vitreous hemorrhage, or occlusion of the central retinal artery.

Symptoms and Approaches to Them	Examples/Interpretations
• **Is it troublesome only with close work or only at distances?**	Difficulty with close work suggests *hyperopia* (farsightedness) or *presbyopia* (aging vision); with distances, *myopia* (near-sightedness).
• **Is the entire visual field blurred, or are only parts of it? If the defect is partial, is it central or peripheral in the visual field, or does it involve only one side of it?**	Slow central loss in nuclear cataract (p. 216), macular degeneration (p. 194); peripheral loss in advanced open-angle glaucoma (p. 188); one-sided loss in hemianopsia and quadrantic defects (p. 212)
• **Are there specks in the vision or spots where the patient cannot see (*scotomas*)? If so, do they move around in the visual field when the patient shifts gaze, or are they fixed?**	Moving specks or strands suggest vitreous floaters; fixed defects (scotomas) suggest lesions in the retinas or visual pathways.
• **Has the patient seen lights flashing across the field of vision?** This symptom may be accompanied by vitreous floaters.	Flashing lights or new vitreous floaters suggest detachment of vitreous from retina. Prompt eye consultation is indicated.
• **Does the patient wear glasses?**	
Continue with questions about *pain* **in or around the eyes,** *redness,* **and** *excessive tearing or watering.*	See Table 7-5, Red Eyes, p. 215.
Ask about double vision (*diplopia*). If diplopia is present, find out whether the images are side-by-side (*horizontal diplopia*) or on top of each other (*vertical diplopia*). Does diplopia persist with one eye closed? With which eye is it seen? One kind of horizontal diplopia is physiologic. Hold one finger upright about 6 inches in front of your face, a second at arm's length. When you focus on either finger, the image of the other is double. A patient who notices this phenomenon can be reassured.	Diplopia indicates a weakness or paralysis of one or more extraocular muscles (pp. 170, 189–190, 218). Horizontal diplopia implicates the 3rd or 6th cranial nerve; vertical diplopia, the 3rd or 4th cranial nerve. Diplopia in one eye, with the other closed, suggests a problem in the cornea or lens.

The Ears

Opening questions for the ears are "How is your hearing?" and "Have you had any trouble with your ears?" If the patient has noticed a *hearing loss*, does it involve one or both ears? Did it start suddenly or gradually? What are the associated symptoms, if any?	See Table 7-17, Patterns of Hearing Loss, pp. 232–233.
Try to distinguish between two basic types of hearing impairment: *conductive loss*, which results from problems in the external or middle ear, and *sensorineural loss*, which results from problems in the inner ear, the	Persons with sensorineural loss have particular trouble understanding speech, often com-

cochlear nerve, or its central connections in the brain. **Two questions may be helpful here. Does the patient have special difficulty understanding people as they talk? What difference does a noisy environment make?**

Symptoms associated with hearing loss, such as earache or vertigo, help you to assess the likely causes. In addition, inquire specifically about medications that might contribute to the impairment and ask about sustained exposure to loud noise.

Hearing loss or total deafness in infants is usually suspected when the parents note a lack of response to their voices or to environmental sounds. Such concerns deserve thorough investigation. Toddlers with hearing loss often manifest this by a delay in the development of speech.

Tinnitus is a perceived sound that has no external stimulus, commonly heard as a musical ringing or as a rushing or roaring noise. One or both ears may be involved. Tinnitus may accompany hearing loss of any kind and often remains unexplained. Occasionally, popping sounds originate in the temporomandibular joint, or vascular noises from the neck may be audible.

Vertigo refers to the false perception that the patient or the environment is rotating or spinning. These sensations point primarily to a problem in the inner ear, the cochlear nerve, or its central connections in the brain.

Vertigo poses a challenge to the interviewer. **"Are there times when you feel dizzy?" is an appropriate first question,** but patients often have great difficulty describing their sensations. Try to distinguish vertigo from (1) a sense of unsteadiness without the feeling of movement, (2) faintness or an impending loss of consciousness, and (3) a vague lightheadedness. **Get the story without biasing it. You may need a multiple-choice question. Determine whether or not the patient has felt pulled to the ground or off to one side. Does a change in position provoke the dizziness? Ask about nausea and vomiting, and about other associated symptoms. Pay special attention to the timing and course of the problem.**

Further symptoms relevant to the ears include:

- *Discharge* from the ear

- *Pain* in the ear, or *earache*

Inquire about these in your usual manner.

plaining that others mumble. Noisy environments make it worse. In conductive loss, noisy environments may help.

Medications that affect hearing include aminoglycosides, aspirin, NSAIDs, quinine, furosemide, and others.

Tinnitus is a common symptom, increasing in frequency with age. When associated with hearing loss and vertigo it suggests Meniere's disease.

See Table 2-2, Vertigo, p. 79.

A feeling of being pulled suggests true vertigo.

Unusually soft wax, debris from inflammation or rash in the ear canal, or discharge through a perforated eardrum secondary to acute or chronic otitis media.

Pain suggests a problem in the external or middle ear, but may also be referred from other structures in the mouth, throat, or neck.

The Nose and Sinuses

Rhinorrhea refers to a nasal discharge and is often associated with *nasal stuffiness,* a sense of obstruction. These symptoms frequently occur together with *sneezing,* watery eyes, and discomfort in the throat. *Itching* may also be felt in the eyes, nose, and throat. **Assess the chronology of the illness. Does it occur for a week or so, especially when common colds and related syndromes are prevalent, or does it occur seasonally when pollens are in the air? Is it associated with specific contacts or environments? What remedies has the patient used? for how long? and how well do they work?**

Causes include viral infections, allergic rhinitis ("hay fever"), and vasomotor rhinitis. Itching favors an allergic cause.

Relation to seasons or environmental contacts suggests allergy.

Excessive use of decongestants can worsen the symptoms.

Inquire about drugs that might cause stuffiness.

Oral contraceptives, reserpine, guanethidine, and alcohol

Are there other symptoms associated with the nasal ones, such as pain and tenderness in the face, local headache, or fever?

These together suggest sinusitis.

Is the patient's nasal stuffiness limited to one side? If so, you may be dealing with a different problem that requires careful physical examination.

Consider a deviated nasal septum, foreign body, or tumor.

Epistaxis means bleeding from the nose. The blood usually originates from the nose itself, but may come from a paranasal sinus or the nasopharynx. There is usually no difficulty in getting a history of epistaxis. When the patient is lying down, however, or when the bleeding originates in posterior structures, blood may pass into the throat rather than out the nostrils. You must then differentiate it from blood that has been coughed up or regurgitated. **Try to determine the site of the bleeding, its severity, and associated symptoms. Is it a recurrent problem, and has there been easy bruising or bleeding elsewhere in the body?**

Local causes of epistaxis include trauma (especially nose picking), inflammation, drying and crusting of the nasal mucosa, tumors, and foreign bodies.

Bleeding disorders may contribute to epistaxis.

The Mouth, Throat, and Neck

Bleeding from the gums is a common symptom, most often noted when brushing teeth. **Inquire about local lesions and any tendency to bleed or bruise elsewhere.**

Bleeding gums are most often caused by gingivitis (p. 239).

A *sore tongue* may be caused by local lesions as well as by general conditions.

Aphthous ulcers (p. 243); sore smooth tongue of nutritional deficiency (p. 243).

Sore throat is a frequent complaint, usually developing as part of an acute illness with other upper respiratory symptoms.

See Table 7-19, Findings in the Pharynx, Palate, and Oral Mucosa (pp. 236–238).

Hoarseness refers to an altered quality of the voice, often described as husky, rough, or harsh. The pitch may be lower than before. Hoarseness most often results from disease of the larynx, but may also develop as extralaryngeal lesions press on the laryngeal nerves. **Inquire about overuse of the voice, allergy, smoking or other inhaled irritants, and any associated symptoms. Distinguish between an acute and a chronic problem.** Hoarseness lasting 2 or more weeks usually makes visual examination of the larynx advisable.

Overuse of the voice (as in cheering) and acute infections are the most likely causes.

Causes of chronic hoarseness include smoking, allergy, voice abuse, hypothyroidism, chronic infections such as tuberculosis, and tumors.

"Have you noticed any 'swollen glands' or lumps in your neck?" is a useful question, even though "glands" is not the proper technical term for lymph nodes. Ask about an enlarged thyroid gland or *goiter* (although symptoms of thyroid dysfunction will be discussed later in the chapter). You may also wish to include *pain or stiffness in the neck* here, but these are discussed with the musculoskeletal system.

Enlarged, tender lymph nodes commonly accompany pharyngitis. Increased, decreased, or normal thyroid function may accompany a goiter.

The Breasts

Questions about a woman's breasts may be included in the history or deferred to the physical examination. **Does the patient examine her own breasts? How often? Inquire about** *pain, discomfort,* **or** *lumps* **in her breasts.** Approximately 50% of women have palpable lumps or nodularity in their breasts. Premenstrual enlargement and tenderness are common.

Lumps may be physiologic or pathologic. They include cysts, benign tumors, and cancers. See Table 10-2, Differentiation of Common Breast Nodules (p. 353).

Ask too about *discharge from the nipples* **and when it occurs.** Discharge that appears only after squeezing a nipple is considered physiologic. If the discharge is spontaneous (seen on the underwear or nightclothes without local stimulation), **inquire about its color, consistency, and quantity. Is it unilateral or bilateral?**

A milky bilateral discharge (*galactorrhea*) may be due to pregnancy or hormonal imbalance. A nonmilky unilateral discharge suggests local breast disease.

The Chest

Chest pain or discomfort frequently raises concern about heart disease, but it commonly originates in other structures as well.

See Table 2-3, Chest Pain (pp. 80–81).

Chief among the sources of chest pain are the following:

- The myocardium

Myocardial infarction, angina pectoris

- The pericardium

Pericarditis

- The aorta

Dissecting aneurysm

- The trachea and large bronchi

Tracheobronchitis

- The parietal pleura

Pleurisy, pericarditis

- The esophagus

  Reflux esophagitis, esophageal spasm

- The chest wall, including the musculoskeletal system and the skin

  Costochondritis, herpes zoster

- Extrathoracic structures, such as the neck, gallbladder, and stomach

  Cervical arthritis, biliary colic, gastritis

Your initial questions should be as broad as possible. "Do you have discomfort or unpleasant feelings in your chest?" As you proceed to the full history, ask the patient to show you exactly where the discomfort is, and watch for any gestures to describe it. All seven attributes (see p. 9) of the symptom are often needed to differentiate among the various causes of chest pain.

A clenched fist over the sternum suggests angina pectoris; a finger pointing to a tender area on the chest wall suggests musculoskeletal origin; a hand moving up and down from epigastrium to neck suggests heartburn.

Lung tissue itself has no pain fibers. Pain in lung conditions such as pneumonia or pulmonary infarction usually reflects inflammation of the adjacent parietal pleura. Muscle strain produced by coughing may also be responsible. The pericardium has few pain fibers, and the pain of pericarditis usually arises from inflammation of adjacent parietal pleura. Chest pain commonly accompanies anxiety, but the mechanism remains obscure.

Anxiety is the most common cause of chest pain in children. Among systemic causes, costochondritis is most common.

It is important to ask "is the pain related to exertion?" "Does it radiate to the neck, shoulder, back, or down the arm?"

Exertional chest pain with radiation to the left side of the neck and down the left arm often in angina pectoris. Sharp pain radiating to the back or into the neck in aortic dissection

Palpitations are an unpleasant awareness of the heartbeat. Patients report their sensations in various terms such as skipping, racing, fluttering, pounding, or stopping of the heart. Palpitations may result from an irregular heartbeat, from rapid acceleration or slowing of the heart, or from increased forcefulness of cardiac contraction, but the perception also depends on patients' sensitivities to their own body sensations. Palpitations do not necessarily mean heart disease, and the most serious arrhythmias, such as ventricular tachycardia, often do not produce palpitations.

Transient skips and flipflops suggest premature contractions; persisting irregularity, atrial fibrillation; rapid regular beating of sudden onset and offset, paroxysmal supraventricular tachycardia. Sinus tachycardia starts and stops more gradually.

You may ask directly about palpitations, but if the patient does not understand your question, reword it. "Are you sometimes aware of your heartbeat? What is it like?" Ask the patient to tap out the rhythm with a hand or finger. Was it fast or slow? regular or irregular? How long did it last? If there was an episode of rapid heart action, did it start and stop suddenly or gradually?

See Tables 9-1 and 9-2 for selected heart rates and rhythms (pp. 320–321). A rapid regular rate of less than 120 per minute is usually sinus tachycardia.

You may wish to teach selected patients how to make serial measurements of their pulse rates in case they have further episodes.

Dyspnea is a nonpainful but uncomfortable awareness of breathing that is inappropriate to the circumstances. Only the patient can report dyspnea. An observer may notice abnormally rapid or deep breathing, but these cannot be equated with the subjective sensation. Dyspnea commonly results from cardiac or bronchopulmonary disease, but also frequently accompanies anxiety.

See Table 2-4, Dyspnea, pp. 82–83.

Ask if the patient has had any difficulty in breathing. Dyspneic patients may describe shortness of breath, a smothering feeling, inability to get enough air, or difficulty in taking a deep enough breath. **Ask when the symptom occurs, at rest or with exercise, and how much effort produces it.** Because of variations in age, body weight, and physical fitness there is no absolute scale on which to quantify dyspnea. **Instead, try to determine its severity based on the patient's daily activities.**

Episodic dyspnea that occurs at rest as well as with exercise suggests anxiety with hyperventilation. Such patients often report that they cannot get a deep enough breath. Deep sighs are frequently observed.

How many steps or flights of stairs can the patient climb without pausing for breath? How about work? carrying the groceries? mopping the floor or making a bed? Has the symptom altered the patient's activities? How? Carefully determine the timing and setting of dyspnea, any associated symptoms, and factors that aggravate it or relieve it.

Orthopnea is dyspnea that occurs when the patient is lying down and improves upon sitting up. It is classically quantified according to the number of pillows on which the patient sleeps, or the fact that the patient prefers to sleep sitting up. Be sure, however, that the patient uses the extra pillows or sleeps in a sitting position because of dyspnea, not for other reasons.

Orthopnea suggests left ventricular failure or mitral stenosis, but may also accompany obstructive lung disease.

Paroxysmal nocturnal dyspnea describes episodes of sudden dyspnea and orthopnea that waken a patient from sleep, usually 1 or 2 hours after going to bed. The patient typically sits up, stands up, or goes to a window for air. Wheezing and cough may be associated. The episode usually subsides spontaneously but may recur at about the same time on subsequent nights.

Paroxysmal nocturnal dyspnea suggests left ventricular failure or mitral stenosis and may be mimicked by nocturnal asthmatic attacks.

Wheezes are musical respiratory sounds that may be audible both to the patient and to others.

Wheezing suggests partial airway obstruction.

Edema refers to the accumulation of excessive fluid in the interstitial spaces, and appears as swelling. Although questions about edema are typically included in the chest history, it has many other causes and may signify local problems as well as more general ones. **Focus your questions on the distribution and timing of the swelling, and explore the associated symptoms and the setting in which it occurs. "Have you had any swelling anywhere? Where? . . . anywhere else? When does it occur? Is it worse in the morning or at night? Do your shoes get tight? Do the rings on your fingers get too tight? Are your eyelids puffy or**

See Table 16-3, Mechanisms and Patterns of Edema, pp. 480–481.

Dependent edema appears in the lowest body parts—the feet and legs except in bedridden persons. Consider peripheral, cardiac, and other causes. Puffy

swollen in the morning? Have you had to let your belt out? Have your clothes gotten too tight around your middle?" Because several liters of extra fluid may accumulate in a person's body before overt edema appears, it is useful to ask the patient who tends to retain fluid to record daily morning weights.

eyelids and tight rings, when associated with edema elsewhere, suggest renal disease or hypoalbuminemia. An enlarged waistline may indicate *ascites* (fluid in the peritoneal cavity) or fat.

Cough is a frequent symptom that varies in significance from the trivial to the ominous. A person may cough voluntarily, but more typically cough is a reflex response to stimuli that irritate receptors in the larynx, trachea, or large bronchi. These stimuli include both external agents such as irritating dusts, foreign bodies, and even extremely hot or cold air, and internal substances such as mucus, pus, and blood. Inflammation of the respiratory mucosa, and pressure or tension on the air passages as from a tumor or enlarged peribronchial lymph node, may also cause coughing.

See Table 2-5, Cough and Hemoptysis, p. 84.

Although cough typically signals a problem in the respiratory tract, the underlying cause may also be cardiovascular.

Cough is an important symptom of left-sided heart failure.

"Do you have a cough?" may be an adequate opening question, but for some patients, especially those who smoke, a morning cough may be so habitual that they fail to mention it. Further questions here are "Do you have to clear your throat in the morning?" and "Do you have a cigarette cough?" Determine the timing of the cough. Is it a new symptom or more chronic? How frequent is it? When does it occur? Is it seasonal? Are there factors that seem to precipitate or aggravate it? Has a chronic cough changed in any way?

Assess the cough qualitatively by whether it is dry or productive of *sputum* (phlegm). Ask the patient to describe the volume of the sputum and its color, odor, and consistency. Many patients have difficulty describing sputum volume. A multiple-choice question may be helpful. "How much do you think you cough up in 24 hours: a teaspoon, tablespoon, quarter cup, half cup, cupful?" If the patient coughs in your presence, offer a tissue, ask the patient to cough into it, and inspect any phlegm. A specimen from deep in the chest is desirable. Symptoms associated with the cough often lead you to its cause.

Mucoid sputum is translucent, white, or gray. *Purulent* sputum is yellowish or greenish. *Mucopurulent* sputum has components of both. Large volumes of purulent sputum suggest bronchiectasis or lung abscess.

Diagnostically helpful symptoms include fever, chest pain, dyspnea, orthopnea, wheezing.

Hemoptysis is the coughing or "spitting up" of blood, which may vary from blood-streaked phlegm to pure blood. Ask if the patient has ever experienced either of these. Assess the volume of blood produced together with other attributes of the sputum. Focus your further questions on the setting in which the hemoptysis occurred and the associated symptoms.

See Table 2-5, Cough and Hemoptysis, p. 84. Hemoptysis is an extremely rare event in infants, children, and adolescents, seen most often in cystic fibrosis.

Before labeling this symptom as hemoptysis, it is important to identify the origin of the bleeding by history and examination when possible. If the blood or blood-streaked material appears without coughing, it may originate in the mouth or pharynx. If it is vomited rather than coughed, it probably originates in the gastrointestinal tract. Blood from either the nasopharynx or the gastrointestinal tract, however, is occasionally aspirated and then coughed out.

Blood originating in the stomach is usually darker than blood from the respiratory tract and may be mixed with food particles.

The Gastrointestinal Tract

Dysphagia is difficulty in swallowing, the sense that food or liquid is sticking, hesitating, or "won't go down right." The sensation of a lump in the throat or in the retrosternal area, unassociated with swallowing, is not true dysphagia. Dysphagia may result from esophageal disorders or from difficulty in transferring food from the mouth to the esophagus.

For transfer and esophageal dysphagia, see Table 2-6, Dysphagia, p. 85.

Ask the patient to show you where the dysphagia is felt.

Pointing to the chest suggests an esophageal disorder; pointing to the throat may occur in either a transfer or an esophageal disorder.

Timing is helpful in assessing dysphagia. When did it start? Is it intermittent or persistent? Is it progressing, and if so, how quickly?

Determine what precipitates it: relatively solid foods such as meat, softer foods such as ground meat and mashed potatoes, or hot or cold liquids. Has the pattern changed? What are the associated symptoms and medical conditions?

Dysphagia with only solid foods suggests a mechanical narrowing of the esophagus; dysphagia related to both solids and liquids suggests a disorder of esophageal motility.

Odynophagia, pain on swallowing, may occur in two forms. A sharp, burning pain suggests mucosal inflammation, while a squeezing, cramping pain suggests a muscular cause. Odynophagia may accompany dysphagia, but either symptom may occur by itself.

Causes of mucosal inflammation include reflux esophagitis and esophageal infections due to herpesvirus or *Candida*.

Indigestion is a common complaint that generally refers to distress associated with eating, but people use the term for many different symptoms. **Find out just what your patient means.** Possibilities include:

• *Heartburn,* a sense of burning or warmth that is felt retrosternally and may radiate from the epigastrium to the neck. It usually originates in the esophagus. When severe, however, it may raise the question of heart disease, in both your mind and that of the patient. Some patients with coronary artery disease, moreover, describe their pain as burning, "like indigestion." **Pay particular attention to what brings on the discomfort and what relieves it.**

Heartburn points to reflux of gastric acid into the esophagus and is often precipitated by a heavy meal, lying down, or bending forward. Ingested alcohol, citrus juices, or aspirin may also cause it. When it is chronic, consider reflux esophagitis. See Table 2-3, Chest Pains, pp. 80–81.

- *Excessive gas,* as manifested by frequent belching, abdominal bloating or distention, or *flatus* (the passage of gas by rectum). **Inquire about specific foods that seem to produce these symptoms. Start with open-ended questions here, but be sure to discover any relationship to the ingestion of milk or milk products.** (A deficiency in intestinal lactase commonly causes gaseousness after the ingestion of milk or milk products.) A normal person passes roughly 600 ml of gas per rectum daily.

- Unpleasant *abdominal fullness after meals* of normal size or *inability to eat a full meal*

- *Abdominal pain*

- *Nausea and vomiting*

Abdominal pain has several possible mechanisms and clinical patterns and warrants careful clinical assessment. Be familiar with three broad categories of abdominal pain:

1. *Visceral pain* occurs when hollow abdominal organs such as the intestine or biliary tree contract unusually forcefully or when they are distended or stretched. Solid organs such as the liver become painful when their capsules are stretched. Visceral pain is rather poorly localized but is typically, though not necessarily, felt near the midline, at levels that vary according to the structure involved, as illustrated below.

Swallowing air (*aerophagia*) is the normal cause of belching but does not cause bloating or excessive flatus. Consider instead gas-producing foods such as legumes, deficiency in intestinal lactase, and irritable bowel syndrome.

Causes include anticholinergic drugs, obstruction of the gastric outlet, gastric cancer, and gastroparesis (a complication of diabetes mellitus).

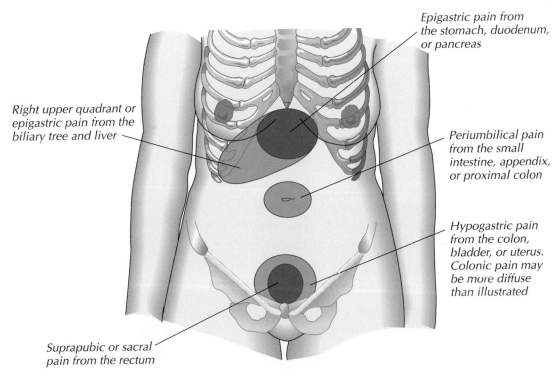

Epigastric pain from the stomach, duodenum, or pancreas

Right upper quadrant or epigastric pain from the biliary tree and liver

Periumbilical pain from the small intestine, appendix, or proximal colon

Hypogastric pain from the colon, bladder, or uterus. Colonic pain may be more diffuse than illustrated

Suprapubic or sacral pain from the rectum

Renal and ureteral pain are illustrated on p. 60.

Visceral pain varies in quality and may be gnawing, burning, cramping, or aching. When it becomes severe, it may be associated with sweating, pallor, nausea, vomiting, and restlessness.

2. *Parietal pain* originates in the parietal peritoneum and is caused by inflammation. It is a steady, aching pain that is usually more severe than visceral pain and more precisely localized over the involved structure. It is typically aggravated by movement or coughing. Patients with this kind of pain usually prefer to lie still.

3. *Referred pain* is felt in more distant sites that are innervated at approximately the same spinal levels as the disordered structure. Referred pain often develops as the initial pain becomes more intense and thus seems to radiate or travel from the initial site. It may be felt superficially or deeply, but usually is well localized.

Pain may also be referred to the abdomen from the chest, spine, or pelvis, thus complicating the assessment of abdominal pain.

After you get the history of abdominal pain in the patient's own words, ask the patient to show you just where it is. If clothes intervene, repeat the question during your examination. Where does the pain start? Does it travel anywhere?

What is the pain like? If the patient has trouble describing it, try a multiple-choice question: "Is it aching, cramping, burning, gnawing, or what?"

How severe is the pain? Is it bearable? Does it interfere with the patient's usual activities? Does it make the patient lie down? The description of the severity of the pain may tell you something about the patient's responses to pain and its impact on the patient's life, but it is not consistently helpful in assessing cause. Sensitivity to abdominal pain varies widely and tends to diminish over the later years, thus masking acute abdominal problems in older people, especially those in or beyond their 70s.

Careful timing of the pain, on the other hand, is particularly helpful. **Did it start suddenly or gradually? When did the pain begin? How long does it last? What is its pattern over a 24-hour period? over weeks and months? Are you dealing with an acute illness or a chronic or recurring one?**

What aggravates or relieves the pain, with special reference to eating, antacids, alcohol, medications (including aspirin-containing and other over-the-counter drugs), emotional factors, and possibly posture? Is the pain related to body functions such as defecation, menstruation, and urination?

Acute appendicitis exemplifies both visceral and parietal pain. Early distention of the inflamed appendix produces periumbilical pain, which is gradually replaced by right lower quadrant pain due to inflammation of the adjacent parietal peritoneum.

Pain of duodenal or pancreatic origin may be referred to the back; pain from the biliary tree, to the right shoulder or the right posterior chest.

The pain of pleurisy or acute myocardial infarction may be referred to the upper abdomen.

See Table 2-7, Abdominal Pain, pp. 86–87.

Cramping (colicky) pain suggests a relationship to peristalsis.

Citrus fruits may aggravate the pain of reflux esophagitis. Abdominal discomfort with milk ingestion suggests lactase deficiency.

What symptoms are associated with the pain, and in what sequence do they occur?

"How is your appetite?" continues the gastrointestinal history but may also lead into other important areas. *Anorexia* refers to loss or lack of appetite. Distinguish it from intolerance to certain foods or reluctance to eat anything because of anticipated discomfort. *Nausea*, which patients often describe as "feeling sick to my stomach," may progress to retching and vomiting. *Retching* describes the spasmodic movements of the chest and diaphragm that precede and culminate in *vomiting*—the forceful expulsion of gastric contents out through the mouth.

Anorexia, nausea, and vomiting accompany gastrointestinal disorders and many other conditions such as pregnancy, responses to prescribed or other drugs, diabetic acidosis, adrenal insufficiency, hypercalcemia, uremia, liver disease, emotional states, and (though without nausea) anorexia/bulimia nervosa.

Regurgitation, the raising of esophageal or gastric contents in the absence of nausea or retching, has implications quite different from vomiting.

Regurgitation may occur when the esophagus is narrowed or when the gastroesophageal sphincter is incompetent.

Assess these symptoms in the usual manner. Ask about any vomitus or regurgitated material, and inspect it yourself if possible. What color is it? What does the vomitus smell like? How much has there been? Ask specifically about blood in the vomitus and try to estimate its amount.

Gastric juice is clear or mucoid. Small amounts of yellowish or greenish bile are common and have no special significance. Brownish or blackish vomitus with small particles that look like coffee grounds suggests blood altered by gastric acid. Both this (when confirmed by chemical testing) and red blood are termed *hematemesis.*

Common causes of hematemesis include duodenal or gastric ulcer, esophageal or gastric varices, and gastritis. A fecal odor suggests obstruction of the ileum or a gastrocolic fistula.

Do the symptoms or setting suggest the complications of vomiting, such as aspiration into the lungs (especially in elderly, debilitated, or obtunded patients), dehydration and electrolyte imbalance (after prolonged vomiting), or significant loss of blood?

Symptoms of blood loss (light-headedness, faintness, syncope) depend on the rate and volume of bleeding and rarely appear before 500 ml or more are lost.

To assess *bowel function*, start with some open-ended questions: "How are your bowel movements? How often do you move your bowels? Do you have any difficulties? Has there been any change in your bowel habits?" The frequency of bowel movements varies in normal adults from about 3 times a day to twice a week. Changes within these limits, however, may be significant in an individual patient.

When asking about the appearance of stools, find out if the patient looks at them. This avoids being misled by confusing or negative responses.

Inquire about the color of the stools and ask about any *black stools* (suggesting *melena*) or *red blood in the stools (hematochezia)*. If either condition is present, how long has the patient noticed it? How often?

See Table 2-8, Black and Bloody Stools, p. 88.

If the blood is red, how much is there? Is it pure blood, mixed in with the stool, or on the surface of it? Is there blood on the toilet paper?

Patients vary widely in their concepts of constipation and diarrhea. **When a person complains of either symptom, determine his or her meaning for the term. What is the *constipation* like: a decrease in the frequency of bowel movements? the passage of hard and perhaps painful stools? the need to strain unusually hard? a sense of incomplete defecation or pressure in the rectum? What do the stools look like? What remedies has the patient tried? Explore the setting in which the constipation has occurred, with particular reference to medications, emotional stress, the person's ideas of normal bowel habits, and the time and conditions available for defecation.** Occasionally constipation becomes complete, with passage of neither feces nor gas. This is termed *obstipation.*

See Table 2-9, Constipation, p. 89.

Obstipation occurs in intestinal obstruction.

Diarrhea is an excessive frequency in the passage of stools that are usually unformed or watery.

Try to determine the size or the volume of the stools as well as their frequency. Are they bulky or small? How often must the patient go to the toilet to pass them?

Consistently large diarrheal stools suggest a disorder in the small bowel or proximal colon; small, frequent stools with urgency to pass them suggest a disorder in the left colon or rectum.

What are the stools like qualitatively? Are they mushy or watery? What color are they? Do they look greasy or oily? frothy? Do they smell unusually foul? Do they float in the toilet (because of excessive gas), and are they therefore difficult to flush? Is mucus, pus, or blood associated?

Large, yellowish or gray, greasy, foul-smelling, and sometimes frothy or floating stools suggest *steatorrhea* (fatty stools), associated with malabsorption.

Assess the course of the diarrhea over time. Is it acute, chronic, or recurrent? Remember, however, that your patient may be experiencing the first acute episode in a chronic or recurrent illness.

See Table 2-10, Diarrhea (pp. 90–91).

Does diarrhea waken the patient at night?

Nocturnal diarrhea suggests an organic cause.

What seems to aggravate and relieve the diarrhea? Does the patient get relief from a bowel movement, or is there an intense urge, with straining, but little or no result (*tenesmus*)?

Relief by moving the bowels or passing gas suggests a disorder in the left colon or rectum. Tenesmus suggests a problem in the rectum near the anal sphincter.

In what setting has the diarrhea occurred, including travel, emotional stress, or a new medication? Do family members or companions have similar symptoms?

What are the associated symptoms?

Jaundice, or *icterus,* refers to the yellowish discoloration of the skin and eyes by an increased amount of bilirubin, a bile pigment derived chiefly from the breakdown of hemoglobin. Normally, liver cells take up this bilirubin, conjugate (combine) it with other substances so that it becomes water soluble, and then excrete it into the bile. Bile passes normally through the biliary tree into the small intestine. Mechanisms of jaundice include:

1. Increased production of bilirubin
2. Decreased uptake of bilirubin by the liver cells
3. Decreased ability of the liver to conjugate the bilirubin, and
4. Decreased excretion of bilirubin into the bile with resulting escape of some bilirubin, now in its conjugated form, back into the blood. The cause may lie *within the liver itself,* as

   a. Hepatocellular jaundice, due to damage to the liver cells, or as
   b. Cholestatic jaundice, a more selective excretory impairment due to damage of liver cells or of intrahepatic bile ducts.

Bilirubin in the blood is predominantly unconjugated in jaundice due to any of the first three mechanisms. Causes include hemolytic anemia (increased production) and Gilbert's syndrome.

When excretion of bilirubin is impaired, the bilirubin in the blood is predominantly conjugated. Causes include: viral hepatitis, cirrhosis; drug-induced cholestasis (oral contraceptives, methyl testosterone, chlorpromazine) or primary biliary cirrhosis.

Alternatively, the cause may lie in *obstruction of the extrahepatic bile ducts.*

Obstruction of the common bile duct by gallstones or cancer of the pancreas

As you interview the jaundiced patient, pay special attention to the associated symptoms and the setting in which the illness occurred.

What color was the urine as the patient became ill? and now? When conjugated bilirubin increases in the blood it may appear in the urine, darkening it into a yellowish brown or tea-like color. Unconjugated bilirubin is not excreted in the urine.

Dark urine stained by bilirubin indicates impaired excretion of bilirubin into the gastrointestinal tract.

How about the color of the stools? When excretion of bile into the intestine is completely obstructed, the stools become light colored and gray (or *acholic,* without bile).

Acholic stools may occur briefly in viral hepatitis and are common in obstructive jaundice.

Does the skin itch without other obvious explanation?

Itching favors cholestatic or obstructive jaundice.

Is there associated pain? What is its pattern? Have there been past and repeated attacks of pain?

Are there factors in the patient's setting that increase the risks of liver disease, such as these?

Consider the aching pain of a distended liver capsule; the persistent pain of pancreatic cancer; and episodes of biliary colic.

1. **Hepatitis: travel in areas of poor sanitation, known contacts with jaundiced persons, sexual contacts with carriers of hepatitis B, ingestion of raw clams or oysters, use of inadequately sterilized needles or syringes (as in drug addiction), treatment with blood transfusions or blood products or exposure to them (as in laboratories, dental offices, or dialysis units)**
2. **Cirrhosis and other alcohol-related liver disease. (Interview the patient carefully about the consumption of alcohol.)**

3. **Toxic liver damage, as from medications and industrial exposure.**
4. **Gallbladder disease, its symptoms, or gallbladder surgery that might have contributed to extrahepatic biliary obstruction**
5. **Hereditary disorders. (Review the family history.)**

The Urinary Tract

Disorders of the urinary tract may cause pain in either the back or the abdomen. *Kidney pain* is felt at or below the costal margin posteriorly, near the costovertebral angle. It may radiate anteriorly toward the umbilicus.

Kidney pain occurs in acute pyelonephritis.

Kidney pain is a visceral pain that is usually produced by sudden distention of the renal capsule and is typically dull, aching, and steady. Dramatically different is *ureteral pain (ureteral or renal colic)*, a severe colicky pain that often originates in the costovertebral angle and radiates around the trunk into the lower quadrant of the abdomen and possibly on into the upper thigh and testicle or labium. Ureteral pain results from sudden distention of the ureter and associated distention of the renal pelvis.

Renal or ureteral colic is caused by sudden obstruction of a ureter, as by urinary stones or blood clots.

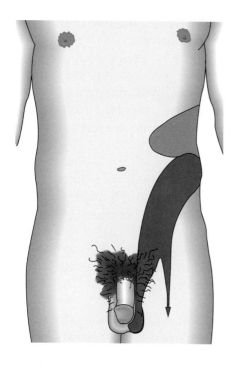 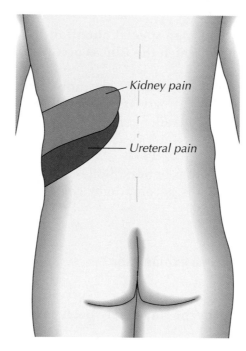

Kidney pain

Ureteral pain

Bladder disorders may cause suprapubic pain. Pain associated with bladder infection, if present at all in the abdomen, is typically dull and steady. Pain associated with sudden overdistention of the bladder is often agonizing, while chronic bladder distention is usually painless. *Prostatic pain* is felt in the perineum and occasionally in the rectum.

Pain of sudden overdistention in acute urinary retention

*Pain on urination** accompanies inflammation or irritation of either the bladder or the urethra, and is usually felt as a burning sensation. Men

Cystitis and urethritis commonly cause painful urination. Consider also stones, foreign bodies or tumors in the bladder, and acute prostatitis. In

---

* Clinicians often refer to painful urination as *dysuria*. Some authorities, however, prefer to define dysuria as any difficulty in voiding.

typically feel it in or proximal to the glans penis, while women perceive it in one of two ways: as an internal urethral discomfort, sometimes described as pressure, or as an external burning caused by urine as it flows across irritated or inflamed labia.

Several symptoms other than pain may accompany voiding. *Urinary urgency* is an unusually intense and immediate desire to void. It sometimes leads to involuntary voiding (*urge incontinence*). In a man with partial obstruction to urinary outflow from the bladder, a cluster of symptoms often develops: *hesitancy* in starting the urinary stream, *straining* to void, *reduced caliber and force of the urinary stream,* and *dribbling* as he tries to complete the voiding process.

Three terms describe important alterations in the patterns of voiding urine. *Polyuria* refers to a significant increase in 24-hour urinary volume, roughly defined as exceeding 3 liters. It must be distinguished from *urinary frequency,* abnormally frequent voiding. Although urinary frequency may be secondary to polyuria and is then associated with a high volume of urine with each voiding, frequency is often associated instead with relatively small volumes at each passage. *Nocturia* refers to urinary frequency at night, sometimes defined as awakening the patient more than once. A change in nocturnal voiding patterns as well as the number of trips to the toilet should be considered in assessing this symptom. Like frequency, nocturia may be associated with large or small volumes of urine. *Polydipsia* is an abnormally high intake of water or other fluids and is commonly associated with polyuria.

Blood in the urine is an important symptom known as *hematuria,* often identified only by urinalysis. When visible to the naked eye it is called *gross hematuria*. Blood may give the urine a pinkish or brownish cast or in larger amounts may make it look frankly bloody. Be sure to distinguish menstrual bleeding from hematuria. If urine is reddish, inquire about ingestion of beets or medications that sometimes discolor the urine. Test the urine with dipstick and microscopic examination before settling on the term hematuria.

Urinary incontinence refers to an involuntary loss of urine that has become a social or hygienic problem. It usually points to a disorder in the urinary bladder or urethra, in the structures that support or surround them, or in the neural regulatory mechanisms that control urination.

The normal adult bladder is a hollow muscular organ that can expand to accommodate roughly 300 ml of urine at relatively low pressures. As distention continues it stimulates the smooth muscle of the bladder (the detrusor muscle) to contract, pressure in the bladder rises, and the urge

women, internal burning suggests cystitis or urethritis; external burning, vulvovaginitis.

Urinary urgency suggests infection or irritation of the bladder. In men, pain on urination without frequency or urgency suggests urethritis.

Polyuria indicates an abnormally high production of urine by the kidneys. Frequency without polyuria (during the day or night) suggests either a disorder of the urinary bladder or impairment to flow at or below the bladder neck.

See Table 2-11, Polyuria, Frequency, and Nocturia, pp. 92–93.

Causes of hematuria include cystitis, malignancy of the bladder or kidney, stones, trauma, tuberculosis, and acute glomerulonephritis. Bilirubin may color the urine yellowish brown.

Drugs that may color the urine reddish include phenolphthalein (common in over-the-counter laxatives) and phenazopyridine (Pyridium).

Incontinence may result when detrusor contractions are too strong (*urge incontinence*), when intraurethral pressure is too

to void becomes conscious. If the setting is inconvenient for voiding, higher centers in the brain can inhibit detrusor contractions until the normal bladder capacity of 400 ml to 500 ml is reached. Pressure within the urethra that exceeds that in the bladder holds the accumulating urine within the bladder reservoir and prevents incontinence. Factors contributing to intraurethral pressure include smooth muscle in the urethra (the internal urethral sphincter), the thickness of normal urethral mucosa, and, in women, sufficient muscular support of the bladder and proximal urethra to maintain the proper geometric relations between them. Striated muscle around the urethra can contract voluntarily to interrupt the voiding process.

low (*stress incontinence*), and when the bladder is grossly enlarged because of outlet obstruction (*overflow incontinence*). Incontinence may also be due to poor general health, to environmental factors (*functional incontinence*), or to medications. See Table 2-12, Urinary Incontinence, pp. 94–95.

Neuroregulatory control of the bladder functions at several levels. In an infant, the bladder empties by a reflex mechanism at the sacral level of the spinal cord. Adult voluntary control of urination depends also on higher centers within the brain and on motor and sensory pathways between the brain and the sacral cord.

General questions for a urinary history include: "Do you have any difficulty passing your urine? How often do you go? Do you get up at night to go? How often? How much do you pass at a time? Is there any pain or burning? Do you have to go so badly that you sometimes have trouble getting to the toilet in time? Do you ever leak any urine? . . . or wet yourself?" If the patient has been incontinent, ask when it happens and how often. Can the patient sense when the bladder is full? and when voiding occurs? Ask women specifically if sudden coughing, sneezing, or laughing makes them lose urine (*stress incontinence*). Roughly half of even young women who have not borne children report this experience.

Unawareness of a full bladder or of wetness suggests a sensory or mental deficit.

Occasional leakage of small amounts of urine is not necessarily significant.

What color is the urine? Has it ever been reddish, or brownish?

Hematuria

If it seems relevant, inquire about pain in the abdomen or back, but in the absence of urinary symptoms you may prefer to cover these topics in your gastrointestinal and musculoskeletal histories.

Renal or ureteral pain

Ask additional questions of middle-aged or elderly men. "Do you have trouble starting your stream? Do you have to stand closer to the toilet than you used to? Have you noticed a change in the force or size of your stream? Do you have to strain down in order to void? Do you hesitate or stop in the middle of voiding? Is there dribbling after you're through?"

The most common cause of these symptoms is partial obstruction of the bladder outlet due to benign prostatic hyperplasia. Urethral stricture may also cause them.

The Genital System—Female

Questions in this section focus on menstruation, pregnancy and related topics, vulvovaginal symptoms, and sexual function.

For the menstrual history, ask the patient how old she was when her monthly, or menstrual, periods began (age at *menarche*). When did her last period start, and, if possible, the one before that? How often do the periods come (as measured by the first day of successive periods)? How regular or irregular are they? How long do they last? How heavy is the flow? What color is it? Flow can be assessed roughly by the number of pads or tampons used daily. Because women vary in their assessments of when sanitary equipment should be changed, however, ask the patient whether she usually soaks a pad or tampon, spots it lightly, or what. Further, does she use more than one at a time? Does she have any bleeding between periods? any bleeding after intercourse or after douching?

The dates of previous periods may alert you to possible pregnancy or menstrual irregularities.

Does the patient have any discomfort or pain before or during her periods? If so, what is it like, how long does it last, and does it interfere with her usual activities? Are other symptoms associated? Ask a middle-aged or older woman if she has stopped menstruating. When? Did any symptoms accompany her change? Has she had any bleeding since?

Unlike the normal dark red menstrual discharge, excessive flow tends to be bright red and may include "clots" (not true fibrin clots).

Questions about menarche, menstruation, and menopause may give you excellent opportunities to explore the patient's need for information and her attitude toward her body. When talking with an adolescent girl, for example, opening questions might include: "How did you first learn about monthly periods? How did you feel when they started? Many girls worry when their periods aren't regular or come late. Has anything like that bothered you?" For a middle-aged woman, "How did (do) you feel about not having your periods any more? Has it affected your life in any way?"

Girls in the United States usually begin to menstruate between the ages of 9 and 16 years, and often take a year or more before they settle into a reasonably regular pattern. Age at menarche varies with several factors, including genetic endowment, socioeconomic status, and nutrition. The interval between periods ranges roughly from 24 to 32 days; the flow lasts from 3 to 7 days.

Amenorrhea refers to the absence of periods. Failure to initiate periods is called *primary amenorrhea*, while the cessation of periods after they have been established is termed *secondary amenorrhea*. Pregnancy, lactation, and menopause are physiologic forms of the secondary type. *Oligomenorrhea* refers to infrequent periods, which may also be irregular. This pattern is common for as long as 2 years after menarche, and it also occurs before menopause.

Other causes of secondary amenorrhea include low body weight from any cause, including malnutrition and anorexia nervosa, stress, chronic illness, and hypothalamic–pituitary–ovarian dysfunctions.

Polymenorrhea means abnormally frequent periods, and *menorrhagia* refers to an increased amount or duration of flow. Bleeding may also occur between periods (variously termed *metrorrhagia* or *intermenstrual bleeding*), after intercourse (*postcoital bleeding*), or after other vaginal contact such as occurs with douches.

Increased frequency, increased flow, or bleeding between periods may have systemic causes or may be dysfunctional. Postcoital bleeding suggests cervical disease (e.g., polyps, cancer) or, in an older woman, atrophic vaginitis.

Menopause, the cessation of menses, usually occurs between the ages of 45 and 52 years, but the range of normal is wider. *Postmenopausal bleeding* is defined as bleeding that occurs after 6 months without periods. The only symptoms clearly associated with menopause are *hot flushes* (or *flashes*), the sweating associated with them, and sometimes the disturbance of sleep that they may cause.

Postmenopausal bleeding raises the question of endometrial cancer, although it also has other causes.

Dysmenorrhea is pain with menstruation, and is usually felt as a bearing down, aching, or cramping sensation in the lower abdomen and pelvis. *Premenstrual syndrome (PMS)* refers to several symptoms noted by some women during the 4 to 10 days before a period. These include tension, nervousness, irritability, depression, and mood swings; weight gain, abdominal bloating, edema, and tenderness of the breasts; and headaches. Though usually mild, the symptoms may be severe and disabling.

Standard questions related to pregnancies include: "Have you ever been (or how often have you been) pregnant? Have you ever had a miscarriage or an abortion? How often? How many living children do you have?" Inquire about any difficulties with the pregnancies and the timing and circumstances of any abortion (spontaneous or induced). What kind of birth control methods, if any, have the patient and her partner used, and how satisfied is she with them?

If amenorrhea suggests a pregnancy now, inquire about its possibility (history of intercourse) and about common early symptoms: tenderness, tingling, or increased size of the breasts; urinary frequency; nausea and vomiting; easy fatigability; and feelings that the baby is moving (the last usually noted at about 20 weeks). Be alert to the patient's feelings in discussing all these topics, and explore them as seems indicated. (See Chapter 14, The Pregnant Woman.)

Amenorrhea followed by heavy bleeding suggests a threatened abortion or dysfunctional uterine bleeding related to lack of ovulation.

The most common vulvovaginal symptoms are *vaginal discharge* and local *itching*. **Follow your usual approach. If the patient reports a discharge, inquire about its amount, color, consistency, and odor. Ask too about any local *sores* or *lumps* in the vulvar area. Are they painful or not? Because patients vary in their understanding of anatomic terms here, be prepared with some alternative phrasing: "Any itching (or other symptom) near your vagina? . . . between your legs? . . . where you urinate?"**

See Table 13-5, Vaginitis, p. 427.

See Table 13-1, Lesions of the Vulva, p. 423.

Local symptoms or findings on physical examination may raise the possibility of sexually transmitted diseases. After establishing the usual attributes of any symptoms, identify the patient' sexual preference as to partners (male, female, or both). Inquire about sexual contacts and establish the number of sexual partners in the prior month. Ask if the patient desires HIV testing or has current or past partners

at risk. Review the past history of venereal disease. "Have you ever had herpes? . . . any other problems such as gonorrhea? . . . syphilis? . . . pelvic infections?" Continue with the more general questions suggested on pp. 19–20.

If the patient seems to have a sexual problem, ask her to tell you about it. Direct questions help you to assess each phase of the sexual response: desire, arousal, and orgasm. "Have you maintained an interest in (appetite for) sex?" inquires about the desire phase. For the orgasmic phase, "Are you able to reach a climax (reach an orgasm or "come")? Is it important for you to reach a climax?" For arousal, "Do you get sexually aroused? Do you lubricate easily (get wet or slippery)? Do you stay too dry?"

Further, "Are you satisfied with your sex life as it is now? Has there been any significant change in the last few years? Are you satisfied with your ability to perform sexually? How satisfied do you think your partner is? Do you feel that your partner is satisfied with the frequency of sexual activity?"

In addition to ascertaining the nature of a sexual problem, ask about its onset, severity (persistent or sporadic), setting, and factors, if any, that make it better or worse. What does the patient think is the cause of the problem, what has she tried to do about it, and what does she hope for? The setting of a sexual dysfunction is an important but complicated topic, involving the patient's general health, medications and drugs including alcohol, her partner's and her own knowledge of sexual practices and techniques, her attitudes, values, and fears, the relationship and communication between her and her partner(s), and the environment in which sexual activity takes place.

Ask also about any discomfort or pain on intercourse (*dyspareunia*). If she has had it, try to localize the symptom. Is it near the outside, occurring at the start of intercourse, or does she feel it farther in, when her partner's penis (or other object) is pushing deeper? *Vaginismus* refers to an involuntary spasm of the muscles surrounding the vaginal orifice that makes penetration during intercourse painful or impossible.

Because of the risk of AIDS and other sexually transmitted diseases, **ask too about oral and anal sex and, if indicated, about symptoms involving the mouth, throat, anus, or rectum.**

The Genital System—Male

For men, questions about the genital system follow naturally after those dealing with the urinary system. They focus on local symptoms and on sexual function.

Examples/Interpretations

Sexual dysfunctions are classified by the phase of sexual response. A woman may lack desire, she may fail to become aroused and to attain adequate vaginal lubrication, or, despite adequate arousal, she may be unable to reach orgasm much or all of the time. Causes include lack of estrogen, medical illness, and psychiatric illness.

More commonly, however, a sexual problem is related to one or more of the situational or psychosocial factors mentioned on the left.

Superficial pain suggests local inflammation, atrophic vaginitis, or inadequate lubrication; deeper pain may be due to pelvic disorders or pressure on a normal ovary. The cause of vaginismus may be physical or psychological.

Ask about any *discharge from the penis*, dripping, or staining of the underwear. If discharge is present, ascertain the amount, its color and consistency, and any associated symptoms. Inquire about *sores* or *growths on the penis* and any *swelling* or *pain in the scrotum*. These symptoms raise the question of sexually transmitted diseases. Ask about previous symptoms or a past history of diseases such as herpes, gonorrhea, and syphilis. When risk factors for HIV infection are present, ask about sexual preference, desire for HIV testing, and partners at risk. Continue with the more general questions suggested on pp. 19–20.

A penile discharge suggests urethritis.

See Table 12-1; Abnormalities of the Penis (p. 399) and Table 12-2, Abnormalities in the Scrotum (pp. 400–401). Many skin conditions other than sexually transmitted diseases affect the genitalia, and a sexually transmitted disease may be present without symptoms or signs.

Because sexually transmitted diseases may involve other parts of the body, additional questions are often indicated. An introductory explanation may be useful. **"Sexually transmitted diseases can involve any body opening where you have sex. It's important for you to tell me which openings you use."** And further, as needed, **"Do you have oral sex? . . . anal sex?"** If the answers to these questions are affirmative, ask about symptoms such as diarrhea, rectal bleeding, anal itching or pain, and sore throat.

Infections from oral–penile transmission include gonorrhea, *Chlamydia*, syphilis, and herpes. Symptomatic or asymptomatic proctitis caused by one or more microorganisms may follow anal intercourse.

If the patient seems to have a sexual problem, ask him to tell you about it. Direct questions help you to assess each phase of the sexual response. **"Have you maintained an interest in (appetite for) sex?"** asks about the desire phase. If there is a problem in this (or a later phase), explore its timing, severity, setting, and any other factors that may have contributed to it.

Lack of desire may be psychogenic or due to medications or medical problems such as lack of androgen.

To assess the arousal phase, ask, **"Are you able to achieve and maintain an erection?"** If there seems to be a problem here, ask the patient how firm the penis becomes. Is the problem constant or sporadic? Are there circumstances in which erection is normal: with other partners? on awakening during the night or in the morning? with masturbation? Were there any changes in his relationship with his partner or in his life situation at the time when the problem began? A firm erection in any circumstance (especially likely early in the morning) suggests that the erectile dysfunction is psychogenic.

In an erectile disorder, a man cannot attain and maintain an erection that is adequate to complete the sexual activity. Causes are systemic, psychogenic, or both. Consider medications, other drugs, or endocrine, vascular, and neurologic problems.

Other questions relate to the phase of ejaculation and orgasm. For ejaculation that is premature (too soon and out of control), ask, **"About how long does intercourse last? Do you come too soon? Do you feel you have any control over it? Do you think your partner would like intercourse to last longer?"** For reduced or absent ejaculation, **"Do you sometimes find that you can't come (ejaculate, have an orgasm) even though your erection is all right?"** If there seems to be a problem, find out whether it involves the pleasurable sensation of orgasm, the ejaculation of seminal fluid, or both. Inquire about the frequency and setting of the problem, medications, surgery, and neurologic symptoms.

Premature ejaculation is very common, especially in young men. Reduced or absent ejaculation of semen is less common and usually affects middle-aged and older men. It may be due to medications, surgery, neurologic deficits, or lack of androgen. Lack of orgasm with ejaculation is usually psychogenic.

Further, "Are you satisfied with your sex life as it is now? Has there been any significant change over the last few years? How satisfied do you think your partner is? Do you feel that your partner is satisfied with the frequency of sexual activity?"

As with women, inquire about the onset, severity, and setting of any problem. What does the patient think has caused it, what has he tried to do about it, and what does he hope for?

The Peripheral Vascular System

Pain in the arms and legs may arise from the skin, the peripheral vascular system, the musculoskeletal system, or the nervous system. In addition, visceral pain, such as that from myocardial infarction, may be referred to the extremities.

Symptoms associated with the pain often give clues to its vascular nature. *Swelling of the feet and legs,* for example, may signify venous disease, although it has many other causes, and *coldness* and *numbness* often accompany arterial disorders. The *redness, swelling,* and *tenderness* of local inflammation are seen in some vascular disorders as well as in other conditions that may mimic them. In contrast, relatively brief leg cramps that commonly occur at night in otherwise healthy people do not indicate a circulatory problem, and cold hands and feet are so common in healthy people that they have relatively little predictive value.

See Table 2-13, Painful Peripheral Vascular Disorders and Their Mimics, pp. 96–97. Local inflammation is seen in superficial thrombophlebitis, lymphangitis, cellulitis, and erythema nodosum. The origin of the common leg cramp is poorly understood.

For most patients, inquiry about two symptoms suffices for screening: swelling of the feet and legs, and pain or discomfort in the legs. "Do your fingertips change color in the cold? How?" may also be useful.

Severe pallor of the fingers, often followed by cyanosis and then redness, indicates Raynaud's disease or phenomenon.

With middle-aged and older people you should also ask about *intermittent claudication,* a specific pattern of pain that accompanies impairment of arterial flow. "How far can you walk without stopping to rest?" is a good opening question. Then determine what makes the patient stop and how quickly relief is felt.

Aching, cramping, and possibly numbness or severe fatigue that appear with walking and disappear promptly with rest typify intermittent claudication.

The Musculoskeletal System

"Have you had any *pains in your joints?*" turns the interview explicitly to the musculoskeletal system. An affirmative answer may indicate a problem not only in the joints but also in bones, muscles, and tissues around the joints. Either now or during the examination, ask the patient to show you as clearly as possible where the pain is felt. Where did it start? What then? Pain originating in the small joints of the hands and feet is more sharply localized than that from the larger joints. Pain from the hip joint is especially deceptive. Although it is typically felt in the groin or the buttock, it is sometimes felt in the anterior thigh or partly or solely in the knee.

Problems in tissues around joints include inflammation of bursae (*bursitis*), tendons (*tendinitis*), or tendon sheaths (*tenosynovitis*), and stretching or tearing of ligaments (*sprains*).

"Hip pain" near the greater trochanter of the femur suggests trochanteric bursitis.

Determine whether the pain has involved one joint or its adjacent tissues, or whether several joints have been affected. If the latter, in what pattern has the involvement spread? Has the pain disappeared from the one or more joints initially involved only to migrate to others, or has the initial pain persisted while pain has progressed to other joints? Is the involvement symmetrical, affecting similar joints on both sides of the body?

Pain in only one joint area suggests bursitis, tendinitis, monoarticular arthritis, or an injury. Rheumatic fever and early gonococcal arthritis often have a migratory pattern of spread; rheumatoid arthritis typically shows a progressive or additive pattern and is symmetrical.

Assess the quality and severity of the joint pain.

Timing is particularly important. Did the pain develop rapidly over the course of a few hours, or insidiously over weeks or even months? Has there been slow progression, or periods of improvement and worsening? How long has the pain lasted? What is it like over the course of a day? in the morning? and as the day wears on?

Unusually severe and rapidly developing pain in a swollen joint, not explained by injury, suggests acute gouty or septic arthritis. In children, especially consider osteomyelitis that involves bone contiguous to a joint.

What aggravates and relieves the pain, with special reference to exercise, rest, and treatments? In what setting did the pain develop? Was there an acute injury or excessive use of the body part?

What symptoms are associated? Here there are three relevant categories. First, are there *other symptoms in the involved joint(s)*—specifically, swelling, stiffness, limitation of motion, tenderness, warmth, or redness? Pains in the joints without objective evidence of arthritis such as swelling, tenderness, or warmth are called *arthralgias*. Pains in the muscles are called *myalgias*. **Inquire about *swelling* in your usual manner, trying to localize it as accurately as possible.**

See Table 2-14, Patterns of Chronic Pain In and Around the Joints, pp. 98–99.

For *limitation of motion,* ask about activities that have been altered due to problems with the involved joint. When relevant, specifically inquire about the patient's ability to walk, stand, lean over, sit, sit up, rise from a sitting position, climb, pinch, grasp, turn a page, open a door or jar, and care for bodily needs such as combing hair, brushing teeth, feeding, dressing, and washing, including washing hard-to-reach areas such as the perineum.

Stiffness is often difficult to assess because people use the term in different ways. Stiffness in the musculoskeletal interview refers to the subjective perception of tightness or resistance to movement, the opposite of feeling limber. It is often associated with discomfort or pain. If the patient has not volunteered a sense of stiffness, ask about it. **Two good questions are "What time do you get up in the morning?" and "What time do you feel about as loose as you are going to get?"** Then calculate the duration of the patient's stiffness. Stiffness, together with muscular soreness, is felt by healthy people after unusually strenuous muscular exertion and peaks in intensity around the second day after exertion.

Stiffness after inactivity is common in degenerative joint disease but usually lasts only a few minutes. This is sometimes called *gelling*. Stiffness in rheumatoid arthritis and other inflammatory arthritides often lasts 30 minutes or longer. Stiffness also accompanies the fibromyalgia syndrome and polymyalgia rheumatica.

Tenderness, warmth, and *redness* are often best detected on examination, but patients can sometimes give you this information and guide you to points of tenderness.

Tenderness, warmth, and redness in a joint suggest acute gout, septic arthritis, or possibly rheumatic fever.

The second category of associated symptoms includes *generalized symptoms* such as *fever, chills, fatigue, anorexia, weight loss,* and *weakness.*

Generalized symptoms are common in rheumatoid and other inflammatory arthritides. High fever and chills suggest an infectious cause.

Third, are there *symptoms elsewhere in the body that give important clues as to the nature of the problem?* These include:

*   *Skin conditions such as*

    A butterfly rash on the cheeks — Systemic lupus erythematosus

    The scaly rash and pitted nails of psoriasis — Psoriatic arthritis

    A few papules, pustules, or vesicles on reddened bases, located on the distal extremities — Gonococcal arthritis

    An expanding erythematous patch early in an illness — Lyme disease

    Hives — Serum sickness, drug reaction

    Erosions or scales on the penis and crusted scaling papules on the soles and palms — Reiter's syndrome, which also includes arthritis, urethritis, and conjunctivitis

    The maculopapular rash of rubella — Arthritis of rubella

    Clubbing of the fingernails (see p. 158) — Hypertrophic osteoarthropathy

*   Red, burning, and itchy eyes (*conjunctivitis*) — Reiter's syndrome

*   Preceding *sore throat* — Acute rheumatic fever or gonococcal arthritis

*   *Diarrhea* and *abdominal pain* — Arthritis with ulcerative colitis or regional enteritis

*   Symptoms of *urethritis* — Reiter's syndrome or possibly gonococcal arthritis

Even if the patient denies joint pain, specifically ask about *backache,* **a very common symptom. Use your usual interviewing method to develop a clear picture of the problem. If pain radiates into the legs, ask about numbness, tingling, or weakness that may be associated.**

See Table 2-15, Low Back Pain, p. 100.

Associated numbness, tingling, or weakness suggests involvement of nerve roots.

Pain in the neck is also common. Approach it in the same manner. When neck pain is chronic, be alert for manifestations of pressure on the spinal cord: weakness, loss of sensation, and, in late stages, loss of bladder and bowel control.

See Table 2-16, Pains in the Neck, p. 101.

The Nervous System

"Have you ever fainted or passed out?" turns the discussion to *loss of consciousness.* Get as complete and unbiased a description of the event as you can. Try to determine what seems to have precipitated the attack(s) and what kind of warning, if any, the patient felt before passing out. Was the patient standing, sitting, or lying down when the attack started? How long did the episode last? Did the patient black out completely, or could voices be heard throughout the episode (indicating some consciousness)? Could voices be heard while passing out and coming to?

In young people who lose consciousness temporarily, consider vasodepressor syncope, hyperventilation, and tonic–clonic seizures. Voices heard when passing out and coming to suggest one of the first two. Cardiac syncope (common in older patients) has sudden onset, sudden offset.

Did anyone observe the episode? If so, what did the patient look like before losing consciousness, during the episode, and afterward? If not, what has the patient been told about any previous attacks? How did the patient feel after recovery?

Appearance before, during, and after the episode, and the feelings after it, help to distinguish a seizure from other conditions.

Syncope is the sudden but temporary loss of consciousness that occurs when blood flow to the brain becomes insufficient. It is commonly described as fainting. The symptoms of an impending faint, including muscular weakness, lightheadedness, and other premonitory feelings without actual loss of consciousness, are called *near syncope* or *pre-syncope.* These are assessed in the usual manner. Syncope must be distinguished from generalized seizures—a task sometimes made difficult by the fact that a severe syncopal attack can occasionally produce a few clonic movements and even urinary incontinence. Syncope is not usually associated, however, with a fully developed tonic–clonic (grand mal) seizure, with fecal incontinence, or with a postictal state.

See Table 2-17, Syncope and Similar Disorders, pp. 102–103.

In contrast with syncope, a tonic–clonic (grand mal) seizure usually starts more quickly, lasts longer, is more likely to involve injury and incontinence, and is followed by a slower recovery.

A *seizure* is a paroxysmal disorder that may or may not involve a loss of consciousness, and may also involve abnormal sensations, movements, feelings, or thought processes. It is caused by a sudden, excessive electrical discharge in the cerebral cortex or its underlying structures. "Have you ever had any seizures or spells? . . . any fits or convulsions?" opens the discussion. As with syncope, get as full a description as possible, including precipitating circumstances, warnings, behavior and feelings during the attack, duration of the attack, and feelings after it. Ask about age at onset, the frequency of seizures, any recent change in frequency, and use of medications. Is there a history of prior head injury or other conditions that may be causally related?

See Table 2-18, Seizure Disorders, pp. 104–105.

To assess motor performance, ask about *weakness* of any part of the body and about *paralysis,* an inability to move a part. Did the weakness start slowly or suddenly? Has it progressed, and how? What

Local weakness may result from abnormalities in the central or peripheral nervous system, the

body parts are involved? Does the weakness affect one or both sides? What movements are affected? Try to distinguish between distal and proximal weakness. For distal weakness in the arms, inquire about hand movements such as opening a jar or can or using hand tools such as scissors, pliers, or a screwdriver. For distal weakness in the legs, ask about frequent tripping. For proximal weakness, ask about combing hair, trying to reach something on a high shelf, and difficulty in rising from a chair or taking a high step up. Does the weakness increase with repeated effort and improve after rest? Are there associated sensory or other symptoms?

neuromuscular junctions, or the muscles themselves. Bilateral, predominantly distal weakness suggests a polyneuropathy; bilateral proximal weakness, a myopathy. Weakness made worse with repeated effort and improved with rest suggests myasthenia gravis and related syndromes.

Tremors and other *involuntary movements* occur with or without additional neurologic manifestations. **Ask about trembling, shakiness, or body movements that the patient seems unable to control.**

See Table 18-3, Involuntary Movements, pp. 610–611.

Pain may stem from neurologic causes and is usually reported in other sections of the systems review, such as the head and musculoskeletal system.

Other sensory symptoms include lost or altered sensation. **Ask about numbness, tingling, pins-and-needles sensations, or other peculiar or unpleasant feelings in the body. If a patient reports numbness, try to determine the real meaning—a *loss of sensation,* an inability to move the part, or an altered sensation. Use your usual style of questioning, paying particular attention to location.**

Loss of sensation, paresthesias, and dysesthesias occur with lesions involving the peripheral nerves, sensory roots, spinal cord, and higher centers. Paresthesias in the hands and around the mouth commonly accompany hyperventilation.

Paresthesias are peculiar sensations of various kinds that have no obvious stimulus. They include tingling, prickling, and feelings of warmth, coldness, and pressure. Paresthesias are what everyone feels when an arm or a leg "goes to sleep" after the compression of a nerve. *Dysesthesias* are distorted sensations in response to a stimulus, and may last longer than the stimulus itself. For example, a person may perceive a light touch or a pinprick as an unpleasant burning or tingling sensation.

Distinct from these symptoms is an almost indescribable *restlessness of the legs* that typically develops at rest and is accompanied by an urge to move about. Walking gives relief.

These symptoms suggest the common but often overlooked restless legs syndrome.

The Hematologic System

The assessment of hematologic disorders depends heavily on physical examination and the laboratory, but symptoms too have some value. Anemia must become moderate or severe before producing symptoms. It then decreases exercise tolerance and leads to dyspnea and palpitations. In persons with atherosclerosis, it may decrease the threshold for angina pectoris or intermittent claudication. Patients with severe anemia may report a variety of symptoms that may lead you astray: headache, dizziness, vertigo, syncope, anorexia, nausea, intolerance to cold, amenorrhea, menorrhagia, loss of libido, and impotence.

Spontaneous bleeding and bleeding disproportionate to an injury suggest a generalized bleeding disorder. It may be congenital or acquired. Normal hemostasis depends on three mechanisms: (1) vasoconstriction following a vascular injury, (2) formation of a platelet plug, and (3) formation of a fibrin clot. The most common bleeding disorders result from deficits in the last two categories. Platelet plugs are essential for prompt hemostasis, especially in the capillaries of the skin and mucous membranes. Fibrin clots are especially important as a second line of defense, particularly in larger vessels such as arterioles or venules.

Congenital bleeding disorders, involving the clotting mechanism, are most common in males. The family history is often positive.

A platelet disorder, therefore, is likely to cause capillary bleeding into the skin or mucous membranes. When the bleeding is initiated by injury, it tends to occur without delay. In contrast, a clotting disorder tends to cause bleeding deep in the tissues. After an injury, bleeding tends to appear several hours later. Bleeding due to a vascular defect tends to resemble that of a platelet disorder and may be associated with it.

Petechiae (see p. 156) in the skin and mucous membranes and small bruises are common in platelet disorders. Large bruises, deep *hematomas* (local masses of extravasated blood), and *hemarthroses* (blood in the joints) are seen in clotting disorders.

"Do you bleed or bruise easily?" opens this discussion. Further, "Have you ever bled a lot (or too much) after having a tooth pulled? . . . or after an operation? How about nosebleeds?" If there is a history of bleeding, try to distinguish between a localized problem and a more general bleeding tendency. If the latter is present, determine the sites of bleeding, timing in relation to possible injury, duration, frequency, and severity. Has the patient needed blood transfusions? Ask about medications, including aspirin and "blood thinners," and, if you have not already specifically done so, carefully review the family history for bleeding problems. Are there reasons to suspect a deficiency in vitamin C or K?

Spontaneous bleeding, bleeding with minor trauma, and bleeding in several sites suggest a general disorder.

Inadequate diet, malabsorption

The Endocrine System

The assessment of endocrine function depends not so much on additional symptoms as on pulling together the data already gathered and recognizing the underlying pattern of an endocrine disorder. When you begin to recognize such a pattern, ask about symptoms that you know might be relevant but try to avoid leading the patient. When you suspect Addison's disease, for example, "Have you noticed any change in the color of your skin?" is better than "Has your skin become darker?" There are, however, a few additional symptoms that are important in an endocrine evaluation. These relate primarily to diabetes mellitus and to thyroid dysfunction.

Obesity, weakness, fatigue, easy bruising, ankle edema, and decreased or absent menstrual periods suggest Cushing's syndrome (adrenal cortical hyperfunction), while weakness, weight loss, nausea, vomiting, darkened skin, and symptoms of postural hypotension suggest Addison's disease (adrenal insufficiency).

Polyuria, already described in the section on the urinary tract, is a frequent symptom of diabetes mellitus. It is then typically associated with excessive *thirst* and with *polydipsia* (an increased intake of fluid). *Polyphagia* (increased food intake) may also occur.

Other symptoms that often accompany the onset of diabetes mellitus include weakness, fatigue, weight loss, and blurred vision.

An assessment of thyroid function involves questions concerning *temperature intolerance* and *sweating*. **Opening questions include "Do you prefer hot or cold weather? Do you generally dress more warmly or less warmly than most people? Do you use more blankets or fewer blankets than others at home? Do you sweat (or perspire) more or less than most people?"** As people grow older, they sweat less, tolerate cold less well, and tend to prefer warmer environments. For other symptoms that may be related to abnormal thyroid function, see Table 7-22, Thyroid Enlargement and Function (p. 244).

Intolerance to cold, preferences for warm clothing and many blankets, and decreased sweating suggest hypothyroidism; the opposites suggest hyperthyroidism.

Episodic sweating and heat intolerance often occur during menopause.

Screening for Mental Status

In the course of the interview you often identify clues to emotional or other psychiatric problems. It is usually wise to inquire about these when the patient mentions them. A few screening questions about *nervousness, tensions, mood*, and possibly *memory* should be included in most histories. In younger patients, be alert to problems of substance abuse; in older patients, memory deficits and behavior change may portend early dementia. This subject is sufficiently important, however, to warrant its own chapter—Chapter 3.

Table 2-1   Headaches

TABLE 2-1 *Headaches*

Problem	Process	Location	Quality and Severity	Timing	
				Onset	*Duration*
Tension Headaches	Unclear	Usually bilateral; may be generalized or localized to the back of the head and upper neck or to the frontotemporal area	Mild and aching or a nonpainful tightness and pressure	Gradual	Variable: hours or days, but often weeks or months
Migraine Headaches (*"Classic migraine" is distinguished from "common migraine" by visual or neurologic symptoms during the half hour before the headache.*)	Dilatation of arteries outside or inside the skull, possibly of biochemical origin; often familial	Typically frontal or temporal, one or both sides, but also may be occipital or generalized. "Classic migraine" is typically unilateral.	Throbbing or aching, variable in severity	Fairly rapid, reaching a peak in 1–2 hr	Several hours to 1–2 dy
Toxic Vascular Headaches *due to fever, toxic substances, or drug withdrawal*	Dilatation of arteries, mainly inside the skull	Generalized	Aching, of variable severity	Variable	Depends on cause
Cluster Headaches	Unclear	One-sided; high in the nose, and behind and over the eye	Steady, severe	Abrupt, often 2–3 hr after falling asleep	Roughly 1–2 hr
Headaches With Eye Disorders					
Errors of Refraction (*farsightedness and astigmatism, but not nearsightedness*)	Probably the sustained contraction of the extraocular muscles, and possibly of the frontal, temporal, and occipital muscles	Around and over the eyes, may radiate to the occipital area	Steady, aching, dull	Gradual	Variable
Acute Glaucoma	Sudden increase in intraocular pressure (see p. 215)	In and around one eye	Steady, aching, often severe	Often rapid	Variable, may depend on treatment

Blanks appear in these tables when the categories are not applicable or are not usually helpful in assessing the problem.

Table 2-1 Headaches

Course	Associated Symptoms	Factors That Aggravate or Provoke	Factors That Relieve	Convenient Categories of Thought
Often recurrent or persistent over long periods	Symptoms of anxiety, tension, and depression may be present.	Sustained muscular tension, as in driving or typing; emotional	Possible massage, relaxation	The two most common kinds of headache
Often begins between childhood and early adulthood. Typically recurrent at intervals of weeks, months, or years, usually decreasing with pregancy and advancing age	Often nausea and vomiting. A minority of patients have preceding visual disturbances (local flashes of light, blind spots) or neurologic symptoms (local weakness, sensory disturbances, and other symptoms).	May be provoked by alcohol, certains foods, or tension. More common premenstrually. Aggravated by noise and bright light	Quiet, dark room; sleep; sometimes transient relief from pressure on the involved artery, if early in the course	
Depends on cause	Depends on cause	Fever, carbon monoxide, hypoxia, withdrawal of caffeine, other causes	Depends on cause	Vascular headaches
Typically clustered in time, with several each day or week and then relief for weeks or months	Unilateral stuffy, runny nose, and reddening and tearing of the eye	During a cluster, may be provoked by alcohol		
Variable	Eye fatigue, "sandy" sensations in the eyes, redness of the conjunctiva	Prolonged use of the eyes, particularly for close work	Rest of the eyes	
Variable, may depend on treatment	Diminished vision, sometimes nausea and vomiting	Sometimes provoked by drops that dilate the pupils		Face pains

(Table continues on next page) ➡

75

Table 2-1   Headaches

TABLE 2 - 1   *(continued)*

Problem	Process	Location	Quality and Severity	Timing	
				Onset	*Duration*
Headaches With Acute Paranasal Sinusitis	Mucosal inflammation of the paranasal sinuses and their openings	Usually above the eye (frontal sinus) or in the cheekbone area (maxillary sinus), one or both sides	Aching or throbbing, variable in severity	Variable	Often several hours at a time, recurring over days or longer
Trigeminal Neuralgia	Mechanism variable, often unknown	Cheek, jaws, lips, or gums (second and third divisions of the trigeminal nerve)	Sharp, short, brief, lightninglike jabs; very severe	Abrupt	Each jab is transient, but jabs recur in clusters at intervals of seconds or minutes
Giant Cell Arteritis	Chronic inflammation of the cranial arteries, cause unknown, often associated with polymyalgia rheumatica	Localized near the involved artery (most often the temporal, also the occipital); may become generalized	Aching, throbbing, or burning, often severe	Gradual or rapid	Variable
Chronic Subdural Hematoma	Bleeding into the subdural space after trauma, followed by slow accumulation of fluid that compresses the brain	Variable	Steady, aching	Gradual onset weeks to months after the injury	Often depends on surgical intervention
Postconcussion Syndrome	Mechanism unclear	May be localized to the injured area, but not necessarily	Variable	Within a few hours of the injury	Weeks, months, or even years
Meningitis	Infection of the meninges that surround the brain	Generalized	Steady or throbbing, very severe	Fairly rapid	Variable, usually days
Subarachnoid Hemorrhage	Bleeding, most often from a ruptured intra-cranial aneurysm	Generalized	Very severe, "the worst of my life"	Usually abrupt. Prodromal symptoms may occur	Variable, usually days
Brain Tumor	Displacement of or traction on pain-sensitive arteries and veins or pressure on nerves, all within the skull	Varies with the location of the tumor	Aching, steady, variable in intensity	Variable	Often brief

Table 2-1   *Headaches*

Course	Associated Symptoms	Factors That Aggravate or Provoke	Factors That Relieve	Convenient Categories of Thought
Often recurrent in a repetitive daily pattern: starting in the morning (frontal) or in the afternoon (maxillary)	Local tenderness, nasal congestion, discharge, and fever	May be aggravated by coughing, sneezing, or jarring the head	Nasal decongestants	Face pains
Pain may be troublesome for months, then disappears for months, but often recurs. It is uncommon at night.	Exhaustion from recurrent pain	Typically triggered by touching certain areas of the lower face or mouth, or by chewing, talking, or brushing teeth		
Recurrent or persistent over weeks to months	Tenderness of the adjacent scalp; fever, malaise, fatigue, and anorexia; muscular aches and stiffness; visual loss or blindness			Consider these three in older adults.
Progressively severe but may be obscured by clouded consciousness	Alterations in consciousness, changes in personality, and hemiparesis (weakness on one side of the body). The injury is often forgotten.			Headaches following head trauma
Tends to diminish over time	Poor concentration, giddiness or vertigo, irritability, restlessness, tenseness, and fatigue	Mental and physical exertion, straining, stooping, emotional excitement, alcohol	Rest	
A persistent headache in an acute illness	Fever, stiff neck			Acute illnesses with very severe headaches
A persistent headache in an acute illness	Nausea, vomiting, possibly loss of consciousness, neck pain			
Often intermittent, but progressive	Neurologic and mental symptoms and nausea and vomiting may develop.	May be aggravated by coughing, sneezing, or sudden movements of the head		An underlying concern of patient and clinician alike

Table 2-2   Vertigo

TABLE 2-2   *Vertigo*

Problem	Timing			Hearing	Tinnitus	Other Associated Symptoms
	Onset	*Duration*	*Course*			
Benign Positional Vertigo	Sudden, on rolling over onto the affected side or tilting the head up	Brief, a few seconds to minutes	Persists a few weeks, may recur	Not affected	Absent	Sometimes nausea and vomiting
Vestibular Neuronitis *(acute labyrinthitis)*	Sudden	Hours to days, up to 2 wk	May recur over 12–18 mo	Not affected	Absent	Nausea, vomiting
Meniere's Disease	Sudden	Several hours to a day or more	Recurrent	Sensorineural hearing loss that improves and recurs, eventually progresses; one or both sides*	Present, fluctuating*	Nausea, vomiting, pressure or fullness in the affected ear
Drug Toxicity *(as from aminoglycosides or alcohol intoxication)*	Insidious or acute	May or may not be reversible. Partial adaptation occurs.		May be impaired, both sides	May be present	Nausea, vomiting
Tumor, Pressing on the 8th Nerve	Insidious**	Variable	Variable	Impaired, one side	Present	Those of pressure on Cranial Nerves V, VI, and VII

Additional disorders of the brainstem or cerebellum may also cause vertigo. These include ischemia secondary to atherosclerosis, tumors, and multiple sclerosis. Additional neurologic symptoms and signs are usually present.

*Hearing impairment, tinnitus, and rotary vertigo do not always develop concurrently. Time is often required to make this diagnosis.

**Persistent unsteadiness is more common, but vertigo may occur.

Table 2-3   Chest Pain

TABLE 2-3   *Chest Pain*

Problem	Process	Location	Quality	Severity
Angina Pectoris	Temporary myocardial ischemia, usually secondary to narrowed arteries due to coronary atherosclerosis	Retrosternal or across the anterior chest, sometimes radiating to the shoulders, arms, neck, lower jaw, or upper abdomen	Pressing, squeezing, tight, heavy, occasionally burning	Mild to moderate, sometimes perceived as discomfort rather than pain
Myocardial Infarction	Prolonged myocardial ischemia, resulting in irreversible muscle damage (necrosis)	Same as in angina	Same as in angina	Often but not always a severe pain
Pericarditis	1. Irritation of parietal pleura adjacent to the pericardium	Precordial, may radiate to the tip of the shoulder and to the neck	Sharp, knifelike	Often severe
	2. Mechanism unclear	Retrosternal	Crushing	Severe
Dissecting Aortic Aneurysm	A splitting within the layers of the aortic wall, allowing the passage of blood to dissect a channel	Anterior chest, radiating to the neck, back, or abdomen	Ripping, tearing	Very severe
Tracheobronchitis	Inflammation of the trachea and large bronchi	Upper sternal or on either side of the sternum	Burning	Mild to moderate
Pleural Pain	Inflammation of the parietal pleura, as from pleurisy, pneumonia, pulmonary infarction, or neoplasm	Chest wall overlying the process	Sharp, knifelike	Often severe
Reflex Esophagitis	Inflammation of the esophageal mucosa by reflux of gastric acid	Retrosternal, may radiate to the back	Burning, may be squeezing	Mild to severe
Diffuse Esophageal Spasm	Motor dysfunction of the esophageal muscle	Retrosternal, may radiate to the back, arms, and jaw	Usually squeezing	Mild to severe
Chest Wall Pain	Variable, often unclear	Often below the left breast or along the costal cartilages, also elsewhere	Stabbing, sticking, or dull, aching	Variable
Anxiety	Unclear	Precordial, below the left breast, or across the anterior chest	Stabbing, sticking, or dull, aching	Variable

Note: Remember that chest pain may be referred from extrathoracic structures such as the neck (arthritis) and abdomen (biliary colic, acute cholecystitis). Pleural pain may be due to abdominal conditions such as subdiaphragmatic abscess.

Table 2-3   Chest Pain

Timing	Factors That Aggravate	Factors That Relieve	Associated Symptoms
Usually 1–3 min but up to 10 min. Prolonged episodes up to 20 min	Exertion, especially in the cold; meals; emotional stress. May occur at rest	Rest, nitroglycerin	Sometimes dyspnea, nausea, sweating
20 min to several hr			Nausea, vomiting, sweating, weakness
Persistent	Breathing, changing position, coughing, lying down, sometimes swallowing	Sitting forward may relieve it.	Of the underlying illness
Persistent			Of the underlying illness
Abrupt onset, early peak, persistent for hours or more	Hypertension		Syncope, hemiplegia, paraplegia
Variable	Coughing		Cough
Persistent	Breathing, coughing, movements of the trunk	Lying on the involved side may relieve it.	Of the underlying illness
Variable	Large meal; bending over, lying down	Antacids, sometimes belching	Sometimes regurgitation, dysphagia
Variable	Swallowing of food or cold liquid; emotional stress	Sometimes nitroglycerin	Dysphagia
Fleeting to hours or days	Movement of chest, trunk, arms		Often local tenderness
Fleeting to hours or day	May follow effort, emotional stress		Breathlessness, palpitations, weakness, anxiety

Table 2-4   Dyspnea

TABLE 2-4   *Dyspnea*

Problem	Process	Timing
Left-Sided Heart Failure (*left ventricular failure or mitral stenosis*)	Elevated pressure in the pulmonary capillary bed with transudation of fluid into the interstitial spaces and alveoli, decreased compliance (increased stiffness) of the lungs, and increased work of breathing	Dyspnea may progress slowly, or suddenly as in acute pulmonary edema.
Chronic Bronchitis*	Excessive mucus production in the bronchi, followed by chronic obstruction of the airways	Chronic productive cough followed by slowly progressive dyspnea
Pulmonary Emphysema*	Overdistention of the air spaces distal to the terminal bronchioles, with destruction of the alveolar septa and chronic obstruction of the airways	Slowly progressive dyspnea; relatively mild cough later
Asthma	Bronchial hyperresponsiveness involving release of inflammatory mediators, increased airway secretions, and bronchoconstriction	Acute episodes, separated by symptom-free periods. Nocturnal episodes are common.
Diffuse Interstitial Lung Diseases (*such as sarcoidosis, widespread neoplasms, asbestosis, and idiopathic pulmonary fibrosis*)	Abnormal and widespread infiltration of cells, fluid, and collagen into the interstitial spaces between the alveoli. Many causes	Progressive dyspnea, which varies in its rate of development with the cause
Pneumonia	Inflammation of the lung parenchyma from the respiratory bronchioles to the alveoli	An acute illness, the timing of which varies with the causative agent
Spontaneous Pneumothorax	Leakage of air into the pleural space through blebs on the visceral pleura, with resulting partial or complete collapse of the lung	Sudden onset of dyspnea
Acute Pulmonary Embolism	Sudden occlusion of all or part of the pulmonary arterial tree by a blood clot that usually originates in the deep veins of the legs or pelvis	Sudden onset of dyspnea
Anxiety With Hyperventilation	Overbreathing, with resultant respiratory alkalosis and fall in the partial pressure of carbon dioxide in the blood	Episodic, often recurrent

* Chronic bronchitis and emphysema often coexist. *Chronic obstructive pulmonary disease (COPD) may result from either or both.*

Table 2-4   Dyspnea

Factors That Aggravate	Factors That Relieve	Associated Symptoms	Setting
Exertion, lying down	Rest, sitting up, though dyspnea may become persistent	Often cough, orthopnea, paroxysmal nocturnal dyspnea; sometimes wheezing	History of heart disease or its predisposing factors
Exertion, inhaled irritants, respiratory infections	Expectoration; rest, though dyspnea may become persistent	Chronic productive cough, recurrent respiratory infections; wheezing may develop	History of smoking, air pollutants, recurrent respiratory infections
Exertion	Rest, though dyspnea may become persistent	Cough, with scant mucoid sputum	History of smoking, air pollutants, sometimes a familial deficiency in alpha$_1$-antitrypsin
Variable, including allergens, irritants, respiratory infections, exercise, and emotion	Separation from aggravating factors	Wheezing, cough, tightness in chest	Environmental and emotional conditions
Exertion	Rest, though dyspnea may become persistent	Often weakness, fatigue. Cough less common than in other lung diseases	Varied. Exposure to one of many substances may be causative.
		Pleuritic pain, cough, sputum, fever, though not necessarily present	Varied
		Pleuritic pain, cough	Often a previously healthy young adult
		Often none. Retrosternal oppressive pain if the occlusion is massive. Pleuritic pain, cough, and hemoptysis may follow an embolism if pulmonary infarction ensues. Symptoms of anxiety (see below).	Postpartum or postoperative periods; prolonged bed rest; congestive heart failure, chronic lung disease, and fractures of hip or leg; deep venous thrombosis (often not clinically apparent)
More often occurs at rest than after exercise. An upsetting event may not be evident.	Breathing in and out of a paper or plastic bag sometimes helps the associated symptoms.	Sighing, lightheadedness, numbness or tingling of the hands and feet, palpitations, chest pain	Other manifestations of anxiety may be present.

Table 2-5 Cough and Hemoptysis

TABLE 2-5 *Cough and Hemoptysis**

Problem	Cough and Sputum	Associated Symptoms and Setting
Acute Inflammations		
Laryngitis	Dry cough (without sputum), may become productive of variable amounts of sputum	An acute, fairly minor illness with hoarseness. Often associated with viral nasopharyngitis
Tracheobronchitis	Dry cough, may become productive (as above)	An acute, often viral illness, with burning retrosternal discomfort
Mycoplasma and Viral Pneumonias	Dry hacking cough, often becoming productive of mucoid sputum	An acute febrile illness, often with malaise, headache, and possibly dyspnea
Bacterial Pneumonias	Pneumococcal: sputum mucoid or purulent; may be blood-streaked, diffusely pinkish, or rusty	An acute illness with chills, high fever, dyspnea, and chest pain. Often is preceded by acute upper respiratory infection.
	Klebsiella: similar; or sticky, red, and jellylike	Typically occurs in older alcoholic men
Chronic Inflammations		
Postnasal Drip	Chronic cough; sputum mucoid or mucopurulent	Repeated attempts to clear the throat. Postnasal discharge may be sensed by the patient or seen in the posterior pharynx. Associated with chronic rhinitis, with or without sinusitis
Chronic Bronchitis	Chronic cough; sputum mucoid to purulent, may be blood-streaked or even bloody	Often longstanding cigarette smoking. Recurrent superimposed infections. Wheezing and dyspnea may develop.
Bronchiectasis	Chronic cough; sputum purulent, often copious and foul-smelling; may be blood-streaked or bloody	Recurrent bronchopulmonary infections common; sinusitis may coexist
Pulmonary Tuberculosis	Cough dry or sputum that is mucoid or purulent; may be blood-streaked or bloody	Early, no symptoms. Later, anorexia, weight loss, fatigue, fever, and night sweats
Lung Abscess	Sputum purulent and foul-smelling; may be bloody	A febrile illness. Often poor dental hygiene and a prior episode of impaired consciousness
Asthma	Cough, with thick mucoid sputum, especially near the end of an attack	Episodic wheezing and dyspnea, but the cough may occur alone. Often a history of allergy
Gastroesophageal Reflux	Chronic cough, especially at night or early in the morning	Wheezing, especially at night (often mistaken for asthma), early morning hoarseness, and repeated attempts to clear the throat. Often a history of heartburn and regurgitation
Neoplasm		
Cancer of the Lung	Cough dry to productive; sputum may be blood-streaked or bloody	Usually a long history of cigarette smoking. Associated manifestations are numerous.
Cardiovascular Disorders		
Left Ventricular Failure or Mitral Stenosis	Often dry, especially on exertion or at night; may progress to the pink frothy sputum of pulmonary edema or to frank hemoptysis	Dyspnea, orthopnea, paroxysmal nocturnal dyspnea
Pulmonary Emboli	Dry to productive; may be dark, bright red, or mixed with blood	Dyspnea, anxiety, chest pain, fever; factors that predispose to deep venous thrombosis
Irritating Particles, Chemicals, or Gases	Variable. There may be a latent period between exposure and symptoms.	Exposure to irritants. Eyes, nose, and throat may be affected.

* Characteristics of hemoptysis are printed in red.

Table 2-6   Dysphagia

T A B L E   2 - 6   *Dysphagia*

Process and Problem	Timing	Factors That Aggravate	Factors That Relieve	Associated Symptoms and Conditions
Transfer Dysphagia, *due to motor disorders affecting the pharyngeal muscles*	Acute or gradual onset and a variable course, depending on the underlying disorder	Attempts to start the swallowing process		Aspiration into the lungs or regurgitation into the nose with attempts to swallow. Neurologic evidence of stroke, bulbar palsy, or other neuromuscular condition

Esophageal Dysphagia

Mechanical Narrowing

Process and Problem	Timing	Factors That Aggravate	Factors That Relieve	Associated Symptoms and Conditions
• Mucosal rings and webs	Intermittent	Solid foods	Regurgitation of the bolus of food	Usually none
• Esophageal stricture	Intermittent, may become slowly progressive	Solid foods	Regurgitation of the bolus of food	A long history of heartburn and regurgitation
• Esophageal cancer	May be intermittent at first; progressive over months	Solid foods, with progression to liquids	Regurgitation of the bolus of food	Pain in the chest and back and weight loss, especially late in the course of illness

Motor Disorders

Process and Problem	Timing	Factors That Aggravate	Factors That Relieve	Associated Symptoms and Conditions
• Diffuse esophageal spasm	Intermittent	Solids or liquids	Maneuvers described below; sometimes nitroglycerin	Chest pain that mimics angina pectoris or myocardial infarction and lasts minutes to hours; possibly heartburn
• Scleroderma	Intermittent, may progress slowly	Solids or liquids	Repeated swallowing, movements such as straightening the back, raising the arms, or a Valsalva maneuver (straining down against a closed glottis)	Heartburn. Other manifestations of scleroderma
• Achalasia	Intermittent, may progress	Solids or liquids		Regurgitation, often at night when lying down, with nocturnal cough; possibly chest pain precipitated by eating

Table 2-7 Abdominal Pain

TABLE 2-7 *Abdominal Pain*

Problem	Process	Location	Quality
Peptic Ulcer and Dyspepsia (*These disorders cannot be reliably differentiated by symptoms and signs.*)	Peptic ulcer refers to a demonstrable ulcer, usually in the duodenum or stomach. Dyspepsia causes similar symptoms but no ulceration. Infection by *Helicobacter pylori* is often present.	Epigastric, may radiate to the back	Variable: gnawing burning, boring, aching, pressing, or hungerlike
Cancer of the Stomach	A malignant neoplasm	Epigastric	Variable
Acute Pancreatitis	An acute inflammation of the pancreas	Epigastric, may radiate to the back or other parts of the abdomen; may be poorly localized	Usually steady
Chronic Pancreatitis	Fibrosis of the pancreas secondary to recurrent inflammation	Epigastric, radiating through to the back	Steady, deep
Cancer of the Pancreas	A malignant neoplasm	Epigastric and in either upper quadrant; often radiates to the back	Steady, deep
Biliary Colic	Sudden obstruction of the cystic duct or common bile duct by a gallstone	Epigastric or right upper quadrant; may radiate to the right scapula and shoulder	Steady, aching; *not* colicky
Acute Cholecystitis	Inflammation of the gallbladder, usually from obstruction of the cystic duct by a gallstone	Right upper quadrant or upper abdominal; may radiate to the right scapular area	Steady, aching
Acute Diverticulitis	Acute inflammation of a colonic diverticulum, a saclike mucosal outpouching through the colonic muscle	Left lower quadrant	May be cramping at first, but becomes steady
Acute Appendicitis	Acute inflammation of the appendix with distention or obstruction	1. Poorly localized *periumbilical pain,* followed usually by 2. *Right lower quadrant pain*	1. Mild but increasing, possibly cramping 2. Steady and more severe
Acute Mechanical Intestinal Obstruction	Obstruction of the bowel lumen, most commonly caused by (1) adhesions or hernias (small bowel), or (2) cancer or diverticulitis (colon)	1. *Small bowel:* periumbilical or upper abdominal 2. *Colon:* lower abdominal or generalized	1. Cramping 2. Cramping
Mesenteric Ischemia	Blood supply to the bowel and mesentery blocked from thrombosis or embolus (acute arterial occlusion), or reduced from hypoperfusion	May be periumbilical at first, then diffuse	Cramping at first, then steady

Table 2-7   Abdominal Pain

Timing	Factors That May Aggravate	Factors That May Relieve	Associated Symptoms and Setting
Intermittent. Duodenal ulcer is more likely than gastric ulcer or dyspepsia to cause pain that (1) wakes the patient at night, and (2) occurs intermittently over a few weeks, then disappears for months, and then recurs.	Variable	Food and antacids may bring relief, but not necessarily in any of these disorders and least commonly in gastric ulcer.	Nausea, vomiting, belching, bloating; heartburn (more common in duodenal ulcer); weight loss (more common in gastric ulcer). Dyspepsia is more common in the young (20–29 yr), gastric ulcer in the older (over 50 yr), and duodenal ulcer in those from 30–60 yr.
The history of pain is typically shorter than in peptic ulcer. The pain is persistent and slowly progressive.	Often food	*Not* relieved by food or antacids	Anorexia, nausea, easy satiety, weight loss, and sometimes bleeding. Most common in ages 50–70
Acute onset, persistent pain	Lying supine	Leaning forward with trunk flexed	Nausea, vomiting, abdominal distention, fever. Often a history of previous attacks and of alcohol abuse or gallstones
Chronic or recurrent course	Alcohol, heavy or fatty meals	Possibly leaning forward with trunk flexed; often intractable	Symptoms of decreased pancreatic function may appear: diarrhea with fatty stools (steatorrhea) and diabetes mellitus.
Persistent pain; relentlessly progressive illness		Possibly leaning forward with trunk flexed; often intractable	Anorexia, nausea, vomiting, weight loss, and jaundice. Emotional symptoms, including depression
Rapid onset over a few minutes, lasts one to several hours and subsides gradually. Often recurrent			Anorexia, nausea, vomiting, restlessness
Gradual onset; course longer than in biliary colic	Jarring, deep breathing		Anorexia, nausea, vomiting, and fever
Often a gradual onset			Fever, constipation. There may be initial brief diarrhea.
1. Lasts roughly 4–6 hr 2. Depends on intervention	1. 2. Movement or cough	1. 2. If it subsides temporarily, suspect perforation of the appendix.	Anorexia, nausea, possibly vomiting, which typically follow the onset of pain; low fever
1. Paroxysmal; may decrease as bowel mobility is impaired 2. Paroxysmal, though typically milder			1. Vomiting of bile and mucus (high obstruction) or fecal material (low obstruction). Obstipation develops. 2. Obstipation early. Vomiting late if at all. Prior symptoms of underlying cause.
Usually abrupt in onset, then persistent			Vomiting, diarrhea (sometimes bloody), constipation, shock

Table 2-8 *Black and Bloody Stools*

TABLE 2-8 *Black and Bloody Stools*

Problem	Selected Causes	Associated Symptoms and Setting
Melena Melena refers to the passage of black, tarry (sticky and shiny) stools. Tests for occult blood are positive. Melena signifies the loss of at least 60 ml of blood into the gastrointestinal tract (less in infants and children), usually from the esophagus, stomach, or duodenum. Less commonly, when intestinal transit is slow, the blood may originate in the jejunum, ileum, or ascending colon. In infants, melena may result from swallowing blood during the birth process.	Peptic ulcer	Often, but not necessarily, a history of epigastric pain
	Gastritis or stress ulcers	Recent ingestion of alcohol, aspirin, or other anti-inflammatory drugs; recent bodily trauma, severe burns, surgery, or increased intracranial pressure
	Esophageal or gastric varices	Cirrhosis of the liver or other cause of portal hypertension
	Reflux esophagitis	History of heartburn
	Mallory–Weiss tear, a mucosal tear in the esophagus due to retching and vomiting	Retching, vomiting, often recent ingestion of alcohol
Black, Nonsticky Stools Black stools may result from other causes and then usually give negative results when tested for occult blood. (Ingestion of iron or other substances, however, may cause a positive test result in the absence of blood.) These stools have no pathologic significance.	Ingestion of iron, bismuth salts as in Pepto-Bismol, licorice, or even commercial chocolate cookies	
Red Blood in the Stools Red blood usually originates in the colon, rectum, or anus, and much less frequently in the jejunum or ileum. Upper gastrointestinal hemorrhage, however, may also cause red stools. The amount of blood lost is then usually large (more than a liter). Transit time through the intestinal tract is accordingly rapid, giving insufficient time for the blood to turn black.	Cancer of the colon	Often a change in bowel habits
	Benign polyps of the colon	Often no other symptoms
	Diverticula of the colon	Often no other symptoms
	Inflammatory conditions of the colon and rectum	
	• Ulcerative colitis	See Table 2-10, Diarrhea.
	• Infectious dysenteries	See Table 2-10, Diarrhea.
	• Proctitis (various causes) in men or women who have had frequent anal intercourse	Rectal urgency, tenesmus
	Ischemic colitis	Lower abdominal pain and sometimes fever or shock in persons over age 50 yr
	Hemorrhoids	Blood on the toilet paper, on the surface of the stool, or dripping into the toilet
	Anal fissure	Blood on the toilet paper or on the surface of the stool; anal pain
Reddish But Nonbloody Stools	The ingestion of beets	Pink urine, which usually precedes the reddish stool

Table 2-9   Constipation

TABLE 2-9 *Constipation*

Problem	Process	Setting and Associated Symptoms
Life Activities and Habits		
Inadequate Time or Setting for the Defecation Reflex	Ignoring the sensation of a full rectum inhibits the defecation reflex.	Hectic schedules, unfamiliar surroundings, bed rest
False Expectations of Bowel Habits	Expectations of "regularity" or more frequent stools than a person's norm	Beliefs, treatments, and advertisements that promote the use of laxatives
Diet Deficient in Fiber	Decreased fecal bulk	Other factors such as debilitation and constipating drugs may contribute.
Irritable Bowel Syndrome	A common disorder of bowel motility	Small, hard stools, often with mucus. Periods of diarrhea. Cramping abdominal pain. Stress may aggravate.
Mechanical Obstruction		
Cancer of the Rectum or Sigmoid Colon	Progressive narrowing of the bowel lumen	Change in bowel habits; often diarrhea, abdominal pain, and bleeding. In rectal cancer, tenesmus and pencil-shaped stools
Fecal Impaction	A large, firm, immovable fecal mass, most often in the rectum	Rectal fullness, abdominal pain, and diarrhea around the impaction. Common in debilitated, bedridden, and often elderly patients
Other Obstructing Lesions (such as diverticulitis, volvulus, intussusception, or hernia)	Narrowing or complete obstruction of the bowel	Colicky abdominal pain, abdominal distention, and in intussesception, often "currant jelly" stools (red blood and mucus)
Painful Anal Lesions	Pain may cause spasm of the external sphincter and voluntary inhibition of the defecation reflex.	Anal fissures, painful hemorrhoids, perirectal abscesses
Drugs	A variety of mechanisms	Opiates, anticholinergics, antacids containing calcium or aluminum, and many others
Depression	A disorder of mood. See Table 3-2, Disorders of Mood.	Fatigue, feelings of depression, and other somatic symptoms
Neurologic Disorders	Interference with the autonomic innervation of the bowel	Spinal cord injuries, multiple sclerosis, Hirschsprung's disease, and other conditions
Metabolic Conditions	Interference with bowel motility	Pregnancy, hypothyroidism, hypercalcemia

Table 2-10 Diarrhea

TABLE 2-10 *Diarrhea*

Problem	Process	Characteristics of Stool
Acute Diarrhea		
Noninflammatory Infections	Infection by viruses, toxin-producing bacteria (such as *Escherichia coli, Staphylococcus aureus*), or *Giardia lamblia*	Watery, without blood, pus, or mucus
Inflammatory Infections	Invasion of the intestinal mucosa by organisms such as *Shigella, Salmonella, Campylobacter, Yersinia,* and invasive *E. coli*	Loose to watery, often with blood, pus, or mucus
Drug-Induced Diarrhea	Action of many drugs, such as magnesium-containing antacids, antibiotics, antineoplastic agents, and laxatives	Loose to watery
Chronic or Recurrent Diarrhea		
Nonspecific Diarrheal Syndromes		
• Irritable bowel syndrome	A disorder of bowel motility	Loose; may show mucus but no blood. Small, hard stools with constipation
• Cancer of the sigmoid colon	Partial obstruction by a malignant neoplasm	May be blood-streaked
Inflammatory Diarrheas		
• Ulcerative colitis	Inflammation of the mucosa and submucosa of the rectum and colon with ulceration; cause unknown	From soft to watery, often containing blood
• Crohn's disease of the small bowel (regional enteritis) or colon (granulomatous colitis)	Chronic inflammation of the bowel wall, typically involving the terminal ileum and/or proximal colon	Small, soft to loose or watery, usually free of gross blood (enteritis) or with less bleeding than ulcerative colitis (colitis)
Voluminous Diarrheas		
• Malabsorption syndromes	Defective absorption of fat and other substances, including fat-soluble vitamins, with excessive excretion of fat (steatorrhea); many causes	Typically bulky, soft, light yellow to gray, mushy, greasy or oily, and sometimes frothy; particularly foul-smelling; usually float in the toilet
• Osmotic diarrheas Lactose intolerance	Deficiency in intestinal lactase	Watery diarrhea of large volume
Abuse of osmotic purgatives	Laxative habit, often surreptitious	Watery diarrhea of large volume
• Secretory diarrheas, associated with a number of uncommon conditions, such as the Zollinger–Ellison syndrome	Variable	Watery diarrhea of large volume

Table 2-10   Diarrhea

Timing	Associated Symptoms	Setting, Persons at Risk
Duration of a few days, possibly longer. Lactase deficiency may lead to a longer course.	Nausea, vomiting, periumbilical cramping pain. Temperature normal or slightly elevated	Often travel, a common food source, or an epidemic
An acute illness of varying duration	Lower abdominal cramping pain and often rectal urgency, tenesmus; fever	Travel, contaminated food or water. Men and women who have had frequent anal intercourse.
Acute, recurrent, or chronic	Possibly nausea; usually little if any pain	Prescribed or over-the-counter medications
Often worse in the morning. Diarrhea rarely wakes the patient at night.	Crampy lower abdominal pain, abdominal distention, flatulence, nausea, constipation	Young and middle-aged adults, especially women
Variable	Change in usual bowel habits, crampy lower abdominal pain, constipation	Middle-aged and older adults, especially over 55 yr
Onset ranges from insidious to acute. Typically recurrent, may be persistent. Diarrhea may wake the patient at night.	Crampy lower or generalized abdominal pain, anorexia, weakness, fever	Often young people
Insidious onset, chronic or recurrent. Diarrhea may wake the patient at night.	Crampy periumbilical or right lower quadrant (enteritis) or diffuse (colitis) pain, with anorexia, low fever, and/or weight loss. Perianal or perirectal abscesses and fistulas	Often young people, especially in the late teens, but also in the middle years. More common in Jews
Onset of illness typically insidious	Anorexia, weight loss, fatigue, abdominal distention, often crampy lower abdominal pain. Symptoms of nutritional deficiencies such as bleeding (vitamin K), bone pain and fractures (vitamin D), glossitis (vitamin B), and edema (protein)	Variable, depending on cause
Follows the ingestion of milk and milk products; is relieved by fasting	Crampy abdominal pain, abdominal distention, flatulence	African Americans, Asians, Native Americans
Variable	Often none	Persons with anorexia nervosa or bulimia nervosa
Variable	Weight loss, dehydration, nausea, vomiting, and cramping abdominal pain	Variable depending on cause

Table 2-11   Polyuria, Frequency, and Nocturia

TABLE 2-11   *Polyuria, Frequency, and Nocturia*

Problem	Mechanisms	Selected Causes	Associated Symptoms
Polyuria	Deficiency in antidiuretic hormone (diabetes insipidus)	A disorder of the posterior pituitary and hypothalamus	Thirst and polydipsia, often severe and persistent; nocturia
	Renal unreponsiveness to antidiuretic hormone (nephrogenic diabetes insipidus)	A number of kidney diseases, including hypercalcemic and hypokalemic nephropathy; drug toxicity, e.g., from lithium	Thirst and polydipsia, often severe and persistent; nocturia
	Solute diuresis		
	• Electrolytes, such as sodium salts	Large saline infusions, potent diuretics, certain kidney diseases	Variable
	• Nonelectrolytes, such as glucose	Uncontrolled diabetes mellitus	Thirst, polydipsia, and nocturia
	Excessive water intake	Primary polydipsia	Polydipsia tends to be episodic. Thirst may not be present. Nocturia is usually absent.
Frequency Without Polyuria	Decreased capacity of the bladder		
	• Increased bladder sensitivity to stretch because of inflammation	Infection, stones, tumor, or foreign body in the bladder	Burning on urination, urinary urgency, sometimes gross hematuria
	• Decreased elasticity of the bladder wall	Infiltration by scar tissue or tumor	Symptoms of associated inflammation (see above) are common.
	• Decreased cortical inhibition of bladder contractions	Motor disorders of the central nervous system, such as a stroke	Urinary urgency; neurologic symptoms such as weakness and paralysis
	Impaired emptying of the bladder, with residual urine in the bladder		
	• Partial mechanical obstruction of the bladder neck or proximal urethra	Most commonly, benign prostatic hyperplasia; also urethral stricture and other obstructive lesions of the bladder or prostate	Prior obstructive symptoms: hesitancy in starting the urinary stream, straining to void, reduced size and force of the stream, and dribbling during or at the end of urination
	• Loss of peripheral nerve supply to the bladder	Neurologic disease affecting the sacral nerves or nerve roots, e.g., diabetic neuropathy	Weakness or sensory defects

(Table continues on next page)   ➡

Table 2-11 Polyuria, Frequency, and Nocturia

Problem	Mechanisms	Selected Causes	Associated Symptoms
Nocturia			
With High Volumes	Most types of polyuria (see p. 92)		
	Decreased concentrating ability of the kidney with loss of the normal decrease in nocturnal urinary output	Chronic renal insufficiency due to a number of diseases	Possibly other symptoms of renal insufficiency
	Excessive fluid intake before bedtime	Habit, especially involving alcohol and coffee	
	Fluid-retaining, edematous states. Dependent edema accumulates during the day and is excreted when the patient lies down at night.	Congestive heart failure, nephrotic syndrome, hepatic cirrhosis with ascites, chronic venous insufficiency	Edema and other symptoms of the underlying disorder. Urinary output during the day may be reduced as fluid reaccumulates in the body. See Table 16-3, Mechanisms and Patterns of Edema.
With Low Volumes	Frequency without polyuria (see p. 92)		
	Voiding while up at night without a real urge, a "pseudo-frequency"	Insomnia	Variable

Table 2-12   Urinary Incontinence

TABLE 2-12   *Urinary Incontinence*

Problem	Mechanisms
Stress Incontinence The urethral sphincter is weakened so that transient increases in intraabdominal pressure raise the bladder pressure to levels that exceed urethral resistance.	In women, most often a weakness of the pelvic floor with inadequate muscular support of the bladder and proximal urethra and a change in the angle between the bladder and the urethra. Suggested causes include childbirth and surgery. Local conditions affecting the internal urethral sphincter, such as postmenopausal atrophy of the mucosa and urethral infection, may also contribute. In men, stress incontinence may follow prostatic surgery.
Urge Incontinence Detrusor contractions are stronger than normal and overcome the normal urethral resistance. The bladder is typically small.	1. Decreased cortical inhibition of detrusor contractions, as by strokes, brain tumors, dementia, and lesions of the spinal cord above the sacral level 2. Hyperexcitability of sensory pathways, caused by, for example, bladder infections, tumors, and fecal impaction 3. Deconditioning of voiding reflexes, caused by, for example, frequent voluntary voiding at low bladder volumes
Overflow Incontinence Detrusor contractions are insufficient to overcome urethral resistance. The bladder is typically large, even after an effort to void.	1. Obstruction of the bladder outlet, as by benign prostatic hyperplasia or tumor 2. Weakness of the detrusor muscle associated with peripheral nerve disease at the sacral level 3. Impaired bladder sensation that interrupts the reflex arc, as from diabetic neuropathy
Functional Incontinence This is a functional inability to get to the toilet in time because of impaired health or environmental conditions.	Problems in mobility resulting from weakness, arthritis, poor vision, or other conditions. Environmental factors such as an unfamiliar setting, distant bathroom facilities, bedrails, or physical restraints
Incontinence Secondary to Medications Drugs may contribute to any type of incontinence listed.	Sedatives, tranquilizers, anticholinergics, sympathetic blockers, and potent diuretics

Patients may have more than one kind of incontinence. Many women with stress incontinence also have some degree of urge incontinence, for example, and an elderly person may be incontinent for several different reasons.

Table 2-12   Urinary Incontinence

Symptoms	Physical Signs
Momentary leakage of small amounts of urine concurrent with stresses such as coughing, laughing, and sneezing while the person is in an upright position. A desire to urinate is not associated with pure stress incontinence.	The bladder is not detected on abdominal examination. Stress incontinence may be demonstrable, especially if the patient is examined before voiding and in a standing position. Atrophic vaginitis may be evident.
Incontinence preceded by an urge to void. The volume tends to be moderate. Urgency Frequency and nocturia with small to moderate volumes If acute inflammation is present, pain on urination Possibly "pseudo-stress incontinence"—voiding 10–20 sec after stresses such as a change of position, going up or down stairs, and possibly coughing, laughing, or sneezing	The bladder is not detectable on abdominal examination. When cortical inhibition is decreased, mental deficits or motor signs of central nervous system disease are often, though not necessarily, present. When sensory pathways are hyperexcitable, signs of local pelvic problems or a fecal impaction may be present.
A continuous dripping or dribbling incontinence Decreased force of the urinary stream Prior symptoms of partial urinary obstruction or other symptoms of peripheral nerve disease may be present.	An enlarged bladder is often found on abdominal examination and may be tender. Other possible signs include prostatic enlargement, motor signs of peripheral nerve disease, a decrease in sensation including perineal sensation, and diminished to absent reflexes.
Incontinence on the way to the toilet or only in the early morning	The bladder is not detectable on physical examination. Look for physical or environmental clues to the likely cause.
Variable. A careful history and chart review are important.	Variable

Table 2-13   *Painful Peripheral Vascular Disorders and Their Mimics*

TABLE 2-13   *Painful Peripheral Vascular Disorders and Their Mimics*

Problem	Process	Location of Pain
Arterial Disorders		
Arteriosclerosis Obliterans		
• Intermittent claudication	Episodic muscular ischemia induced by exercise, due to obstruction of large or middle-sized arteries by atherosclerosis	Usually the calf, but may also be felt in the buttock, hip, thigh, or foot, depending on the level of obstruction
• Rest pain	Ischemia even at rest	Distal pain, in the toes or forefoot
Acute Arterial Occlusion	Embolism or thrombosis, possibly superimposed on arteriosclerosis obliterans	Distal pain, usually involving the foot and leg
Venous Disorders		
Superficial Thrombophlebitis	Clot formation and acute inflammation in a superficial vein	Pain in a local area along the course of a superficial vein, most often in the saphenous system
Deep Venous Thrombosis	Clot formation in a deep vein	Pain, if present, is usually in the calf, but the process more often is painless.
Chronic Venous Insufficiency (Deep)	Chronic venous engorgement secondary to venous occlusion or incompetency of venous valves	Diffuse aching of the leg(s)
Acute Lymphangitis	Acute bacterial infection (usually streptococcal) spreading up the lymphatic channels from a portal of entry such as an injured area or an ulcer	An arm or a leg
Thromboangiitis Obliterans (*Buerger's disease*)	Inflammatory and thrombotic occlusions of small arteries and also of veins, occurring in smokers	1. Intermittent claudication, particularly in the arch of the foot 2. Rest pain in the fingers or toes
Raynaud's Disease (*and phenomenon*)	Episodic spasm of the small arteries and arterioles, without organic occlusion. When the syndrome is secondary to other conditions (and then called Raynaud's phenomenon), occlusion may occur.	Distal portions of one or more fingers. Pain is usually not prominent unless fingertip ulcers develop. Numbness and tingling are common.
Mimics*		
Acute Cellulitis	Acute bacterial infection of the skin and subcutaneous tissues	Arms, legs, or elsewhere
Erythema Nodosum	Subcutaneous inflammatory lesions associated with a variety of systemic conditions such as pregnancy, sarcoidosis, tuberculosis, and streptococcal infections	Anterior surfaces of both lower legs

* Mistaken primarily for acute superficial thrombophlebitis.

Table 2-13   Painful Peripheral Vascular Disorders and Their Mimics

Timing	Factors That Aggravate	Factors That Relieve	Associated Manifestations
Fairly brief; pain usually forces the patient to rest.	Exercise such as walking	Rest usually stops the pain in 1–3 min.	Local fatigue, numbness, diminished pulses, often signs of arterial insufficiency (see p. 478)
Persistent, often worse at night	Elevation of the feet, as in bed	Sitting with legs dependent	Numbness, tingling, trophic signs and color changes of arterial insufficiency (see p. 478)
Sudden onset; associated symptoms may occur without pain.			Coldness, numbness, weakness, absent distal pulses
An acute episode lasting days or longer			Local redness, swelling, tenderness, a palpable cord, possibly fever
Often hard to determine because of lack of symptoms			Possibly swelling of the foot and calf and local calf tenderness; often nothing
Chronic, increasing as the day wears on	Prolonged standing	Elevation of the leg(s)	Chronic edema, pigmentation, possibly ulceration (see pp. 478, 479)
An acute episode lasting days or longer			Red streak(s) on the skin, with tenderness, enlarged, tender lymph nodes, and fever
1. Fairly brief but recurrent 2. Chronic, persistent, may be worse at night	1. Exercise	1. Rest. Permanent cessation of smoking helps both kinds of pain (but patients seldom stop).	Distal coldness, sweating, numbness, and cyanosis; ulceration and gangrene at the tips of fingers or toes; migratory thrombophlebitis
Relatively brief (minutes) but recurrent	Exposure to cold, emotional upset	Warm environment	Color changes in the distal fingers: severe pallor (essential for the diagnosis) followed by cyanosis and then redness
An acute episode lasting days or longer			A local area of diffuse swelling, redness, and tenderness with enlarged, tender lymph nodes and fever; no palpable cord
Pain associated with a series of lesions over several weeks			Raised, red, tender swellings recurring in crops; often malaise, joint pains, and fever

Table 2-14   Patterns of Chronic Pain In and Around the Joints

TABLE 2-14   *Patterns of Chronic Pain In and Around the Joints*

Problem	Process	Common Locations	Pattern of Spread	Onset	Progression and Duration
Rheumatoid Arthritis	Chronic inflammation of synovial membranes with secondary erosion of adjacent cartilage and bone, and damage to ligaments and tendons	Hands (proximal interphalangeal and metacarpo-phalangeal joints), feet (metatarsopha-langeal joints), wrists, knees, elbows, ankles	Symmetrically additive: progresses to other joints while persisting in the initial ones	Usually insidious	Often chronic, with remissions and exacerbations
Osteoarthritis (*degenerative joint disease*)	Degeneration and progressive loss of cartilage within the joints, damage to underlying bone, and formation of new bone at the margins of the cartilage	Knees, hips, hands (distal, sometimes proximal inter-phalangeal joints), cervical and lumbar spine, and wrists (first carpometacarpal joint); also joints previously injured or diseased	Additive; however, only one joint may be involved.	Usually insidious	Slowly progressive, with temporary exacerbations after periods of overuse
Gouty Arthritis					
Acute Gout	An inflammatory reaction to microcrystals of sodium urate	Base of the big toe (the first metatarso-phalangeal joint), the instep or dorsum of feet, the ankles, knees, and elbows	Early attacks are usually confined to one joint.	Sudden, often at night, often after injury, surgery, fasting, or excessive food or alcohol intake	Occasional isolated attacks lasting days up to 2 wk; they may get more frequent and severe, with per-sisting symptoms.
Chronic Tophaceous Gout	Multiple local accumulations of sodium urate in the joints and other tissues (tophi), with or without inflammation	Feet, ankles, wrists, fingers, and elbows	Additive, not so symmetrical as rheumatoid arthritis	Gradual development of chronicity with repeated attacks	Chronic symptoms with acute exacerbations
Polymyalgia Rheumatica	A disease of unclear nature seen in people over age 50 yr, especially women; may be associated with giant cell arteritis	Muscles of the hip girdle and shoulder girdle; symmetrical		Insidious or abrupt, even appearing overnight	Chronic but ultimately self-limiting
Fibromyalgia Syndrome	Widespread musculoskeletal pain and tender points. May accompany other diseases. Mechanisms unclear	"All over," but especially in the neck, shoulders, hands, low back, and knees	Shifts unpredict-ably or worsens in response to immobility, excessive use, or chilling	Variable	Chronic, with "ups and downs"

The vagueness of these characteristics is in itself a clue to the fibromyalgia syndrome.

Table 2-14   Patterns of Chronic Pain In and Around the Joints

Associated Symptoms

Swelling	Redness, Warmth, and Tenderness	Stiffness	Limitation of Motion	Generalized Symptoms
Frequent swelling of synovial tissue in joints or tendon sheaths; also subcutaneous nodules	Tender, often warm, but seldom red	Prominent, often for an hour or more in the mornings, also after inactivity	Often develops	Weakness, fatigue, weight loss, and low fever are common.
Small effusions in the joints may be present, especially in the knees; also bony enlargement.	Possibly tender, seldom warm, and rarely red	Frequent but brief (usually 5–10 min), in the morning and after inactivity	Often develops	Usually absent
Present, within and around the involved joint	Exquisitely tender, hot, and red	Not evident	Motion is limited primarily by pain.	Fever may be present.
Present, as tophi, in joints, bursae, and subcutaneous tissues	Tenderness, warmth, and redness may be present during exacerbations.	Present	Present	Possibly fever; patient may also develop symptoms of renal failure and renal stones.
None	Muscles often tender, but not warm or red	Prominent, especially in the morning	Usually none	Malaise, a sense of depression, possibly anorexia, weight loss, and fever, but no true weakness
None	Multiple specific and symmetric tender points, often not recognized until the examination	Present, especially in the morning	Absent, though stiffness is greater at the extremes of movement	A disturbance of sleep, usually associated with morning fatigue

Table 2-15   Low Back Pain

TABLE 2-15   *Low Back Pain*

Patterns	Possible Causes	Possible Physical Signs
Common Low Back Pain Acute, often recurrent, or possibly chronic aching pain in the lumbosacral area, possibly radiating into the posterior thighs but not below the knees. The pain is often precipitated or aggravated by moving, lifting, or twisting motions and is relieved by rest. Spinal movements are typically limited by pain. This is the back pain common from the teenage years through the 40s.	The exact cause cannot usually be proven. Intervertebral disc disease is probably involved in many cases. Congenital disorders of the spine, such as spondylolisthesis, may be present in a small percentage. In older women or in persons on long-term corticosteroid therapy, consider osteoporosis complicated by a collapsed vertebra.	Local tenderness, muscle spasm, pain on movement of the back, and loss of the normal lumbar lordosis, but no motor or sensory loss or reflex abnormalities. In osteoporosis there may be a thoracic kyphosis, percussion tenderness over a spinous process, or fractures elsewhere such as in the thoracic spine or in a hip.
Sciatica A radicular (nerve root) pain, usually superimposed on low back pain. The sciatic pain is shooting and radiates down one or both legs, usually to below the knee(s) in a dermatomal distribution, often with associated numbness and tingling and possibly local weakness. The pain is usually worsened by spinal movement such as bending and by sneezing, coughing, or straining.	A herniated intervertebral disc with compression or traction of nerve root(s) is the most common cause in persons under age 50 yr. The nerve roots of L5 or S1 are most often affected. Spinal cord tumors or abscesses are much less common causes. Compared to a disc, they tend to affect more nerve roots and to produce more neurologic deficits.	Pain on straight leg raising (see pp. 540), tenderness of the sciatic nerve, loss of sensation in a dermatomal distribution, local muscular weakness and atrophy, and decreased to absent reflex(es), especially affecting the ankle jerks. Dermatomal signs and reflex changes may be absent when only a single root is affected.
Back Pain or Sciatica With Pseudoclaudication Pseudoclaudication is a pain in the back or legs that worsens with walking and improves with flexing of the spine, as by sitting or bending forward.	Lumbar stenosis, which is a combination of degenerative disc disease and osteoarthritis that narrows the spinal canal and impinges on the spinal nerves. It is a common cause of pain after age 60.	The posture may become flexed forward.
Chronic Persistent Low Back Stiffness	Ankylosing spondylitis, a chronic inflammatory polyarthritis, most common in young men	Loss of the normal lumbar lordosis, muscle spasm, and limitation of anterior and lateral flexion
	Diffuse idiopathic skeletal hyperostosis (DISH), which affects middle-aged and older men	Flexion and immobility of the spine
Aching Nocturnal Back Pain, Unrelieved by Rest	Consider metastatic malignancy in the spine, as from cancer of the prostate, breast, lung, thyroid, and kidney, and multiple myeloma.	Variable with the source. Local bone tenderness may be present.
Back Pain Referred From the Abdomen or Pelvis Usually a deep, aching pain, the level of which varies with the source	Peptic ulcer, pancreatitis, pancreatic cancer, chronic prostatitis, endometriosis, dissecting aortic aneurysm, retroperitoneal tumor, and other causes	Spinal movements are not painful and range of motion is not affected. Look for signs of the primary disorder.

Table 2-16   Pains in the Neck

TABLE 2-16   *Pains in the Neck*

Classifications of neck pain vary considerably, partly because pathologic or other presumably definitive criteria are usually lacking. While "simple stiff neck" is very common, for example, people who have it seldom seek care for it.

Patterns	Possible Causes	Possible Physical Signs
"Simple Stiff Neck" Acute, episodic, localized pain in the neck, often appearing on awakening and lasting 1–4 dy. No dermatomal radiation	The mechanisms are not understood.	Local muscular tenderness and pain on certain movements
Aching Neck A persistent dull aching in the back of the neck, often spreading to the occiput. This is common with postural strain, as with prolonged typing or studying, and may also accompany tension and depression.	Poorly understood; may be related to sustained muscle contraction	Local muscular tenderness. When areas of pain and tenderness are also present elsewhere in the body, consider the fibromyalgia syndrome (see Table 2-14, Patterns of Chronic Pain In and Around the Joints).
"Cervical Sprain" Acute and often recurrent neck pains that are often more severe and last longer than simple stiff neck. There may be a precipitating factor such as a whiplash injury, heavy lifting, or a sudden movement, but there is no dermatomal radiation.	Poorly understood	Local tenderness and pain on movement
Neck Pain With Dermatomal Radiation Neck pain as in cervical sprain, but with radiation of the pain to the shoulder, back, or arm in a dermatomal distribution. This radicular pain is typically sharp, burning, or tingling in quality.	Compression of one or more nerve roots caused by either a herniated cervical disc or degenerative disease of the intervertebral discs with bony spurring*	Muscle tenderness and spasm, a limited range of neck motion, increase in the pain on coughing or straining, and possible sensory loss, weakness, muscular atrophy, and decreased reflexes in the areas involved
Neck Pain With Symptoms Suggesting Compression of the Cervical Spinal Cord Associated here is weakness or paralysis of the legs, often with a decrease in or loss of sensation. These symptoms may occur in addition to the radicular symptoms or by themselves. The neck pain may be mild or even absent.	Compression of the spinal cord in the neck caused by either a herniated cervical disc or degenerative disease of the intervertebral discs with bony spurring. Trauma may also be the cause.*	Limited range of motion in the neck, weakness or paralysis in the legs of the central nervous system type, Babinski responses, loss of position and vibration sense in the legs, and, less commonly, loss of pain and temperature sensation. Radicular signs in the arms may also be present.

* Tumors or abscesses of the cervical spinal cord, though less common, should also be considered.

Table 2-17   Syncope and Similar Disorders

TABLE 2-17   *Syncope and Similar Disorders*

Problem	Mechanism	Precipitating Factors
Vasodepressor Syncope (*the common faint*)	Sudden peripheral vasodilatation, especially in the skeletal muscles, without a compensatory rise in cardiac output. Blood pressure falls.	A strong emotion such as fear or pain
Postural (*orthostatic*) **Hypotension**	1. *Inadequate vasoconstrictor reflexes* in both arterioles and veins, with resultant venous pooling, decreased cardiac output, and low blood pressure	1. Standing up
	2. *Hypovolemia,* a diminished blood volume insufficient to maintain cardiac output and blood pressure, especially in the upright position	2. Standing up after hemorrhage or dehydration
Cough Syncope	Several possible mechanisms associated with increased intrathoracic pressure	Severe paroxysm of coughing
Micturition Syncope	Unclear	Emptying the bladder after getting out of bed to void
Cardiovascular Disorders		
Arrhythmias	Decreased cardiac output secondary to rhythms that are too fast (usually more than 180) or too slow (less than 35–40)	A sudden change in rhythm
Aortic Stenosis and Hypertrophic Cardiomyopathy	Vascular resistance falls with exercise, but cardiac output cannot rise.	Exercise
Myocardial Infarction	Sudden arrhythmia or decreased cardiac output	Variable
Massive Pulmonary Embolism	Sudden hypoxia or decreased cardiac output	Variable
Disorders Resembling Syncope		
Hypocapnia (decreased carbon dioxide) Due to Hyperventilation	Constriction of cerebral blood vessels secondary to hypocapnia that is induced by hyperventilation	Possibly a stressful situation
Hypoglycemia	Insufficient glucose to maintain cerebral metabolism; secretion of epinephrine contributes to symptoms.	Variable, including fasting
*Hysterical Fainting Due to a Conversion Reaction**	The symbolic expression of an unacceptable idea through body language	Stressful situation

* Important diagnostic observations in hysterical fainting include normal skin color and normal vital signs, sometimes bizarre and purposive movements, and occurrence in the presence of other people.

Table 2-17 Syncope and Similar Disorders

Predisposing Factors	Prodromal Manifestations	Postural Associations	Recovery
Fatigue, hunger, a hot, humid environment	Restlessness, weakness, pallor, nausea, salivation, sweating, yawning	Usually occurs when standing, possibly when sitting	Prompt return of consciousness when lying down, but pallor, weakness, nausea, and slight confusion may persist for a time.
1. Peripheral neuropathies and disorders affecting the autonomic nervous system; drugs such as antihypertensives and vasodilators; prolonged bed rest	1. Often none	1. Occurs soon after the person stands up	1. Prompt return to normal when lying down
2. Bleeding from the GI tract or trauma, potent diuretics, vomiting, diarrhea, polyuria	2. Lightheadedness and palpitations (tachycardia) on standing up	2. Usually occurs soon after the person stands up	2. Improvement on lying down
Chronic bronchitis in a muscular man	Often none except for cough	May occur in any position	Prompt return to normal
Nocturia, usually in elderly or adult men	Often none	Standing to void	Prompt return to normal
Organic heart disease and old age decrease the tolerance to abnormal rhythms.	Often none	May occur in any position	Prompt return to normal unless brain damage has resulted
The cardiac disorders	Often none. Onset is sudden.	Occurs with or after exercise	Usually a prompt return to normal
Coronary artery disease	Often none	May occur in any position	Variable
Deep venous thrombosis	Often none	May occur in any position	Variable
A predisposition to anxiety attacks and hyperventilation	Dyspnea, palpitations, chest discomfort, numbness and tingling of the hands and around the mouth lasting for several minutes. Consciousness is often maintained.	May occur in any position	Slow improvement as hyperventilation ceases
Insulin therapy and a variety of metabolic disorders	Sweating, tremor, palpitations, hunger; headache, confusion, abnormal behavior, coma. True syncope is uncommon.	May occur in any position	Variable, depending on severity and treatment
Hysterical personality traits	Variable	A slump to the floor, often from a standing position without injury	Variable, may be prolonged, often with fluctuating responsiveness

Table 2-18   Seizure Disorders

TABLE 2-18   *Seizure Disorders*

Partial seizures are those that start with focal manifestations. They are further divided into *simple partial seizures,* which do not impair consciousness, and *complex partial seizures,* which do. Each of these two types may remain localized or progress into a third type, *partial seizures that become generalized.* Partial seizures of all kinds usually indicate a structural lesion in the cerebral cortex, such as a scar, tumor, or infarction. The quality of such seizures helps the clinician to localize the causative lesion in the brain.

Problem	Clinical Manifestations	Postictal *(Postseizure)* State
Partial Seizures		
Simple Partial Seizures		
• With motor symptoms		
Jacksonian	Tonic and then clonic movements that start unilaterally in the hand, foot, or face and spread to other body parts on the same side	Normal consciousness
Other motor	Turning of the head and eyes to one side, or tonic and clonic movements of an arm or leg without the Jacksonian spread	Normal consciousness
• With sensory symptoms	Numbness, tingling; simple visual, auditory, or olfactory hallucinations such as flashing lights, buzzing, or odors	Normal consciousness
• With autonomic symptoms	A "funny feeling" in the epigastrium, nausea, pallor, flushing, lightheadedness	Normal consciousness
• With psychic symptoms	Anxiety or fear; feelings of familiarity (déjà vu) or unreality; dreamy states; fear or rage; flashback experiences; more complex hallucinations	Normal consciousness
Complex Partial Seizures May start with simple partial seizures or with impaired consciousness. Automatisms may develop.	The seizure may or may not start with the autonomic or psychic symptoms that are outlined above. Consciousness is impaired and the person appears confused. Automatisms include automatic motor behaviors such as chewing, smacking the lips, walking about, and unbuttoning clothes; also more complicated and skilled behaviors such as driving a car.	The patient may remember initial autonomic or psychic symptoms (which are then termed an *aura*), but is amnesic for the rest of the seizure. Temporary confusion and headache may occur.
Partial Seizures That Become Generalized	Partial seizures that become generalized resemble tonic–clonic seizures (see p. 105). Unfortunately, the patient may not recall the focal onset and observers may overlook it.	As in a tonic–clonic seizure, described on the next page. Two attributes indicate a partial seizure that has become generalized: (1) the recollection of an aura, and (2) a unilateral neurologic deficit during the postictal period.

(Table continues on next page) ➡

Table 2-18 Seizure Disorders

Generalized seizures, in contrast to partial ones, begin with either bilateral bodily movements or impairment of consciousness, or both. They suggest a widespread, bilateral cortical disturbance that may be either hereditary or acquired. When generalized seizures of the tonic–clonic (grand mal) variety start in childhood or young adulthood, they are often hereditary. When tonic–clonic seizures begin after the age of 30, suspect either a partial seizure that has become generalized or a general seizure caused by a toxic or metabolic problem. Toxic and metabolic causes include withdrawal from alcohol or other sedative drugs, uremia, hypoglycemia, hyperglycemia, hyponatremia and water intoxication, and bacterial meningitis.

Problem	Clinical Manifestations	Postictal (*Postseizure*) State
Generalized Seizures		
*Tonic–Clonic Convulsion (grand mal)**	The person loses consciousness suddenly, sometimes with a cry, and the body stiffens into tonic extensor rigidity. Breathing stops and the person becomes cyanotic. A clonic phase of rhythmic muscular contraction follows. Breathing resumes and is often noisy, with excessive salivation. Injury, tongue biting, and urinary incontinence may occur.	Confusion, drowsiness, fatigue, headache, muscular aching, and sometimes the temporary persistence of bilateral neurologic deficits such as hyperactive reflexes and Babinski responses. The person has amnesia for the seizure and recalls no aura.
Absence	A sudden brief lapse of consciousness, with momentary blinking, staring, or movements of the lips and hands but no falling. Two subtypes are recognized. *Petit mal absences* last less than 10 sec and stop abruptly. *Atypical absences* may last more than 10 sec.	No aura recalled. In petit mal absences, a prompt return to normal; in atypical absences, some postictal confusion
Atonic Seizure, or Drop Attack	Sudden loss of consciousness with falling but no movements. Injury may occur.	Either a prompt return to normal or a brief period of confusion
Myoclonus	Sudden, brief, rapid jerks, involving the trunk or limbs. Associated with a variety of disorders	Variable
Pseudoseizures May mimic seizures but are due to a conversion reaction (a psychological disorder).	The movements may have personally symbolic significance and often do not follow a neuroanatomic pattern. Injury is uncommon.	Variable

* *Febrile convulsions* that resemble brief tonic–clonic seizures may occur in infants and young children. They are usually benign but occasionally may be the first manifestation of a seizure disorder.

Mental Status

CHAPTER 3

Components of Mental Function

When assessing each body system, clinicians use selected attributes to evaluate the system's structure and function, to distinguish a healthy from a pathologic state, and to diagnose disease. Just as symptoms, pressures, and pulse waves serve these purposes in the cardiovascular system, for example, specific components of mental function do so for the mind. Although these components do not encompass all the aspects of human thought and feeling, they serve as useful clinical tools.

Level of consciousness refers to alertness and a person's state of awareness of the environment. *Attention* refers to the ability to focus or concentrate over time on one task or activity. An inattentive or distractible person whose consciousness is impaired has difficulty giving a history or responding to questions. *Memory,* too, contributes importantly to such responses. A person first must register or record material in the mind—a function usually tested by asking for immediate repetition of material. Information must then be stored or retained in memory. *Recent* (or *short-term) memory* refers to memory over an interval of minutes, hours, or days, while *remote* (or *long-term) memory* refers to intervals of years. *Orientation* depends on both memory and attention. It refers to people's awareness of who or what they are in relation to time, place, and other people.

A person becomes aware of objects in the environment and their qualities and interrelationships through sensory *perceptions*. While most perceptions are initiated by external stimuli, others, like dreams and hallucinations, arise in the mind itself.

Thought processes refer to the sequence, logic, coherence, and relevance of a person's thought as it leads to selected goals. While thought processes describe how people think, *thought content* refers to what they think about. Thought includes insight and judgment. In the context of a mental status examination, *insight* refers to a person's awareness that his or her symptoms or disturbed behaviors are abnormal. One person may realize that the hallucinations experienced are mental figments, for example, while another, lacking this insight, is convinced that they are real external phenomena. In making *judgments,* a person compares and evaluates alternatives for purposes of deciding on a course of action. Inherent in judgment is a set of values that may or may not be based on reality and may or may not conform to societal norms.

In contrast to thought, affect and mood describe how people feel. *Affect* is an immediately observable, usually episodic feeling tone expressed through voice, facial expression, or demeanor, while *mood* is a more sustained emotion that may color a person's view of the world. As weather is to climate, so affect is to mood.

People communicate with each other through *language,* a complex symbolic system of expressing, receiving, and comprehending words. Like consciousness, attention, and memory, language is essential to other mental functions; significant impairment here makes assessment of certain other functions difficult or even impossible.

Higher cognitive functions include a person's *vocabulary,* fund of *information,* and abilities to *think abstractly, calculate numbers,* and *copy or construct objects* that have two or three dimensions.

Recognizing the interplay of body and mind in relation to these attributes is very important but not always easy. Mental disorders such as anxiety or depression often manifest themselves as physical illnesses and, in turn, physical illnesses cause mental and emotional responses. Especially in elderly people, a physical illness may severely impair mental function without causing typical symptoms or signs such as fever or pain. When you detect mental dysfunction, you should therefore look carefully for physical (and pharmacologic) causes while you also try to understand the context and emotional meaning of the changes in mental status.

This chapter does not deal with personality, psychodynamics, or personal experiences. These are explored during the interview. By integrating and correlating all the relevant data, the clinician tries to understand the person as a whole.

Changes With Age

Adolescence marks a time of continuing intellectual maturation—information, vocabulary, and reasoning continue to grow, processes that began in childhood. At approximately 12 years of age, adolescents begin to think abstractly—to use generalizations, make hypotheses, develop theories, reason logically, and consider future plans, risks, and possibilities. Given intelligence, education, and experience, among other requisites, judgment develops along with an underlying set of values. This maturational process, however, like height, weight, and puberty, varies in its time of onset, pace, and duration and cannot be predicted by chronologic age alone. Some individuals never achieve the levels customarily defined as normal adult function.

Lack of ability to think abstractly and to weigh consequences affects health-related behaviors such as sexual activity, the use of tobacco, alcohol, or other drugs, and taking risks that lead to injuries. In a society giving emphasis to such behaviors in the media and elsewhere, they have become prevalent among adolescents. In addition, psychological problems may appear during the teenage years. These include concerns about change in appearance and body contour, panic attacks, rage reactions, depression, suicidal behaviors, and psychotic disorders, including schizophrenia.

Aging. Age-related losses may take their toll on the mental function of an elderly person. These include the deaths of loved ones and friends, retirement from valued employment, diminution in income, decreased physical capacities including impairments in vision and hearing, and perhaps decreased stimulation or growing isolation. In addition, biological changes affect the aging brain. Brain volume and the number of cortical brain cells decrease, and both microanatomic and biochemical changes have been identified. Nevertheless, most men and women adapt well to getting older. They maintain their self-esteem, they alter their activities in ways that are appropriate to their changing capacities and circumstances, and eventually they ready themselves for death.

Most elderly people do well on a mental status examination but functional impairments may become evident, especially at advanced ages. Many older people complain of their memories. "Benign forgetfulness" is the usual explanation and may occur at any age. This term refers to a difficulty in recalling the names of people or objects or certain details of specific events. Naming this common phenomenon, when appropriate, may help to reassure a person who is worried that it signifies Alzheimer's disease. In addition to this circumscribed forgetfulness, elderly people retrieve and process data more slowly, and they take more time to learn new material. Their motor responses may slow, and their ability to perform complex tasks may become impaired.

The clinician must often try to distinguish these age-related changes from the manifestations of specific mental disorders, some of which are more prevalent in old age. Dementia has been estimated to affect a third or more of people who are 85 or older. Depressive symptoms occur in about 15% of noninstitutionalized people over 65 years of age, but are more common among those who live in institutional settings. Diagnosing depression, however, may be difficult. Its symptoms may be mixed with those of physical ailments, and both patients and clinicians may attribute all somatic complaints to physical causes without considering a possible mood disturbance. Cognitive deficits in older patients may further impair the recognition and reporting of mood symptoms, which, if identified, might be treatable. Delirium is an important disorder among the aged. Elderly people are especially susceptible to this temporary confusional state, and the clinician must recognize it promptly in order to treat it properly and protect the patient from harm. Further, delirium may be the first clue to a physical illness, such as a myocardial infarction or pneumonia.

Techniques of Examination

Most of the mental status examination should be done in the context of the interview. As you talk to the patient and listen to the story, you should assess level of consciousness, general appearance and affect, and ability to pay attention, remember, understand, and speak. By noting the patient's vocabulary and general fund of information in the context of cultural and educational background, you can often make a rough estimate of intelligence, while the patient's responses to illness and circumstance often tell you much about insight and judgment. If the patient has unusual thoughts, preoccupations, beliefs, or perceptions, you should explore them as the subject arises. Moreover, if you suspect a problem in orientation or memory, you can check these too as part of the interview. "Let's see, your last clinic appointment was when? . . . and the date today. . . ?" The more you can integrate your exploration of mental status into a sensitive history of the patient's experience, the less it will seem like an interrogation.

For some patients, you need to go further. All patients with documented or suspected brain lesions, those with psychiatric symptoms, and those in whom family members or friends have reported vague behavioral symptoms need further careful, specific assessment. Patients who seem unable to take their medications properly, whose attention to home or business responsibilities seems to be slipping, and who are losing interest in their usual activities may be showing signs of dementia. The patient who is behaving strangely after surgery or during an acute illness may be delirious. Each problem should be identified as expeditiously as possible. Mental function, moreover, importantly influences a person's ability to find and hold a job and thus may constitute the critical component in evaluating disability.

For these kinds of patients, and others as well, you will need to supplement your interview with questions in specific areas. In doing so, give simple introductory explanations, be tactful, and show the same acceptance and respect for the patient as in other portions of the examination.

Students may feel uneasy about performing mental status examinations and reluctant to do them. They may worry about upsetting patients, invading their privacy, and labeling their thoughts or behavior as pathologic. Such concerns are understandable and indeed appropriate. An insensitive examination of mental status may, in fact, offend or frighten a patient; even a skillful examination may expose to the patient embarrassing or alarming deficits that he or she was trying to ignore. It may be helpful to discuss these concerns or some of the issues they raise with your instructor or other experienced clinicians. As in other parts of the assessment process, your skills and confidence will improve with practice and rewards will follow. Many patients will appreciate an understanding listener, and some will owe their health, their safety, or even their lives to your attention.

The format that follows should help to organize your observations, but it is not intended as a step-by-step guide. When a full examination is indicated, you should be flexible in your approach while thorough in your coverage. In some situations, however, sequence is important. If during your initial interview the patient's consciousness, attention, comprehension of words, or ability to speak seems impaired, assess this attribute promptly. A person so impaired cannot give a reliable history and you will not be able to test most of the other mental functions.

Appearance and Behavior

Use here all the relevant observations made throughout the course of your history and examination. Include these areas:

Level of Consciousness. Is the patient awake and alert? Does the patient seem to understand your questions and respond appropriately and reasonably quickly, or is there a tendency to lose track of the topic and fall silent or even asleep?

See the table, Level of Consciousness (Arousal), p. 600.

If the patient does not respond to your questions, escalate the stimulus in steps:

• Speak to the patient by name and in a loud voice.

Lethargic patients are drowsy but open their eyes and look at you, respond to questions, and then fall asleep.

• Shake the patient gently, as if awakening a sleeper.

Obtunded patients open their eyes and look at you, but respond slowly and are somewhat confused.

If there is no response to these stimuli, promptly assess the patient for stupor or coma—severe reductions in the level of consciousness (see p. 600).

Posture and Motor Behavior. Does the patient lie in bed, or prefer to walk about? Note body posture and the patient's ability to relax. Observe the pace, range, and character of movements. Do they seem to be under voluntary control? Are certain parts immobile? Do posture and motor activity change with topics under discussion or with activities or people around the patient?

Tense posture, restlessness, and fidgetiness of anxiety; crying, pacing, and handwringing of agitated depression; hopeless, slumped posture and slowed movements of depression; singing, dancing, and expansive movements of a manic episode.

Dress, Grooming, and Personal Hygiene. How is the patient dressed? Is clothing clean, pressed, and properly fastened? How does it compare with clothing worn by people of comparable age and social group? Note the patient's hair, nails, teeth, skin, and, if present, beard. How are they groomed? How do the person's grooming and hygiene compare

Grooming and personal hygiene may deteriorate in depression, schizophrenia, and dementia. Excessive fastidiousness may be seen in an

with those of other people of comparable age, lifestyle, and socioeconomic group? Compare one side of the body with the other.

Facial Expression. Observe the face, both at rest and when the patient is interacting with others. Watch for variations in expression with topics under discussion. Are they appropriate? Or is the face relatively immobile throughout?

Manner, Affect, and Relationship to Persons and Things. Using your observations of facial expressions, voice, and body movements, assess the patient's affect. Does it vary appropriately with topics under discussion, or is the affect labile, blunted, or flat? Does it seem inappropriate or extreme at certain points? If so, how? Note the patient's openness, approachability, and reactions to others and to the surroundings. Does the patient seem to hear or see things that you do not or seem to be conversing with someone who is not there?

Speech and Language

Throughout the interview, note the characteristics of the patient's speech, including the following:

Quantity. Is the patient talkative or relatively silent? Are comments spontaneous or only responsive to direct questions?

Rate. Is speech fast or slow?

Loudness

Articulation of Words. Are the words spoken clearly and distinctly? Is there a nasal quality to the speech?

Fluency, which involves the rate, flow, and melody of speech and the content and use of words. Be alert for abnormalities of spontaneous speech such as these:

• Hesitancies and gaps in the flow and rhythm of words

• Disturbed inflections, such as a monotone

• Circumlocutions, in which phrases or sentences are substituted for a word the person cannot think of, such as "what you write with" for "pen"

• Paraphasias, in which words are malformed ("I write with a den"), wrong ("I write with a bar"), or invented ("I write with a dar")

Examples of Abnormalities:

obsessive–compulsive disorder. One-sided neglect may result from a lesion in the opposite parietal cortex, usually the nondominant side.

Expressions of anxiety, depression, apathy, anger, elation. Facial immobility of parkinsonism

Anger, hostility, suspiciousness, or evasiveness of paranoid patients. Elation and euphoria of the manic syndrome. Flat affect and remoteness of schizophrenia. Apathy (dulled affect with detachment and indifference) in dementia. Anxiety, depression

Slow speech of depression; rapid, loud speech in a manic syndrome

Dysarthria refers to defective articulation. *Aphasia* refers to a disorder of language. See Table 3-1, Disorders of Speech, p. 123.

These abnormalities suggest aphasia. The patient may have so much difficulty in talking or in understanding others that you may not be able to obtain a history. You may also falsely suspect a psychotic disorder.

If the patient's speech lacks meaning or fluency, proceed with further testing as outlined in the following table.

Testing for Aphasia	
Word Comprehension	Ask the patient to follow a one-stage command, such as "Point to your nose." Try a two-stage command: "Point to your mouth, then your knee."
Repetition	Ask the patient to repeat a phrase of one-syllable words (the most difficult repetition task): "No ifs, ands, or buts."
Naming	Ask the patient to name the parts of a watch.
Reading Comprehension	Ask the patient to read a paragraph aloud.
Writing	Ask the patient to write a sentence.

These tests help you to decide what kind of aphasia the patient may have. Remember that deficiencies in vision, hearing, intelligence, and education may also affect performance. Two common kinds of aphasia—Wernicke's and Broca's—are compared in Table 3-1, Disorders of Speech, p. 123.

A person who can write a correct sentence does not have aphasia.

Mood

Assess mood during the interview by exploring the patient's own perceptions of it. Find out about the patient's usual mood level and how it has varied with life events. "How did you feel about that?", for example, or, more generally, "How are your spirits?" The reports of relatives and friends may be of great value in making this assessment.

Moods include sadness and deep melancholy; contentment, joy, euphoria, and elation; anger and rage; anxiety and worry; and detachment and indifference.

What has the patient's mood been like? How intense has it been? Has it been labile or fairly unchanging? How long has it lasted? Is it appropriate to the patient's circumstances? In case of depression, have there also been episodes of an elevated mood, suggesting a bipolar disorder?

For depressive and bipolar disorders, see Table 3-2, Disorders of Mood, p. 124.

If you suspect depression, assess its depth and any associated risk of suicide. A series of questions such as the following is useful, proceeding as far as the patient's positive answers warrant.

Do you get pretty discouraged (or depressed or blue)?
How low do you feel?
What do you see for yourself in the future?
Do you ever feel that life isn't worth living? Or that you would just as soon be dead?
Have you ever thought of doing away with yourself?
How did (do) you think you would do it?
What would happen after you were dead?

Asking about suicidal thoughts does not implant the idea in the patient's mind, and it may be the only way to get the information. Although many student clinicians feel uneasy about exploring this topic, most patients can discuss their thoughts and feelings about it freely with you, sometimes with considerable relief. By such discussion, you demonstrate your interest and concern for what may well be the patient's most serious and threatening problem. By avoiding the issue, you may miss the most important feature of the patient's illness.

Thought and Perceptions

Thought Processes. Assess the logic, relevance, organization, and coherence of the patient's thought processes as they are revealed in words and speech throughout the interview. Does speech progress in a logical manner toward a goal? Here you are using the patient's speech as a window into the patient's mind. Listen for patterns of speech that suggest disorders of thought processes, as outlined in the table below.

Variations and Abnormalities in Thought Processes

Circumstantiality	Speech characterized by indirection and delay in reaching the point because of unnecessary detail, although the components of the description have a meaningful connection. Many people without mental disorders speak circumstantially.	Observed in obsessional persons
Derailment (Loosening of Associations)	Speech in which a person shifts from one subject to others that are unrelated or only obliquely related without realizing that the subjects are not meaningfully connected. Ideas slip off the track between clauses, not within them.	Observed in schizophrenia, manic episodes, and other psychiatric disorders
Flight of Ideas	An almost continuous flow of accelerated speech in which a person changes abruptly from topic to topic. Changes are usually based on understandable associations, plays on words, or distracting stimuli, but the ideas do not progress to sensible conversation.	Most frequently noted in manic episodes
Neologisms	Invented or distorted words, or words with new and highly idiosyncratic meanings	Observed in schizophrenia, other psychotic disorders, and aphasia
Incoherence	Speech that is largely incomprehensible because of illogic, lack of meaningful connections, abrupt changes in topic, or disordered grammar or word use. Shifts in meaning occur within clauses. Flight of ideas, when severe, may produce incoherence.	Observed in severely disturbed psychotic persons (usually schizophrenic)
Blocking	Sudden interruption of speech in mid-sentence or before completion of an idea. The person attributes this to losing the thought. Blocking occurs in normal people.	Blocking may be striking in schizophrenia.
Confabulation	Fabrication of facts or events in response to questions, to fill in the gaps in an impaired memory	Common with amnesia
Perseveration	Persistent repetition of words or ideas	Occurs in schizophrenia and other psychotic disorders
Echolalia	Repetition of the words and phrases of others	Occurs in manic episodes and schizophrenia
Clanging	Speech in which a person chooses a word on the basis of sound rather than meaning, as in rhyming and punning speech. For example, "Look at my eyes and nose, wise eyes and rosy nose. Two to one, the ayes have it!"	Occurs in schizophrenia and manic episodes

Thought Content. You should ascertain most of the information relevant to thought content during the interview. Follow appropriate leads as they occur rather than using stereotyped lists of specific questions. For example, "You mentioned a few minutes ago that a neighbor was responsible for your entire illness. Can you tell me more about that?" Or, in another situation, "What do you think about at times like these?"

You may need to make more specific inquiries. If so, couch them in tactful and accepting terms. "When people are upset like this, they sometimes can't keep certain thoughts out of their minds," or "... things seem unreal. Have you experienced anything like this?"

In these ways find out about any of the patterns shown in the following table.

Abnormalities of Thought Content	
Compulsions	Repetitive behaviors or mental acts that a person feels driven to perform in order to produce or prevent some future state of affairs, although expectation of such an effect is unrealistic
Obsessions	Recurrent, uncontrollable thoughts, images, or impulses that a person considers unacceptable and alien
Phobias	Persistent, irrational fears, accompanied by a compelling desire to avoid the stimulus
Anxieties	Apprehensions, fears, tensions, or uneasiness that may be focused (phobia) or free floating (a general sense of ill-defined dread or impending doom)
Feelings of Unreality	A sense that things in the environment are strange, unreal, or remote
Feelings of Depersonalization	A sense that one's self is different, changed, or unreal, or has lost identity or become detached from one's mind or body
Delusions	False, fixed, personal beliefs that are not shared by other members of the person's culture or subculture. Examples include: • *Delusions of persecution* • *Grandiose delusions* • *Delusional jealousy* • *Delusions of reference*, in which a person believes that external events, objects, or people have a particular and unusual personal significance (e.g., that the radio or television might be commenting on or giving instructions to the person) • *Delusions of being controlled* by an outside force • *Somatic delusions* of having a disease, disorder, or physical defect • *Systematized delusions*, a single delusion with many elaborations or a cluster of related delusions around a single theme, all systematized into a complex network

Compulsions, obsessions, phobias, and anxieties are often associated with neurotic disorders. See Table 3-3, Anxiety Disorders (p. 126).

Delusions and feelings of unreality or depersonalization are more often associated with psychotic disorders. See Table 3-4, Psychotic Disorders (p. 126). Delusions may also occur in delirium, severe mood disorders, and dementia.

Perceptions. Inquire about false perceptions in a manner similar to that used for thought content. For example, "When you heard the voice speaking to you, what did it say? How did it make you feel?" Or, "After you've been drinking a lot, do you ever see things that aren't really there?" Or, "Sometimes after major surgery like this, people hear peculiar or frightening things. Have you experienced anything like that?" In these ways find out about the following abnormal perceptions.

Abnormalities of Perception	
Illusions	Misinterpretations of real external stimuli
Hallucinations	Subjective sensory perceptions in the absence of relevant external stimuli. The person may or may not recognize the experiences as false. Hallucinations may be auditory, visual, olfactory, gustatory, tactile, or somatic. (False perceptions associated with dreaming, falling asleep, and awakening are not classified as hallucinations.)

Illusions may occur in grief reactions, delirium, acute and posttraumatic stress disorders, and schizophrenia.

Hallucinations may occur in delirium, dementia (less commonly), posttraumatic stress disorder, and schizophrenia.

Insight and Judgment. These attributes are usually best assessed during the interview.

Insight. Some of your very first questions of the patient often yield important information about insight: "What brings you to the hospital?" "What seems to be the trouble?" "What do you think is wrong?" More specifically, note whether or not the patient is aware that a particular mood, thought, or perception is abnormal or part of an illness.

Patients with psychotic disorders often lack insight into their illness. Denial of impairment may accompany some neurologic disorders.

Judgment. You can usually assess judgment by noting the patient's responses to family situations, jobs, use of money, and interpersonal conflicts. "How do you plan to get the help you'll need after leaving the hospital?" "How are you going to manage if you lose your job?" "If your husband starts to abuse you again, what will you do?" "Who will attend to your financial affairs while you are in the nursing home?"

Judgment may be poor in delirium, dementia, mental retardation, and psychotic states. Judgment is affected also by anxiety, mood disorders, intelligence, education, socioeconomic options, and cultural values.

Note whether decisions and actions are based on reality or, for example, on impulse, wish fulfillment, or disordered thought content. What values seem to underlie the patient's decisions and behavior? Allowing for cultural variations, how do these compare with mature adult standards? Because judgment is part of the maturational response, it may be variable and unpredictable during adolescence.

Cognitive Functions

Orientation. By skillful questioning you can often determine the patient's orientation in the context of the interview. For example, you can ask quite naturally for specific dates and times, the patient's address and telephone number, the names of family members, or the route taken to the hospital. At times—when rechecking the status of a delirious patient, for example—simple, direct questions may be indicated.

Disorientation occurs especially when memory or attention is impaired, as in delirium.

"Can you tell me what time it is now . . . and what day is it?" In either of these ways, determine the patient's orientation for the following:

- *Time* (e.g., the time of day, day of the week, month, season, date and year, duration of hospitalization)
- *Place* (e.g., the patient's residence, the names of the hospital, city, and state)
- *Person* (e.g., the patient's own name, and the names of relatives and professional personnel)

Attention. These tests of attention are commonly used:

Digit Span. Explain that you would like to test the patient's ability to concentrate, perhaps adding that people tend to have trouble with that when they are in pain, or ill, or feverish. Recite a series of digits, starting with two at a time and speaking each number clearly at a rate of about one per second. Ask the patient to repeat the numbers back to you. If this repetition is accurate, try a series of three numbers, then four, and so on as long as the patient responds correctly. Jotting down the numbers as you say them helps to ensure your own accuracy. If the patient makes a mistake, try once more with another series of the same length. Stop after a second failure in a single series.

Causes of poor performance include delirium, dementia, mental retardation, and performance anxiety.

In choosing digits you may use street numbers, zip codes, telephone numbers, and other numerical sequences that are familiar to you, but avoid consecutive numbers, easily recognized dates, and sequences that possibly are familiar to the patient.

Now, starting again with a series of two, ask the patient to repeat the numbers to you backward.

Normally, a person should be able to repeat correctly at least five digits forward and four backward.

Serial 7s. Instruct the patient, "Starting from a hundred, subtract 7, and keep subtracting 7. . . ." Note the effort required and the speed and accuracy of the responses. (Writing down the answers helps you keep up with the arithmetic.) Normally, a person can complete serial 7s in 1½ minutes, with fewer than four errors. If the patient cannot do serial 7s, try 3s or counting backward.

Poor performance may be due to delirium, the late stage of dementia, mental retardation, loss of calculating ability, anxiety, or depression. Also consider the possibility of limited education.

Spelling Backward can substitute for serial 7s. Say a five-letter word, spell it, e.g., W-O-R-L-D, and ask the patient to spell it backward.

Remote Memory. Inquire about birthdays, anniversaries, social security number, names of schools attended, jobs held, or past historical events such as wars relevant to the patient's past.

Remote memory may be impaired in the late stage of dementia.

Recent Memory (e.g., the events of the day). Ask questions with answers that you can check against other sources so that you will know whether or not the patient is confabulating (making up facts to compensate for a defective memory). These might include the day's weather, today's appointment time, and medications or laboratory tests

Recent memory is impaired in dementia and delirium. See Table 3-5. Delirium and Dementia, p. 127. *Amnestic disorders* impair memory or new

taken during the day. (Asking what the patient had for breakfast may be a waste of time unless you can check the accuracy of the answer.)

New Learning Ability. Give the patient three or four words such as "83 Water Street and blue," or "table, flower, green, and hamburger." Ask the patient to repeat them so that you know that the information has been heard and registered. (This step, like digit span, tests registration and immediate recall.) Then proceed to other parts of the examination. After about 3 to 5 minutes, ask the patient to repeat the words. Note the accuracy of the response, awareness of whether or not it is correct, and any tendency to confabulate. Normally, a person should be able to remember the words.

learning ability significantly and reduce a person's social or occupational functioning, but they do not have the global features of delirium or dementia. Anxiety, depression, and mental retardation may also impair recent memory.

Higher Cognitive Functions

Information and Vocabulary

Information and vocabulary, when observed clinically, enable a rough estimate of a person's intelligence. Assess them during the interview. Ask a student, for example, about favorite courses, or inquire about a person's work, hobbies, reading, favorite television programs, or current events. Explore such topics first with simple questions, then with more difficult ones. Note the person's grasp of information, the complexity of the ideas expressed, and the vocabulary used.

More directly, you can ask about specific facts, such as these:

The name of the president, vice president, or governor
The names of the last four or five presidents
The names of five large cities in the country

If considered in the context of cultural and educational background, information and vocabulary are fairly good indicators of intelligence. They are relatively unaffected by any but the most severe psychiatric disorders, and may be helpful in distinguishing mentally retarded adults (whose information and vocabulary are limited) from those with mild or moderate dementia (whose information and vocabulary are fairly well preserved).

Calculating Ability. Test the patient's ability to do arithmetical calculations, starting at the rote level with simple addition ("What is 4 + 3? . . . 8 + 7?") and multiplication ("What is 5 × 6? . . . 9 × 7?"). The task can be made more difficult by using two-digit numbers ("15 + 12" or "25 × 6") or longer, written examples.

Alternatively, pose practical and functionally important questions, such as "If something costs 78 cents and you give the clerk one dollar, how much should you get back?"

Poor performance may be a useful sign of dementia or may accompany aphasia, but it must be assessed in terms of the patient's intelligence and education.

Abstract Thinking. The capacity to think abstractly can be tested in two ways.

Proverbs. Ask the patient what people mean when they use some of the following proverbs:

A stitch in time saves nine.
Don't count your chickens before they're hatched.
The proof of the pudding is in the eating.
A rolling stone gathers no moss.
The squeaking wheel gets the grease.

Concrete responses are often given by persons with mental retardation, delirium, or dementia, but may also be simply a function of limited education. Schizophrenics may respond concretely or with personal, bizarre interpretations.

Note the relevance of the answers and their degree of concreteness or abstractness. For example, "You should sew a rip before it gets bigger" is concrete, while "Prompt attention to a problem prevents trouble" is abstract. Average patients should give abstract or semi-abstract responses.

Similarities. Ask the patient to tell you how the following are alike:

An orange and an apple   A church and a theater
A cat and a mouse   A piano and a violin
A child and a dwarf   Wood and coal

Note the accuracy and relevance of the answers and their degree of concreteness or abstractness. For example, "A cat and a mouse are both animals" is abstract, "They both have tails" is concrete, and "A cat chases a mouse" is not relevant.

Constructional Ability. The task here is to copy figures of increasing complexity onto a piece of blank unlined paper. Show each figure one at a time and ask the patient to copy it as well as possible.

The three diamonds below are rated poor, fair, and good (but not excellent).

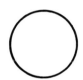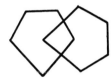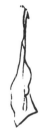

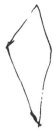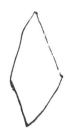

(Strub RL, Black FW: The Mental Status Examination in Neurology, 2nd ed. Philadelphia, FA Davis, 1985)

In another approach, ask the patient to draw a clock face complete with numbers and hands. The example below is rated excellent.

These three clocks are poor, fair, and good.

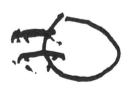

(Strub RL, Black FW: The Mental Status Examination in Neurology, 2nd ed. Philadelphia, FA Davis, 1985)

If vision and motor ability are intact, poor constructional ability suggests dementia or parietal lobe damage. Mental retardation may also impair performance.

Special Technique

Mini-Mental State Examination (MMSE). This brief test of cognitive functions is useful in screening for dementia and following its course over time. The maximum score for each question or task is shown in parentheses.

- "Can you tell me the date?" Ask for any parts omitted: year, season, date, day, month. (5)

  Subtract 1 for each part not given.

- "Where are you?" Ask for any items omitted: state, county, town, hospital, floor. (5)

  Subtract 1 for each item not given.

- Name three objects slowly and clearly, and ask the patient to repeat them. (3)

  Subtract 1 for each item not registered.

- Ask the patient to do serial 7s. Stop after five answers. Alternatively, ask the patient to spell WORLD backward. (5)

  Subtract 1 for each wrong number or out-of-order letter.

- Ask for the names of the three objects repeated above. (3)

  Subtract 1 for each object not recalled.

- Show the patient a watch and ask for its name. Repeat with a pencil. (2)

  Subtract 1 for each item not named correctly.

- Ask the patient to repeat "No ifs, ands, or buts." (1)

  Score 0 or 1 on the first trial.

- Offer the patient a piece of plain, blank paper, and say "Take this paper in your right hand, fold it in half, and put it on the floor." (3)

  Subtract 1 for each of the three actions not performed.

- Show the patient a piece of paper on which is printed in large letters CLOSE YOUR EYES. Ask the patient to read it and do it. (1)

  Subtract 1 if the patient's eyes do not close.

- Ask the patient to write a sentence of his or her own. (1)

  Subtract 1 for absence of subject, verb, or sensible meaning.

- Ask the patient to copy a pair of intersecting pentagons onto a piece of blank paper. (1)

  Subtract 1 for fewer than ten angles or two intersecting lines.

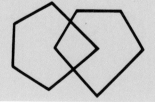

Out of the maximum score of 30, 24 to 30 is considered normal.

Scores of less than 24 increase the likelihood of dementia.

Adapted from Folstein MF, Folstein SE, McHugh PR: "Mini-Mental State": A practical method for grading the cognitive state of patients for the clinician. J Psychiatr Res 12:196–198, 1975, with kind permission from Pergamon Press Ltd, Headington Hill Hall, Oxford OX3 OBW, U.K. For further interpretation, see the bibliography.

Health Promotion and Counseling

Up to a third of all primary care visits involve mental health—depressed mood, anxiety, somatic concerns, and more serious disorders of mood and mental function. The burden of suffering imposed by these disorders is great. For the general population, focus health promotion and counseling on depression, suicidality, and dementia, three important conditions often overlooked.

The lifetime prevalence of major depression meeting formal diagnostic criteria is 5% to 10% in men and 10% to 20% in women. Primary-care providers fail to diagnose major depression in up to 50% of affected patients, often missing early clues such as low self-esteem, anhedonia (failure to find pleasure in daily activities), sleep disorders, and difficulty in concentrating or making decisions. Routine general screening has not been shown to improve outcomes; rather, target diagnosis and treatment of patients who are symptomatic. Watch carefully for depressive symptoms, especially in patients who are young, female, single, divorced, separated, seriously or chronically ill, or bereaved. Patients with a prior history of depression or positive family history are also at risk. Failure to diagnose depression can have consequences that are fatal—suicide rates in patients with major depression are eight times higher than in the general population.[*]

Clinicians must be adept at eliciting suicidal ideation or intent (see Chap. 1, p. 21). Suicide rates are highest among men over age 65, but have been increasing in teenagers and young adults. Risk factors include any history of psychiatric illness (especially if linked to a hospital admission), substance abuse, personality disorder, prior suicide attempt, or family history of suicide. Clinicians should ask about domestic firearms and screen for alcohol dependence: guns are present in the home of more than half of all suicide victims, and alcohol intoxication is associated with nearly 25% of suicide deaths. Any evidence of suicidal ideation must be further assessed. Has a weapon been obtained? Is there a plan or a note? Such patients should be promptly referred for mental health and psychiatric care and for treatment of any related problems of alcohol or drug abuse.

Dementia, a "global impairment of cognitive function that interferes with normal activities,"[†] affects 16% of Americans over 65. Prominent features include short- and long-term memory deficits and impaired judgment. Thought processes are impoverished and speech may be hesitant due to difficulty in finding words. Loss of orientation to place may make navigating by foot or car problematic or even dangerous. Most dementias represent Alzheimer's disease (~50%–85%) or vascular

[*]U.S. Preventive Services Task Force: Chapter 49: "Screening for Depression." In *Guide to Clinical Preventive Services*. Baltimore: Williams and Wilkins, 1996, pp. 541–546.
[†]U.S. Preventive Services Task Force: Ch. 48: "Screening for Dementia." In *Guide to Clinical Preventive Services*. Baltimore: Williams and Wilkins, 1996, pp. 531–541.

multi-infarct dementia (~10%–20%). Be watchful for Alzheimer's disease in individuals with a positive family history, since their risk is three times higher than in the general population.

Dementia often has a slow, insidious onset and may escape detection by both families and clinicians, especially in its initial stages. Currently there are no reliable screening tests to help you detect dementia early in its course. Clinicians should be alert to evidence of change in cognitive function or activities of daily living, and to family complaints about new or unusual patient behaviors. Use of the Mini-Mental State Examination is helpful for assessing cognitive impairment (although scores may be affected by level of education and cultural variables such as language; see p. 120). Once cognitive change is identified, be sure to address the possible role of medications, depression, or metabolic abnormalities. For demented patients and affected families, counseling about the potential for disruptive behavior, accidents and falls, and termination of driving privileges is warranted. Clinicians can foster discussion of legal matters such as power of attorney and advanced directives while the patient is still able to contribute to decision-making.

Table 3-1   Disorders of Speech

TABLE 3-1   *Disorders of Speech*

Disorders of speech fall into three groups, those affecting (1) the voice, (2) the articulation of words, and (3) the production and comprehension of language.

Aphonia refers to a loss of voice that accompanies disease affecting the larynx or its nerve supply. *Dysphonia* refers to less severe impairment in the volume, quality, or pitch of the voice. For example, a person may be hoarse or only able to speak in a whisper. Causes include laryngitis, laryngeal tumors, and a unilateral vocal cord paralysis (Cranial Nerve X).

Dysarthria refers to a defect in the muscular control of the speech apparatus (lips, tongue, palate, or pharynx). Words may be nasal, slurred, or indistinct, but the central symbolic aspect of language remains intact. Causes include motor lesions of the central or peripheral nervous system, parkinsonism, and cerebellar disease.

Aphasia refers to a disorder in producing or understanding language. It is often caused by lesions in the dominant cerebral hemisphere (usually the left).

Compared below are two common types of aphasia, (1) Wernicke's, a fluent (receptive) aphasia, and (2) Broca's, a nonfluent (or expressive) aphasia. There are other less common kinds of aphasia, which may be distinguished from each other by differing responses on the specific tests listed. Neurologic consultation is usually indicated.

	Wernicke's Aphasia	**Broca's Aphasia**
Qualities of Spontaneous Speech	Fluent; often rapid, voluble, and effortless. Inflection and articulation are good, but sentences lack meaning and words are malformed (paraphasias) or invented (neologisms). Speech may be totally incomprehensible.	Nonfluent; slow, with few words and laborious effort. Inflection and articulation are impaired but words are meaningful, with nouns, transitive verbs, and important adjectives. Small grammatical words are often dropped.
Word Comprehension	Impaired	Fair to good
Repetition	Impaired	Impaired
Naming	Impaired	Impaired, though the patient recognizes objects
Reading Comprehension	Impaired	Fair to good
Writing	Impaired	Impaired
Location of Lesion	Posterior superior temporal lobe	Posterior inferior frontal lobe

While it is important to recognize aphasia early in your encounter with a patient, its full diagnostic meaning does not become clear until you integrate this information with your neurologic examination.

Tables 3-2 through 3-5 summarize the manifestations of selected disorders. They show how the data collected can be used diagnostically, and will help you to recognize and think about certain patterns of illness.

Tables 3-2, 3-3, and 3-4 are based, with permission, on the *Diagnostic and Statistical Manual of Mental Disorders*, Fourth Edition, Washington, D.C., American Psychiatric Association, 1994. For further details and criteria, the reader should consult this manual, its successor, or comprehensive textbooks of psychiatry.

Table 3-2   Disorders of Mood

TABLE 3-2   *Disorders of Mood*

Mood disorders may be either depressive or bipolar. A bipolar disorder includes manic or hypomanic features as well as depressive ones. Four types of *episodes,* described below, are combined in different ways in diagnosis of *mood disorders.* A major depressive disorder includes only one or more major depressive episodes. A *bipolar I disorder* includes one or more manic or mixed episodes, usually accompanied by major depressive episodes. A *bipolar II disorder* includes one or more major depressive episodes accompanied by at least one hypomanic episode.

Dysthymic and *cyclothymic disorders* are chronic and less severe conditions that do not meet the criteria of the other disorders. *Mood disorders due to general medical conditions or substance abuse* are classified separately.

Major Depressive Episode

At least five of the symptoms listed below (including one of the first two) must be present during the same 2-week period. They must also represent a change from the person's previous state.

- Depressed mood (may be an irritable mood in children and adolescents) most of the day, nearly every day
- Markedly diminished interest or pleasure in almost all activities most of the day, nearly every day
- Significant weight gain or loss (not dieting) or increased or decreased appetite nearly every day
- Insomnia or hypersomnia nearly every day
- Psychomotor agitation or retardation nearly every day
- Fatigue or loss of energy nearly every day
- Feelings of worthlessness or inappropriate guilt nearly every day
- Inability to think or concentrate or indecisiveness nearly every day
- Recurrent thoughts of death or suicide, or a specific plan for or attempt at suicide

The symptoms cause significant distress or impair social, occupational, or other important functions. In severe cases, hallucinations and delusions may occur.

Mixed Episode

A mixed episode, which must last at least 1 week, meets the criteria for both manic and major depressive episodes.

Dysthymic Disorder

A depressed mood and symptoms for most of the day, for more days than not, over at least 2 years (1 year in children and adolescents). Freedom from symptoms lasts no more than 2 months at a time.

Manic Episode

A distinct period of abnormally and persistently elevated, expansive, or irritable mood must be present for at least a week (any duration if hospitalization is necessary). During this time, at least three of the symptoms listed below have been persistent and significant. (Four of the these symptoms are required if the mood is only irritable).

- Inflated self-esteem or grandiosity
- Decreased need for sleep (e.g., feels rested after sleeping 3 hours)
- More talkative than usual or pressure to keep talking
- Flight of ideas or racing thoughts
- Distractibility
- Increased goal-directed activity (either socially at work or school, or sexually) or psychomotor agitation
- Excessive involvement in pleasurable high-risk activities (e.g., buying sprees, foolish business ventures, sexual indiscretions)

The disturbance is severe enough to impair social or occupational functions or relationships. It may necessitate hospitalization for the protection of self or others. In severe cases, hallucinations and delusions may occur.

Hypomanic Episode

The mood and symptoms resemble those in a manic episode but are less impairing, do not require hospitalization, do not include hallucinations or delusions, and have a shorter minimum duration—4 days.

Cyclothymic Episode

Numerous periods of hypomanic and depressive symptoms that last for at least 2 years (1 year in children and adolescents). Freedom from symptoms lasts no more than 2 months a time.

Table 3-3   Anxiety Disorders

TABLE 3-3   *Anxiety Disorders*

Anxiety disorders cause great distress and impair function, but those affected are not psychotic. The disorders are distinguished by the symptoms, the entities feared, or the stressors.

Panic Disorder	A panic disorder is defined by recurrent, unexpected panic attacks, at least one of which has been followed by a month or more of persistent concern about further attacks, worry over their implications or consequences, or a significant change in behavior in relation to the attacks. A *panic attack* is a discrete period of intense fear or discomfort that develops abruptly and peaks within 10 minutes. It involves at least four of the following symptoms: (1) palpitations, pounding heart, or accelerated heart rate, (2) sweating, (3) trembling or shaking, (4) shortness of breath or a sense of smothering, (5) a feeling of choking, (6) chest pain or discomfort, (7) nausea or abdominal distress, (8) feeling dizzy, unsteady, lightheaded, or faint, (9) feelings of unreality or depersonalization, (10) fear of losing control or going crazy, (11) fear of dying, (12) paresthesias (numbness or tingling), (13) chills or hot flushes. Panic disorder may occur with or without agoraphobia.
Agoraphobia	Agoraphobia is an anxiety about being in places or situations where escape may be difficult or embarrassing or help for sudden symptoms unavailable. Such situations are avoided, require a companion, or cause marked anxiety.
Specific Phobia	A specific phobia is a marked, persistent, and excessive or unreasonable fear that is cued by the presence or anticipation of a specific object or situation, such as dogs, injections, or flying. The person recognizes the fear as excessive or unreasonable, but exposure to the cue provokes immediate anxiety. Avoidance or fear impairs the person's normal routine, occupational or academic functioning, or social activities or relationships.
Social Phobia	A social phobia is a marked, persistent fear of one or more social or performance situations that involve exposure to unfamiliar people or to scrutiny by others. Those afflicted fear that they will act in embarrassing or humiliating ways, as by showing their anxiety. Exposure creates anxiety and possibly a panic attack, and the person avoids precipitating situations. He or she recognizes the fear as excessive or unreasonable. Normal routines, occupational or academic functioning, or social activities or relationships are impaired.
Obsessive– Compulsive Disorder	This disorder involves obsessions or compulsions that cause marked anxiety or distress. While they are recognized at some point as excessive or unreasonable, they are very time consuming and interfere with the person's normal routine, occupational functioning, or social activities or relationships.
Acute Stress Disorder	The person has been exposed to a traumatic event that involved actual or threatened death or serious injury to self or others and responded with intense fear, helplessness, or horror. During or immediately after this event, the person has at least three of these dissociative symptoms: (1) a subjective sense of numbing, detachment, or absence of emotional responsiveness; (2) a reduced awareness of surroundings, as in a daze; (3) feelings of unreality; (4) feelings of depersonalization; and (5) amnesia for an important part of the event. The event is persistently reexperienced, as in thoughts, images, dreams, illusions, and flashbacks, or distress from reminders of the event. The person is very anxious or shows increased arousal and tries to avoid stimuli that evoke memories of the event. The disturbance causes marked distress or impairs social, occupational, or other important functions. The symptoms occur within 4 wk of the event and last from 2 days to 4 weeks.
Posttraumatic Stress Disorder	The event, the fearful response, and the persistent reexperiencing of the traumatic event resemble those in acute stress disorder. Hallucinations may occur. The person has increased arousal, tries to avoid stimuli related to the trauma, and has numbing of general responsiveness. The disturbance causes marked distress, impairs social, occupational, or other important functions, and lasts for more than a month.
Generalized Anxiety Disorder	This disorder lacks a specific traumatic event or focus for concern. Excessive anxiety and worry, which the person finds hard to control, are about a number of events or activities. At least three of the following symptoms are associated: (1) feeling restless, keyed up, or on edge, (2) being easily fatigued, (3) difficulty in concentrating or mind going blank, (4) irritability, (5) muscle tension, (6) difficulty in falling or staying asleep, or restless, unsatisfying sleep. The disturbance causes significant distress or impairs social, occupational, or other important functions.

Table 3-4 Psychotic Disorders

TABLE 3-4 Psychotic Disorders

Psychotic disorders involve grossly impaired reality testing. Specific diagnoses depend on the nature and duration of the symptoms and on a cause when it can be identified. Seven disorders are outlined below.

Schizophrenia	Schizophrenia impairs major functioning, as at work or school or in interpersonal relations or self care. For this diagnosis, performance of one or more of these functions must have decreased for a significant time to a level markedly below prior achievement. In addition, the person must manifest at least two of the following for a significant part of 1 month: (1) delusions, (2) hallucinations, (3) disorganized speech, (4) grossly disorganized or catatonic behavior,* and (5) negative symptoms such as a flat affect, alogia (lack of content in speech), or avolition (lack of interest, drive, and ability to set and pursue goals). Continuous signs of the disturbance must persist for at least 6 months.
	Subtypes of this disorder include paranoid, disorganized, and catatonic schizophrenia.
Schizophreniform Disorder	A schizophreniform disorder has symptoms similar to those of schizophrenia but they last less than 6 months, and the functional impairment seen in schizophrenia need not be present.
Schizoaffective Disorder	A schizoaffective disorder has features of both a major mood disturbance and schizophrenia. The mood disturbance (depressive, manic, or mixed) is present during most of the illness and must, for a time, be concurrent with symptoms of schizophrenia (listed above). During the same period of time, there must also be delusions or hallucinations for at least 2 weeks without prominent mood symptoms.
Delusional Disorder	A delusional disorder is characterized by nonbizarre delusions that involve situations in real life, such as having a disease or being deceived by a lover. The delusion has persisted for at least a month, but the person's functioning is not markedly impaired and behavior is not obviously odd or bizarre. The symptoms of schizophrenia except for tactile and olfactory hallucinations related to the delusion have not been present.
Brief Psychotic Disorder	In this disorder, at least one of the following psychotic symptoms must be present: delusions, hallucinations, disordered speech such as frequent derailment or incoherence, or grossly disorganized or catatonic behavior. The disturbance lasts at least 1 day but less than 1 month, and the person returns to his or her prior functional level.
Psychotic Disorder Due to a General Medical Condition	Prominent hallucinations or delusions may be experienced during a medical illness. For this diagnosis, they should not occur exclusively during the course of delirium. The medical condition should be documented and judged to be causally related to the symptoms.
Substance-Induced Psychotic Disorder	Prominent hallucinations or delusions may be induced by intoxication or withdrawal from a substance such as alcohol, cocaine, or opioids. For this diagnosis, these symptoms should not occur exclusively during the course of delirium. The substance should be judged to be causally related to the symptoms.

*Catatonic behaviors are psychomotor abnormalities that include stupor, mutism, negativistic resistance to instructions or attempts to move the person, rigid or bizarre postures, and excited, apparently purposeless activity.

Table 3-5   Delirium and Dementia

TABLE 3-5   *Delirium and Dementia*

Delirium and dementia are common and very important disorders that affect multiple aspects of mental status. Both have many possible causes. Some clinical features of these two conditions and their effects on mental status are compared below. A delirium may be superimposed on dementia.

	Delirium	Dementia
Clinical Features		
Onset	Acute	Insidious
Course	Fluctuating, with lucid intervals; worse at night	Slowly progressive
Duration	Hours to weeks	Months to years
Sleep/Wake Cycle	Always disrupted	Sleep fragmented
General Medical Illness or Drug Toxicity	Either or both present	Often absent, especially in Alzheimer's disease
Mental Status		
Level of Consciousness	Disturbed. Person less clearly aware of the environment and less able to focus, sustain, or shift attention	Usually normal until late in the course of the illness
Behavior	Activity often abnormally decreased (somnolence) or increased (agitation, hypervigilance)	Normal to slow; may become inappropriate
Speech	May be hesitant, slow or rapid, incoherent	Difficulty in finding words, aphasia
Mood	Fluctuating, labile, from fearful or irritable to normal or depressed	Often flat, depressed
Thought Processes	Disorganized, may be incoherent	Impoverished. Speech gives little information.
Thought Content	Delusions common, often transient	Delusions may occur.
Perceptions	Illusions, hallucinations, most often visual	Hallucinations may occur.
Judgment	Impaired, often to a varying degree	Increasingly impaired over the course of the illness
Orientation	Usually disoriented, especially for time. A known place may seem unfamiliar.	Fairly well maintained, but becomes impaired in the later stages of illness
Attention	Fluctuates. Person easily distracted, unable to concentrate on selected tasks	Usually unaffected until late in the illness
Memory	Immediate and recent memory impaired	Recent memory and new learning especially impaired
Examples of Cause	Delirium tremens (due to withdrawal from alcohol)	*Reversible:* Vitamin B$_{12}$ deficiency, thyroid disorders
	Uremia	
	Acute hepatic failure	*Irreversible:* Alzheimer's disease, vascular dementia (from multiple infarcts), dementia due to head trauma
	Acute cerebral vasculitis	
	Atropine poisoning	

Physical Examination: Approach and Overview

General Approach

Most patients view a physical examination with at least some anxiety. They feel vulnerable, physically exposed, apprehensive about possible pain, and uneasy about what the clinician may find. At the same time, they often appreciate detailed concern for their problems and may enjoy the attention they receive.

Mindful of such feelings, the skillful clinician is thorough without wasting time, systematic without being rigid, gentle yet not afraid to cause discomfort if this should be required. By listening, looking, touch, or smell, the skillful clinician examines each region of the body and at the same time senses the whole patient, notes the wince or worried glance, and calms, explains, and reassures.

Early in their experience students, like patients, are apprehensive. They feel uneasy in their ambiguous roles as student-professionals and uncertain of their newfledged competencies. Touching intimate areas of a patient's body and making a patient uncomfortable often cause special concern. Anxieties are unavoidable.

Over time, however, competence and self-confidence grow. Through study and repetitive practice the flow of the examination becomes smooth, and you can gradually shift your attention from where to place your hands or instruments to what you hear, see, and feel. At the same time you become accustomed to the physical contact, skilled in minimizing discomfort, and more conscious of the patient's reactions than of your own feelings. Before long, you will be able to accomplish in 5 to 10 minutes what first took an hour or two. Continuing progress should be a lifetime goal.

Despite inevitable insecurities as you begin to examine patients, you should take command of your own demeanor. Try to look calm, organized, and competent, even when you do not exactly feel that way. If you forget a portion of your examination, as you undoubtedly will, do not get flustered. Simply do that part out of sequence—smoothly. If you have already left the patient, return and ask if you can check one more thing. Avoid expressions of disgust, alarm, distaste, or other negative reactions. They have no place at the bedside, even when you come upon an ominous mass, a deep and smelly ulcer, or a pubic louse.

As in the interview, be sensitive to the patient's feelings. The patient's facial expression or an apparently casual question such as "Is it okay?" may give you clues to previously unexpressed worries. Ascertain them when you can. Also consider the patient's physical comfort and needs. Adjust the slant of the bed or examining table accordingly, and use pillows for comfort or blankets for warmth as necessary. Assure as much privacy as possible by using drapes appropriately and closing doors.

As an examiner you too should be comfortable, because awkward positions may impair your perceptions. Adjust the bed to a convenient height, and ask the patient to move toward you if this will help you examine a body region more comfortably.

Good lighting and a quiet environment contribute importantly to what you see and hear but may be remarkably hard to arrange. Do the best you can. If a nearby patient's television interferes with hearing your patient's heart sounds, politely ask the neighbor to lower the volume. Most people cooperate readily. Remember to thank them when you are through.

Keep the patient informed as you proceed with your examination, especially when you anticipate possible embarrassment or discomfort. Patients vary considerably in their knowledge of examination procedures and in their need for information. Some people want to know what you are doing when you listen to the lungs or feel for a liver, while others already know or do not care. By words or gestures, be as clear as possible in your instructions. When telling patients what to do, be courteous. "I would like to examine your heart now. Would you please lie down."

Clinicians differ in how and when they report their findings to their patients. Beginning students should avoid almost all such interpretive statements because they do not yet carry the primary responsibility for the patient and may give conflicting or erroneous information. As experience and responsibility increase, however, sharing findings with the patient becomes appropriate. If you know or suspect that the patient has specific concerns, it may be helpful to make a reassuring comment as you finish examining the relevant area. A steady series of reassuring comments, however, presents at least one potential problem: what to say when you find an unexpected abnormality. You may wish you had maintained judicious silence earlier.

Regardless of differing approaches, all students should develop one habit that will help them avoid alarming patients needlessly. Beginners spend much more time than experienced clinicians on techniques such as ophthalmoscopic examination or cardiac auscultation. Whenever you do this, pause and explain. "I would like to spend a long time examining your heart so I can listen carefully to each of the heart sounds. It does not mean that I hear anything wrong." Be forthright with the patient about your status as a student. Such openness will clarify your relationship and probably reduce anxieties on both sides.

How Complete Should an Examination Be? There is no simple answer to this common question. The outline below summarizes a fairly comprehensive examination suitable for an adult patient who needs a thorough checkup. It also summarizes a clinician's basic repertory of examining skills.

For patients who have symptoms restricted to a specific body system or region, a more limited examination may be more appropriate. Here, as in the history, select the methods relevant to assessing the problem as precisely and efficiently as possible. The patient's symptoms and demographic characteristics such as age and sex all influence this selection and help you decide what to do. So does your knowledge of disease patterns. Out of all the patients with sore throat, for example, you will need to decide who may have infectious mononucleosis and warrants careful palpation of the liver and spleen and who, in contrast, has a common cold and does not need this examination. The clinical thinking that underlies and guides such decisions is discussed in Chapter 20.

The need for a periodic physical examination for screening, detection, and prevention of disease in men and women has sometimes been challenged. Many of the techniques of the physical examination have yet to be shown to reduce subsequent morbidity and mortality. Clinical studies have validated blood pressure assessment, the clinical breast examination, listening to the heart for evidence of valvular disease, and the pelvic examination with Papanicolaou smears. The list of recommended examinations has been further expanded based on consensus panels and expert opinion.

A thorough examination does more than prevent sickness and prolong the lives of healthy men and women. Most people who seek health care have health-related worries or symptoms. The physical examination may help both to identify such concerns and to explain the symptoms. It gives information with which to answer the patient's questions and provides baseline data for future use. The physical examination also provides important opportunities for health promotion through education and counseling, and increases both the credibility and the conviction of the clinician's advice or reassurance. The physical contact involved often enhances the clinician–patient relationship. Furthermore, students must repeatedly perform such examinations to gain proficiency, and clinicians must do them periodically to maintain their skills. How best to divide one's usually limited time with a patient between listening, discussion, or counseling on the one hand and the physical examination on the other requires judgment and experience.

Sequence. The sequence of the comprehensive examination is designed to minimize the patient's need to change positions and maximize the examiner's efficiency. Variations in order are possible, of course, and you may wish to develop a method of your own. In general, it is helpful to move "from head to toe." Avoid moving from a patient's feet, genitalia, or rectum to the face or mouth or from rectum to vagina.

The Examiner's Position and Handedness. This book recommends examining a supine patient from the patient's right side, moving to the foot of the bed or to the other side as necessary. Working chiefly from one side helps you to master skills more quickly and promotes the efficiency of your examination.

The right side has several advantages over the left: the jugular veins on the right are more reliable for estimating venous pressure, the palpating hand rests more comfortably on the apical impulse, the right kidney is more frequently palpable than the left, and examining tables are sometimes placed against one wall to favor this right-handed approach.

Left-handed students may find this position awkward at first but are encouraged to practice it. Unless they are reasonably ambidextrous, however, most will find it easier to use the left hand for percussing or for holding instruments such as an otoscope or a reflex hammer.

Examining the Supine Patient. Under certain circumstances, the sequence of the examination must differ from the one described on the following pages. Some patients, for example, are unable to sit up in bed or stand. You can examine the head, neck, and anterior chest of such persons as they lie supine. Then roll the patient onto each side to listen to the lungs, examine the back, and inspect the skin. The remainder of the examination is completed with the patient supine.

Tangential Lighting. Tangential lighting is recommended to inspect structures such as the jugular venous pulse, the thyroid gland, and the apical impulse of the heart. This is a method of casting light along a surface in order to maximize shadows. As shown below, these shadows help to reveal any elevations or indentations—moving or stationary—on that surface.

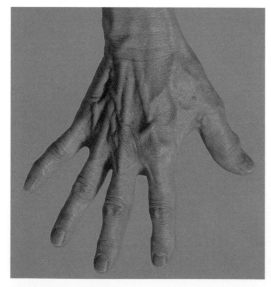

TANGENTIAL LIGHTING

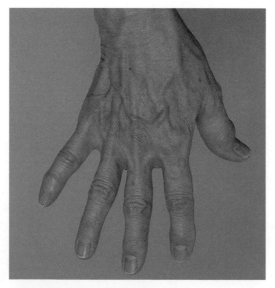

PERPENDICULAR LIGHTING

When light is perpendicular to the surface or diffuse, as shown on the right, shadows are reduced and subtle undulations in the surface are lost.

Experiment with focused, tangential lighting across the tendons and veins on the back of your hand, and try to see the pulsations of the radial artery at your wrist.

Overview of a Comprehensive Examination

To get an overview of the physical examination, skim the following outline now. Later chapters deal with individual body regions or systems. After you have completed the study and practice involved in one or more chapters, reread this overview to see how each segment of the examination fits into an integrated whole.

General Survey. Observe the patient's general state of health, height, build, and sexual development. Weigh the patient, if possible. Note posture, motor activity, and gait; dress, grooming, and personal hygiene; and any odors of body or breath. Watch the patient's facial expressions and note manner, affect, and reactions to persons and things in the environment. Listen to the patient's manner of speaking and note state of awareness or level of consciousness.

The survey continues throughout the history and examination.

Vital Signs. Count the pulse and respiratory rate. Measure the blood pressure and, if indicated, the body temperature.

Skin. Observe the skin of the face and its characteristics. Identify any lesions, noting their location, distribution, arrangement, type, and color. Inspect and palpate the hair and nails. Study the patient's hands. Continue your assessment of the skin as you examine the other body regions.

The patient is sitting on the edge of the bed or examining table, unless this position is contraindicated. You should be standing in front of the patient, moving to either side as needed.

Head. Examine the hair, scalp, skull, and face.

Eyes. Check visual acuity and screen the visual fields. Note the position and alignment of the eyes. Observe the eyelids and inspect the sclera and conjunctiva of each eye. With oblique lighting, inspect each cornea, iris, and lens. Compare the pupils and test their reactions to light. Assess the extraocular movements. With an ophthalmoscope, inspect the ocular fundi.

The room should be darkened for the ophthalmoscopic examination.

Ears. Inspect the auricles, canals, and drums. Check auditory acuity. If acuity is diminished, check lateralization (Weber test) and compare air and bone conduction (Rinne test).

Nose and Sinuses. Examine the external nose, and with the aid of a light and speculum inspect the nasal mucosa, septum, and turbinates. Palpate for tenderness of the frontal and maxillary sinuses.

Mouth and Pharynx. Inspect the lips, oral mucosa, gums, teeth, tongue, palate, tonsils, and pharynx.

Neck. Inspect and palpate the cervical lymph nodes. Note any masses or unusual pulsations in the neck. Feel for any deviation of the trachea. Observe the sound and effort of the patient's breathing. Inspect and palpate the thyroid gland.

Back. Inspect and palpate the spine and muscles of the back. Check for costovertebral angle tenderness.

Posterior Thorax and Lungs. Inspect, palpate, and percuss the chest. Identify the level of diaphragmatic dullness on each side. Listen to the breath sounds, identify any adventitious sounds, and, if indicated, listen to the transmitted voice sounds.

Breasts, Axillae, and Epitrochlear Nodes. In a woman, inspect the breasts with her arms relaxed, then elevated, and then with her hands pressed on her hips. In either sex, inspect the axillae and feel for the axillary nodes. Feel for the epitrochlear nodes.

Move behind the sitting patient to feel the thyroid gland and to examine the back, posterior thorax, and lungs.

Move to the front again.

By this time you have made some preliminary observations of the musculoskeletal system. You have inspected the hands, surveyed the upper back, and, at least in women, made a fair estimate of the shoulders' range of motion. Use these and subsequent observations to decide whether a full musculoskeletal examination is warranted.

Musculoskeletal System. If indicated, examine the hands, arms, shoulders, neck, and temporomandibular joint while the patient is still sitting. Inspect and palpate the joints and check their range of motion.

Breasts. Palpate the breasts, while at the same time continuing your inspection.

Anterior Thorax and Lungs. Inspect, palpate, and percuss the chest. Listen to the breath sounds, any adventitious sounds, and, if indicated, transmitted voice sounds.

Cardiovascular System. Inspect and palpate the carotid pulsations. Listen for carotid bruits. Observe the jugular venous pulsations, and measure the jugular venous pressure in relation to the sternal angle.

Inspect and palpate the precordium. Note the location, diameter, amplitude, and duration of the apical impulse. Listen at the apex and the lower sternal border with the bell of a stethoscope. Listen at each auscultatory area with the diaphragm. Listen for physiologic splitting of the second heart sound and for any abnormal heart sounds or murmurs.

Ask the patient to lie down. You should stand at the right side of the patient's bed.

Elevate the head of the bed to about 30° for the cardiovascular examination, adjusting it as necessary to see the jugular venous pulsations. Ask the patient to roll partly onto the left side while you listen at the apex. Then have the patient lie back while you listen to the rest of the heart. The patient should sit, lean forward, and exhale while you listen for the murmur of aortic regurgitation.

Abdomen. Inspect, auscultate, and percuss the abdomen. Palpate lightly, then deeply. Assess the liver and spleen by percussion and then palpation. Try to feel the kidneys, and palpate the aorta and its pulsations.

Lower the head of the bed to the flat position. The patient should be supine.

Rectal Examination in Men. Inspect the sacrococcygeal and perianal areas. Palpate the anal canal, rectum, and prostate. If the patient cannot stand, examine the genitalia before doing the rectal examination.

The patient is lying on his left side for the rectal examination.

Genitalia and Rectal Examination in Women. Examine the external genitalia, vagina, and cervix. Obtain Pap smears. Palpate the uterus and the adnexa. Do a rectovaginal and rectal examination.

The patient is supine in the lithotomy position. You should be seated at first, then standing at the foot of the examining table.

Legs. Examine the legs, assessing three systems while the patient is still supine. Each of these systems will be examined further when the patient stands.

The patient is supine.

Peripheral Vascular System. Note any swelling, discoloration, or ulcers. Palpate for pitting edema. Feel the dorsalis pedis, posterior tibial, and femoral pulses, and, if indicated, the popliteal pulses. Palpate the inguinal lymph nodes.

Musculoskeletal System. Note any deformities or enlarged joints. If indicated, palpate the joints and check their range of motion.

Neurologic System. Observe the muscle bulk, the position of the limbs, and any abnormal movements.

Examination With Patient Standing. Assess the following:

The patient is standing. You should sit on a chair or stool.

Peripheral Vascular System. Inspect for varicose veins.

Musculoskeletal System. Examine the alignment of the spine and its range of motion, the alignment of the legs, and the feet.

Genitalia and Hernias in Men. Examine the penis and scrotal contents and check for hernias.

Nervous System. Observe the patient's gait and ability to walk heel-to-toe, walk on the toes, walk on the heels, hop in place, and do shallow knee bends. Do a Romberg test and check for a pronator drift.

Additional Neurologic Examination, as indicated:

The patient is sitting or supine.

Mental Status. If indicated and not done during the interview, assess the patient's mood, thought processes, thought content, abnormal perceptions, insight and judgment, memory and attention, information and vocabulary, calculating abilities, abstract thinking, and constructional ability.

Cranial Nerves not already examined: sense of smell, strength of the temporal and masseter muscles, corneal reflexes, facial movements, gag reflex, and strength of the trapezii and sternomastoid muscles

Motor. Muscle tone, muscle strength, rapid alternating movements, and point-to-point movements

Sensory. Pain, temperature, light touch, position, vibration, and discrimination. Compare right with left sides and distal with proximal areas on the limbs.

Reflexes

When you have completed your examination, tell the patient what to do and what to expect next. If you are examining a hospitalized patient, rearrange the immediate environment to suit the patient. If you initially found the bedrails up, put them back in this position unless you are sure that they are not necessary. Lower the bed so that the patient can get in and out easily without risking falls. When you have finished, wash your hands and clean your equipment or dispose of it properly.

The General Survey

CHAPTER 5

Anatomy and Physiology

This section deals briefly with the general topics of body height, weight, and build, and introduces the concept of sexual maturity ratings.

In all these attributes, people vary according to socioeconomic status, nutrition, genetic makeup, early illnesses, gender, the region of the world where they live, and the era in which they were born. The apparent shortening of aging Americans, for example, is partly illusory. Although people do shrink with age, their heights also vary according to the year of their birth. Young adults today on the average have grown taller than their parents, and the parents taller than the grandparents. Clinicians should be cautious in applying the norms of one group to a person of another.

Height, Growth, and Build. When height is charted from birth to late adolescence, one can readily discern an *adolescent growth spurt.* In girls this peaks relatively early in puberty, at about the age of 12, and in boys relatively late, at about 14. Musculoskeletal proportions change during this growth spurt, with variations in degree and timing according to gender. A boy's shoulders, for example, broaden more than a girl's, while a girl's hips widen more than a boy's. These changes are summarized in the illustration on the next page.

Toward the other end of the lifespan, other changes occur. People decrease in height, and posture may become somewhat stooped as the thoracic spine becomes more convex and the knees and hips fail to extend fully. Fat tends to concentrate near the hips and lower abdomen and, together with weakening of the abdominal muscles, may produce a potbelly. The figure on p. 139 illustrates some of the changes occurring in persons ranging in age from 78 to 94. These and other changes with age are further detailed in subsequent chapters.

Sexual Maturity Ratings. Changes in an adolescent's reproductive organs and secondary sex characteristics are closely related to the growth spurt. Later chapters describe sexual maturity ratings for assessing sexual development: in breasts and pubic hair of girls and in genitalia and pubic hair of boys. The interrelationships between these sexual characteristics and the adolescent growth spurt give the clinician a biological yardstick with which to assess an adolescent's growth and development and to identify significant deviations from normal patterns. They also

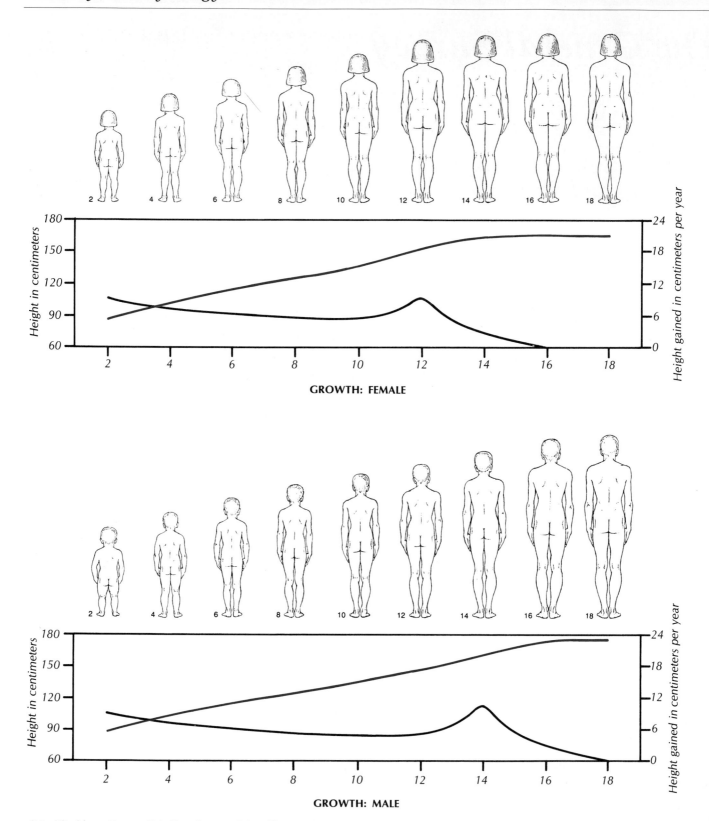

GROWTH: FEMALE

GROWTH: MALE

(Modified from Tanner JM: Growing up. Scientific American 229:36–37, September 1973)

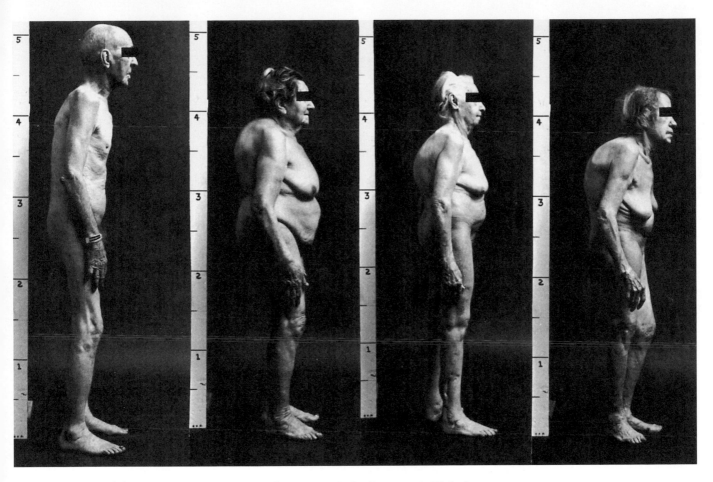

A man, age 82, and three women, ages 78, 79, and 94, respectively. (Rossman I: Clinical Geriatrics, 3rd ed. Philadelphia, JB Lippincott, 1986)

help the clinician to interpret for the adolescent whether growth and sexual maturation are proceeding normally and to predict what further changes may be expected.

During your initial survey of the adolescent patient, you measure only one of these variables—height. You may also make a few preliminary observations of breast and muscular development, pitch of voice, and facial hair. The full meaning of these observations, however, does not emerge until you correlate them with other data: the patient's body build, growth pattern over time, muscular development, sexual maturity ratings, and psychosexual feelings, attitudes and knowledge. During the assessment process, you will bring these interrelated variables together and try to understand the patient's development and any related problems as well as you can.

Weight. Definitions of appropriate weights for adults remain controversial. The height/weight table on p. 140 is based on the body weights for each height that were associated with the lowest mortality. Note that these weights vary according to gender and the size of the frame.

Height (Without Shoes)	Weight in Pounds (Without Clothing)		
	Small Frame	*Medium Frame*	*Large Frame*
Men			
5'1"	105–113	111–122	119–134
5'2"	108–116	114–126	122–137
5'3"	111–119	117–129	125–141
5'4"	114–122	120–132	128–145
5'5"	117–126	123–136	131–149
5'6"	121–130	127–140	135–154
5'7"	125–134	131–145	140–159
5'8"	129–138	135–149	144–163
5'9"	133–143	139–153	148–167
5'10"	137–147	143–158	152–172
5'11"	141–151	147–163	157–177
6'0"	145–155	151–168	161–182
6'1"	149–160	155–173	168–187
6'2"	153–164	160–178	171–192
6'3"	157–168	165–183	175–197
Women			
4'9"	90–97	94–106	102–118
4'10"	92–100	97–109	106–121
4'11"	95–103	100–112	108–124
5'0"	98–106	103–116	111–127
5'1"	101–109	106–118	114–130
5'2"	104–112	109–122	117–134
5'3"	107–115	112–126	121–138
5'4"	110–119	116–131	125–142
5'5"	114–123	120–136	129–146
5'6"	118–127	124–139	133–150
5'7"	122–131	128–143	137–154
5'8"	126–136	132–147	141–159
5'9"	130–140	136–151	145–164
5'10"	134–144	140–155	149–169

Height and Weight Tables for Adults Age 25 and Over

From Clinician's Handbook of Preventive Services. Washington, DC: U.S. Department of Health and Human Services, 1994:142–143.

The data are derived from an insured population. Note that body frame is not easily measured and must be derived visually. Lower weights may be advisable for patients at risk for cardiovascular disease and diabetes mellitus.

Techniques of Examination

Begin your observations from the first moment you see the patient and continue them throughout your interaction. Does the patient hear you when called in the waiting room? rise with ease? walk easily or stiffly? If hospitalized when you first meet, what is the patient doing: sitting up and enjoying television? or lying in bed? What occupies the bedside table: a magazine? a flock of "get well" cards? a Bible or rosary? an emesis basin? or nothing at all? Each of these observations should raise one or more tentative hypotheses and guide your further assessments.

Level of Consciousness. Is the patient awake, alert, and responsive to you and others in the environment?

If not, promptly assess the level of consciousness (see p. 600).

Signs of Distress. For example, does the patient show evidence of these problems:

- Cardiorespiratory insufficiency

Labored breathing, wheezing, cough

- Pain

Wincing, sweating, protectiveness of a painful part

- Anxiety

Anxious face, fidgety movements, cold moist palms

Apparent State of Health. Try to make this general judgment based on observations made throughout your encounter. Support it with the significant details.

Acutely or chronically ill, frail, feeble, robust, vigorous

Skin Color and Obvious Lesions. See Chapter 6 for details.

Pallor, cyanosis, jaundice, rashes, bruises

Height and Build. If possible, measure the patient's height in stocking feet. Is the patient unusually short or tall? Is the build slender and lanky, muscular, or stocky? Is the body symmetrical? Note the general body proportions and look for any deformities.

Very short stature in Turner's syndrome and childhood renal failure, and in achondroplastic and hypopituitary dwarfism; long limbs in proportion to the trunk in hypogonadism and Marfan's syndrome

Sexual Development. Are the voice, facial hair, and breast size appropriate to the patient's age and gender?

Delayed or precocious puberty, hypogonadism, virilism

Weight. Is the patient emaciated, slender, plump, obese, or somewhere in between? If the patient is obese, is the fat distributed rather evenly or does it concentrate in the trunk?

Generalized fat in simple obesity; truncal fat with relatively thin limbs in Cushing's syndrome

If possible, weigh the patient. Weight provides one index of caloric sufficiency, and changes over time give other valuable diagnostic data. Remember that weight may rise or fall with changes in body fluids as well as in fat or muscle.

Causes of weight loss include malignancy, diabetes mellitus, hyperthyroidism, chronic infection, depression, diuresis, and successful dieting

Posture, Gait, and Motor Activity. What is the patient's preferred posture?

Preference for sitting up in left-sided heart failure, and for leaning forward with arms braced in chronic obstructive pulmonary disease

Is the patient restless or quiet? How often does the patient move about? How fast are the movements?

Fast, frequent movements of hyperthyroidism; slowed activity of myxedema

Are there apparently involuntary motor activities, or are some body parts immobile? What parts are involved?

Tremors or other involuntary movements; paralyses. See Table 18-3, Involuntary Movements (pp. 610–611)

Does the patient walk easily, with comfort, self-confidence, and good balance, or is there a limp, discomfort on walking, fear of falling, loss of balance, or abnormality in motor pattern?

See Table 18-6, Abnormalities of Gait and Posture (pp. 616–617).

Dress, Grooming, and Personal Hygiene. How is the patient dressed? Is clothing appropriate to the temperature and weather? Is it clean, properly buttoned, and zipped? How does it compare with clothing worn by people of comparable age and social group?

Dress may reflect the cold intolerance of hypothyroidism, the hiding of a skin rash or needle marks, or personal preferences in lifestyle.

Glance at the patient's shoes. Have holes been cut in them? Are the laces tied? Or is the patient wearing slippers?

Cut-out holes or slippers may indicate gout, bunions, or other painful foot conditions. Untied laces or slippers also suggest edema.

Is the patient wearing any unusual jewelry?

Copper bracelets are sometimes worn for arthritis.

Note the patient's hair, fingernails, and use of cosmetics. They may reflect the patient's personality, mood, or lifestyle. Nail polish and hair coloring that have "grown out" may be due to decreased interest in personal appearance.

"Grown-out" hair and nail polish may help you estimate the length of an illness when the patient can't give a history.

Do personal hygiene and grooming seem appropriate to the patient's age, lifestyle, occupation, and socioeconomic group? There are, of course, wide variations in norms.

Unkempt appearance may be seen in depression and dementia, but this appearance must be compared with the patient's probable norm.

Techniques of Examination	*Examples of Abnormalities*

Odors of Body or Breath. Although odors give important diagnostic clues, never assume that alcohol on a patient's breath explains neurologic or mental status findings. Alcoholics may have other serious and potentially correctable problems such as hypoglycemia or subdural hematoma, and an alcoholic scent may not mean alcoholism.

Breath odors of alcohol, acetone (diabetes), pulmonary infections, uremia, or liver failure

Facial Expression. Observe facial expression at rest, during conversation about specific topics, during the physical examination, and in interaction with others.

The stare of hyperthyroidism; the immobile face of parkinsonism

Vital Signs. Note the pulse, blood pressure, respiratory rate, and temperature. You may make these measurements at the beginning of the examination or integrate them with your cardiovascular and thoracic assessments. If you do them first, count the radial pulse. Then, with your fingers still on the patient's wrist, count the respiratory rate without the patient's realizing it. (Breathing may change when a person becomes conscious that someone is watching.) Check the blood pressure; if it is high, repeat your measurement later in the examination.

See Table 9-3, Abnormalities of the Arterial Pulse and Pressure Waves (p. 322). See Table 8-1, Abnormalities in Rate and Rhythm of Breathing (p. 269).

Although you may omit measuring temperature in many ambulatory patients, take it if symptoms or signs suggest a possible abnormality. Oral temperatures are more convenient for patients than rectal ones. However, it is unwise to take oral temperatures when patients are unconscious, restless, or unable to close their mouths. Temperature readings may be inaccurate and thermometers may be broken by unexpected movements of the patient's mouth.

Fever or *pyrexia* refers to an elevated body temperature. *Hyperpyrexia* refers to extreme elevation in temperature, above 41.1°C (106°F), while *hypothermia* refers to an abnormally low temperature, below 35°C (95°F) rectally.

Oral temperatures can be taken with glass or electronic thermometers. When using a glass thermometer, shake the thermometer down to below 35.5°C (96°F), insert it under the tongue, instruct the patient to close both lips, and wait 3 to 5 minutes. Then read the thermometer, reinsert it for a minute, and read it again. If the temperature is still rising, repeat this procedure until the reading remains stable. If using an electronic thermometer, carefully place the disposable cover over the probe and insert the thermometer under the tongue. Ask the patient to close both lips, and then watch closely for the digital readout. An accurate temperature recording usually takes about 10 seconds.

Causes of fever include infections, trauma (such as surgery or crushing injury), malignancies, infarctions, blood disorders (such as acute hemolytic anemia), various drugs, and immune disorders (such as collagen diseases).

Whether an oral temperature is taken with a glass or an electronic thermometer, drinking hot or cold liquids may alter it artifactually. Wait 10 to 15 minutes before measurement.

To take a *rectal temperature,* select a rectal thermometer (with a stubby tip), lubricate it, and insert it about 3 cm to 4 cm (1½ inches) into the anal canal, in a direction pointing toward the umbilicus. Remove and read it after 3 minutes. Alternatively, use an electronic thermometer after careful lubrication of the probe cover. Wait about 10 seconds for the digital temperature recording to appear.

The chief cause of hypothermia is exposure to cold. Other predisposing causes include decreased muscular movement (as from paralysis), interference with vasoconstriction (as from alcohol and sepsis), starvation, hypothyroidism, and hypoglycemia. Elderly people are especially susceptible to hypothermia and are less likely to develop fever.

The average oral temperature, usually quoted at 37°C (98.6°F), fluctuates considerably and must be interpreted accordingly. In the early morning hours it may be as low as 35.8°C (96.4°F), in the late afternoon or evening as high as 37.3°C (99.1°F). Rectal temperatures average 0.4° to 0.5°C (0.7° to 0.9°F) higher than oral readings, but this difference varies considerably.

Another alternative is use of special electronic thermometers to measure the *tympanic membrane temperatare*. This method is quick and safe and measures core body temperature; therefore, the measurement is approximately 0.8°C (1.4°F) higher than the normal oral temperature. Place the probe in the ear canal for 2 to 3 seconds until the digital temperature reading appears.

Rapid respiratory rates tend to increase the discrepancy between oral and rectal temperatures. Rectal measurements are then more reliable.

The Skin

CHAPTER 6

Anatomy and Physiology

The skin functions in many important ways. It holds body fluids within its boundaries; it protects the underlying tissues from microorganisms, harmful substances, and radiation; it synthesizes vitamin D; and it helps to modulate body temperature.

The skin is composed of three layers: the epidermis, the dermis, and the subcutaneous tissues.

The most superficial layer, the *epidermis*, is thin, devoid of blood vessels, and itself divided into two layers: an outer horny layer of dead keratinized cells, and an inner cellular layer where both melanin and keratin are formed.

The epidermis depends on the underlying *dermis* for its nutrition. The dermis is well supplied with blood. It contains connective tissue, the sebaceous glands, and some of the hair follicles. It merges below with the *subcutaneous tissues*, which contain fat, the sweat glands, and the remainder of the hair follicles.

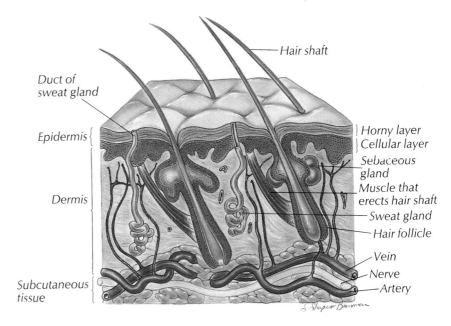

Hair shaft
Duct of sweat gland
Epidermis {
Horny layer
Cellular layer
Sebaceous gland
Muscle that erects hair shaft
Dermis
Sweat gland
Hair follicle
Vein
Nerve
Subcutaneous tissue {
Artery

Hair, nails, and sebaceous and sweat glands are considered appendages of the skin. Adults have two types of hair: *vellus hair*, which is short, fine, inconspicuous, and unpigmented, and *terminal hair*, which is coarser, thicker, more conspicuous, and usually pigmented. Scalp hair and eyebrows are examples of terminal hair.

Nails protect the distal ends of the fingers and toes. The firm, rectangular, and usually curving *nail plate* gets its pink color from the vascular *nail bed* to which the plate is firmly attached. Note the whitish moon (*lunula*) and the free edge of the nail plate. Roughly a fourth of the nail plate (the *nail root*) is covered by the *proximal nail fold*. The *cuticle* extends from this fold and, functioning as a seal, protects the space between the fold and the plate from external moisture. *Lateral nail folds* cover the sides of the nail plate. Note that the angle between the proximal nail fold and the nail plate is normally less than 180°.

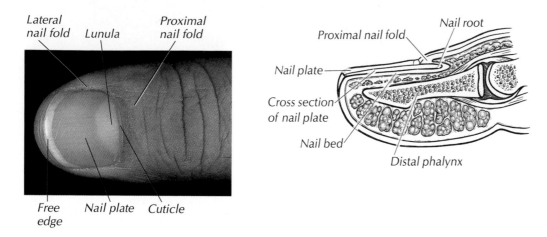

Fingernails grow at about 0.1 mm daily; toenails grow more slowly.

Sebaceous glands secrete a protective fatty substance which gains access to the skin surface through the hair follicles. These glands are present on all skin surfaces except the palms and soles. *Sweat glands* are of two types: eccrine and apocrine. The *eccrine glands* are widely distributed, open directly onto the skin surface, and by their sweat production help to control body temperature. In contrast, the *apocrine glands* are found chiefly in the axillary and genital regions, usually open into hair follicles, and are stimulated by emotional stress. Bacterial decomposition of apocrine sweat is responsible for adult body odor.

The color of normal skin depends primarily on four pigments: melanin, carotene, oxyhemoglobin, and deoxyhemoglobin. The amount of *melanin,* the brownish pigment of the skin, is genetically determined and is increased by sunlight. *Carotene* is a golden yellow pigment that exists in subcutaneous fat and in heavily keratinized areas such as the palms and soles.

Hemoglobin, which circulates in the red cells and carries most of the oxygen of the blood, exists in two forms. *Oxyhemoglobin,* a bright red pigment, predominates in the arteries and capillaries. An increase in blood flow through the arteries to the capillaries of the skin causes a reddening of the skin, while the opposite change usually produces pallor. The skin of light-colored persons is normally redder on the palms, soles, face, neck, and upper chest.

As blood passes through the capillary bed, some of the oxyhemoglobin loses its oxygen to the tissues and changes to *deoxyhemoglobin*—a darker and somewhat bluer pigment. An increased concentration of deoxyhemoglobin in cutaneous blood vessels gives the skin a bluish cast known as *cyanosis.*

Cyanosis is of two kinds, depending on the oxygen level in the arterial blood. If this level is low, cyanosis is *central*. If it is normal, cyanosis is *peripheral*. Peripheral cyanosis occurs when cutaneous blood flow decreases and slows, and tissues extract more oxygen than usual from the blood. Peripheral cyanosis may be a normal response to anxiety or a cold environment.

Skin color is affected not only by pigments but also by the scattering of light as it is reflected back through the turbid superficial layers of the skin or vessel walls. This scattering makes the color look more blue and less red. The bluish color of a subcutaneous vein is due to this effect; it is much bluer than the venous blood obtained on venipuncture.

Changes With Age

Adolescence. During the pubertal years coarse, or terminal, hair appears in new places: the face in boys, and the axillae and pubic areas in both sexes. Hair on the trunk and limbs increases through and after puberty, more obviously in men. During puberty apocrine glands enlarge, axillary sweating increases, and the characteristic adult body odor appears.

Aging. As people age their skin wrinkles, becomes lax, and loses turgor. The vascularity of the dermis decreases and the skin of white persons tends to look paler and more opaque. Comedones (blackheads) often appear on the cheeks or around the eyes. Where skin has been exposed to the sun it looks weatherbeaten: thickened, yellowed, and deeply furrowed. Skin on the backs of the hands and forearms appears thin, fragile, loose, and transparent, and may show whitish, depigmented patches known as pseudoscars. Well demarcated, vividly purple macules or patches, termed actinic purpura, may also appear in the same areas, fading after several weeks. These purpuric spots come from blood that has leaked through poorly supported capillaries and has spread within the dermis. Dry skin (asteatosis)—a common problem—is flaky, rough, and often itchy. It is frequently shiny, especially on the legs, where a network of shallow fissures often creates a mosaic of small polygons.

Some common benign lesions often accompany aging: cherry angiomas (p. 156), which often appear early in adulthood, seborrheic keratoses (p. 157), and, in sun-exposed areas, actinic lentigines or "liver spots" (p. 160) and actinic keratoses (p. 157). Elderly people may also develop two fairly common skin cancers: basal cell carcinoma and squamous cell carcinoma (p. 157)

Nails lose some of their luster with age and may yellow and thicken, especially on the toes.

Hair on the scalp loses its pigment, producing the well-known graying. As early as 20, a man's hairline may start to recede at the temples; hair loss at the vertex follows. Many women show a less severe loss of hair in a similar pattern. Hair loss in this distribution is genetically determined.

In both sexes, the number of scalp hairs decreases in a generalized pattern, and the diameter of each hair diminishes.

Less familiar, but probably more important clinically, is the normal hair loss elsewhere on the body: the trunk, pubic areas, axillae, and limbs. These changes will be discussed in later chapters. Coarse facial hairs appear on the chin and upper lip of many women by about the age of 55, but do not increase further thereafter.

Many of the observations described here pertain to lighter-skinned persons and do not necessarily apply to others. For example, Native American men have relatively little facial and body hair compared to that of white men and should be evaluated according to their own norms.

Techniques of Examination

Observe the skin and related structures during the general survey and throughout the rest of your examination. The entire skin surface should be inspected in good light, preferably natural light or artificial light that resembles it. Correlate your findings with observations of the mucous membranes. Diseases may manifest themselves in both areas, and both are necessary for assessing skin color. Techniques of examining these membranes are described in later chapters.

Artificial light often distorts colors and masks jaundice.

To make your observations more astute, acquaint yourself now with some of the skin lesions and colors that you may encounter.

See Table 6-1, Basic Types of Skin Lesions (pp. 153–154), and Table 6-2, Skin Colors (p. 155).

Skin. Inspect and palpate the skin. Note these characteristics:

Color. Patients may notice a change in their skin color before the clinician does. Ask about it. Look for increased pigmentation (brownness), loss of pigmentation, redness, pallor, cyanosis, and yellowing of the skin.

The red color of oxyhemoglobin and the pallor due to a lack of it are best discerned where the horny layer of the epidermis is thinnest and causes the least scatter: the fingernails, the lips, and the mucous membranes, particularly those of the mouth and the palpebral conjunctiva. In dark-skinned persons, inspecting the palms and soles may also be useful.

Pallor due to decreased redness is seen in anemia and in decreased blood flow, as in fainting or arterial insufficiency.

Central cyanosis is best identified in the lips, oral mucosa, and tongue. The lips, however, may turn blue in the cold, and melanin in the lips may simulate cyanosis in darker-skinned people.

Cyanosis of the nails, hands, and feet may be central or peripheral in origin. Peripheral cyanosis may be due to anxiety or a cold examining room.

Causes of central cyanosis include advanced lung disease, congenital heart disease, and abnormal hemoglobins. Cyanosis in congestive heart failure is usually peripheral, reflecting decreased blood flow, but in pulmonary edema it may also be central. Venous obstruction may cause peripheral cyanosis.

Look for the yellow color of jaundice in the sclera. Jaundice may also appear in the palpebral conjunctiva, lips, hard palate, undersurface of the tongue, and skin. To see jaundice more easily in the lips, blanch out the red color by pressure with a glass slide.

Jaundice suggests liver disease or excessive hemolysis of red blood cells.

For the yellow color that accompanies high levels of carotene, look at the palms, soles, and face.

Carotenemia

Moisture. Examples are dryness, sweating, and oiliness.

Dryness in hypothyroidism; oiliness in acne

Temperature. Use the backs of your fingers to make this assessment. In addition to identifying generalized warmth or coolness of the skin, note the temperature of any red areas.

Generalized warmth in fever, hyperthyroidism; coolness in hypothyroidism. Local warmth of inflammation or cellulitis

Texture. Examples are roughness and smoothness.

Roughness in hypothyroidism

Mobility and Turgor. Lift a fold of skin and note the ease with which it lifts up (mobility) and the speed with which it returns into place (turgor).

Decreased mobility in edema, scleroderma; decreased turgor in dehydration

Lesions. Observe any lesions of the skin, noting their characteristics:

- Their *anatomic location and distribution* over the body. Are they generalized or localized? Do they, for example, involve the exposed surfaces, the intertriginous (skin fold) areas, or areas exposed to specific allergens or irritants such as wrist bands, rings, or industrial chemicals?

Many skin diseases have typical distributions. Acne affects the face, upper chest, and back; psoriasis, the knees and elbows (among other areas); and *Candida* infections, the intertriginous areas.

- Their *arrangement.* For example, are they linear, clustered, annular (in a ring), arciform (in an arc), or dermatomal (covering a skin band that corresponds to a sensory nerve root; see pp. 586–587)?

Vesicles in a unilateral dermatomal pattern are typical of herpes zoster.

- The *type(s) of skin lesions* (e.g., macules, papules, vesicles). If possible, find representative and recent lesions that have not been traumatized by scratching or otherwise altered. Inspect them carefully and feel them.

See Table 6-1, Basic Types of Skin Lesions (pp. 153–154); Table 6-3, Vascular and Purpuric Lesions of the Skin (p. 156); and Table 6-4, Skin Tumors (p. 157).

- Their *color.*

Nails. Inspect and palpate the fingernails and toenails. Note their color and shape, and any lesions. Longitudinal bands of pigment may be seen in the nails of normal people who have darker skin.

See Table 6-5, Findings In or Near the Nails (pp. 158–159).

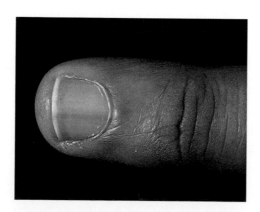

Hair. Inspect and palpate the hair. Note its quantity, distribution, and texture.

Alopecia refers to hair loss—diffuse, patchy, or total.

Sparse hair in hypothyroidism; fine silky hair in hyperthyroidism

After familiarizing yourself with the basic types of lesions, review their appearances in Table 6-6 and in a well illustrated textbook of dermatology. Whenever you see a skin lesion, look it up in such a text. The type of lesions, their location, and their distribution, together with other information from the history and the examination, should equip you well for this search and, in time, for arriving at specific dermatologic diagnoses.

See Table 6-6, Skin Lesions in Context (pp. 160–161).

Health Promotion and Counseling

Clinicians play an important role in counseling patients about protective measures for skin care and the hazards of excessive sun exposure. Basal cell and squamous cell carcinomas are the most common cancers in the United States and are found most frequently in sun-exposed areas, particularly the head, neck, and hands. Malignant melanoma, although rare, is the most rapidly increasing U.S. malignancy, doubling in incidence in the 1980s. Although melanoma often arises in non–sun-exposed areas, it is associated with intermittent and intense sun exposure and blistering sunburns in childhood. Other risk factors include family history of melanoma, light skin, presence of atypical moles (dysplastic nevi) or ≥ 50 common moles, and immunosuppression.

Protective measures are three-fold: avoiding unnecessary sun exposure, using sunscreen, and inspecting the skin. Caution patients to minimize direct sun exposure, especially at midday when ultraviolet B rays (UV-B), the most common cause of skin cancer, are most intense. Sunscreens fall into two categories—thick pastelike ointments that block all solar rays, and light-absorbing sunscreens rated by "sun protective factor" (SPF). The SPF is a ratio of the number of minutes for treated versus untreated skin to redden with exposure to UV-B. An SPF of at least 15 is recommended and protects against 93% of UV-B. (There is no scale for UV-A, which causes photoaging, or UV-C, the most carcinogenic ray but blocked in the atmosphere by ozone.) Water-resistant sunscreens that remain on the skin for prolonged periods are preferable.

Detection of skin cancer rests on visual inspection, preferably of the total body surface. Current detection rates are higher for clinicians than patients, but the benefits of self-examination are not well studied. Recommendations about screening intervals are variable. The American Cancer Society recommends monthly self-examination, clinician screening at 3-year intervals for persons aged 20 to 39, and annual clinical examination for persons over age 40. Clinicians and patients should know the "ABCDEs" for melanoma: **A** for *a*symmetry, **B** for irregular *b*orders, **C** for *c*olor variation or change (especially blue or black), **D** for *d*iameter larger than 6 mm, and **E** for *e*levation. Look in sun-exposed areas for ulcerated nodules with translucent or pearly surfaces (seen in squamous cell carcinoma) and roughened patches of skin with accompanying erythema (common in basal cell carcinoma). Patients with suspicious lesions should be referred to a dermatologist for further evaluation and biopsy.

Table 6-1   *Basic Types of Skin Lesions*

TABLE 6-1   *Basic Types of Skin Lesions*

Primary Lesions (*May Arise From Previously Normal Skin*)

Circumscribed, Flat, Nonpalpable Changes in Skin Color

Macule—Small spot. Examples: freckle, petechia

Patch—Larger than macule. Example: vitiligo

Palpable Elevated Solid Masses

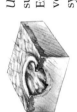

Papule—Up to 0.5 cm. Example: an elevated nevus

Plaque—A flat, elevated surface larger than 0.5 cm, often formed by the coalescence of papules

Nodule—larger than 0.5 cm; often deeper and firmer than a papule

Tumor—A large nodule

Wheal—A somewhat irregular, relatively transient, superficial area of localized skin edema. Examples: mosquito bite, hive

Circumscribed Superficial Elevations of the Skin Formed by Free Fluid in a Cavity Within the Skin Layers

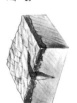

Vesicle—Up to 0.5 cm; filled with serous fluid. Example: herpes simplex

Bulla—Greater than 0.5 cm; filled with serous fluid. Example: 2nd-degree burn

Pustule—Filled with pus. Examples: acne, impetigo

Secondary Lesions (*Result From Changes in Primary Lesions*)

Loss of Skin Surface

Erosion—Loss of the superficial epidermis; surface is moist but does not bleed. Example: moist area after the rupture of a vesicle, as in chickenpox

Ulcer—A deeper loss of skin surface; may bleed and scar. Examples: stasis ulcer of venous insufficiency, syphilitic chancre

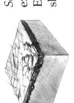

Fissure—A linear crack in the skin. Example: athlete's foot

Material on the Skin Surface

Scale—A thin flake of exfoliated epidermis. Examples: dandruff, dry skin, psoriasis

Crust—The dried residue of serum, pus, or blood. Example: impetigo

Continued

Table 6-1   Basic Types of Skin Lesions

TABLE 6-1 (continued)

Miscellaneous Lesions

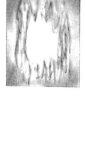

Lichenification—Thickening and roughening of the skin with increased visibility of the normal skin furrows. Example: atopic dermatitis

Scar—Replacement of destroyed tissue by fibrous tissue. May be thick and pink (hypertrophic) or thin and white (atrophic), but does not extend beyond the injured area

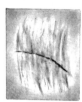

Atrophy—Thinning of the normal skin furrows; the skin looks shinier and more translucent than normal. Example: arterial insufficiency

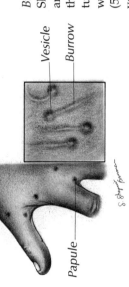

Vesicle
Burrow
Papule

Excoriation—An abrasion or scratch mark. It may be linear, as illustrated, or rounded, as in a scratched insect bite.

Burrow of Scabies—A person with scabies has intense itching. Skin lesions include small papules, pustules, lichenified areas, and excoriations. With a magnifying lens, look for the *burrow* of the mite that causes it. A burrow is a minute, slightly raised tunnel in the epidermis and is commonly found on the finger webs and on the sides of the fingers. It looks like a short (5–15 mm), linear or curved, gray line and may end in a tiny vesicle.

Several additional terms deserve mention. A *comedo* is the common blackhead and marks the plugged opening of a sebaceous gland. Comedones are one of the hallmarks of acne. *Telangiectasias* are dilated small vessels that look either red or bluish. They can appear by themselves or as parts of other lesions such as a basal cell carcinoma or radiodermatitis (skin injury from ionizing radiation). The common mole—a flat to slightly elevated, round, evenly pigmented lesion—is technically called a *nevus*, although there are other nevi that look quite different.

Table 6-2 *Skin Colors*

TABLE 6-2 Skin Colors

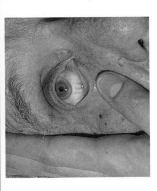

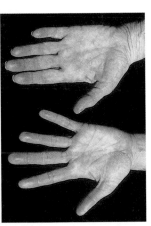

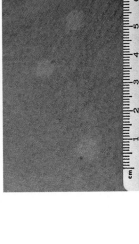

Cyanosis

Cyanosis is the somewhat bluish color that is visible in these toenails and toes. Compare this color with the normally pink fingernails and fingers of the same patient. Impaired venous return in the leg caused this example of peripheral cyanosis. Cyanosis, especially when slight, may be hard to distinguish from normal skin color.

Carotenemia

The yellowish palm of carotenemia, shown on the left, is compared with a normally pink palm—a useful technique for a sometimes subtle finding. Unlike jaundice, carotenemia does not affect the sclera, which remains white. The cause is a diet high in carrots and other yellow vegetables or fruits. Carotenemia is not harmful, but indicates the need for assessing dietary intake.

Jaundice

Jaundice makes the skin diffusely yellow. Note this patient's skin color, contrasted with the examiner's hand. The color of jaundice is seen most easily and reliably in the sclera, as shown here. It may also be visible in mucous membranes. Causes include liver disease and hemolysis of red blood cells.

Changes in Melanin

A widespread increase in melanin may be due to Addison's disease (hypofunction of the adrenal cortex) or to some pituitary tumors. More common are local areas of increased or decreased pigment:

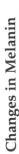

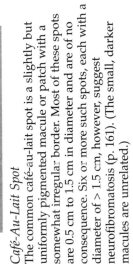

Café-Au-Lait Spot

The common café-au-lait spot is a slightly but uniformly pigmented macule or patch with a somewhat irregular border. Most of these spots are 0.5 cm to 1.5 cm in diameter and are of no consequence. Six or more such spots, each with a diameter of > 1.5 cm, however, suggest neurofibromatosis (p. 161). (The small, darker macules are unrelated.)

Vitiligo

In vitiligo, depigmented macules appear on the face, hands, feet, and other regions and may coalesce into extensive areas that lack melanin. The brown pigment on this woman's legs is her normal skin color; the pale areas are due to vitiligo. The condition may be hereditary. These changes may be distressing to the patient.

Tinea Versicolor

More common than vitiligo is this superficial fungus infection of the skin. It causes hypopigmented, slightly scaly macules on the trunk, neck, and upper arms. They are easier to see in darker skin and may become more obvious after tanning. In lighter skin, the macules may look reddish or tan instead of pale. The macules may be much more numerous than in this example.

Table 6-3   Vascular and Purpuric Lesions of the Skin

TABLE 6-3   Vascular and Purpuric Lesions of the Skin

	Vascular			Purpuric	
	Spider Angioma	Spider Vein	Cherry Angioma	Petechia/Purpura	Ecchymosis
Color	Fiery red	Bluish	Bright or ruby red; may become brownish with age	Deep red or reddish purple, fading away over time	Purple or purplish blue, fading to green, yellow, and brown with time
Size	From very small to 2 cm	Variable, from very small to several inches	1–3 mm	Petechia, 1–3 mm; purpura, larger	Variable, larger than petechiae
Shape	Central body, sometimes raised, surrounded by erythema and radiating legs	Variable. May resemble a spider or be linear, irregular, cascading	Round, flat or sometimes raised, may be surrounded by a pale halo	Rounded, sometimes irregular; flat	Rounded, oval, or irregular; may have a central subcutaneous flat nodule (a hematoma)
Pulsatility	Often demonstrable in the body of the spider, when pressure with a glass slide is applied	Absent	Absent	Absent	Absent
Effect of Pressure	Pressure on the body causes blanching of the spider.	Pressure over the center does not cause blanching, but diffuse pressure blanches the veins.	May show partial blanching, especially if pressure is applied with the edge of a pinpoint	None	None
Distribution	Face, neck, arms, and upper trunk; almost never below the waist	Most often on the legs, near veins; also on the anterior chest	Trunk; also extremities	Variable	Variable
Significance	Liver disease, pregnancy, vitamin B deficiency; also occurs in some normal people	Often accompanies increased pressure in the superficial veins, as in varicose veins	None; increase in size and numbers with aging	Blood outside the vessels; may suggest a bleeding disorder or, if petechiae, emboli to skin	Blood outside the vessels; often secondary to trauma; also seen in bleeding disorders

(Sources of photos: *Spider Angioma*—Marks R: Skin Disease in Old Age. Philadelphia, JB Lippincott, 1987; *Petechia/Purpura*—Kelley WN: Textbook of Internal Medicine. Philadelphia, JB Lippincott, 1989)

Table 6-4   Skin Tumors

TABLE 6-4   Skin Tumors

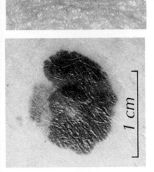

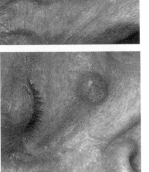

Basal Cell Carcinoma

A basal cell carcinoma, though malignant, grows slowly and seldom metastasizes. It is most common in fair-skinned adults over age 40, and usually appears on the face. An initial translucent nodule spreads, leaving a depressed center and a firm, elevated border. Telangiectatic vessels are often visible, as in this lesion on the eyelid.

Squamous Cell Carcinoma

Squamous cell carcinoma usually appears on sun-exposed skin of fair-skinned adults over 60. It may develop in an actinic keratosis. It usually grows more quickly than a basal cell carcinoma, is firmer, and looks redder. The face and the back of the hand are often affected, as shown here.

Kaposi's Sarcoma in AIDS

When Kaposi's sarcoma, a malignant tumor, accompanies AIDS, it may appear in many forms: macules, papules, plaques, or nodules almost anywhere in the body. Lesions are often multiple and may involve internal structures. On the left are ovoid, pinkish red plaques that typically lengthen along the skin lines. They may become pigmented. On the right is a purplish red nodule on the foot.

Malignant Melanoma

Noticeable growth or color change in a benign nevus (mole) warns of possible malignant melanoma, a highly malignant tumor most common in fair-skinned people. Additional suggestive signs are asymmetry, an irregular border, diameter more than 6 mm, and an elevated irregular surface. Two forms are illustrated: superficial spreading (left) and nodular (right).

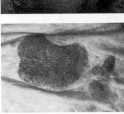

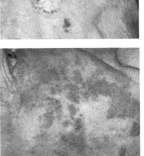

Actinic Keratosis

Actinic keratoses are superficial, flattened papules covered by a dry scale. Often multiple, they may be round or irregular, and are pink, tan, or grayish. They appear on sun-exposed skin of older, fair-skinned persons. Though themselves benign, these lesions may give rise to squamous cell carcinoma (suggested by rapid growth, induration, redness at the base, and ulceration). Keratoses on face and hand, typical locations, are shown.

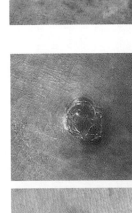

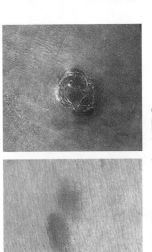

Seborrheic Keratosis

Seborrheic keratoses are common, benign, yellowish to brown, raised lesions that feel slightly greasy and velvety or warty. Typically multiple and symmetrically distributed on the trunk of older people, they may also appear on the face and elsewhere. In black people, often younger women, they may appear as small, deeply pigmented papules on the cheeks and temples (dermatosis papulosa nigra).

(Sources of photos: *Basal Cell Epithelioma, Squamous Cell Carcinoma, Actinic Keratosis,* and *Seborrheic Keratosis*—Sauer GC: Manual of Skin Diseases, 5th ed. Philadelphia, JB Lippincott, 1985; *Malignant Melanoma*—Balch CM, Milton GW [eds]: Cutaneous Melanoma Philadelphia, JB Lippincott, 1985; *Kaposi's Sarcoma in AIDS*—DeVita VT Jr, Hellman S, Rosenberg SA [eds]: AIDS: Etiology, Diagnosis, Treatment, and Prevention. Philadelphia, JB Lippincott, 1985)

Table 6-5   Findings In or Near the Nails

TABLE 6-5   Findings In or Near the Nails

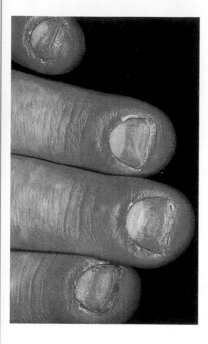

Clubbing of the Fingers

In clubbing, the distal phalanx of each finger is rounded and bulbous. The nail plate is more convex, and the angle between the plate and the proximal nail fold increases to 180° or more. The proximal nail fold, when palpated, feels spongy or floating. Causes are many, including chronic hypoxia and lung cancer.

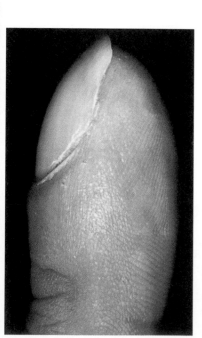

Onycholysis

Onycholysis refers to a painless separation of the nail plate from the nail bed. It starts distally, enlarging the free edge of the nail to a varying degree. Several or all nails are usually affected. Causes are many.

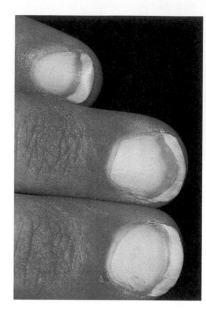

Paronychia

A paronychia is an inflammation of the proximal and lateral nail folds. It may be acute or, as illustrated, chronic. The folds are red, swollen, and often tender. The cuticle may not be visible. People who frequently immerse their nails in water are especially susceptible. Multiple nails are often affected.

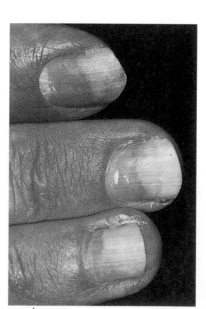

Terry's Nails

Terry's nails are mostly whitish with a distal band of reddish brown. The lunulae of the nails may not be visible. These nails may be seen with aging and in people with chronic diseases such as cirrhosis of the liver, congestive heart failure, and non–insulin-dependent diabetes.

Table 6-5   Findings In or Near the Nails

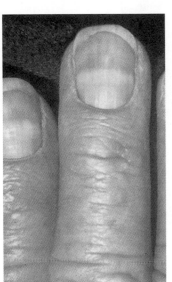

White Spots (*Leukonychia*)

Trauma to the nails is commonly followed by white spots that grow slowly out with the nail. Spots in the pattern illustrated are typical of overly vigorous and repeated manicuring. The curves in this example resemble the curve of the cuticle and proximal nail fold.

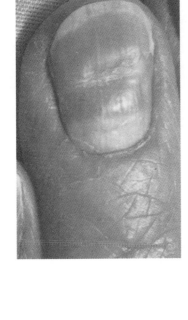

Transverse White Lines (*Mees' Lines*)

These are transverse lines, not spots, and their curves are similar to those of the lunula, not the cuticle. These uncommon lines may follow an acute or severe illness. They emerge from under the proximal nail folds and grow out with the nails.

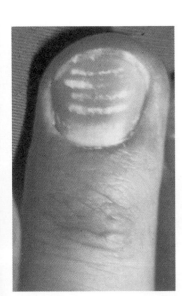

Psoriasis

Small pits in the nails may be early signs of psoriasis but are not specific for it. Additional findings, not shown here, include onycholysis and a circumscribed yellowish tan discoloration known as an "oil spot" lesion. Marked thickening of the nails may develop.

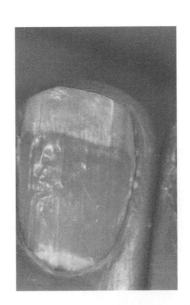

Beau's Lines

Beau's lines are transverse depressions in the nails associated with acute severe illness. The lines emerge from under the proximal nail folds weeks later and grow gradually out with the nails. As with Mees' lines, clinicians may be able to estimate the timing of a causal illness.

(Sources of photos: *Clubbing of the Fingers, Paronychia, Onycholysis, Terry's Nails*—Habit TP: Clinical Dermatology: A Color Guide to Diagnosis and Therapy, 2nd ed. St. Louis, CV Mosby, 1990; *White Spots,* 1990; *White Spots, Transverse White Lines, Psoriasis, Beau's Lines*—Sams WM Jr, Lynch PJ: Principles and Practice of Dermatology. New York, Churchill Livingstone, 1990)

Table 6-6   Skin Lesions in Context

TABLE 6-6   Skin Lesions in Context

This table shows a variety of primary and secondary skin lesions. Try to identify them, including those indicated by letters, before reading the accompanying text.

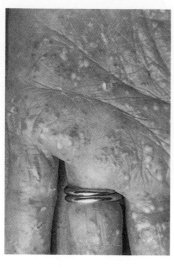

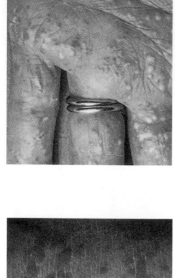

Pustules on the palm (in pustular psoriasis)

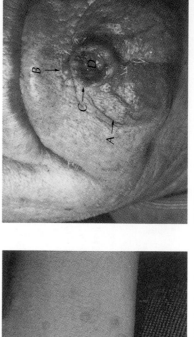

(A) Telangiectasia, (B) nodule, (C) tumor, (D) ulcer (in squamous cell carcinoma)

Papules on the knee (in lichen planus)

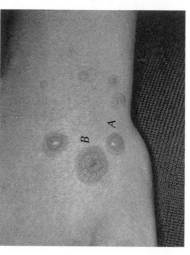

(A) Bulla and (B) target (or iris) lesion (in erythema multiforme)

Macules on the dorsum of the hand, wrist, and forearm (actinic lentigines)

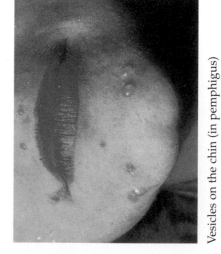

Vesicles on the chin (in pemphigus)

Table 6-6   Skin Lesions in Context

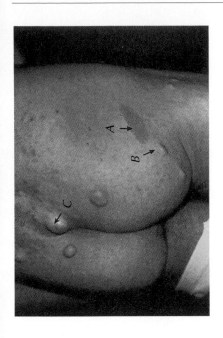

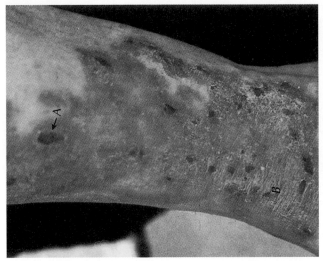

Wheals (urticaria) in a drug eruption in an infant

(A) Patch, (B) nodule, (C) tumor—a combination typical of neurofibromatosis. This patch is a café-au-lait spot.

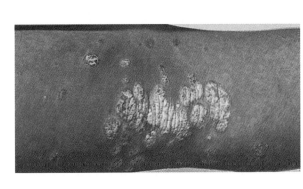

Plaques with scales on the front of a knee (in psoriasis)

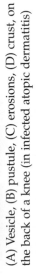

(A) Excoriation and (B) lichenification on the leg (in atopic dermatitis)

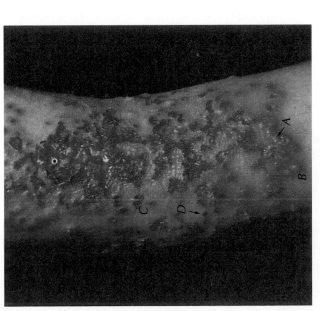

(A) Vesicle, (B) pustule, (C) erosions, (D) crust, on the back of a knee (in infected atopic dermatitis)

(Source of all photos except for *Macules*: Sauer GC: Manual of Skin Diseases, 5th ed. Philadelphia, JB Lippincott, 1985)

The Head and Neck

Anatomy and Physiology

The Head

Regions of the head take their names from the underlying bones (e.g., frontal area). Knowledge of this anatomy helps to locate and describe physical findings.

Two paired salivary glands lie near the mandible: the *parotid gland*, superficial to and behind the mandible (both visible and palpable when enlarged), and the *submandibular gland*, located deep to the mandible. Feel for the latter as you press your tongue against your upper incisors. Its lobular surface can often be felt against the tightened muscle. The openings of the parotid and submandibular ducts are visible within the oral cavity (see p. 177).

The *superficial temporal artery* passes upward just in front of the ear, where it is readily palpable. In many normal people, especially thin and elderly ones, the tortuous course of one of its branches can be traced across the forehead.

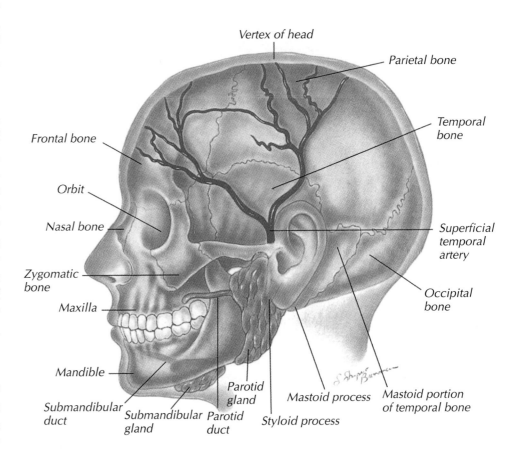

The Eye

Gross Anatomy. Identify the structures illustrated. Note that the upper eyelid covers a portion of the iris but does not normally overlap the pupil. The opening between the eyelids is called the *palpebral fissure.* The

163

white *sclera* may look somewhat buff-colored at its extreme periphery. Do not mistake this color for jaundice, which is a deeper yellow.

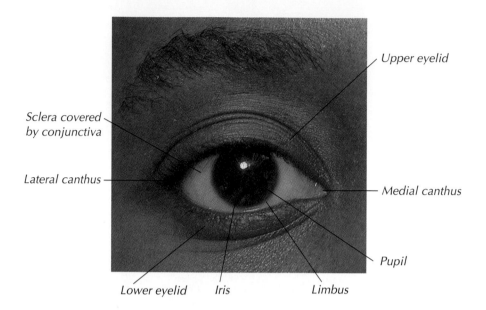

The *conjunctiva* is a clear mucous membrane with two easily visible components. The bulbar conjunctiva covers most of the anterior eyeball, adhering loosely to the underlying tissue. It meets the cornea at the *limbus*. The palpebral conjunctiva lines the eyelids. The two parts of the conjunctiva merge in a folded recess that permits the eyeball to move.

Within the *eyelids* lie firm strips of connective tissue called *tarsal plates*. Each plate contains a parallel row of *meibomian glands*, which open on the lid margin. The *levator palpebrae muscle*, which raises the upper eyelid, is innervated by the oculomotor nerve (Cranial Nerve III). Smooth muscle, innervated by the sympathetic nervous system, contributes to raising this lid.

A film of *tear fluid* protects the conjunctiva and cornea from drying, inhibits microbial growth, and gives a smooth optical surface to

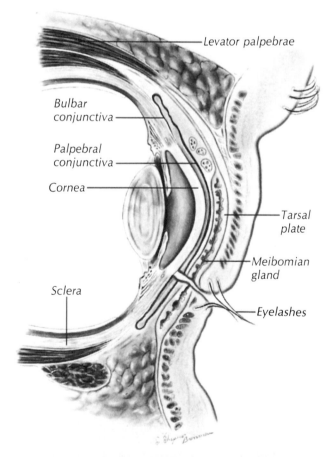

SAGITTAL SECTION OF ANTERIOR EYE WITH LIDS CLOSED

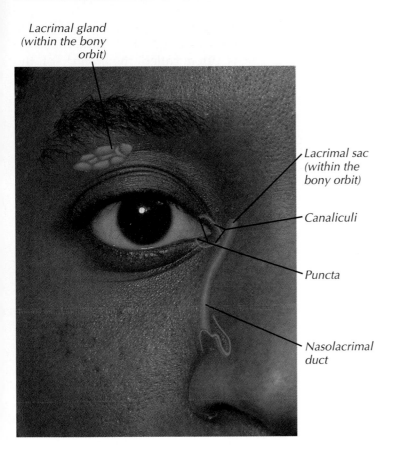

Lacrimal gland
(within the bony
orbit)

Lacrimal sac
(within the
bony orbit)

Canaliculi

Puncta

Nasolacrimal
duct

the cornea. This fluid comes from three sources: meibomian glands, conjunctival glands, and the lacrimal gland. The *lacrimal gland* lies mostly within the bony orbit, above and lateral to the eyeball. The tear fluid spreads across the eye and drains medially through two tiny holes called *lacrimal puncta.* The tears then pass into the *lacrimal sac* and on into the nose through the *nasolacrimal duct.* (You can easily find a punctum atop the small elevation of the lower lid medially. You cannot detect the lacrimal sac, which rests in a small depression inside the bony orbit.)

The eyeball is a spherical structure that focuses light on the neurosensory elements within the retina. The muscles of the *iris* control pupillary size. Muscles of the *ciliary body* control the thickness of the lens, allowing the eye to focus on near or distant objects.

A clear liquid called *aqueous humor* fills the anterior and posterior chambers of the eye. Aqueous humor is produced by the ciliary body, circulates from the posterior chamber through the pupil into the anterior chamber, and drains out through the canal of Schlemm. This circulatory system helps to control the pressure inside the eye.

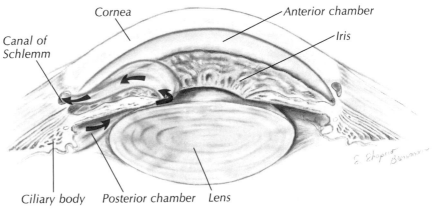

Cornea

Anterior chamber

Iris

Canal of
Schlemm

Ciliary body   Posterior chamber   Lens

CIRCULATION OF AQUEOUS HUMOR

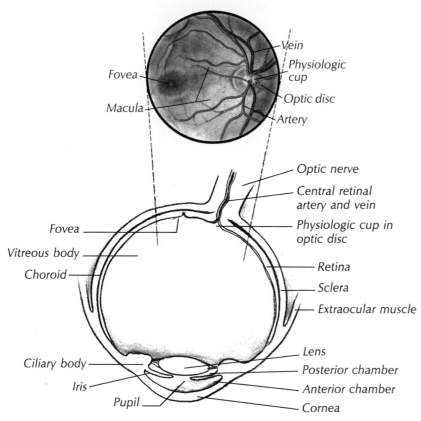

CROSS SECTION OF THE RIGHT EYE FROM ABOVE SHOWING A PORTION OF THE FUNDUS COMMONLY SEEN WITH THE OPHTHALMOSCOPE

The posterior part of the eye that is seen through an ophthalmoscope is often called the *fundus* of the eye. Structures here include the retina, choroid, fovea, macula, optic disc, and retinal vessels. The optic nerve with its retinal vessels enters the eyeball posteriorly. You can find it with an ophthalmoscope at the *optic disc.* Lateral and slightly inferior to the disc, there is a small depression in the retinal surface that marks the point of central vision. Around it is a darkened circular area called the *fovea.* The roughly circular *macula* (named for a microscopic yellow spot) surrounds the fovea but has no discernible margins. It does not quite reach the optic disc. You do not usually see the normal *vitreous body,* a transparent mass of gelatinous material that fills the eyeball behind the lens. It helps to maintain the shape of the eye.

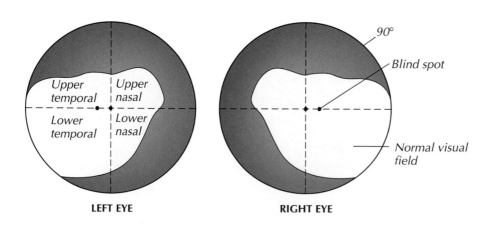

LEFT EYE   **RIGHT EYE**

Visual Fields. A *visual field* is the entire area seen by an eye when it looks at a central point. Fields are conventionally diagrammed on circles from the patient's point of view. The center of the circle represents the focus of gaze. The circumference is 90° from the line of gaze. Each visual field, shown by the white areas on the left, is divided into quadrants. Note that the fields extend farthest on the temporal sides. Visual fields are normally limited by the brows above, by the cheeks below, and by the nose medially. A lack of retinal receptors at the optic disc produces an oval blind spot in the normal field of each eye, 15° temporal to the line of gaze.

When a person is using both eyes, the two visual fields overlap in an area of binocular vision. Laterally, vision is monocular.

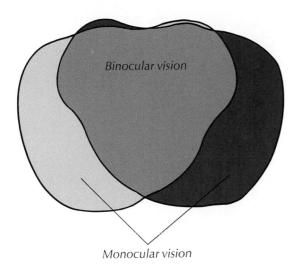

Binocular vision

Monocular vision

Visual Pathways. For an image to be seen, light reflected from it must pass through the pupil and be focused on sensory neurons in the retina. The image projected there is upside down and reversed right to left. An image from the upper nasal visual field thus strikes the lower temporal quadrant of the retina.

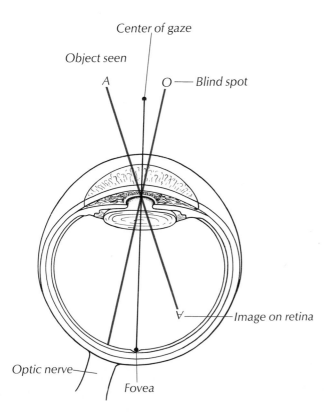

Center of gaze

Object seen

A   O —— Blind spot

V ———— Image on retina

Optic nerve ——

Fovea

Nerve impulses, stimulated by light, are conducted through the retina, optic nerve, and optic tract on each side, and then on through a curving tract called the *optic radiation.* This ends is the visual cortex, a part of the occipital lobe.

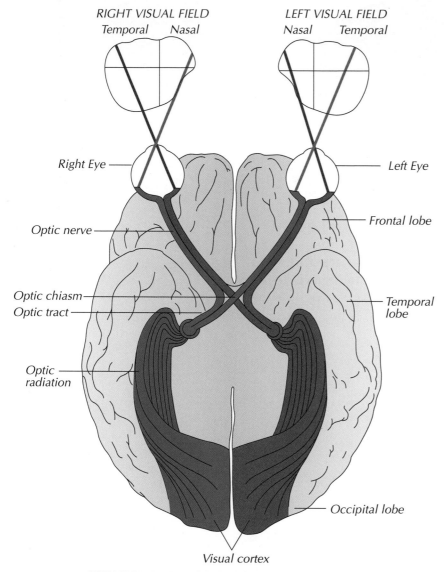

RIGHT VISUAL FIELD
Temporal   Nasal

LEFT VISUAL FIELD
Nasal   Temporal

Right Eye

Left Eye

Optic nerve

Frontal lobe

Optic chiasm
Optic tract

Temporal lobe

Optic radiation

Occipital lobe

Visual cortex

VIEW FROM BASE (INFERIOR SURFACE) OF THE BRAIN

Pupillary Reactions. Pupillary size changes in response to light and to the effort of focusing on a near object.

The Light Reaction. A light beam shining onto one retina causes pupillary constriction in both that eye (the *direct reaction* to light) and the opposite eye (the *consensual reaction*). The initial sensory pathways are similar to those described for vision: retina, optic nerve, and optic tract. The pathways diverge in the midbrain, however, and impulses are transmitted through the oculomotor nerve to the constrictor muscles of the iris of each eye.

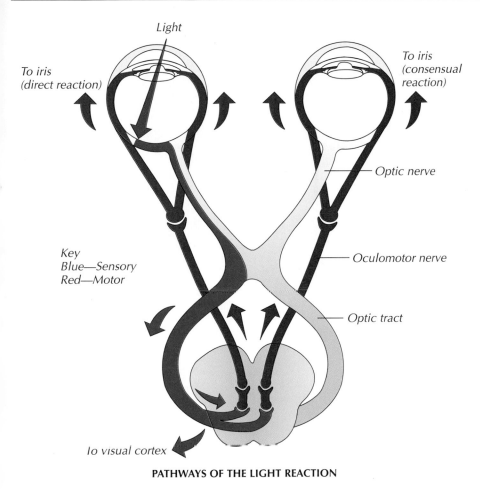

Key
Blue—Sensory
Red—Motor

To iris
(direct reaction)

Light

To iris
(consensual
reaction)

Optic nerve

Oculomotor nerve

Optic tract

To visual cortex

PATHWAYS OF THE LIGHT REACTION

The Near Reaction. When a person shifts gaze from a far object to a near one, the pupils constrict. This response, like the light reaction, is mediated by the oculomotor nerve. Coincident with this pupillary reaction (but not part of it) are (1) *convergence of the eyes,* an extraocular movement, and (2) *accommodation,* an increased convexity of the lenses caused by contraction of the ciliary muscles. This change in shape of the lenses brings near objects into focus but is not visible to the examiner.

Autonomic Nerve Supply to the Eyes. Fibers traveling in the oculomotor nerve and producing pupillary constriction are part of the parasympathetic nervous system. The iris is also supplied by sympathetic fibers. When these are stimulated, the pupil dilates and the upper eyelid rises a little, as if from fear. The sympathetic pathway starts in the hypothalamus and passes down through the brainstem and cervical cord into the neck. From there, it follows the carotid artery or its branches into the orbit. A lesion anywhere along this pathway may impair sympathetic effects on the pupil.

Extraocular Movements. The movement of each eye is controlled by the coordinated action of six muscles, the four rectus and two oblique muscles. You can test the function of each muscle and the nerve that supplies it by asking the patient to move the eye in the direction controlled by that muscle. There are six such *cardinal directions,* indicated by the red lines on p. 170. When a person looks down and to the right, for example, the right inferior rectus (Cranial Nerve III) is principally responsible for

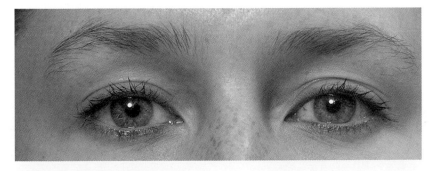

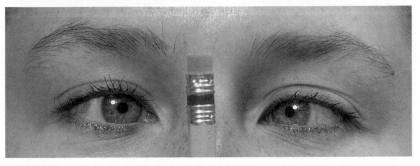

moving the right eye, while the left superior oblique (Cranial Nerve IV) is principally responsible for moving the left. If one of these muscles is paralyzed, the eye will deviate from its normal position in that direction of gaze and the eyes will no longer appear conjugate, or parallel.

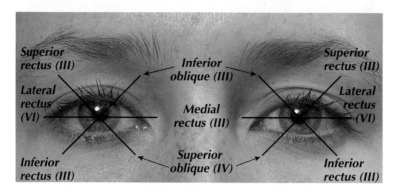

CARDINAL DIRECTIONS OF GAZE

The Ear

Anatomy. The ear has three compartments: the external ear, the middle ear, and the inner ear.

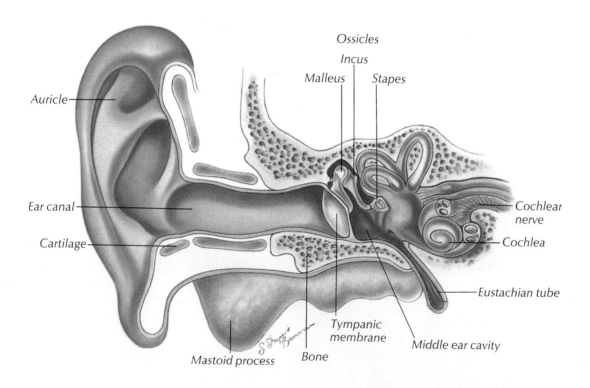

The *external ear* comprises the auricle and ear canal. The *auricle* consists chiefly of cartilage covered by skin and has a firm, elastic consistency.

The *ear canal* opens behind the tragus and curves inward about 24 mm. Its outer portion is surrounded by cartilage. The skin in this outer portion is hairy and contains glands that produce cerumen (wax). The inner portion of the canal is surrounded by bone and lined by thin, hairless skin. Pressure on this latter area causes pain—a point to remember when you examine the ear.

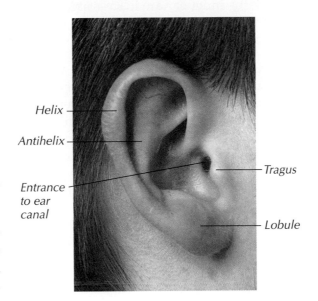

The bone behind and below the ear canal is the mastoid part of the temporal bone. The lowest portion of this bone, the mastoid process, is palpable behind the lobule.

At the end of the ear canal lies the *tympanic membrane* (eardrum), marking the lateral limits of the middle ear. The *middle ear* is an air-filled cavity that transmits sound by way of three tiny bones, the ossicles. It is connected by the eustachian tube to the nasopharynx.

The eardrum is an oblique membrane held inward at its center by one of the ossicles, the *malleus*. Find the *handle* and the *short process* of the malleus—the two chief landmarks. From the *umbo*, where the eardrum meets the tip of the malleus, a light reflection called the *cone of light* fans downward and anteriorly. Above the short process lies a small portion of the eardrum called the *pars flaccida*. The remainder of the drum is the *pars tensa*. Anterior and posterior malleolar folds, which extend obliquely upward from the short process, separate the pars flaccida from the pars tensa but are usually invisible unless the eardrum is retracted. A second ossicle, the incus, can sometimes be seen through the drum.

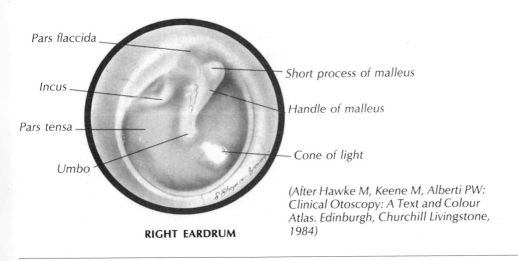

RIGHT EARDRUM

(After Hawke M, Keene M, Alberti PW: *Clinical Otoscopy: A Text and Colour Atlas.* Edinburgh, Churchill Livingstone, 1984)

Much of the middle ear and all of the inner ear are inaccessible to direct examination. Some inferences concerning their condition can be made, however, by testing auditory function.

Pathways of Hearing. Vibrations of sound pass through the air of the external ear and are transmitted through the eardrum and ossicles of the middle ear to the cochlea, a part of the inner ear. The cochlea senses and codes the vibrations, and nerve impulses are sent to the brain through the cochlear nerve. The first part of this pathway—from the external ear through the middle ear—is known as the *conductive* phase, and a disorder here causes conductive hearing loss. The second part of the pathway, involving the cochlea and the cochlear nerve, is called the *sensorineural* phase; a disorder here causes sensorineural hearing loss.

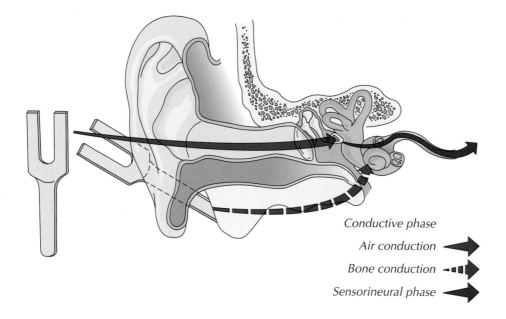

Conductive phase

Air conduction

Bone conduction

Sensorineural phase

Air conduction describes the normal first phase in the hearing pathway. An alternate pathway, known as *bone conduction,* bypasses the external and the middle ear and is used for testing purposes. A vibrating tuning fork, placed on the head, sets the bone of the skull into vibration and stimulates the cochlea directly. In a normal person, air conduction is more sensitive.

Equilibrium. The labyrinth within the inner ear senses the position and movements of the head and helps to maintain balance.

The Nose and Paranasal Sinuses

Review the terms used to describe the external anatomy of the nose.

Approximately the upper third of the nose is supported by bone, the lower two thirds by cartilage. Air enters the nasal cavity by way of the *anterior naris* on either side, then passes into a widened area known as the *vestibule* and on through the narrow nasal passage to the nasopharynx. The medial wall of each nasal cavity is formed by the *nasal septum* which, like the external nose, is supported by both bone and cartilage. It is covered by a mucous membrane well supplied with blood. The vestibule, unlike the rest of the nasal cavity, is lined with hair-bearing skin, not mucosa.

Laterally, the anatomy is more complex. Curving bony structures, the *turbinates,* covered by a highly vascular mucous membrane, protrude into the nasal cavity. Below each turbinate is a groove, or meatus, each named according to the turbinate above it. Into the inferior meatus drains the nasolacrimal duct; into the middle meatus drain most of the paranasal sinuses. Their openings are not usually visible.

The additional surface area provided by the turbinates and the mucosa covering them aids the nasal cavities in their principal functions: cleansing, humidification, and temperature control of inspired air.

Inspection of the nasal cavity through the anterior naris is usually limited to the vestibule, the anterior portion of the septum, and the lower and middle turbinates. Examination with a nasopharyngeal mirror is required for detection of posterior abnormalities. This technique is beyond the scope of this book.

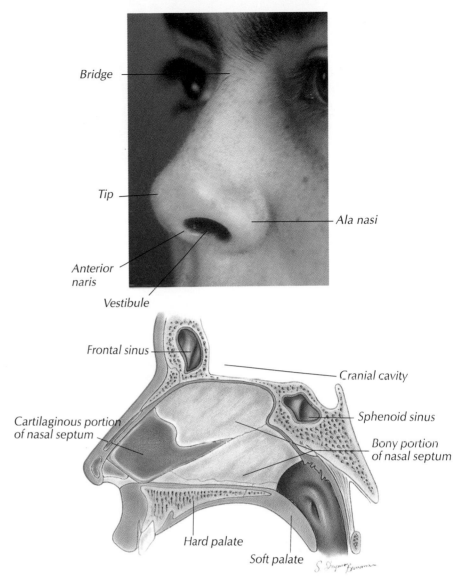

Bridge

Tip

Anterior naris

Vestibule

Ala nasi

Frontal sinus

Cranial cavity

Sphenoid sinus

Cartilaginous portion of nasal septum

Bony portion of nasal septum

Hard palate

Soft palate

MEDIAL WALL—LEFT NASAL CAVITY (MUCOSA REMOVED)

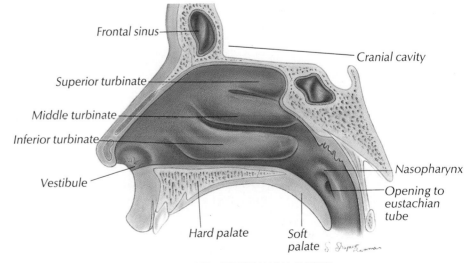

Frontal sinus

Cranial cavity

Superior turbinate

Middle turbinate

Inferior turbinate

Vestibule

Nasopharynx

Opening to eustachian tube

Hard palate

Soft palate

LATERAL WALL—RIGHT NASAL CAVITY

The *paranasal sinuses* are air-filled cavities within the bones of the skull. Like the nasal cavities into which they drain, they are lined with mucous membrane. Their locations are diagrammed below. Only the frontal and maxillary sinuses are readily accessible to clinical examination.

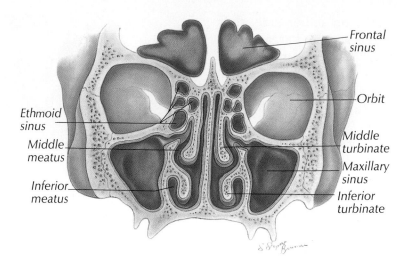

CROSS SECTION OF NASAL CAVITY—ANTERIOR VIEW

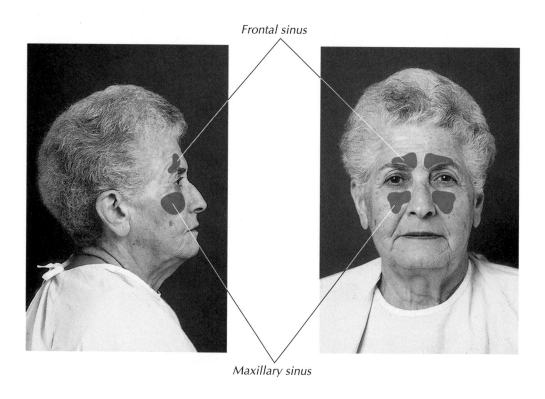

Frontal sinus

Maxillary sinus

The Mouth and Pharynx

The *lips* are muscular folds that surround the entrance to the mouth. When opened, the gums (gingiva) and teeth are visible. Note the scalloped shape of the *gingival margins* and the pointed *interdental papillae*.

The *gingiva* is firmly attached to the teeth and to the maxilla or mandible in which they are seated. In lighter-skinned people, the gingiva is pale or coral pink and lightly stippled. In darker-skinned and some other

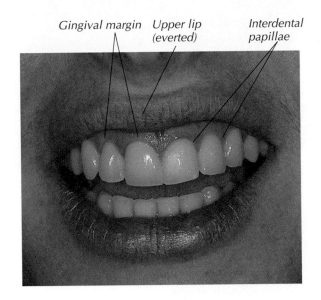

Gingival margin Upper lip (everted) Interdental papillae

people, it may be diffusely or partly brown as shown below. A midline mucosal fold, called a *labial frenulum*, connects each lip with the gingiva. A shallow *gingival sulcus* between the gum's thin margin and each tooth is not readily visible (but is probed and measured by dentists). Adjacent to the gingiva is the *alveolar mucosa*, which merges with the *labial mucosa* of the lip.

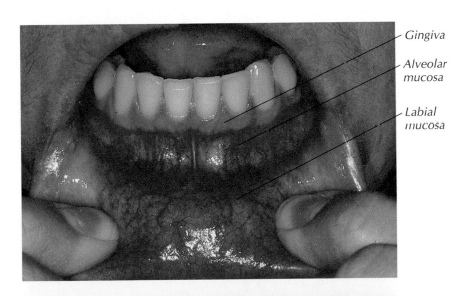

Gingiva

Alveolar mucosa

Labial mucosa

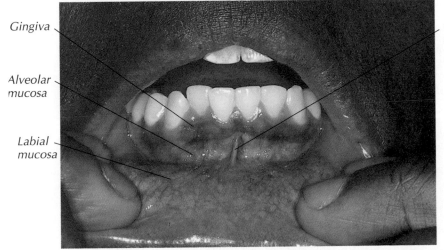

Gingiva

Alveolar mucosa

Labial mucosa

Labial frenulum

Each *tooth*, composed mostly of dentin, lies rooted in a bony socket with only its enamel-covered crown exposed. Small blood vessels and nerves enter the tooth through its apex and pass into the pulp canal and pulp chamber.

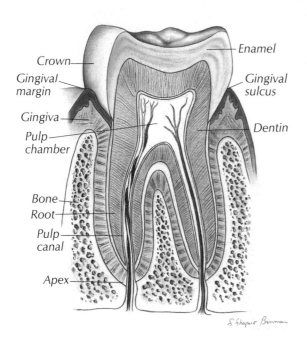

The 32 adult teeth (16 in each jaw) are identified below.

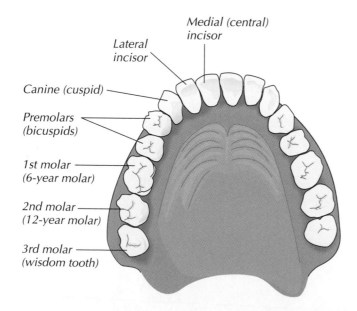

The dorsum of the *tongue* is covered with papillae, giving it a rough surface. Some of these papillae look like red dots, which contrast with the thin white coat that often covers the tongue. The undersurface of the tongue has no papillae. Note the midline *lingual frenulum* that connects the tongue to the floor of the mouth. At the base of the tongue the *ducts of the submandibular gland* (Wharton's ducts) pass forward and medially. They open on papillae that lie on each side of the lingual frenulum.

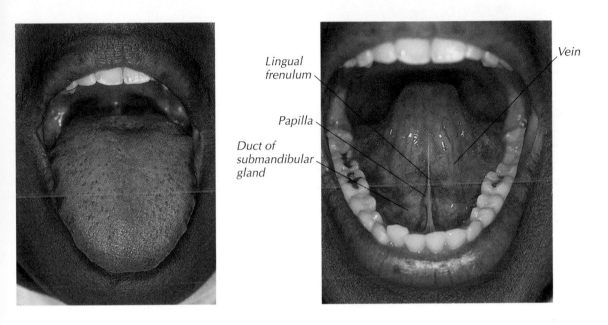

Lingual frenulum
Vein
Papilla
Duct of submandibular gland

Each *parotid duct* (Stensen's duct) empties into the mouth near the upper 2nd molar, where its location is frequently marked by a small papilla. The *buccal mucosa* lines the cheeks.

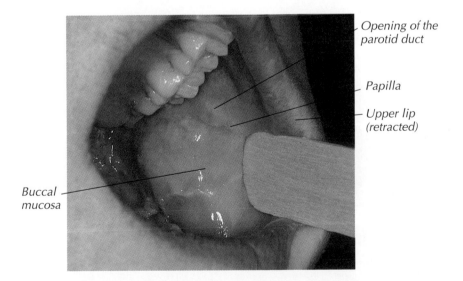

Opening of the parotid duct
Papilla
Upper lip (retracted)
Buccal mucosa

Above and behind the tongue rises an arch formed by the *anterior* and *posterior pillars, soft palate*, and *uvula*. In the following example, the right *tonsil* can be seen in its fossa (cavity) between the anterior and posterior pillars. In adults, tonsils are often small or absent, as exemplified on the left side here. A meshwork of small blood vessels may web the soft palate. Between the soft palate and tongue the *pharynx* is visible.

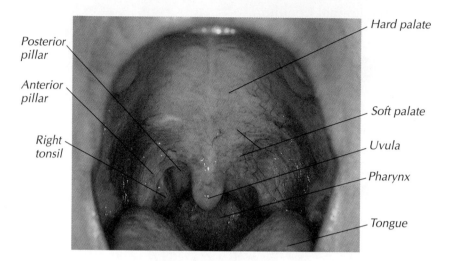

The Neck

For descriptive purposes, each side of the neck is divided into two triangles by the sternomastoid (sternocleidomastoid) muscle. The *anterior triangle* is bounded above by the mandible, laterally by the sternomastoid, and medially by the midline of the neck. The *posterior triangle* extends from the sternomastoid to the trapezius and is bounded below by

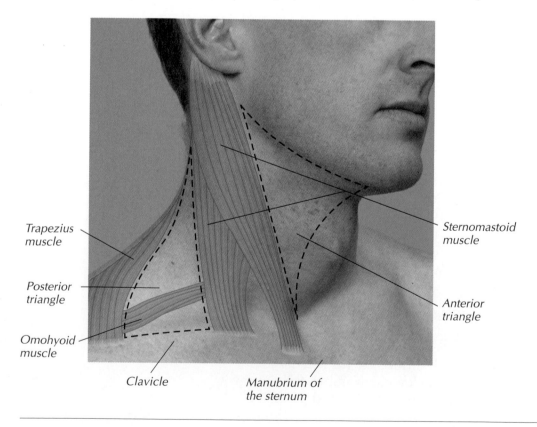

the clavicle. A portion of the omohyoid muscle crosses the lower portion of the posterior triangle and can be mistaken by the uninitiated for a lymph node or mass.

Deep to the sternomastoids run the great vessels of the neck: the *carotid artery* and *internal jugular vein*. The *external jugular vein* passes diagonally over the surface of the sternomastoid.

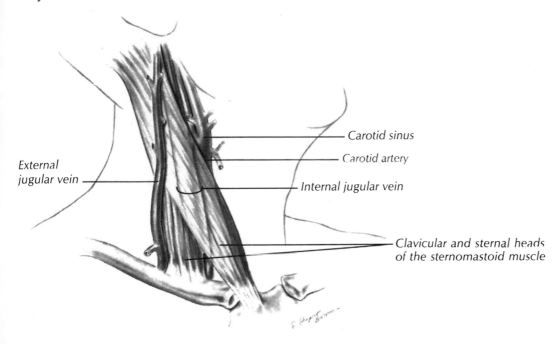

the thyroid gland. The isthmus of the thyroid gland lies across the

Now identify the following midline structures: (1) the mobile *hyoid bone* just below the mandible, (2) the *thyroid cartilage*, readily identified by the notch on its superior edge, (3) the *cricoid cartilage*, (4) the *tracheal rings*, and (5) the *thyroid gland*. The isthmus of the thyroid gland lies across the

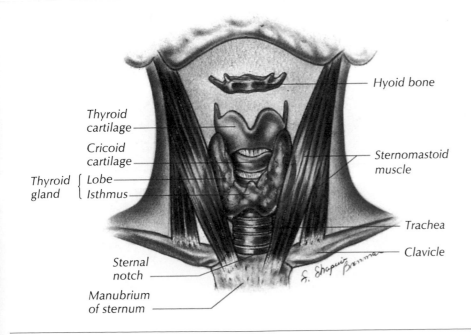

trachea below the cricoid. The lateral lobes of this gland curve posteriorly around the sides of the trachea and the esophagus. Except in the midline, the thyroid gland is covered by thin straplike muscles, among which only the sternomastoids are visible.

Women have larger and more easily palpable glands than men.

The *lymph nodes* of the head and neck have been classified in a variety of ways. One classification is shown here, together with the directions of lymphatic drainage. The deep cervical chain is largely obscured by the overlying sternomastoid muscle, but at its two extremes the tonsillar node and supraclavicular nodes may be palpable. The submandibular nodes lie superficial to the submandibular gland, from which they should be differentiated. Nodes are normally round or ovoid, smooth, and smaller than the gland. The gland is larger and has a lobulated, slightly irregular surface (see p. 163).

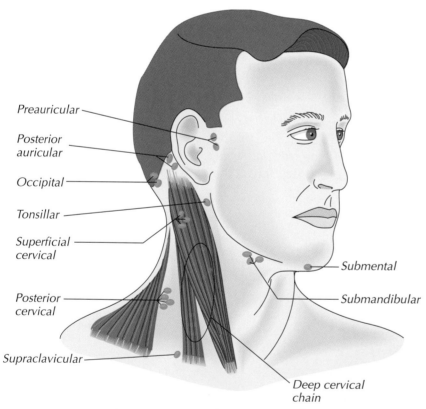

LYMPH NODES OF THE HEAD AND NECK

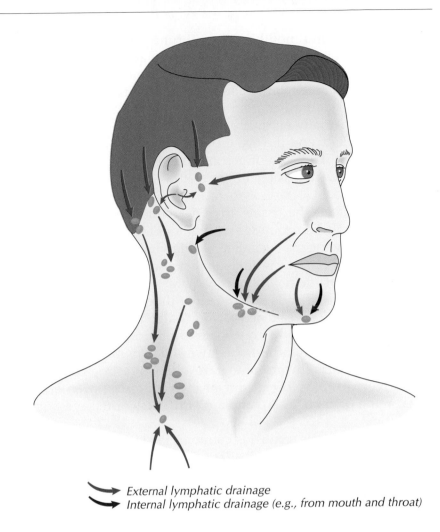

External lymphatic drainage
Internal lymphatic drainage (e.g., from mouth and throat)

Note that the tonsillar, submandibular, and submental nodes drain portions of the mouth and throat as well as the face.

Knowledge of the lymphatic system is important to a sound clinical habit: whenever a malignant or inflammatory lesion is observed, look for involvement of the regional lymph nodes that drain it; whenever a node is enlarged or tender, look for a source such as infection in the area that it drains.

Changes With Age

Adolescence. Several changes in the head and neck accompany adolescence. In boys the voice begins to deepen and the thyroid cartilage enlarges perceptibly. Facial hair appears on the upper lip, then on the cheeks and the lower lip, and finally on the chin. The facial contours of both boys and girls change subtly as they mature. Lengthening of the eyeballs in their anteroposterior diameter may cause or accentuate myopia (near-sightedness). The comedones (blackheads) and pustules of acne commonly appear on the face. Lymphoid tissues, which grow rapidly in late childhood (see p. 621), are still relatively prominent in adolescents, and cervical lymph nodes are readily palpable in most teenagers.

Aging. Tonsils, which are also composed of lymphoid tissue, become gradually smaller after the age of 5 years. In adulthood, they become inconspicuous or invisible. The frequency of palpable cervical nodes gradually diminishes with age, and according to one study falls below 50% sometime between the ages of 50 and 60. In contrast to the lymph nodes, the submandibular glands become easier to feel in older people.

The eyes, ears, and mouth bear the brunt of old age. Visual acuity remains fairly constant between the ages of 20 and 50 and then diminishes, gradually until about age 70 and then more rapidly. Nevertheless, most elderly people retain good to adequate vision—20/20 to 20/70 as measured by standard charts. Near vision, however, begins to blur noticeably for virtually everyone. From childhood on, the lens gradually loses its elasticity and the eye grows progressively less able to focus on nearby objects. This loss of accommodative power, called presbyopia, usually becomes noticeable in one's 40s.

Aging also affects the tissues in and around the eyes. In some elderly people the fat that surrounds and cushions the eye within the bony orbit atrophies, allowing the eyeball to recede somewhat in the orbit. The skin of the eyelids becomes wrinkled, occasionally hanging in loose folds. Fat may push the fascia of the eyelids forward, creating soft bulges, especially in the lower lids and the inner third of the upper ones (p. 213). Combinations of a weakened levator palpebrae, relaxation of the skin, and increased weight of the upper eyelid may cause a senile ptosis (drooping). More important, the lower lid may fall outward away from the eyeball or turn inward onto it, resulting in ectropion and entropion, respectively (p. 213). Because their eyes produce fewer lacrimal secretions, aging patients may complain of dryness of the eyes.

Corneal arcus (arcus senilis) is common in elderly persons and in them has no clinical significance (p. 216). The corneas lose some of their luster. The pupils become smaller—a characteristic that makes it more difficult to examine the fundi of elderly people. The pupils may also become slightly irregular but should continue to respond to light and near effort. Except for possible impairment in upward gaze, extraocular movements should remain intact.

Lenses thicken and yellow with age, impairing the passage of light to the retinas, and elderly people need more light to read and do fine work. When the lens of an elderly person is examined with a flashlight it frequently looks gray, as if it were opaque, when in fact it permits good visual acuity and looks clear on ophthalmoscopic examination. Do not depend on your flashlight alone, therefore, to make a diagnosis of cataract—a true opacity of the lens (p. 216). Cataracts do become relatively common, however, affecting 1 out of 10 people in their 60s and 1 out of 3 in their 80s. Because the lens continues to grow over the years, it may push the iris forward, narrowing the angle between iris and cornea and increasing the risk of narrow-angle glaucoma (p. 188).

Ophthalmoscopic examination reveals fundi that have lost their youthful shine and light reflections. The arteries look narrowed, paler, straighter, and less brilliant (p. 226). Drusen (colloid bodies) may be seen (p. 223). On a more anterior plane you may be able to see some vitreous floaters—degenerative changes that may cause annoying specks or webs in the field of vision. You may also find evidence of other, more serious, conditions that occur more often in elderly people than in younger ones: macular degeneration, glaucoma, retinal hemorrhages, or possibly retinal detachment.

Acuity of hearing, like that of vision, usually diminishes with age. Early losses, which start in young adulthood, involve primarily the high-pitched sounds beyond the range of human speech and have relatively little functional significance. Gradually, however, loss extends to sounds in the middle and lower ranges. When a person fails to catch the upper tones of words while hearing the lower ones, words sound distorted and are difficult to understand, especially in noisy environments. Hearing loss associated with aging, known as presbycusis, becomes increasingly evident, usually after the age of 50.

Diminished salivary secretions and a decreased sense of taste have been attributed to aging, but medications or various diseases probably account for most of these changes. Teeth may wear down or become abraded over time, or they may be lost to dental caries or other conditions (pp. 240–241). Periodontal disease is the chief cause of tooth loss in most adults (p. 239). If a person has no teeth, the lower portion of the face looks small and sunken, with accentuated "purse-string" wrinkles radiating out from the mouth. Overclosure of the mouth may lead to maceration of the skin at the corners—angular cheilitis (p. 234). The bony ridges of the jaws that once surrounded the tooth sockets are gradually resorbed, especially in the lower jaw.

Techniques of Examination

The Head

Because abnormalities covered by the hair are easily missed, ask if the patient has noticed anything wrong with the scalp or hair. If you note a hairpiece or wig, ask the patient to remove it.

Examine:

The Hair. Note its quantity, distribution, texture, and pattern of loss if any. Be alert for nits—tiny white ovoid granules that adhere to hairs. Do not mistake them for the loose flakes of dandruff.

Fine hair in hyperthyroidism; coarse hair in hypothyroidism. Nits are the eggs of lice.

The Scalp. Part the hair in several places and look for scaliness, lumps, or other lesions.

Redness and scaling in seborrheic dermatitis, psoriasis; pilar cysts (wens)

The Skull. Observe the general size and contour of the skull. Note any deformities, lumps, or tenderness. Familiarize yourself with the irregularities in a normal skull, such as those near the suture lines between the parietal and occipital bones.

Enlarged skull in hydrocephalus, Paget's disease of bone. Tenderness after trauma

The Face. Note the patient's facial expression and contours. Observe for asymmetry, involuntary movements, edema, and masses.

See Table 7-1, Selected Facies (p. 211).

The Skin. Observe the skin, noting its color, pigmentation, texture, thickness, hair distribution, and any lesions.

Acne in many adolescents. Hirsutism (excessive facial hair) in some women

The Eyes

Visual Acuity. To test the acuity of central vision use a Snellen eye chart, if possible, and light it well. Position the patient 20 feet from the chart. Patients who use glasses other than reading glasses should wear them. Ask the patient to cover one eye with a card (to prevent peeking through the fingers) and to read the smallest line of print possible. Coaxing to attempt the next line may improve performance. A patient who cannot read the largest letter should be positioned closer to the chart, with the distance from it noted. Determine the smallest line of print from which the patient can identify more than half the letters. Record the visual acuity designated at the side of this line, along with the use of glasses, if any. Visual acuity is expressed as two numbers (e.g., 20/30), in which the first indicates the distance of patient from chart, and the second, the distance at which a normal eye can read the line of letters.

Vision of 20/200 means that at 20 feet the patient can read print that a person with normal vision could read at 200 feet. The larger the second number, the worse the vision. "20/40 corrected" means the patient could read the 40 line with glasses (a correction).

Myopia is impaired far vision.

Testing near vision with a special hand-held card helps to identify the need for reading glasses or bifocals in patients over age 45. You can also use this card to test visual acuity at the bedside. Held 14 inches from the patient's eyes, the card simulates a Snellen chart. You may, however, let patients choose their own distance.

Presbyopia is the impaired near vision found in middle-aged and older people. A presbyopic person often sees better when the card is farther away.

If you have no charts, screen visual acuity with any available print. If patients cannot read even the largest letters, test their ability to count your upraised fingers and distinguish light (such as your flashlight) from dark.

In the United States, a person is usually considered legally blind when vision in the better eye, corrected by glasses, is 20/200 or less. Legal blindness also results from a constricted field of vision: 20° or less in the better eye.

Visual Fields by Confrontation

Screening. Screening starts in the temporal fields because most defects involve these areas. Imagine the patient's visual fields projected onto a glass bowl that encircles the front of the patient's head. Ask the patient to look with both eyes into your eyes. While you return the patient's gaze, place your hands about 2 feet apart, lateral to the patient's ears. Instruct the patient to point to your fingers as soon as they are seen. Then slowly move the wiggling fingers of both your hands along the imaginary bowl and toward the line of gaze until the patient identifies them. Repeat this pattern in the upper and lower temporal quadrants.

Field defects that are all or partly temporal include homonymous hemianopsia,

bitemporal hemianopsia,

and quadrantic defects.

Review these patterns in Table 7-2, Visual Field Defects, p. 212.

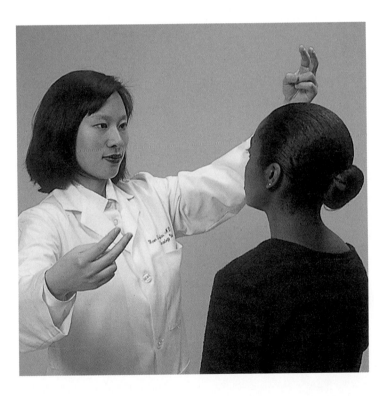

Normally, a person sees both sets of fingers at the same time. If so, fields are usually normal.

Further Testing. If you find a defect, try to establish its boundaries. Test one eye at a time. If you suspect a temporal defect in the left visual field, for example, ask the patient to cover the right eye and, with the left one, to look into your eye directly opposite. Then slowly move your wiggling fingers from the defective area toward the better vision, noting where the patient first responds. Repeat this at several levels to define the border.

When the patient's left eye repeatedly does not see your fingers until they have crossed the line of gaze, a left temporal

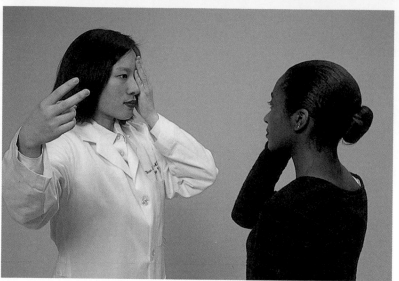

LEFT   **RIGHT**

hemianopsia is present. It is diagrammed from the patient's viewpoint.

A temporal defect in the visual field of one eye suggests a nasal defect in the other eye. To test this hypothesis, examine the other eye in a similar way, again moving from the anticipated defect toward the better vision.

A left homonymous hemianopsia may thus be established.

LEFT   **RIGHT**

Small visual field defects and enlarged blind spots require a finer stimulus. Using a small red object such as a red-headed matchstick or the red eraser on a pencil, test one eye at a time. As the patient looks into your eye directly opposite, move the object about in the visual field. The normal blind spot can be found 15° temporal to the line of gaze. (Find your own blind spots for practice.)

An enlarged blind spot occurs in conditions affecting the optic nerve, e.g., glaucoma, optic neuritis, and papilledema.

Position and Alignment of the Eyes. Stand in front of the patient and survey the eyes for position and alignment with each other. If one or both eyes seem to protrude, assess them from above (see p. 206).

Inward or outward deviation of the eyes; abnormal protrusion in Graves' disease or ocular tumors

Eyebrows. Inspect the eyebrows, noting their quantity and distribution and any scaliness of the underlying skin.

Scaliness in seborrheic dermatitis; lateral sparseness in hypothyroidism

Eyelids. Note the position of the lids in relation to the eyeballs. Inspect for the following:

- Width of the palpebral fissures
- Edema of the lids
- Color of the lids (e.g., redness)
- Lesions

See Table 7-3, Variations and Abnormalities of the Eyelids (p. 213). *Blepharitis* is an inflammation of the eyelids along the lid margins, often with crusting or scales.

- Condition and direction of the eyelashes
- Adequacy with which the eyelids close. Look for this especially when the eyes are unusually prominent, when there is facial paralysis, or when the patient is unconscious.

Lacrimal Apparatus. Briefly inspect the regions of the lacrimal gland and lacrimal sac for swelling.

Look for excessive tearing or dryness of the eyes. Assessment of dryness may require special testing by an ophthalmologist. To test for naso-lacrimal duct obstruction, see p. 206.

Failure of the eyelids to close exposes the corneas to serious damage.

See Table 7-4, Lumps and Swellings In and Around the Eyes (p. 214).

Excessive tearing may be due to increased production or impaired drainage of tears. In the first group, causes include conjunctival inflammation and corneal irritation; in the second, ectropion (p. 213) and naso-lacrimal duct obstruction.

Conjunctiva and Sclera. Ask the patient to look up as you depress both lower lids with your thumbs, exposing the sclera and conjunctiva. Inspect the sclera and palpebral conjunctiva for color, and note the vascular pattern against the white scleral background. Look for any nodules or swelling.

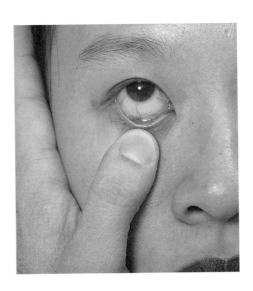

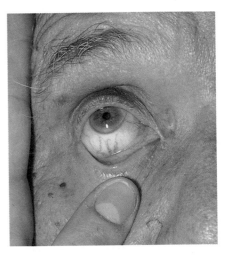

A yellow sclera indicates jaundice.

If you need a fuller view of the eye, rest your thumb and finger on the bones of the cheek and brow, respectively, and spread the lids.

Ask the patient to look to each side and down. This technique gives you a good view of the sclera and bulbar conjunctiva, but not of the palpebral conjunctiva of the upper lid. For this purpose, you need to evert the lid (see p. 207).

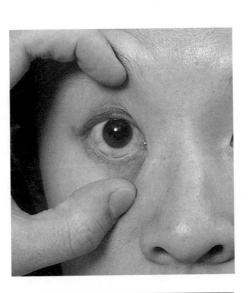

The local redness below is due to nodular episcleritis:

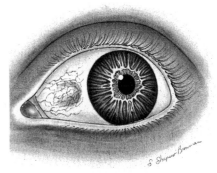

For comparisons, see Table 7-5, Red Eyes (p. 215).

Cornea and Lens. With oblique lighting, inspect the cornea of each eye for opacities and note any opacities in the lens that may be visible through the pupil.

See Table 7-6, Opacities of the Cornea and Lens (p. 216).

Iris. At the same time, inspect each iris. The markings should be clearly defined. With your light shining directly from the temporal side, look for a crescentic shadow on the medial side of the iris. Since the iris is normally fairly flat and forms a relatively open angle with the cornea, this lighting casts no shadow.

Occasionally the iris bows abnormally far forward, forming a very narrow angle with the cornea. The light then casts a crescentic shadow. This narrow

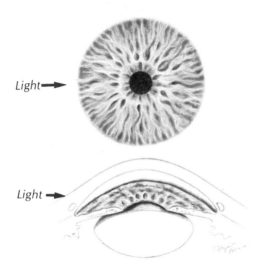
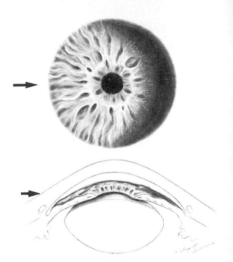

In open-angle glaucoma—the common form of glaucoma—the normal spatial relation between iris and cornea is preserved and the iris is fully lit.

angle increases the risk of acute narrow-angle glaucoma—a sudden increase in intraocular pressure when drainage of aqueous humor is blocked.

Pupils. Inspect the *size, shape,* and *symmetry* of the pupils. If the pupils are large (>5 mm), small (<3 mm), or unequal, measure them. A card with black circles of varying sizes facilitates measurement.

Miosis refers to constriction of the pupils, *mydriasis* to dilation.

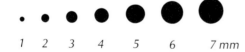

1 2 3 4 5 6 7 mm

Pupillary inequality of less than 0.5 mm (*anisocoria*) is visible in about 20% of normal people. If pupillary reactions are normal, anisocoria is considered benign.

Compare benign anisocoria with Horner's syndrome, oculomotor nerve paralysis, and tonic pupil. See Table 7-7, Pupillary Abnormalities (p. 217).

Test the *pupillary reactions to light.* Ask the patient to look into the distance, and shine a bright light obliquely into each pupil in turn. (Both the distant gaze and the oblique lighting help to prevent a near reaction.) Look for:

- The direct reaction (pupillary constriction in the same eye)
- The consensual reaction (pupillary constriction in the opposite eye)

Always darken the room and use a bright light before deciding that a light reaction is absent.

If the reaction to light is impaired or questionable, test the *near reaction* in normal room light. Testing one eye at a time makes it easier to concentrate on pupillary responses, without the distraction of extraocular movement. Hold your finger or pencil about 10 cm from the patient's eye. Ask the patient to look alternately at it and into the distance directly behind it. Watch for pupillary constriction with near effort.

Testing the near reaction is helpful in diagnosing Argyll Robertson and tonic (Adie's) pupils (see p. 217).

Extraocular Muscles. From about 2 feet directly in front of the patient, shine a light onto the patient's eyes and ask the patient to look at it. *Inspect the reflections in the corneas.* They should be visible slightly nasal to the center of the pupils.

Asymmetry of the corneal reflections indicates a deviation from normal ocular alignment. A temporal light reflection on one cornea, for example, indicates a nasal deviation of that eye. See Table 7-8, Deviations of the Eyes, p. 218.

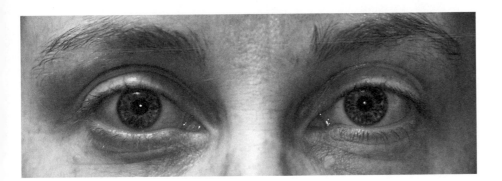

A *cover–uncover test* may reveal a slight or latent muscle imbalance not otherwise seen (see p. 218).

Now *assess the extraocular movements,* looking for:

- The normal *conjugate movements* of the eyes in each direction, or any *deviation* from normal

See Table 7-8, Deviations of the Eyes (p. 218).

- *Nystagmus,* a fine rhythmic oscillation of the eyes. A few beats of nystagmus on extreme lateral gaze are within normal limits. If you see it, bring your finger in to within the field of binocular vision and look again.

Sustained nystagmus within the binocular field of gaze is seen in a variety of neurologic conditions. See Table 18-1, Nystagmus (pp. 606–607).

- A *lid lag* as the eyes move from above downward.

Lid lag of hyperthyroidism.

To make these observations, *ask the patient to follow your finger or pencil* as you sweep through the six cardinal directions of gaze. Making a wide H in the air, lead the patient's gaze (1) to the patient's extreme right, (2) to the right and upward, and (3) down on the right; then (4) without pausing in the middle, to the extreme left, (5) to the left and upward, and (6) down on the left. Pause during upward and lateral gaze to detect nystagmus. Move your finger or pencil at a comfortable distance from the patient. Because middle-aged or older people may have difficulty focusing on near objects, make this distance greater for them than for young people. Some patients move their heads to follow your finger. If necessary, hold the head in the proper midline position.

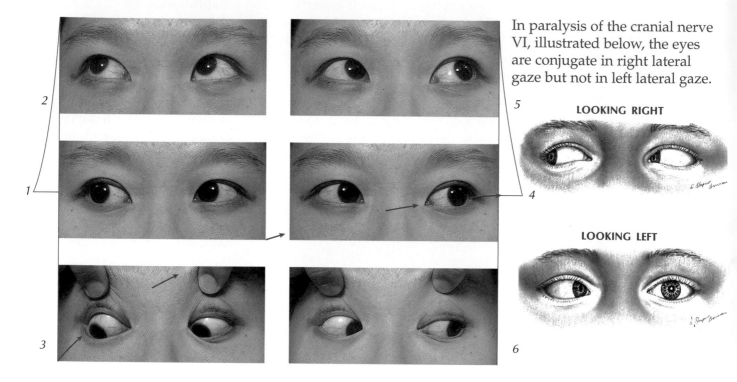

In paralysis of the cranial nerve VI, illustrated below, the eyes are conjugate in right lateral gaze but not in left lateral gaze.

LOOKING RIGHT

LOOKING LEFT

If you suspect a lid lag or hyperthyroidism, ask the patient to follow your finger again as you move it slowly from up to down in the midline. The lid should overlap the iris slightly throughout this movement.

In the lid lag of hyperthyroidism, a rim of sclera is seen between the upper lid and iris; the lid seems to lag behind the eyeball.

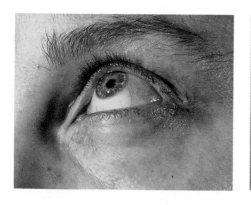
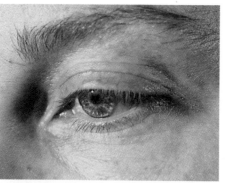
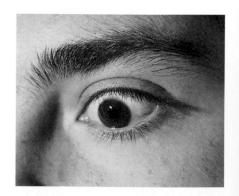

Finally, test for *convergence.* Ask the patient to follow your finger or pencil as you move it in toward the bridge of the nose. The converging eyes normally follow the object to within 5 cm to 8 cm of the nose.

Poor convergence in hyperthyroidism

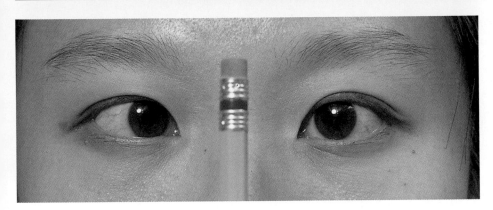

CONVERGENCE

Ophthalmoscopic Examination. In general health care, you should usually examine your patients' eyes without dilating their pupils. Your view is therefore limited to the posterior structures of the retinal surface. To see more peripheral structures, to evaluate the macula well, or to investigate unexplained visual loss, the pupils should be dilated with mydriatic drops unless this is contraindicated.

Contraindications for mydriatic drops include (1) head injury and coma, in which continuing observations of pupillary reactions are essential, and (2) any suspicion of narrow-angle glaucoma.

Using the Ophthalmoscope. Remove your glasses unless you have marked nearsightedness or severe astigmatism. If patients have such refractive errors and you cannot focus clearly on their fundi, it may be easier to examine them with their glasses on. Both of you may leave contact lenses in place.

Darken the room. Switch on the ophthalmoscope light, and adjust it to the large round beam of white light.* By shining this light on the back of your hand, you can check both the type of light and the ophthalmoscope's electrical charge.

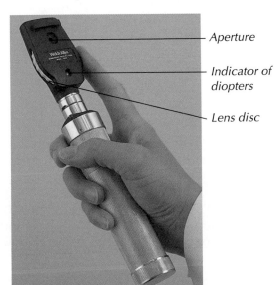

Aperture

Indicator of diopters

Lens disc

Turn the lens disc to 0 diopters (a lens that neither converges nor diverges the light rays). Keep your index finger on the lens disc so that you can focus the ophthalmoscope during the examination.

*Some clinicians like to use the large round beam for large pupils, the small round beam for small pupils. The other beams are rarely helpful. The slitlike beam is sometimes used to assess elevations or concavities in the retina, the green (or red-free) beam to detect small red lesions, and the grid to make measurements. Ignore the last three lights and practice with the large round white beam.

Use your *right hand* and *right eye* for the patient's *right eye*; your *left hand* and *left eye* for the patient's *left eye*. You thereby avoid facing your patient nose to nose, and your examination is closer, more mobile, and less intimate. Initially you will have difficulty using your nondominant eye, but persist. Hold your ophthalmoscope firmly braced up under the medial aspect of your bony orbit. Keep the handle tilted laterally at about a 20° slant from the vertical. You should be able to see clearly through the aperture. Ask the patient to look slightly up and over your shoulder and gaze at a specific point on the wall.

From a position about 15 inches away from the patient and about 15° lateral to the patient's line of vision, shine the light beam on the pupil. Note the orange glow in the pupil—the *red reflex*. Also note any opacities interrupting the red reflex.

Absence of a red reflex suggests an opacity of the lens (cataract) or possibly of the vitreous. Less commonly, a detached retina or, in children, a retinoblastoma may obscure this reflex. Do not be fooled by an artificial eye, which of course has no red reflex either.

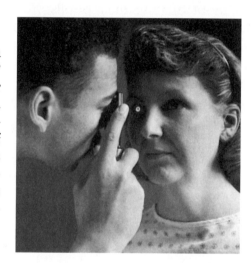

Keeping the light beam focused on the red reflex, move in on the 15° line toward the pupil until your ophthalmoscope is very close to it, almost touching the patient's eyelashes. By placing the thumb of your other hand on the patient's eyebrow you gain extra proprioceptive guidance as you come closer to the patient, but this technique is not essential.

Try to keep both eyes open. Keep your eyes relaxed, as if gazing into the distance. This will help to minimize the fluctuating blurriness as your eyes attempt to accommodate. Some patients find the light of modern ophthalmoscopes too bright. Lowering the light's intensity often improves their comfort without impairing your observations.

Finding the Optic Disc. You should now be seeing the retina in the vicinity of the *optic disc*—a yellowish orange to creamy pink oval or round structure. The disc may fill your field of gaze or even exceed it. If you do not see it, follow a blood vessel centrally until you do. You can tell which direction is central by noting the angles at which vessels branch and the progressive enlargement of vessel size at each junction as you approach the disc.

When the lens has been removed surgically, its magnifying effect is lost. Retinal structures then look much smaller than usual, and you can see a much larger expanse of fundus.

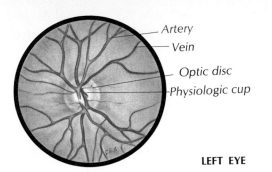
Artery
Vein
Optic disc
Physiologic cup

LEFT EYE

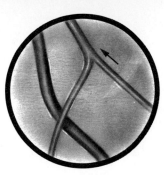

Now *bring the optic disc into sharp focus* by adjusting the lens of your ophthalmoscope. If both you and the patient have no refractive errors, the ophthalmoscope should focus on the retina at 0 diopters.† If structures are blurred, use trial and error to find the best focus. For a myopic (nearsighted) patient, you will need to rotate the lens disc counterclockwise to the minus diopters. For a hyperopic (farsighted) patient, rotate the disc clockwise to the plus diopters. You can correct your own refractive error in the same way.

In a refractive error, light rays from a distance do not focus on the retina. In myopia, they focus anterior to it; in hyperopia, posterior to it. Retinal structures in a myopic eye look larger than normal.

Inspecting the Optic Disc. Inspect the optic disc, noting:

- The clarity of the disc outline. The nasal outline may be normally somewhat blurred.
- The color of the disc, normally yellowish orange to creamy pink
- The possible presence of normal white or pigmented rings or crescents around the disc
- The size of the central physiologic cup, if present. This cup is normally yellowish white. Its horizontal diameter is usually less than half the horizontal diameter of the disc.
- The symmetry of the eyes in terms of these observations

See Table 7-9, Normal Variations of the Optic Disc (p. 219), and Table 7-10, Abnormalities of the Optic Disc (p. 220).

An enlarged cup suggests chronic open-angle glaucoma.

In a normal person, you may or may not see pulsations of the veins as they emerge from the disc. These are normal, but their absence has no clinical significance.

The presence of venous pulsations at the disc suggests but does not prove that cerebrospinal fluid pressure is normal.

Inspecting the Retina. Identify the *arteries and veins*. They may be distinguished by the features listed in the following table.

	Arteries	Veins
Color	Light red	Dark red
Size	Smaller (⅔ to ⅘ the diameter of veins)	Larger
Light Reflex *(reflection)*	Bright	Inconspicuous or absent

†A diopter is a unit that measures the power of a lens to converge or diverge light.

Follow the vessels peripherally in each of four directions, noting their relative sizes and the character of the arteriovenous crossings. Identify any lesions of the surrounding *retina* and note their size, shape, color, and distribution. As you search the retina, move your head and instrument as a unit, using the patient's pupil as an imaginary fulcrum. At first, you may repeatedly lose your view of the retina because your light falls out of the pupil. You will improve with practice.

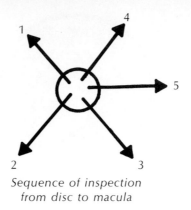

Sequence of inspection from disc to macula

LEFT EYE

See Table 7-11, Retinal Arteries and Arteriovenous Crossings: Normal and Hypertensive (p. 221).

See Table 7-12, Red Spots and Streaks in the Fundi (p. 222).

See Table 7-13, Light-Colored Spots in the Fundi (pp. 223–224).

See Table 7-14, Ocular Fundi (pp. 225–226).

Finally, by directing your light beam laterally or by asking the patient to look directly into the light, inspect the *fovea* and surrounding *macula.* Except in older people, the tiny bright reflection at the center of the fovea helps to orient you. Shimmering light reflections in the macular area are common in young people.

Macular degeneration of aging is an important cause of poor central vision in elderly people. It takes many forms, including hemorrhages, exudates, cysts, and "holes." A common form with altered pigmentation is illustrated here.

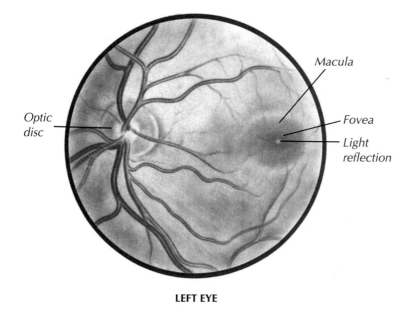

Optic disc

Macula

Fovea

Light reflection

LEFT EYE

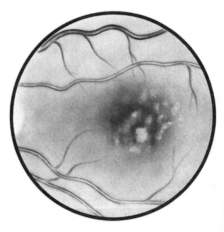

MACULAR DEGENERATION OF AGING

Inspecting Anterior Structures. Look for opacities in the *vitreous* or *lens* by rotating the lens disc progressively to diopters of around +10 or +12. This technique focuses on more anterior structures in the eye.

Vitreous floaters may be seen as dark specks or strands between the fundus and the lens. Cataracts are densities in the lens (see p. 216).

Measurement Within the Eye. Lesions of the retina can be located in relation to the optic disc and are measured as "disc diameters." Among the cotton wool patches illustrated on the right, there is an irregular one between 1 and 2 o'clock, less than ½ disc diameter from the disc. It measures about 1 by ½ disc diameters.

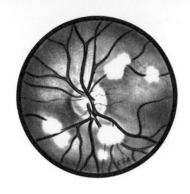

The elevated optic disc of papilledema can be measured by noting the differences in diopters of the two lenses used to focus clearly on the disc and on the uninvolved retina.

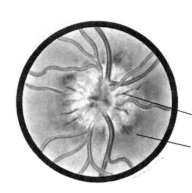

Clear focus here at +3 diopters
Clear focus here at −1 diopter

$$+3 - (-1) = +4,$$ therefore a disc elevation of 4 diopters

For Interest. On ophthalmoscopic examination, the normal retina is magnified about 15 times, the normal iris about 4 times. The optic disc actually measures about 1.5 mm. At the retina, 3 diopters of elevation = 1 mm.

The Ears

The Auricle. Inspect each auricle and surrounding tissues for deformities, lumps, or skin lesions.

See Table 7-15, Lumps On or Near the Ear (pp. 228–229).

If ear pain, discharge, or inflammation is present, move the auricle up and down, press the tragus, and press firmly just behind the ear.

Ear Canal and Drum. To see the ear canal and drum, use an otoscope with the largest ear speculum that the canal will accommodate. Position the patient's head so that you can see comfortably through the instrument. To straighten the ear canal, grasp the auricle firmly but gently and pull it upward, backward, and slightly away from the head.

Movement of the auricle and tragus is painful in acute *otitis externa* (inflammation of the ear canal), but not in *otitis media* (inflammation of the middle ear). Tenderness behind the ear may be present in otitis media.

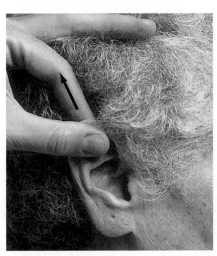

Holding the otoscope handle between your thumb and fingers, brace your hand against the patient's face. Your hand and instrument thus follow unexpected movements by the patient. (If you are uncomfortable switching hands for the left ear, as shown below, you may reach over that ear to pull it up and back with your left hand and rest your otoscope-holding right hand on the head behind the ear.)

Insert the speculum gently into the ear canal, directing it somewhat down and forward and through the hairs, if any.

Nontender nodular swellings covered by normal skin deep in the ear canals suggest *exostoses.* These are nonmalignant overgrowths, which may obscure the drum.

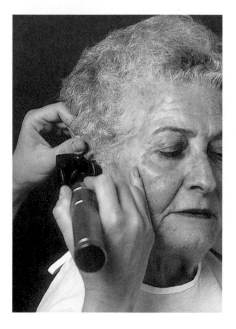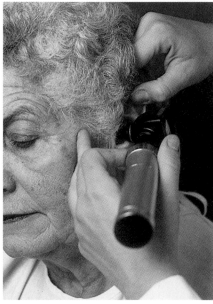

Inspect the ear canal, noting any discharge, foreign bodies, redness of the skin, or swelling. Cerumen, which varies in color and consistency from yellow and flaky to brown and sticky or even to dark and hard, may wholly or partly obscure your view.

In acute otitis externa, shown below, the canal is often swollen, narrowed, moist, pale, and tender. It may be reddened.

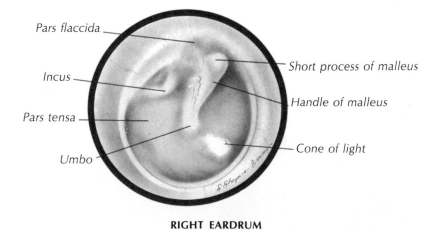

Pars flaccida

Short process of malleus

Incus

Handle of malleus

Pars tensa

Cone of light

Umbo

RIGHT EARDRUM

(After Hawke M, Keene M, Alberti PW: Clinical Otoscopy: A Text and Colour Atlas. Edinburgh, Churchill Livingstone, 1984)

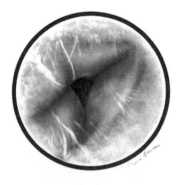

In chronic otitis externa, the skin of the canal is often thickened, red, and itchy.

Inspect the eardrum, noting its color and contour. The cone of light—usually easy to see—helps to orient you.

Red bulging drum of acute purulent otitis media, amber drum of a serous effusion

Identify the *handle of the malleus,* noting its position, and inspect the *short process of the malleus.*

An unusually prominent short process and a prominent handle that looks more horizontal suggest a retracted drum.

Gently move the speculum so that you can see as much of the drum as possible, including the pars flaccida superiorly and the margins of the pars tensa. Look for any perforations. The anterior and inferior margins of the drum may be obscured by the curving wall of the ear canal.

See Table 7-16, Abnormalities of the Eardrum (pp. 230–231).

Mobility of the eardrum can be evaluated with a pneumatic otoscope. See p. 195.

A serous effusion, a thickened drum, or purulent otitis media may decrease mobility.

Auditory Acuity. To estimate hearing, test one ear at a time. Ask the patient to occlude one ear with a finger or, better still, occlude it yourself. When auditory acuity on the two sides is different, move your finger rapidly, but gently, in the occluded canal. The noise so produced will help to prevent the occluded ear from doing the work of the ear you wish to test. Then, standing 1 or 2 feet away, exhale fully (so as to minimize the intensity of your voice) and whisper softly toward the unoccluded ear. Choose numbers or other words with two equally accented syllables, such as "nine-four," or "baseball." If necessary, increase the intensity of your voice to a medium whisper, a loud whisper, and then a soft, medium, and loud voice. To make sure the patient does not read your lips, cover your mouth or obstruct the patient's vision.

Air and Bone Conduction. If hearing is diminished, *try to distinguish between conductive and sensorineural hearing loss.* You need a quiet room and a tuning fork, preferably of 512 Hz or possibly 1024 Hz. These frequencies fall within the range of human speech (300 Hz to 3000 Hz)—functionally the most important range. Forks with lower pitches may lead to overestimating bone conduction and can also be felt as vibration.

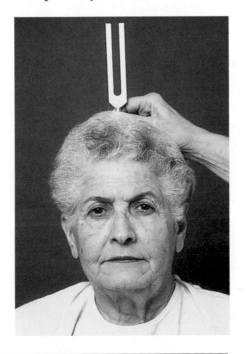

Set the fork into light vibration by briskly stroking it between thumb and index finger ⟶⟵ or by tapping it on your knuckles.

1. *Test for lateralization* (Weber test). Place the base of the lightly vibrating tuning fork firmly on top of the patient's head or on the midforehead.

In unilateral conductive hearing loss, sound is heard in (lateralized to) the impaired ear. Visible explanations include acute otitis media, perforation

Ask where the patient hears it: on one or both sides. Normally the sound is heard in the midline or equally in both ears. If nothing is heard, try again, pressing the fork more firmly on the head.

of the eardrum, and obstruction of the ear canal, as by cerumen.

In unilateral sensorineural hearing loss, sound is heard in the good ear.

2. *Compare air conduction (AC) and bone conduction (BC)* (Rinne test). Place the base of a lightly vibrating tuning fork on the mastoid bone, behind the ear and level with the canal. When the patient can no longer hear the sound, quickly place the fork close to the ear canal and ascertain whether the sound can be heard again. Here the "U" of the fork should face forward, thus maximizing its sound for the patient. Normally the sound is heard longer through air than through bone (AC > BC).

In conductive hearing loss, sound is heard through bone as long as or longer than it is through air (BC = AC or BC > AC). In sensorineural hearing loss, sound is heard longer through air (AC > BC). See Table 7-17, Patterns of Hearing Loss (pp. 232–233).

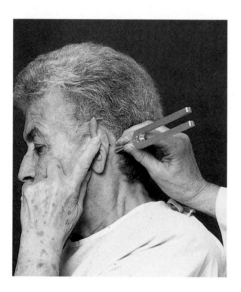
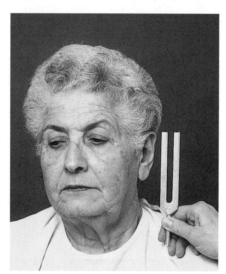

The Nose and Paranasal Sinuses

Inspect the anterior and inferior surfaces of the nose. Gentle pressure on the tip of the nose with your thumb usually widens the nostrils and, with the aid of a penlight or otoscope light, you can get a partial view of each nasal vestibule. If the tip is tender, be particularly gentle and manipulate the nose as little as possible.

Tenderness of the nasal tip or alae suggests local infection such as a furuncle.

Note any asymmetry or deformity of the nose.

Deviation of the lower septum is common and may be easily visible, as illustrated on the next page. Deviation seldom obstructs air flow.

Test for nasal obstruction, if indicated, by pressing on each ala nasi in turn and asking the patient to breathe in.

Inspect the inside of the nose with an otoscope and the largest ear speculum available.‡ Tilt the patient's head back a bit and insert the speculum gently into the vestibule of each nostril, avoiding contact with the sensitive nasal septum. Hold the otoscope handle to one side to avoid the patient's chin and improve your mobility. By directing the speculum posteriorly, then upward in small steps, try to see the inferior and middle turbinates, the nasal septum, and the narrow nasal passage between them. Some asymmetry of the two sides is normal.

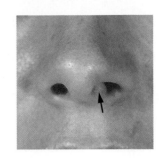

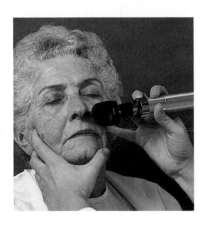
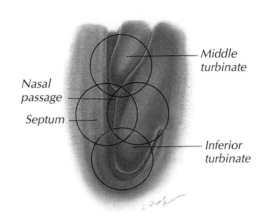

Middle turbinate

Nasal passage

Septum

Inferior turbinate

Observe:

1. The *nasal mucosa* that covers the septum and turbinates. Note its color and any swelling, bleeding, or exudate. If exudate is present, note its character: clear, mucopurulent, or purulent. The nasal mucosa is normally somewhat redder than the oral mucosa.

   In viral rhinitis the mucosa is reddened and swollen; in allergic rhinitis it may be pale, bluish, or red.

2. The *nasal septum*. Note any deviation, inflammation, or perforation of the septum. The lower anterior portion of the septum (where the patient's finger can reach) is a common source of *epistaxis* (nosebleed).

   Fresh blood or crusting may be seen. Causes of septal perforation include trauma, surgery, and the intranasal use of cocaine or amphetamines.

3. Any *abnormalities* such as ulcers or polyps

   Polyps are pale, semitranslucent masses that usually come from the middle meatus. Ulcers may result from nasal use of cocaine.

Make it a habit to place all nasal and ear specula outside your instrument case after use. Then discard them or clean and disinfect them appropriately. (Check with the policies of your institution.)

---

‡A nasal illuminator, equipped with a short wide nasal speculum but lacking an otoscope's magnification, may also be used, but structures look much smaller. Otolaryngologists use special equipment not widely available to others.

Palpate for sinus tenderness. Press up on the *frontal sinuses* from under the bony brows, avoiding pressure on the eyes. Then press up on the *maxillary sinuses.*

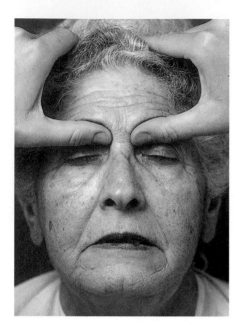
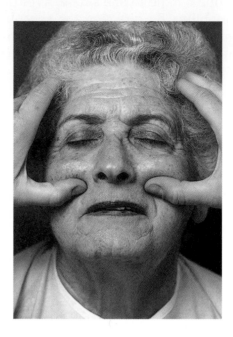

Local tenderness, together with symptoms such as pain, fever, and nasal discharge, suggests acute sinusitis involving the frontal or maxillary sinuses. Transillumination may be diagnostically useful. For this technique, see p. 208.

The Mouth and Pharynx

If the patient wears dentures, offer a paper towel and ask the patient to remove them so that you can see the mucosa underneath. If suspicious ulcers or nodules are observed, put on a glove and palpate the lesion, noting especially any thickening or infiltration of the tissues that might suggest malignancy.

Bright red edematous mucosa underneath a denture suggests denture sore mouth. There may be ulcers or papillary granulation tissue.

Inspect the following:

The Lips. Observe their color and moisture, and note any lumps, ulcers, cracking, or scaliness.

Cyanosis, pallor. See Table 7-18, Abnormalities of the Lips (pp. 234–235).

The Oral Mucosa. Look into the patient's mouth and, with a good light and the help of a tongue blade, inspect the oral mucosa for color, ulcers, white patches, and nodules. The wavy white line on this buccal mucosa developed where the upper and lower teeth meet. Irritation from sucking or chewing may cause or intensify it.

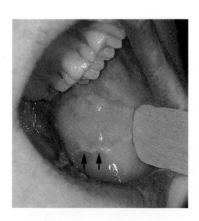

An aphthous ulcer on the labial mucosa is shown by the patient.

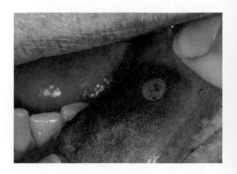

See p. 243 and Table 7-19, Findings in the Pharynx, Palate, and Oral Mucosa (pp. 236–238).

The Gums and Teeth. Note the color of the gums, normally pink. Patchy brownness may be present, especially but not exclusively in black people.

Redness of gingivitis, black line of lead poisoning

Inspect the gum margins and the interdental papillae for swelling or ulceration.

Swollen interdental papillae in gingivitis. See Table 7-20, Findings in the Gums and Teeth (pp. 239–241).

Inspect the teeth. Are any of them missing, discolored, misshapen, or abnormally positioned? You can check for looseness with your gloved thumb and index finger.

The Roof of the Mouth. Inspect the color and architecture of the hard palate.

Torus palatinus, a midline lump (see p. 237)

The Tongue and the Floor of the Mouth. Ask the patient to put out his or her tongue. Inspect it for symmetry—a test of the hypoglossal nerve (Cranial Nerve XII).

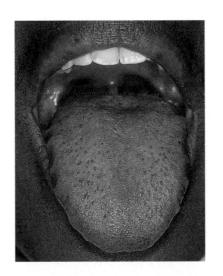

Asymmetric protrusion suggests a lesion of Cranial Nerve XII, as shown below.

Note the color and texture of the dorsum of the tongue.

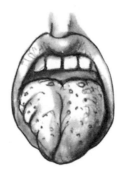

Inspect the sides and undersurface of the tongue and the floor of the mouth. These are the areas where cancer most often develops. Note any white or reddened areas, nodules, or ulcerations. Because cancer of the tongue is more common in men over age 50, especially in those who use tobacco and drink alcohol, palpation is indicated for these patients. Explain what you plan to do and put on gloves. Ask the patient to protrude his tongue. With your right hand, grasp the tip of the tongue with a square of gauze and gently pull it to the patient's left. Inspect the side of the tongue, and then palpate it with your gloved left hand, feeling for any induration (hardness). Reverse the procedure for the other side.

Cancer of the tongue is the second most common cancer of the mouth, second only to cancer of the lip. Any persistent nodule or ulcer, red or white, must be suspect. Induration of the lesion further increases the possibility of malignancy. Cancer occurs most often on the side of the tongue, next most often at its base.

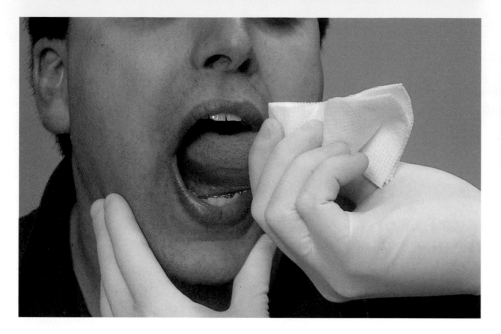

A carcinoma on the left side of a tongue:

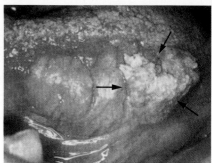

(Photo reprinted by permission of the New England Journal of Medicine, 328: 186, 1993—arrows added)

See Table 7-21, Findings In or Under the Tongue (pp. 242–243).

The Pharynx. Now, with the patient's mouth open but the tongue not protruded, ask the patient to say "ah" or yawn. This action may let you see the pharynx well. If not, press a tongue blade firmly down upon the midpoint of the arched tongue—far enough back to get good visualization of the pharynx but not so far that you cause gagging. Simultaneously, ask for an "ah" or a yawn. Note the rise of the soft palate—a test of the 10th cranial (vagus) nerve.

In 10th nerve paralysis, the soft palate fails to rise and the uvula deviates to the opposite side.

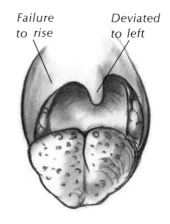

Failure to rise   Deviated to left

Inspect the soft palate, anterior and posterior pillars, uvula, tonsils, and pharynx. Note their color and symmetry and look for exudate, swelling, ulceration, or tonsillar enlargement. If possible, palpate any suspicious area for induration or tenderness. Tonsils have crypts, or deep infoldings of squamous epithelium. Whitish spots of normal exfoliating epithelium may sometimes be seen in these crypts.

See Table 7-19, Findings in the Pharynx, Palate, and Oral Mucosa (pp. 236–238).

Discard your tongue blade after use.

The Neck

Survey. Inspect the neck, noting its symmetry and any masses or scars. Look for enlargement of the parotid or submandibular glands, and note any visible lymph nodes.

A scar of past thyroid surgery may be the clue to unsuspected thyroid disease.

Lymph Nodes. Palpate the lymph nodes. Using the pads of your index and middle fingers, move the skin over the underlying tissues in each area. The patient should be relaxed, with neck flexed slightly forward and, if needed, slightly toward the side of the examination. You can usually examine both sides at once. For the submental node, however, it is helpful to feel with one hand while bracing the top of the head with the other.

Feel in sequence for the following nodes:

1. Preauricular—in front of the ear
2. Posterior auricular—superficial to the mastoid process
3. Occipital—at the base of the skull posteriorly
4. Tonsillar—at the angle of the mandible
5. Submandibular—midway between the angle and the tip of the mandible. These nodes are usually smaller and smoother than the lobulated submandibular gland against which they lie.
6. Submental—in the midline a few cm behind the tip of the mandible
7. Superficial cervical—superficial to the sternomastoid
8. Posterior cervical—along the anterior edge of the trapezius
9. Deep cervical chain—deep to the sternomastoid and often inaccessible to examination. Hook your thumb and fingers around either side of the sternomastoid muscle to find them.
10. Supraclavicular—deep in the angle formed by the clavicle and the sternomastoid

A "tonsillar node" that pulsates is really the carotid artery. A small, hard, tender "tonsillar node" high and deep between the mandible and the sternomastoid is probably a styloid process.

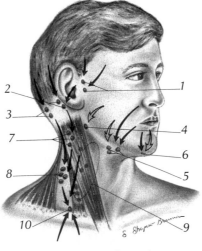

→ *External lymphatic drainage*

⇁ *Internal lymphatic drainage (e.g., from mouth and throat)*

Enlargement of a supraclavicular node, especially on the left, suggests possible metastasis from a thoracic or an abdominal malignancy.

Note their size, shape, delimitation (discrete or matted together), mobility, consistency, and any tenderness. Small, mobile, discrete, nontender nodes are frequently found in normal persons.

Tender nodes suggest inflammation; hard or fixed nodes suggest malignancy.

Enlarged or tender nodes, if unexplained, call for (1) reexamination of the regions they drain, and (2) careful assessment of lymph nodes elsewhere so that you can distinguish between regional and generalized lymphadenopathy.

Occasionally you may mistake a band of muscle or an artery for a lymph node. You should be able to roll a node in two directions: up and down, and side to side. Neither a muscle nor an artery will pass this test.

The Trachea and the Thyroid Gland. To orient yourself to the neck, identify the thyroid and cricoid cartilages and the trachea below them.

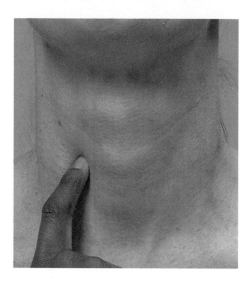

Inspect the trachea for any deviation from its usual midline position. Then *feel for any deviation.* Place your finger along one side of the trachea and note the space between it and the sternomastoid. Compare it with the other side. The spaces should be symmetrical.

Masses in the neck may push the trachea to one side. Tracheal deviation may also signify important problems in the thorax, such as a mediastinal mass, atelectasis, or a large pneumothorax (see p. 275).

Inspect the neck for the thyroid gland. Tip the patient's head back a bit. Using tangential lighting directed downward from the tip of the patient's chin, inspect the region below the cricoid cartilage for the gland. The lower, shadowed border of each thyroid gland shown here is outlined by arrows.

The lower border of this large thyroid gland is outlined by tangential lighting. *Goiter* is a general term for an enlarged thyroid gland.

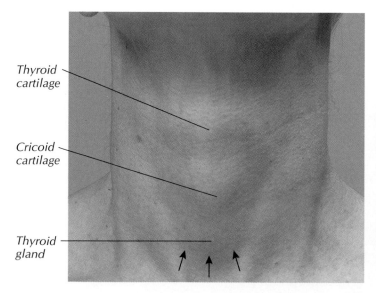

Thyroid cartilage

Cricoid cartilage

Thyroid gland

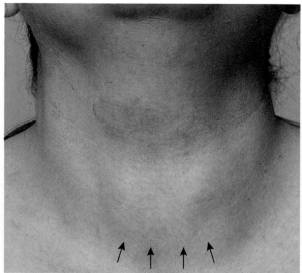

AT REST

Ask the patient to sip some water and to extend the neck again and swallow. Watch for upward movement of the thyroid gland, noting its contour and symmetry. The thyroid cartilage, the cricoid cartilage, and the thyroid gland all rise with swallowing and then fall to their resting positions.

With swallowing, the lower border of this large gland rises and looks less symmetrical.

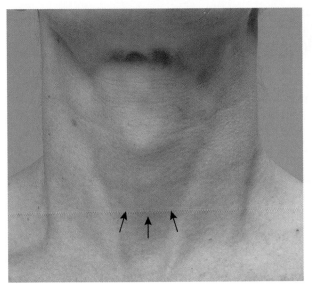 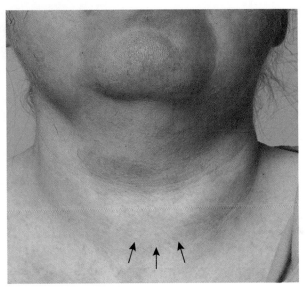

SWALLOWING

Until you become familiar with this examination, check your visual observations with your fingers from in front of the patient. This will orient you to the next step.

Palpate the thyroid gland from behind. Place the fingers of both hands on the patient's neck so that your index fingers are just below the cricoid. Adjust the patient's neck extension to avoid tightened neck muscles that might interfere with your palpation, and ask the patient to sip and swallow water as before. Feel for any glandular tissue rising under your finger pads. The thyroid isthmus is often but not always palpable. The lobes are more lateral than the isthmus and harder to feel. Move your fingers laterally as needed.

Although physical characteristics of the thyroid gland, such as size, shape, and consistency, are diagnostically important, they tell you little if anything about thyroid function. Assessment of thyroid function depends upon symptoms, signs elsewhere in the body, and laboratory tests. See Table 7-22, Thyroid Enlargement and Function (p. 244).

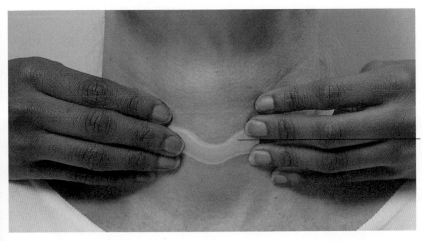

Cricoid cartilage

Note the size, shape, and consistency of the gland and identify any nodules or tenderness. The anterior surface of a lateral lobe is approximately the size of the distal phalanx of the thumb; it feels somewhat rubbery.

Benign and malignant nodules, tenderness in thyroiditis

The thyroid gland is usually easier to feel in a long slender neck than in a short stocky one. In the latter, further extension of the neck may help. In some persons, however, the thyroid gland is partially or wholly substernal.

If the thyroid gland is enlarged, listen over the lateral lobes with a stethoscope to detect a *bruit* (a sound similar to a cardiac murmur but of noncardiac origin).

A localized systolic or continuous bruit may be heard in hyperthyroidism.

The Carotid Arteries and Jugular Veins. You will probably defer a detailed examination of these vessels until the patient lies down for the cardiovascular examination. Jugular venous distention, however, may be visible in the sitting position and should not be overlooked. You should also be alert to unusually prominent arterial pulsations. See Chapter 9 for further discussion.

Special Techniques

For Assessing Prominent Eyes. Inspect unusually prominent eyes from above. Standing behind the seated patient, draw the upper lids gently upward, and then compare the positions of the eyes and note the relationship of the corneas to the lower lids. Further assessment can be made with an exophthalmometer, an instrument that measures the prominence of the eyes from the side. The upper limits of normal for eye prominence are greater in African Americans than in whites.

Exophthalmos is an abnormal protrusion of the eye (see p. 213).

For Nasolacrimal Duct Obstruction. This test helps to identify the cause of excessive tearing. Ask the patient to look up. Press on the lower lid close to the medial canthus, just *inside* the rim of the bony orbit. You are thus compressing the lacrimal sac.

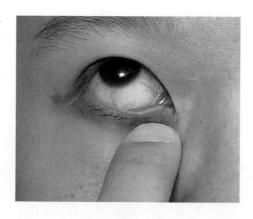

Look for fluid regurgitated out of the puncta into the eye. Avoid this test if the area is inflamed and tender.

Regurgitation of mucopurulent fluid from the puncta suggests an obstructed nasolacrimal duct.

For Inspection of the Upper Palpebral Conjunctiva. Adequate examination of the eye in search of a foreign body requires eversion of the upper eyelid. Follow these steps:

1. Instruct the patient to look down. Get the patient to relax the eyes—by reassurance and by gentle, assured, and deliberate movements. Raise the upper eyelid slightly so that the eyelashes protrude, and then grasp the upper eyelashes and pull them gently down and forward.

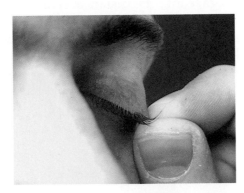

2. Place a small stick such as an applicator or a tongue blade at least 1 cm above the lid margin (and therefore at the upper border of the tarsal plate). Push down on the stick as you raise the edge of the lid, thus everting the eyelid or turning it "inside out." Do not press on the eyeball itself.

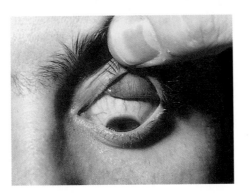

3. Secure the upper lashes against the eyebrow with your thumb and inspect the palpebral conjunctiva. After your inspection, grasp the upper eyelashes and pull them gently forward. Ask the patient to look up. The eyelid will return to its normal position.

This view allows you to see the upper palpebral conjunctiva and look for a foreign body that might be lodged there.

Swinging Flashlight Test. This test helps you to decide whether reduced vision is due to ocular disease or to optic nerve disease. For an adequate test, vision must not be entirely lost. In dim room light, note the size of the pupils. After asking the patient to gaze into the distance, swing the beam of a penlight back and forth from one pupil to the other, each time concentrating on the pupillary size and reaction in the eye that is lit. Normally, each illuminated eye looks or promptly becomes constricted. The opposite eye also constricts consensually.

When the optic nerve is damaged, as in the left eye below, the sensory (afferent) stimulus sent to the midbrain is reduced. The pupil, responding less vigorously, dilates from its prior constricted state. This response is an *afferent pupillary defect* (Marcus Gunn pupil). The opposite eye responds consensually.

When ocular disease, e.g., a cataract, impairs vision, the pupils respond normally.

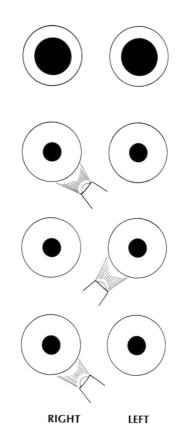

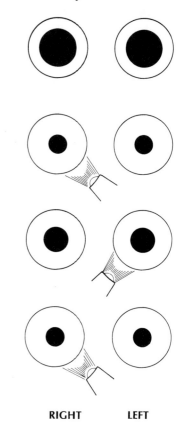

RIGHT   LEFT   RIGHT   LEFT

Transillumination of the Sinuses. When sinus tenderness or other symptoms suggest sinusitis, this test can at times be helpful but is not highly sensitive or specific for diagnosis. The room should be thoroughly darkened. Using a strong, narrow light source, place the light snugly deep under each brow, close to the nose. Shield the light with your hand. Look for a dim red glow as light is transmitted through the air-filled frontal sinus to the forehead.

Absence of glow on one or both sides suggests a thickened mucosa or secretions in the frontal sinus, but it may also result from developmental absence of one or both sinuses.

Ask the patient to tilt his or her head back with mouth opened wide. (An upper denture should first be removed.) Shine the light downward from just below the inner aspect of each eye. Look through the open mouth at the hard palate. A reddish glow indicates a normal air-filled maxillary sinus.

Absence of glow suggests thickened mucosa or secretions in the maxillary sinus. See p. 673 for an alternative method of transilluminating the maxillary sinuses.

Health Promotion and Counseling

Vision and hearing, critical senses for experiencing the world around us, are two areas of special importance for health promotion and counseling. Oral health, often overlooked, also merits clinical attention.

Disorders of vision shift with age. Healthy young adults generally have refractive errors. Up to 25% of adults over 65 have refractive errors; however, cataracts, macular degeneration, and glaucoma become more prevalent. These disorders reduce awareness of the social and physical environment and contribute to falls and injuries. To improve detection of visual defects, test visual acuity lens and with a Snellen chart or hand-held card (pp. 168–169). Examine the fundi for: clouding of the lens (cataracts); mottling of the macula, variations in the retinal pigmentation, subretinal hemorrhage or exudate (macular degeneration); and change in size and color of the optic cup (glaucoma). After diagnosis, review effective treatments—corrective lenses, cataract surgery, photocoagulation for choroidal neovascularization in macular degeneration, and topical medications for glaucoma.

Surveillance for glaucoma is especially important. Glaucoma is the leading cause of blindness in African Americans and the second leading cause of blindness overall. There is gradual loss of vision with damage to the optic nerve, loss of visual fields beginning usually at the periphery, and pallor and increasing size of the optic cup (enlarging to more than half the diameter of the optic disc). Elevated intraocular pressure (IOP) is seen in up to 80% of cases and is linked to damage of the optic nerve. Risk factors include age over 65, African American origin, diabetes mellitus, myopia, family history of glaucoma, and ocular hypertension (IOP ≥ 21 mm Hg). Screening tests include tonometry to measure IOP, ophthalmoscopy or slit-lamp examination of the optic nerve head, and perimetry to map the visual fields. In the hands of general clinicians, however, all three tests lack accuracy, so attention to risk factors and referral to eye specialists remain important tools for clinical care.

Hearing loss can also trouble the later years. More than a third of adults over age 65 have detectable hearing deficits, contributing to emotional isolation and social withdrawal. These losses may go undetected—unlike vision prerequisites for driving and vision, there is no mandate for widespread testing and many seniors avoid use of hearing aids. Questionnaires and hand-held audioscopes work well for periodic screening. Less sensitive are the clinical "whisper test," rubbing fingers, or use of the tuning fork. Groups at risk are those with a history of congenital or familial hearing loss, syphilis, rubella, meningitis, or exposure to hazardous noise levels at work or on the battlefield.

Clinicians should play an active role in promoting oral health: up to half of all children ages 5 to 17 have from one to eight cavities, and the average US adult has 10 to 17 teeth that are decayed, missing, or filled. In adults, the prevalence of gingivitis and periodontal disease is 50% and

80% respectively. In the U.S., more than half of all adults over age 65 have no teeth at all!* Effective screening begins with careful examination of the mouth. Inspect the oral cavity for decayed or loose teeth, inflammation of the gingiva, and signs of periodontal disease (bleeding, pus, recession of the gums, and bad breath). Inspect the mucous membranes, the palate, the oral floor, and the surfaces of the tongue for ulcers and leukoplakia, warning signs for oral cancer and HIV disease.

To improve oral health, counsel patients to adopt daily hygiene measures. Use of flouride-containing toothpastes reduces tooth decay, and brushing and flossing retard periodontal disease by removing bacterial plaques. Urge patients to seek dental care at least annually to receive the benefits of more specialized preventive care such as scaling, planing of roots, and topical fluorides.

Diet, tobacco and alcohol use, changes in salivary flow from medication, and proper use of dentures should also be addressed.** As with children, adults should avoid excessive intake of foods high in refined sugars, such as sucrose, which enhance attachment and colonization of cariogenic bacteria. Use of all tobacco products and excessive alcohol, the principal risk factors for oral cancers, should be avoided.

Saliva cleanses and lubricates the mouth. Many medications reduce salivary flow, increasing risk of tooth decay, mucositis, and gum disease from xerostomia, especially for the elderly. For those wearing dentures, be sure to counsel removal and cleaning each night to reduce bacterial plaque and risk of malodor. Regular massage of the gums relieves soreness and pressure from dentures on the underlying soft tissue.

*U.S. Preventive Services Task Force: *Guide to Clinical Preventive Services,* 2nd ed. Baltimore, Williams & Wilkins, 1996, pp. 711–721.

**Greene JC and Greene AR: Chapter 15: Oral Health. In Woolf SH, Jonas S and Lawrence RS (eds): *Health Promotion and Disease Prevention in Clinical Practice.* Baltimore, Williams & Wilkins, 1996, pp. 315–334.

Table 7-1   Selected Facies

TABLE 7-1   Selected Facies

Acromegaly

The increased growth hormone of acromegaly produces enlargement of both bone and soft tissues. The head is elongated, with bony prominence of the forehead, nose, and lower jaw. Soft tissues of the nose, lips, and ears also enlarge. The facial features appear generally coarsened.

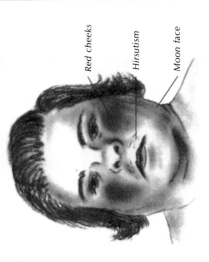

Brow prominent

Soft tissues of nose, ears, lips enlarged

Jaw prominent

Cushing's Syndrome

The increased adrenal hormone production of Cushing's syndrome produces a round or "moon" face with red cheeks. Excessive hair growth may be present in the mustache and sideburn areas and on the chin.

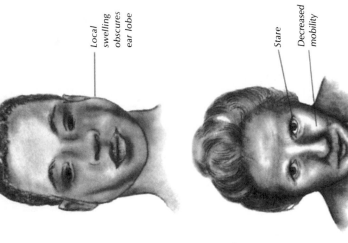

Red cheeks

Hirsutism

Moon face

Myxedema

The patient with severe hypothyroidism (*myxedema*) has a dull, puffy facies. The edema, often particularly pronounced around the eyes, does not pit with pressure. The hair and eyebrows are dry, coarse, and thinned. The skin is dry.

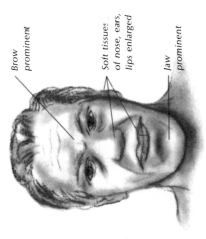

Hair dry, coarse, sparse

Lateral eyebrows thin

Periorbital edema

Puffy dull face with dry skin

Parotid Gland Enlargement

Chronic bilateral asymptomatic parotid gland enlargement may be associated with obesity, diabetes, cirrhosis, and other conditions. Note the swellings anterior to the ear lobes and above the angles of the jaw. Gradual unilateral enlargement suggests neoplasm. Acute enlargement is seen in mumps.

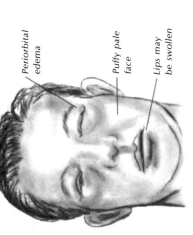

Local swelling obscures ear lobe

Nephrotic Syndrome

The face is edematous and often pale. Swelling usually appears first around the eyes and in the morning. The eyes may become slitlike when edema is severe.

Periorbital edema

Puffy pale face

Lips may be swollen

Parkinson's Disease

Decreased facial mobility blunts expression. A masklike face may result, with decreased blinking and a characteristic stare. Since the neck and upper trunk tend to flex forward, the patient seems to peer upward toward the observer. Facial skin becomes oily, and drooling may occur.

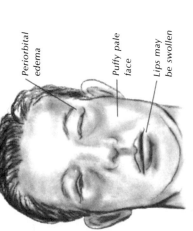

Stare

Decreased mobility

Table 7-2 Visual Field Defects

TABLE 7-2 *Visual Field Defects*

Visual Field Defects

Diagrammed from Patient's Viewpoint

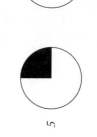

1

2

3

4

5

6

LEFT RIGHT

Visual Field Defects

Horizontal Defect

Occlusion of a branch of the central retinal artery may cause a horizontal (altitudinal) defect. Shown is the lower field defect associated with occlusion of the superior branch of this artery.

Blind Left Eye (left optic nerve)

A lesion of the optic nerve, and of course of the eye itself, produces unilateral blindness.

Bitemporal Hemianopsia (optic chiasm)

A lesion at the optic chiasm may involve only the fibers that are crossing over to the opposite side. Since these fibers originate in the nasal half of each retina, visual loss involves the temporal half of each field.

Right Homonymous Hemianopsia (left optic tract)

A lesion of the optic tract interrupts fibers originating on the same side of both eyes. Visual loss in the eyes is therefore similar (homonymous) and involves half of each field (hemianopsia).

Homonymous Right Upper Quadrantic Defect (left optic radiation, partial)

A partial lesion of the optic radiation may involve only a portion of the nerve fibers, producing, for example, a homonymous quadrantic defect.

Right Homonymous Hemianopsia (left optic radiation)

A complete interruption of fibers in the optic radiation produces a visual defect similar to that produced by a lesion of the optic tract.

Visual Pathways

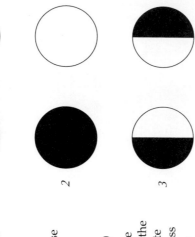

RIGHT VISUAL FIELD
Temporal Nasal

LEFT VISUAL FIELD
Nasal Temporal

Left Eye

Frontal lobe

Temporal lobe

Occipital lobe

Visual cortex

BASE (INFERIOR SURFACE) OF THE BRAIN

Optic radiation

Optic chiasm
Optic tract

Optic nerve

Right Eye

Table 7-3   Variations and Abnormalities of the Eyelids

TABLE 7-3   Variations and Abnormalities of the Eyelids

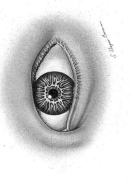

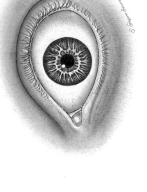

Ptosis

Ptosis is a drooping of the upper lid. Causes include myasthenia gravis, damage to the oculomotor nerve, and damage to the sympathetic nerve supply (*Horner's syndrome*). A weakened muscle, relaxed tissues, and the weight of herniated fat may cause senile ptosis. Ptosis may also be congenital.

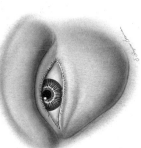
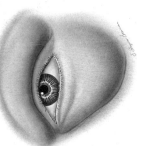
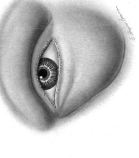

Retracted Lid

A wide-eyed stare suggests retracted eyelids—in this case, the upper lid. Note the rim of sclera between the upper lid and the iris. Retracted lids and a lid lag (p. 190) are often due to hyperthyroidism but may be seen in normal people. The eye does not protrude forward unless exophthalmos coexists.

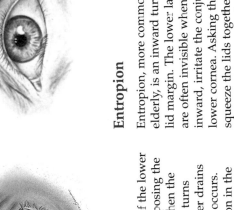

Epicanthus

An epicanthus (epicanthal fold) is a vertical fold of skin that lies over the medial canthus. It is normal among many Asian peoples. These folds are also seen in Down's syndrome and in a few other congenital conditions. They may falsely suggest a convergent strabismus (see p. 218).

Exophthalmos

In exophthalmos the eyeball protrudes forward. When bilateral, it suggests the infiltrative ophthalmopathy of Graves' disease, a form of hyperthyroidism. Edema of the eyelids and conjunctival injection may be associated. Unilateral exophthalmos may be due to Graves' disease or to a tumor or inflammation in the orbit.

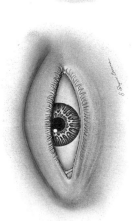

Ectropion

In ectropion the margin of the lower lid is turned outward, exposing the palpebral conjunctiva. When the punctum of the lower lid turns outward, the eye no longer drains satisfactorily and tearing occurs. Ectropion is more common in the elderly.

Entropion

Entropion, more common in the elderly, is an inward turning of the lid margin. The lower lashes, which are often invisible when turned inward, irritate the conjunctiva and lower cornea. Asking the patient to squeeze the lids together and then open them may reveal an entropion that is not obvious.

Periorbital Edema

Because the skin of the eyelids is loosely attached to underlying tissues, edema tends to accumulate there easily. Causes include allergies, local inflammation, cellulitis, myxedema, and fluid-retaining states such as the nephrotic syndrome.

Herniated Fat

Puffy eyelids may be caused by fat. It pushes weakened fascia in the eyelids forward, producing bulges that involve the lower lids, the inner third of the upper ones, or both. These bulges appear more often in elderly people but may affect younger ones.

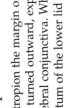

Table 7-4   Lumps and Swellings In and Around the Eyes

TABLE 7-4   Lumps and Swellings In and Around the Eyes

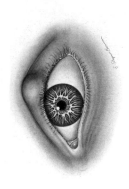

Pinguecula

A yellowish, somewhat triangular nodule in the bulbar conjunctiva on either side of the iris, a pinguecula is harmless. Pingueculae appear frequently with aging, first on the nasal and then on the temporal side.

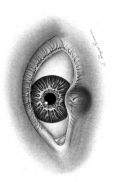

Sty (Acute Hordeolum)

A painful, tender, red infection around a hair follicle of the eyelashes, a sty looks like a pimple or boil pointing on the lid margin.

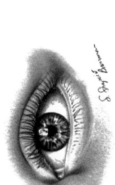
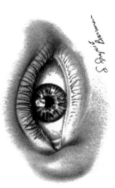

Chalazion

A chalazion is a chronic inflammatory lesion involving a meibomian gland. A beady nodule in an otherwise normal lid, it is usually painless. Occasionally a chalazion becomes acutely inflamed but, unlike a sty, usually points inside the lid rather than on the lid margin.

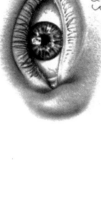
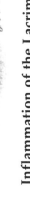

Inflammation of the Lacrimal Sac (Dacryocystitis)

A swelling between the lower eyelid and nose suggests inflammation of the lacrimal sac. An *acute* inflammation is painful, red, and tender. *Chronic* inflammation (illustrated) is associated with obstruction of the nasolacrimal duct. Tearing is prominent, and pressure on the sac produces regurgitation of material through the puncta of the eyelids.

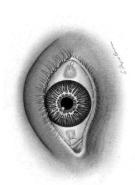

Episcleritis

Episcleritis is a localized ocular redness from inflammation of the episcleral vessels. In natural light, vessels appear salmon pink and are movable over the scleral surface. Usually benign and self-limited, episcleritis may be nodular, as shown here, or may show only redness and dilated vessels.

Xanthelasma

Slightly raised, yellowish, well circumscribed plaques in the skin, xanthelasmas appear along the nasal portions of one or both eyelids. They may accompany lipid disorders (e.g., hypercholesterolemia), but may also occur independently.

Table 7-5 Red Eyes

TABLE 7-5 Red Eyes

	Conjunctivitis	Corneal Injury or Infection	Acute Iritis	Glaucoma	Subconjunctival Hemorrhage
Pattern of Redness	Conjunctival injection: diffuse dilatation of conjunctival vessels with redness that tends to be maximal peripherally	Ciliary injection: dilation of deeper vessels that are visible as radiating vessels or a reddish violet flush around the limbus. Ciliary injection is an important sign of these three conditions but may not be apparent. The eye may be diffusely red instead. Other clues of these more serious disorders are pain, decreased vision, unequal pupils, and a less than perfectly clear cornea.			Leakage of blood outside of the vessels, producing a homogeneous, sharply demarcated, red area that fades over days to yellow and then disappears
Pain	Mild discomfort rather than pain	Moderate to severe, superficial	Moderate, aching, deep	Severe, aching, deep	Absent
Vision	Not affected except for temporary mild blurring due to discharge	Usually decreased	Decreased	Decreased	Not affected
Ocular Discharge	Watery, mucoid, or mucopurulent	Watery or purulent	Absent	Absent	Absent
Pupil	Not affected	Not affected unless iritis develops	May be small and, with time, irregular	Dilated, fixed	Not affected
Cornea	Clear	Changes depending on cause	Clear or slightly clouded	Steamy, cloudy	Clear
Significance	Bacterial, viral, and other infections; allergy; irritation	Abrasions, and other injuries; viral and bacterial infections	Associated with many ocular and systemic disorders	Acute increase in intraocular pressure—an emergency	Often none. May result from trauma, bleeding disorders, or a sudden increase in venous pressure, as from cough

Table 7-6 Opacities of the Cornea and Lens

TABLE 7-6 Opacities of the Cornea and Lens

Corneal Arcus

A corneal arcus is a thin grayish white arc or circle not quite at the edge of the cornea. It accompanies normal aging but may also be seen in younger people, especially African Americans. In young people, a corneal arcus suggests the possibility of hyperlipoproteinemia but does not prove it. Some surveys have revealed no relationship.

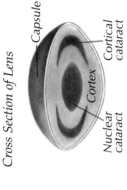

Corneal Scar

A corneal scar is a superficial grayish white opacity in the cornea, secondary to an old injury or to inflammation. Size and shape are variable. It should not be confused with the opaque lens of a cataract, visible on a deeper plane and only through the pupil.

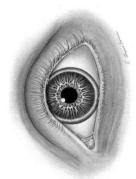

Pterygium

A pterygium is a triangular thickening of the bulbar conjunctiva that grows slowly across the outer surface of the cornea, usually from the nasal side. Reddening may occur intermittently. A pterygium may interfere with vision as it encroaches upon the pupil.

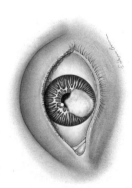
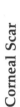

Cataracts

A cataract is an opacity of the lens and is seen through the pupil. Cataracts are classified in many ways, including cause and location. Old age is the most common cause. Two kinds of age-related cataract are illustrated below. In each example, the pupil has been widely dilated.

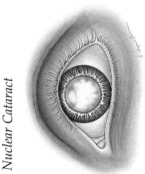

Cross Section of Lens

Capsule

Cortical cataract

Cortex

Nuclear cataract

Nuclear Cataract

A nuclear cataract looks gray when seen by a flashlight. If the pupil is widely dilated, the gray opacity is surrounded by a black rim. Through an ophthalmoscope, the cataract looks black against the red reflex.

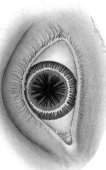

Peripheral Cataract

A peripheral cataract produces spokelike shadows that point inward—gray against black as seen with a flashlight, or black against red with an ophthalmoscope. A dilated pupil, as shown here, facilitates this observation.

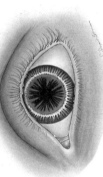

Table 7-7 *Pupillary Abnormalities*

TABLE 7-7 Pupillary Abnormalities

Unequal Pupils (*Anisocoria*)

When anisocoria is greater in bright light than in dim light, the larger pupil cannot constrict properly. Causes include blunt trauma to the eye, open-angle glaucoma (p. 188), and impaired parasympathetic nerve supply to the iris, as in tonic pupil and oculomotor nerve paralysis. When anisocoria is greater in dim light, the smaller pupil cannot dilate properly, as in Horner's syndrome, which is caused by an interruption of the sympathetic nerve supply.

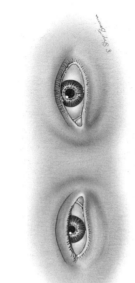

Tonic Pupil (*Adie's Pupil*)

A tonic pupil is large, regular, and usually unilateral. Its reaction to light is severely reduced and slowed, or even absent. The near reaction, though very slow, is present. Slow accommodation causes blurred vision. Deep tendon reflexes are often decreased.

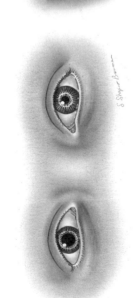

Oculomotor Nerve Paralysis

The dilated pupil (about 6–7 mm) is fixed to light and near effort. Ptosis of the upper eyelid and lateral deviation of the eye, as shown here, are often but not always present. (An even more dilated [8–9 mm] and fixed pupil may be due to local application of atropine-like agents.)

Light

Equal Pupils and One Blind Eye

Unilateral blindness does not cause anisocoria as long as the sympathetic and parasympathetic innervation to both irises is normal. A light directed into the seeing eye produces a direct reaction in that eye and a consensual reaction in the blind eye. A light directed into the blind eye, however, causes no response in either eye.

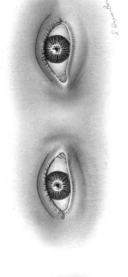

Horner's Syndrome

The affected pupil, though small, reacts briskly to light and near effort. Ptosis of the eyelid is present, perhaps with loss of sweating on the forehead of the same side. In congenital Horner's syndrome, the involved iris is lighter in color than its fellow (*heterochromia*).

Blind eye

Light

Small Irregular Pupils

Small, irregular pupils that do not react to light but do react to near effort indicate *Argyll Robertson pupils*. They are usually but not always caused by central nervous system syphilis.

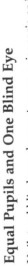

See also Table 18-8, Pupils in Comatose Patients, p. 619.

Table 7-8 Deviations of the Eyes

TABLE 7-8 Deviations of the Eyes

Deviation of the eyes from their normally conjugate position is termed *strabismus* or *squint*. Strabismus may be classified into two groups: (1) *nonparalytic*, in which the deviation is constant in all directions of gaze, and (2) *paralytic*, in which the deviation varies depending on the direction of gaze.

Nonparalytic Strabismus

Nonparalytic strabismus is caused by an imbalance in ocular muscle tone. It has many causes, may be hereditary, and usually appears early in childhood. Deviations are further classified according to direction:

Convergent Strabismus (Esotropia)

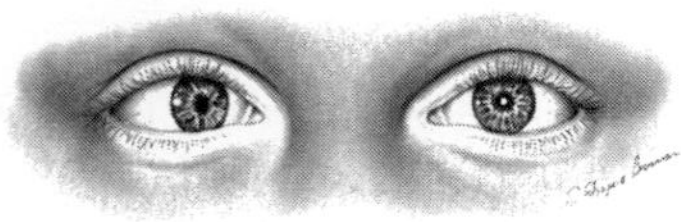

Divergent Strabismus (Exotropia)

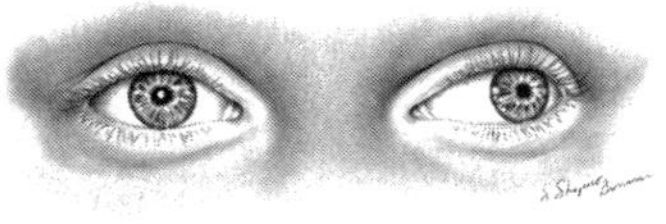

COVER–UNCOVER TEST

A cover–uncover test may be helpful. Here is what you would see in the right monocular esotropia illustrated above.

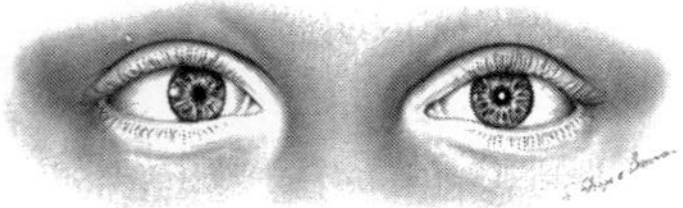

Corneal reflections are asymmetrical.

COVER

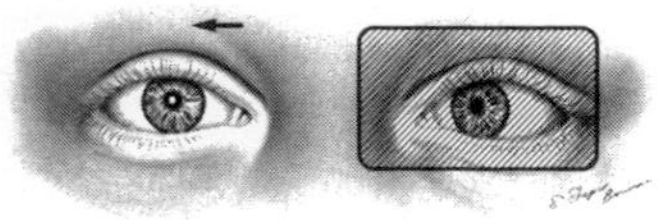

The right eye moves outward to fix on the light. (The left eye is not seen but moves inward to the same degree.)

UNCOVER

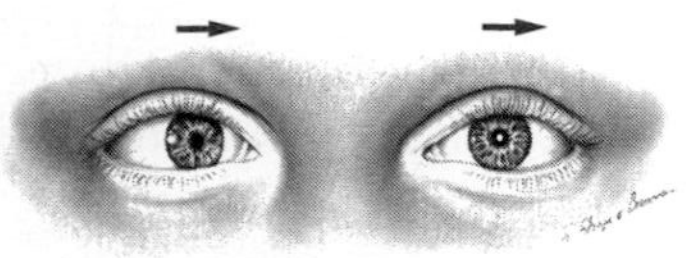

The left eye moves outward to fix on the light. The right eye deviates inward again.

Paralytic Strabismus

Paralytic strabismus is usually caused by weakness or paralysis of one or more extraocular muscles. Determine the direction of gaze that maximizes the deviation. For example:

A Left 6th Nerve Paralysis

LOOKING TO THE RIGHT

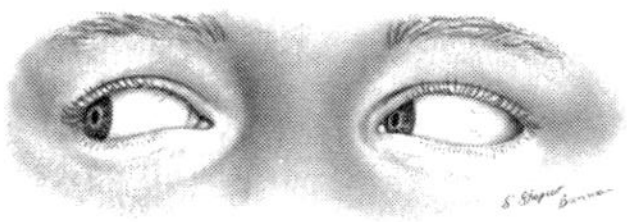

Eyes are conjugate.

LOOKING STRAIGHT AHEAD

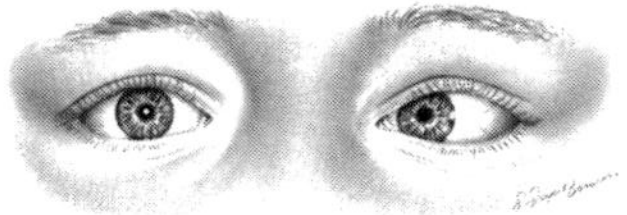

Esotropia appears.

LOOKING TO THE LEFT

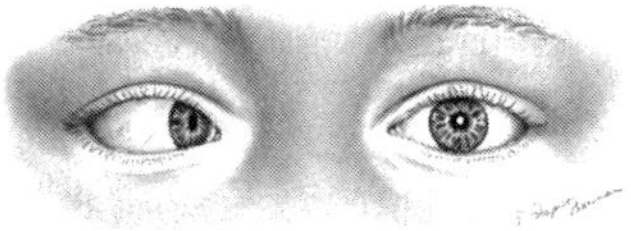

Esotropia is maximum.

A left 4th Nerve Paralysis

LOOKING DOWN AND TO THE RIGHT

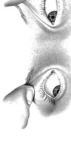

The left eye cannot look down when turned inward. Deviation is maximum in this direction.

A left 3rd Nerve Paralysis

LOOKING STRAIGHT AHEAD

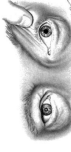

The eye is pulled outward by action of the 6th nerve. Upward, downward, and inward movements are impaired or lost. Ptosis and pupillary dilation may be associated.

Table 7-9   Normal Variations of the Optic Disc

TABLE 7-9   Normal Variations of the Optic Disc

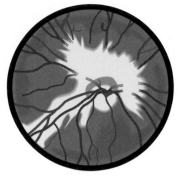

Medullated Nerve Fibers

Medullated nerve fibers are a much less common but dramatic finding. Appearing as irregular white patches with feathered margins, they obscure the disc edge and retinal vessels. They have no pathologic significance.

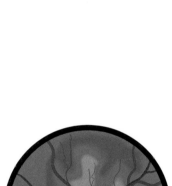

Rings and Crescents

Rings and crescents are often seen around the optic disc. These are developmental variations in which you can glimpse either white sclera, black retinal pigment, or both, especially along the temporal border of the disc. Rings and crescents are not part of the disc itself and should not be included in your estimates of disc diameters.

Central cup

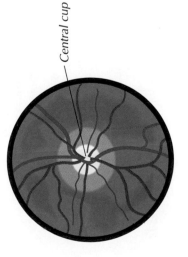

Temporal cup

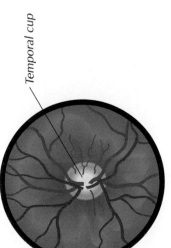

Physiologic Cupping

The physiologic cup is a small whitish depression in the optic disc from which the retinal vessels appear to emerge. Although sometimes absent, the cup is usually visible either centrally or toward the temporal side of the disc. Grayish spots are often seen at its base.

Table 7-10 Abnormalities of the Optic Disc

TABLE 7-10 Abnormalities of the Optic Disc

	Normal	Optic Atrophy	Papilledema	Glaucomatous Cupping
Process	Tiny disc vessels give normal color to the disc.	Death of optic nerve fibers leads to loss of the tiny disc vessels.	Venous stasis leads to engorgement and swelling.	Increased pressure within the eye leads to increased cupping (backward depression of the disc) and atrophy.
Appearance	Color yellowish orange to creamy pink	Color white	Color pink, hyperemic	The base of the enlarged cup is pale.
	Disc vessels tiny	Disc vessels absent	Disc vessels more visible, more numerous, curve over the borders of the disc	
	Disc margins sharp (except perhaps nasally)		Disc swollen with margins blurred	
	The physiologic cup is located centrally or somewhat temporally. It may be conspicuous or absent. Its diameter from side to side is usually less than half that of the disc.		The physiologic cup is not visible.	The physiologic cup is enlarged, occupying more than half of the disc's diameter, at times extending to the edge of the disc. Retinal vessels sink in and under it, and may be displaced nasally.

TABLE 7-11   Retinal Arteries and Arteriovenous Crossings: Normal and Hypertensive

Normal Retinal Artery and Arteriovenous (A-V) Crossing

The normal arterial wall is transparent. Only the column of blood within it can usually be seen. The normal light reflex is narrow—about ¼ the diameter of the blood column.

Because the arterial wall is transparent, a vein crossing beneath the artery can be seen right up to the column of blood on either side.

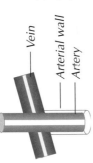

— Arterial wall (invisible)
— Column of blood
— Light reflex

— Vein
— Arterial wall
— Artery

The Retinal Arteries in Hypertension

SPASM AND THICKENING OF ARTERIAL WALLS

— Narrowed column of blood
— Narrowed light reflex

— Focal narrowing

In hypertension, the arteries may show areas of focal or generalized narrowing. The light reflex is also narrowed. Over many months or years, the arterial wall thickens and becomes less transparent.

COPPER WIRE ARTERIES

Sometimes the arteries, especially those close to the disc, become full and somewhat tortuous and develop an increased light reflex with a bright coppery luster. Such a vessel is called a copper wire artery.

SILVER WIRE ARTERIES

Occasionally a portion of a narrowed artery develops such an opaque wall that no blood is visible within it. It is then called a silver wire artery. This change typically occurs in the smaller branches.

Arteriovenous Crossing

When the arterial walls lose their transparency, changes appear in the arteriovenous crossings. Decreased transparency of the retina probably also contributes to the first two changes shown below.

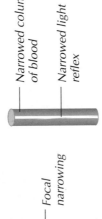

TAPERING

The vein appears to taper down on either side of the artery.

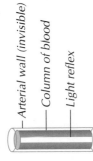

CONCEALMENT OR A-V NICKING

The vein appears to stop abruptly on either side of the artery.

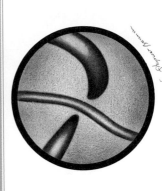

BANKING

The vein is twisted on the distal side of the artery and forms a dark, wide knuckle.

Table 7-12   Red Spots and Streaks in the Fundi

TABLE 7-12   Red Spots and Streaks in the Fundi

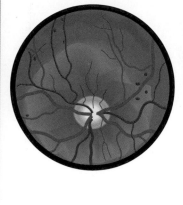

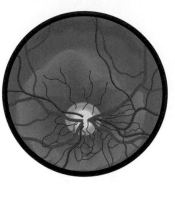

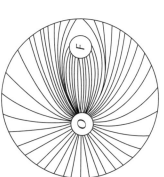

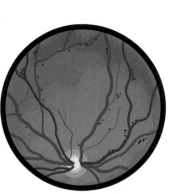

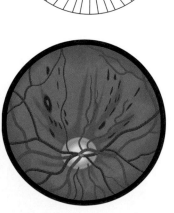

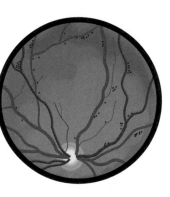

Superficial Retinal Hemorrhages

Superficial retinal hemorrhages are small, linear, flame-shaped, red streaks in the fundi. They are shaped by the superficial bundles of nerve fibers that radiate from the optic disc in the pattern illustrated (O = optic disc; F = fovea). Sometimes the hemorrhages occur in clusters and then simulate a larger hemorrhage, but the linear streaking at the edges shows their true nature. Superficial hemorrhages are seen in severe hypertension, papilledema, and occlusion of the retinal vein, among other conditions.

An occasional superficial hemorrhage has a white center consisting of fibrin. White-centered retinal hemorrhages have many causes.

Deep Retinal Hemorrhages

Deep retinal hemorrhages are small, rounded, slightly irregular red spots that are sometimes called dot or blot hemorrhages. They occur in a deeper layer of the retina than flame-shaped hemorrhages. Diabetes mellitus is a common cause.

Neovascularization

Neovascularization refers to the formation of new blood vessels. They are more numerous, more tortuous, and narrower than other blood vessels in the area and form disorderly-looking red arcades. A common cause is the late, proliferative stage of diabetic retinopathy. The vessels may grow into the vitreous, where retinal detachment or hemorrhage may cause loss of vision.

Preretinal Hemorrhage

A preretinal (subhyaloid) hemorrhage develops when blood escapes into the potential space between retina and vitreous. This hemorrhage is typically larger than retinal hemorrhages. Because it is anterior to the retina, it obscures any underlying retinal vessels. In an erect patient, red cells settle, creating a horizontal line of demarcation between plasma above and cells below. Causes include a sudden increase in intracranial pressure.

Microaneurysms

Microaneurysms are tiny, round, red spots seen commonly but not exclusively in and around the macular area. They are minute dilatations of very small retinal vessels, but the vascular connections are too small to be seen ophthalmoscopically. Microaneurysms are characteristic of diabetic retinopathy but not specific to it.

Table 7-13   Light-Colored Spots in the Fundi

TABLE 7-13   *Light-Colored Spots in the Fundi*

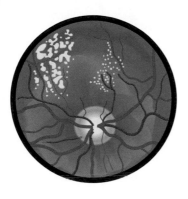

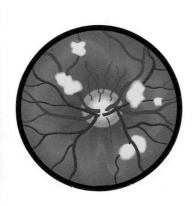

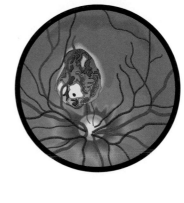

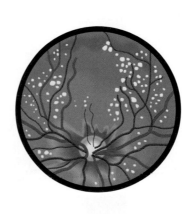

Cotton Wool Patches (*Soft Exudates*)

Cotton wool patches are white or grayish, ovoid lesions with irregular (thus "soft") borders. They are moderate in size but usually smaller than the disc. They result from infarcted nerve fibers and are seen with hypertension and many other conditions.

Hard Exudates

Hard exudates are creamy or yellowish, often bright lesions with well defined (thus "hard") borders. They are small and round (as shown in the lower group of exudates) but may coalesce into larger irregular spots (as shown in the upper group). They often occur in clusters or in circular, linear, or star-shaped patterns. Causes include diabetes and hypertension.

Drusen

Drusen are yellowish round spots that vary from tiny to small. They are haphazardly distributed but may concentrate at the posterior pole. Drusen appear with normal aging but may also accompany various conditions, including age-related macular degeneration.

Healed Chorioretinitis

Here inflammation has destroyed the superficial tissues to reveal a well defined, irregular patch of white sclera marked with dark pigment. Size varies from small to very large. Toxoplasmosis is illustrated. Multiple, small, somewhat similar-looking areas may be due to laser treatments.

Continued

Table 7-13   Light-Colored Spots in the Fundi

TABLE 7-13 (continued)

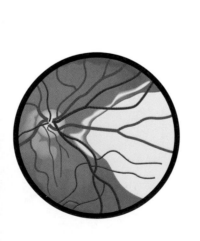

Coloboma

A coloboma of the choroid and retina is a developmental abnormality. A well demarcated, moderate-sized to large, white oval of sclera is visible below the disc, often extending well beyond the limits of your examination. Its borders may be pigmented.

Proliferative Diabetic Retinopathy

Bands or strands of white fibrous tissue develop in the late proliferative stage of diabetic retinopathy. They lie anterior to the retinal vessels and therefore obscure them. Neovascularization (p. 222) is typically associated.

Table 7-14   Ocular Fundi

TABLE 7-14   *Ocular Fundi*

Out of a piece of paper, cut a circle about the size of an optic disc shown below. The circle simulates an ophthalmoscope's light beam. Lay it on each illustration, and inspect each fundus systematically.

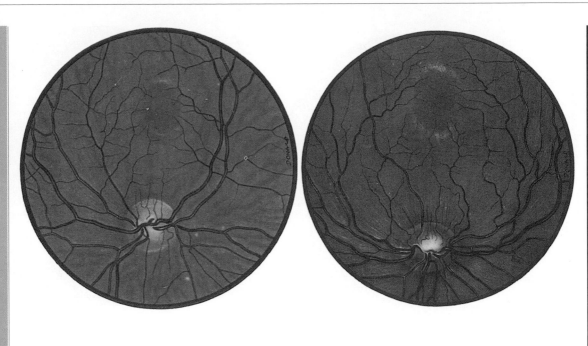

Normal Fundus of a Fair-Skinned Person

Find and inspect the optic disc. Follow the major vessels in four directions, noting their relative sizes and the nature of the arteriovenous crossings—both normal here. Inspect the macular area. The slightly darker fovea is just discernible; no light reflex is visible in this subject. Look for any lesions in the retina. Note the striped, or tessellated, character of the fundus, especially in the lower field. This comes from normal choroidal vessels that are unobscured by pigment.

Normal Fundus of a Dark-Skinned Person

Again, inspect the disc, the vessels, the macula, and the retinal background. The ring around the fovea is a normal light reflection. Compare the color of the fundus to that in the illustration above. It has a grayish brownish, almost purplish cast, which comes from pigment in the retina and the choroid. This pigment characteristically obscures the choroidal vessels, and no tessellation is visible. In contrast to either of these two figures, the fundus of a light-skinned person with brunette coloring is redder.

Continued

Table 7-14   Ocular Fundi

TABLE 7-14 (continued)

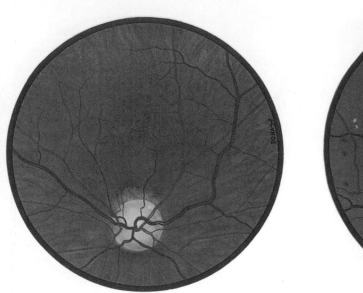

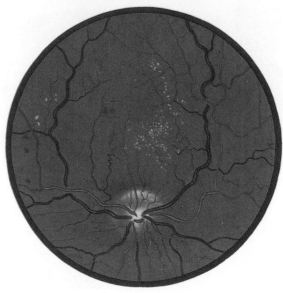

Normal Fundus of an Older Person

Inspect the fundus as before. What differences do you observe? Two characteristics of the aging fundus can be seen in this example. The blood vessels are straighter and narrower than those in younger people, and the choroidal vessels can be seen easily. In this person the optic disc is less pink, and pigment may be seen temporal to the disc and in the macular area.

Hypertensive Retinopathy

Inspect the fundus as before. The nasal border of the optic disc is blurred. The light reflexes from the arteries just above and below the disc are increased. Note the venous tapering—at the A–V crossing, about 1 disc diameter above the disc. Tapering and banking can be seen at 4:30 o'clock, 2 disc diameters from the disc. Punctate hard exudates and a few deep hemorrhages are readily visible.

Table 7-14   Ocular Fundi

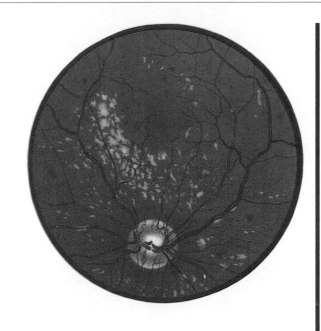

Hypertensive Retinopathy With Macular Star

Punctate exudates are readily visible here. Some are scattered, while others radiate from the fovea to form a macular star. Note the two small, soft exudates about 1 disc diameter from the disc. A number of flame-shaped hemorrhages sweep toward 4 o'clock and 5 o'clock, and a few more may be seen toward 2 o'clock.

The changes shown in both this and the previous illustration of hypertensive retinopathy are typical of accelerated (malignant) hypertension. The other important abnormality that may accompany these changes is papilledema (p. 220).

Diabetic Retinopathy

Punctate exudates have coalesced here into homogeneous, waxy-looking patches that are typical of diabetic retinopathy. What kinds of red spots can you find? Microaneurysms are most easily visible about 1 disc diameter below the disc. A few deep hemorrhages can also be seen, around 2 o'clock and 3 o'clock about 3 disc diameters from the disc.

This picture, with its combination of microaneurysms, deep hemorrhages, and hard exudates, is classified as background (*nonproliferative*) retinopathy. A later stage, known as *proliferative* retinopathy, includes neovascularization (p. 222), proliferating fibrous tissue (p. 224), and vitreous hemorrhages.

(Source of illustrations: Michaelson IC: Textbook of the Fundus of the Eye, 3rd ed. Edinburgh, Churchill Livingstone, 1980)

Table 7-15   Lumps On or Near the Ear

T A B L E 7 - 1 5   *Lumps On or Near the Ear*

Squamous Cell Carcinoma

Squamous cell carcinoma is most common in light-skinned people who have been frequently exposed to sunlight. This location on the helix and the raised, crusted border with central ulceration are both frequently seen. Biopsy confirms the diagnosis. A suture is present here. A squamous cell carcinoma spreads locally. Occasionally it metastasizes, most often to regional lymph nodes.

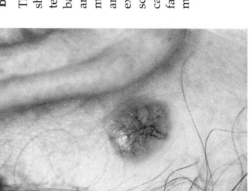

Basal Cell Carcinoma

The raised nodule behind this ear shows the lustrous surface and telangiectatic vessels that suggest basal cell carcinoma, a slow-growing and common malignancy that rarely metastasizes. Ulceration may occur, and in the absence of treatment extends in width and depth. Like squamous cell carcinoma, basal cell carcinoma occurs more frequently in fair-skinned people who have been much exposed to sunlight.

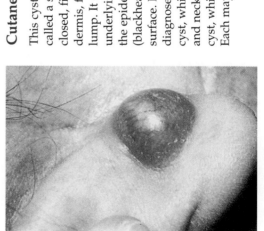

Chondrodermatitis Helicis

This chronic inflammatory lesion starts as a painful, tender papule that is usually on the helix but may be on the antihelix. Typically the lesion is single, but in this case two are visible. The lower papule is an early lesion; the upper lesion illustrates the later stage of ulceration and crusting. Reddening may occur. Older men are usually affected. To distinguish chondrodermatitis from carcinoma, a biopsy is needed.

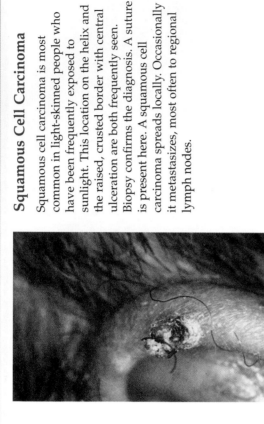

Cutaneous Cyst

This cyst behind the ear used to be called a sebaceous cyst. It is a benign, closed, firm sac that lies in the dermis, forming a dome-shaped lump. It can be moved over underlying tissues but is attached to the epidermis. A dark dot (blackhead) may be visible on its surface. Histologically, one of two diagnoses is likely: (1) *epidermoid* cyst, which is common on the face and neck, and (2) *pilar (trichilemmal)* cyst, which is common in the scalp. Each may become inflamed.

(Sources of photos: *Chondrodermatitis Helicis, Cutaneous Cyst*—Young EM Jr, Newcomer VD, Kligman AM: Geriatric Dermatology: Color Atlas and Practitioner's Guide. Philadelphia, Lea & Febiger, 1993; *Squamous Cell Carcinoma, Basal Cell Carcinoma*—Reprinted, by permission of the New England Journal of Medicine, 326:169–170, 1992)

Table 7-15   Lumps On or Near the Ear

Rheumatoid Nodules

In a patient with chronic arthritis, one or more small lumps on the helix or antihelix may be rheumatoid nodules of rheumatoid arthritis, as shown here. Do not mistake such lumps for tophi. Look for additional nodules elsewhere, e.g., on the hands, along the surface of the ulna distal to the elbow (pp. 546, 547), on the knees, and on the heels. Ulceration may result from repeated small injuries. Rheumatoid nodules may antedate the arthritis.

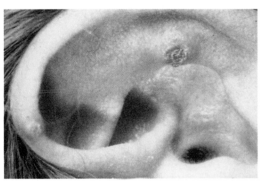

Lepromatous Leprosy

The ear is one of the sites for lepromatous leprosy, a form of Hansen's disease, which results from infection by *Mycobacterium leprae*. The multiple papules and nodules on this auricle are due to this chronic infection. Similar lesions would probably be visible on the face and elsewhere in the body. Now seldom seen in the United States, leprosy is still a worldwide problem. Other forms of the disease have different manifestations.

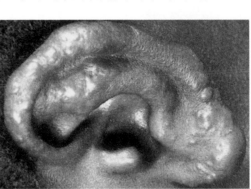

Tophi

A tophus is a deposit of uric acid crystals characteristic of chronic tophaceous gout. Tophi appear as hard nodules in the helix or antihelix and may discharge their chalky white crystals through the skin. Tophi may also appear near the joints, as in the hands (p. 547), feet, and other areas. Tophi usually develop only after years of sustained high blood levels of uric acid. With better control of hyperuricemia by drugs, tophi are becoming less common.

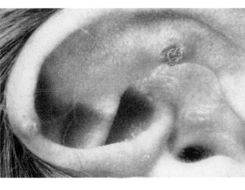

Keloid

A keloid is a firm, nodular, hypertrophic mass of scar tissue that extends beyond the area of injury. It may develop in any scarred area, but is most common on the shoulders and upper chest. A keloid on an earlobe that was pierced for earrings may be especially troublesome because of its cosmetic effects. Darker-skinned people are more likely than lighter ones to develop keloids. Recurrence of the growth may follow treatment.

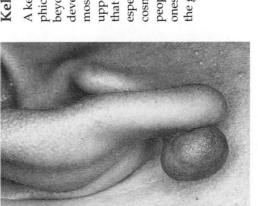

(Sources of photos: *Tophi, Lepromatous Leprosy*—From Atlas of Clinical Dermatology, 2nd ed, by Anthony du Vivier. London, UK, Gower Medical Publishing, 1993; *Rheumatoid Nodules*—Champion RH, Burton JL, Ebling FJG (eds): Rook/Wilkinson/Ebling Textbook of Dermatology, 5th ed. Oxford, Blackwell Scientific Publications Limited, 1992; *Keloid*—Sams WM Jr, Lynch PJ (eds): Principles and Practice of Dermatology. Edinburgh, Churchill Livingstone, 1990)

Table 7-16 Abnormalities of the Eardrum

TABLE 7-16   Abnormalities of the Eardrum

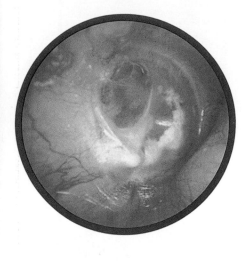

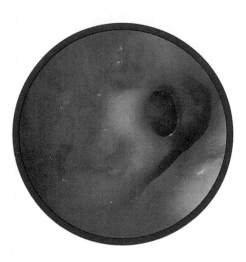

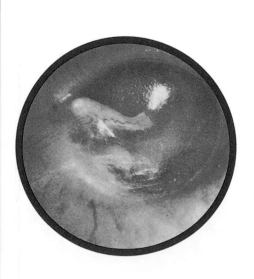

Normal Eardrum

This normal right eardrum (tympanic membrane) is pinkish gray. The handle of the malleus lies in a somewhat oblique position behind the upper part of the drum. The short process of the malleus pushes the membrane laterally, creating a small white elevation. Above the short process lies a small portion of the eardrum called the pars flaccida. The remainder of the drum is the pars tensa. Anterior and posterior malleolar folds, which extend obliquely upward from the short process, separate the pars flaccida from the pars tensa, but they are often invisible unless the eardrum is retracted. From the umbo the bright cone of light fans anteriorly and downward. Other light reflections seen in this photo are artifactual. Posterior to the malleus, part of the incus is visible behind the drum. The small blood vessels that course along the handle of the malleus are within the range of normal and do not indicate inflammation. The ear canal, which surrounds the eardrum, looks flatter than it really is because of distortion inherent in the photographic technique.

Perforation of the Drum

Perforations are holes in the eardrum that usually result from purulent infections of the middle ear. They are classified as *central* perforations, which do not extend to the margin of the drum, and *marginal* perforations, which do involve the margin.

The more common central perforation is illustrated here. In this case a reddened ring of granulation tissue surrounds the perforation, indicating a chronic infectious process. The eardrum itself is scarred and no landmarks are discernible. Discharge from the infected middle ear may drain out through such a perforation, but none is visible here.

A perforation of the eardrum often closes in the healing process, as illustrated in the next photo. The membrane covering the hole may be exceedingly thin and transparent.

Tympanosclerosis

In the inferior portion of this left eardrum there is a large, chalky white patch with irregular margins. It is typical of tympanosclerosis: a deposition of hyaline material within the layers of the tympanic membrane that sometimes follows a severe episode of otitis media. It does not usually impair hearing, and is seldom clinically significant.

Other abnormalities in this eardrum include a *healed perforation* (the large oval area in the upper posterior drum) and signs of a *retracted drum.* A retracted drum is pulled medially, away from the examiner's eye, and the malleolar folds are tightened into sharp outlines. The short process often protrudes sharply, and the handle of the malleus, pulled inward at the umbo, looks foreshortened and more horizontal.

(Sources of photos: *Normal eardrum*—Hawke M, Keene M, Alberti PW: Clinical Otoscopy: A Text and Colour Atlas. Edinburgh, Churchill Livingstone, 1984; *Perforation of the Drum, Tympanosclerosis*—Courtesy of Michael Hawke, M.D., Toronto, Canada)

Table 7-16   Abnormalities of the Eardrum

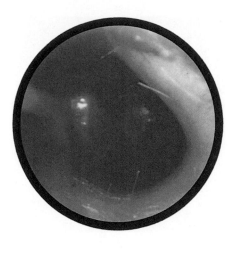

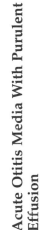

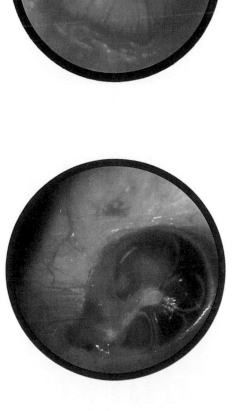

Serous Effusion

Serous effusions are usually caused by viral upper respiratory infections (*otitis media with serous effusion*) or by sudden changes in atmospheric pressure as from flying or diving (*otitic barotrauma*). The eustachian tube cannot equalize the air pressure in the middle ear with that of the outside air. Air is partly or completely absorbed from the middle ear into the bloodstream, and serous fluid accumulates there instead. Symptoms include fullness and popping sensations in the ear, mild conduction hearing loss, and perhaps some pain.

Amber fluid behind the eardrum is characteristic, as in this left drum of a patient with otitic barotrauma. A fluid level, a line between air above and amber fluid below, can be seen on either side of the short process. Air bubbles (not always present) can be seen here within the amber fluid.

Acute Otitis Media With Purulent Effusion

Acute otitis media with purulent effusion is caused by bacterial infection. Symptoms include earache, fever, and hearing loss. The eardrum reddens, loses its landmarks, and bulges laterally, toward the examiner's eye.

In this right ear the drum is bulging and most landmarks are obscured. Redness is most obvious near the umbo, but dilated vessels can be seen in all segments of the drum. A diffuse redness of the entire drum often develops. Spontaneous rupture (perforation) of the drum may follow, with discharge of purulent material into the ear canal.

Moving the auricle and pressing on the tragus do not cause pain in otitis media as they usually do in acute otitis externa. Hearing loss is of the conductive type. Acute purulent otitis media is much more common in children than in adults.

Bullous Myringitis

Bullous myringitis is a viral infection characterized by painful hemorrhagic vesicles that appear on the tympanic membrane, the ear canal, or both. Symptoms include earache, blood-tinged discharge from the ear, and hearing loss of the conductive type.

In this right ear, at least two large vesicles (bullae) are discernible on the drum. The drum is reddened, and its landmarks are obscured. Several different viruses may cause this condition.

(Sources of photos: *Serous Effusion*—Hawke M, Keene M, Alberti PW: Clinical Otoscopy: A Text and Colour Atlas. Edinburgh, Churchill Livingstone, 1984; *Acute Otitis Media, Bullous Myringitis*—The Wellcome Trust, National Medical Slide Bank, London, UK)

Table 7-17 *Patterns of Hearing Loss*

TABLE 7-17 Patterns of Hearing Loss

Hearing loss is of two major types. In *conductive hearing loss*, a disorder of the external or middle ear impairs the conduction of sound to the inner ear. In *sensorineural hearing loss*, a disorder of the inner ear, the cochlear nerve, or its central connections impairs the transmission of nerve impulses to the brain. A *mixed hearing loss* has both deficits.

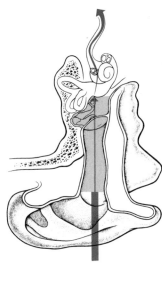

	Conductive Loss	Sensorineural Loss
Distortion of Sounds That Impairs the Understanding of Words	Relatively minor	Often present as the upper tones of words are disproportionately lost
Effect of a Noisy Environment	Hearing may seem to improve.	Hearing typically worsens.
Patient's Own Voice	Tends to be soft: the patient's voice is conducted through bone to a normal inner ear and cochlear nerve.	May be loud: the patient has trouble hearing his or her own voice.
Usual Age of Onset	Most often in childhood and young adulthood, up to age 40	Most often in the middle or later years.
Ear Canal and Drum	An abnormality is usually visible, except in otosclerosis.	The problem is not visible.

Table 7-17 Patterns of Hearing Loss

Weber Test *(in unilateral hearing loss)*

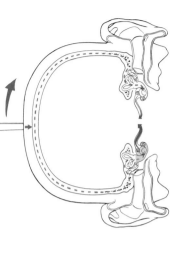 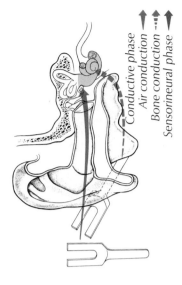

The sound lateralizes to the impaired ear. Because this ear is not distracted by room noise, it can detect the tuning fork's vibrations better than normal. (Test yourself while plugging one ear with your finger.) This lateralization disappears in an absolutely quiet room.

The sound lateralizes to the good ear. The impaired inner ear or cochlear nerve is less able to transmit impulses no matter how the sound reaches the cochlea. The sound is therefore heard in the better ear.

Conductive phase
Air conduction
Bone conduction
Sensorineural phase

Rinne Test

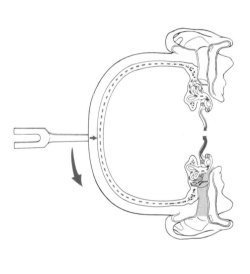 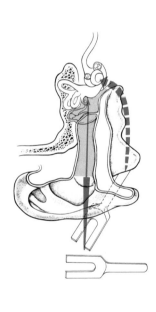

Bone conduction lasts longer than or is equal to air conduction (BC > AC or BC = AC). While air conduction through the external or middle ear is impaired, vibrations through bone bypass the problem to reach the cochlea.

Air conduction lasts longer than bone conduction (AC > BC). The inner ear or cochlear nerve is less able to transmit impulses regardless of how the vibrations reach the cochlea. The normal pattern prevails.

Causes Include:

Obstruction of the ear canal, otitis media, a perforated or relatively immobilized eardrum, and otosclerosis (a fixation of the ossicles by bony overgrowth)

Sustained exposure to loud noise, drugs, infections of the inner ear, trauma, tumors, congenital and hereditary disorders, and aging (presbycusis)

Further evaluation is done by audiometry and other specialized procedures.

Table 7-18   Abnormalities of the Lips

TABLE 7-18   *Abnormalities of the Lips*

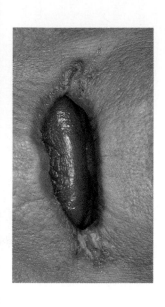

Angular Cheilitis

Angular cheilitis starts with softening of the skin at the angles of the mouth, followed by fissuring. It may be due to nutritional deficiency or, more commonly, to overclosure of the mouth, as in persons with no teeth or with ill-fitting dentures. Saliva wets and macerates the infolded skin, often leading to secondary infection with *Candida*, as in this example.

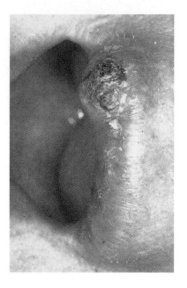

Carcinoma of the Lip

Like actinic cheilitis, carcinoma usually affects the lower lip. It may appear as a scaly plaque, as an ulcer with or without a crust, or as a nodular lesion, illustrated here. Fair skin and prolonged exposure to the sun are common risk factors.

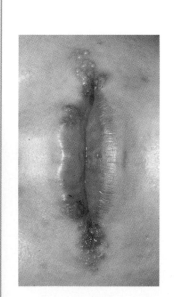

Herpes Simplex (*Cold Sore, Fever Blister*)

The herpes simplex virus (HSV) produces recurrent and painful vesicular eruptions of the lips and surrounding skin. A small cluster of vesicles first develops. As these break, yellow-brown crusts form, and healing ensues within 10 to 14 days. Both of these stages are visible here.

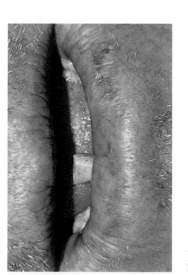

Actinic Cheilitis

Actinic cheilitis results from excessive exposure to sunlight and affects primarily the lower lip. Fair-skinned men who work outdoors are most often affected. The lip loses its normal redness and may become scaly, somewhat thickened, and slightly everted. Because solar damage also predisposes to carcinoma of the lip, be alert to this possibility.

(Sources of photos: *Herpes Simplex, Angular Cheilitis*—From Neville B et al: Color Atlas of Clinical Oral Pathology. Philadelphia, Lea & Febiger, 1991. Used with permission; *Actinic Cheilitis*—From Langlais RP, Miller CS: Color Atlas of Common Oral Diseases. Philadelphia, Lea & Febiger, 1992. Used with permission; *Carcinoma of the Lip*—Tyldesley WR: A Colour Atlas of Orofacial Diseases, 2nd ed. London, Wolfe Medical Publications, 1991)

Table 7-18   Abnormalities of the Lips

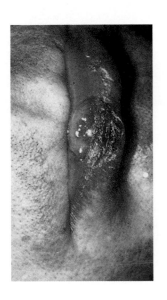

Angioedema

Angioedema is a diffuse, nonpitting, tense swelling of the dermis and subcutaneous tissue. It develops rapidly, and typically disappears over subsequent hours or days. Although usually allergic in nature and sometimes associated with hives, angioedema does not itch.

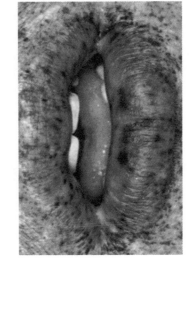

Chancre of Syphilis

This lesion of primary syphilis may appear on the lip rather than on the genitalia. It is a firm, buttonlike lesion that ulcerates and may become crusted. A chancre may resemble a carcinoma or a crusted cold sore. Because it is infectious, use gloves to feel any suspicious lesion.

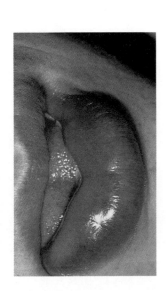

Hereditary Hemorrhagic Telangiectasia

Multiple small red spots on the lips strongly suggest hereditary hemorrhagic telangiectasia. Spots may also be visible on the face and hands and in the mouth. The spots are dilated capillaries and may bleed when traumatized. Affected people often have nosebleeds and gastrointestinal bleeding.

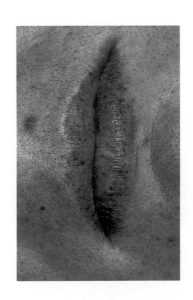

Peutz-Jeghers Syndrome

When pigmented spots on the lips are more prominent than freckling of the surrounding skin, suspect this syndrome. Pigment in the buccal mucosa helps to confirm the diagnosis. Pigmented spots may also be found on the face and hands. Multiple intestinal polyps are often associated.

(Sources of photos: *Angioedema*—From Neville B et al: Color Atlas of Clinical Oral Pathology. Philadelphia, Lea & Febiger, 1991. Used with permission; *Chancre of Syphilis*—Wisdom A: A Colour Atlas of Sexually Transmitted Diseases, 2nd ed. London, Wolfe Medical Publications, 1989; *Hereditary Hemorrhagic Telangiectasia*—From Langlais RP, Miller CS: Color Atlas of Common Oral Diseases. Philadelphia, Lea & Febiger, 1992. Used with permission; *Peutz–Jeghers Syndrome*—Robinson HBG, Miller AS: Colby, Kerr, and Robinson's Color Atlas of Oral Pathology. Philadelphia, JB Lippincott, 1990)

Table 7-19 Findings in the Pharynx, Palate, and Oral Mucosa

T A B L E 7 - 1 9   Findings in the Pharynx, Palate, and Oral Mucosa

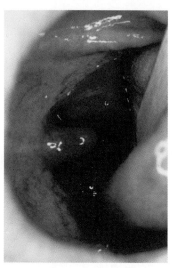

A

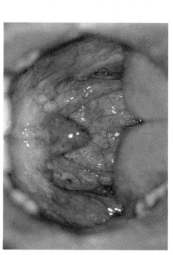

B

Pharyngitis

These two photos show reddened throats without exudate. In *A*, redness and vascularity of the pillars and uvula are mild to moderate. In *B*, redness is diffuse and intense. Each patient would probably complain of a sore throat, or at least a scratchy one. Possible causes include several kinds of viruses and bacteria. If the patient has no fever, exudate, or enlargement of cervical lymph nodes, the chances of infection by either of two common and important causes—group A streptococci and Epstein-Barr virus (infectious mononucleosis)—are very small.

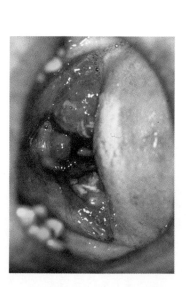

Exudative Tonsillitis

This red throat has a white exudate on the tonsils. This, together with fever and enlarged cervical nodes, increases the probability of group A streptococcal infection, or infectious mononucleosis. Some anterior cervical lymph nodes are usually enlarged in the former, posterior nodes in the latter.

Diphtheria

Diphtheria (an acute infection caused by *Corynebacterium diphtheriae*) is now rare but still important. Prompt diagnosis may lead to life-saving treatment. The throat is dull red, and a gray exudate (pseudomembrane) is present on the uvula, pharynx, and tongue. The airway may become obstructed.

(Sources of photos: *Pharyngitis (A and B)*, *Exudative Tonsillitis*—The Wellcome Trust, National Medical Slide Bank, London, UK; *Diphtheria*—Reproduced with permission from Harnisch JP et al: Diphtheria among alcoholic urban adults. Ann Intern Med 1989;111:77)

Table 7-19   *Findings in the Pharynx, Palate, and Oral Mucosa*

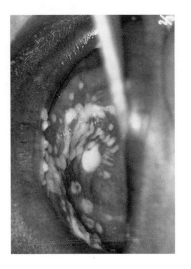

Thrush on the Palate (Candidiasis)

Thrush is a yeast infection due to *Candida*. Shown here on the palate, it may appear elsewhere in the mouth (see p. 242). Thick, white plaques are somewhat adherent to the underlying mucosa. Predisposing factors include (1) prolonged treatment with antibiotics or corticosteroids, and (2) AIDS.

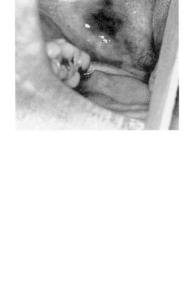

Kaposi's Sarcoma in AIDS

The deep purple color of these lesions, although not necessarily present, strongly suggests Kaposi's sarcoma. The lesions may be raised or flat. Among people with AIDS, the palate, as illustrated here, is a common site for this tumor.

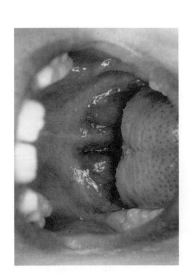

Large Normal Tonsils

Normal tonsils may be large without being infected, especially in children. They may protrude medially beyond the pillars and even to the midline. Here they touch the sides of the uvula and obscure the pharynx. Their color is within normal limits. The white marks are light reflections, not exudate.

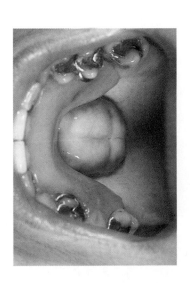

Torus Palatinus

A torus palatinus is a midline bony growth in the hard palate that is fairly common in adults. Its size and lobulation vary. Although alarming at first glance, it is harmless. In this example, an upper denture has been fitted around the torus.

(Sources of photos: *Large Normal Tonsils, Thrush on the Palate*—The Wellcome Trust, National Medical Slide Bank, London, UK; *Kaposi's Sarcoma in AIDS*—Joachim HL: Textbook and Atlas of Disease Associated With Acquired Immune Deficiency Syndrome. London, UK, Gower Medical Publishing, 1989)

➡ *Continued*

Table 7-19   Findings in the Pharynx, Palate, and Oral Mucosa

TABLE 7-19   (continued)

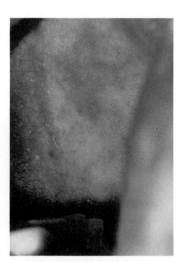

Koplik's Spots

Koplik's spots are an early sign of measles (rubeola). Search for small white specks that resemble grains of salt on a red background. They usually appear on the buccal mucosa near the first and second molars. In this photo, look also in the upper third of the mucosa. The rash of measles appears within a day.

Fordyce Spots *(Fordyce Granules)*

Fordyce spots are normal sebaceous glands that appear as small yellowish spots in the buccal mucosa or on the lips. A worried person who has suddenly noticed them may be reassured. Here they are seen best anterior to the tongue and lower jaw. These spots are usually not so numerous.

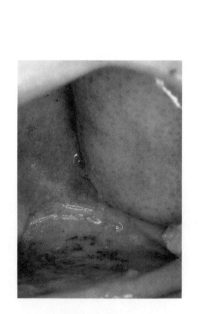

Petechiae

Petechiae are small red spots that result when blood escapes from capillaries into the tissues. Petechiae in the buccal mucosa, as shown, are often caused by accidentally biting the cheek. Oral petechiae may be due to infection or decreased platelets, as well as to trauma.

Leukoplakia

A thickened white patch (leukoplakia) may occur anywhere in the oral mucosa. The extensive example shown on this buccal mucosa resulted from frequent chewing of tobacco, a local irritant. This kind of irritation may lead to cancer.

(Sources of photos: *Koplik's Spots, Petechiae*—The Wellcome Trust, National Medical Slide Bank, London, UK; *Fordyce Spots*—From Neville B et al: Color Atlas of Clinical Oral Pathology. Philadelphia, Lea & Febiger, 1991. Used with permission; *Leukoplakia*—Robinson HBG, Miller AS: Colby, Kerr, and Robinson's Color Atlas of Oral Pathology. Philadelphia, JB Lippincott, 1990)

Table 7-20   Findings in the Gums and Teeth

TABLE 7-20   Findings in the Gums and Teeth

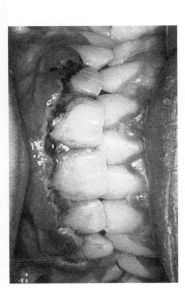

Marginal Gingivitis

Marginal gingivitis is common among teenagers and young adults. The gingival margins are reddened and swollen, and the interdental papillae are blunted, swollen, and red. Brushing the teeth often makes the gums bleed. *Plaque*—the soft white film of salivary salts, protein, and bacteria that covers the teeth and leads to gingivitis—is not readily visible.

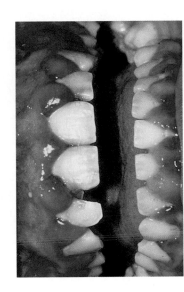

Acute Necrotizing Ulcerative Gingivitis

This uncommon form of gingivitis occurs suddenly in adolescents and young adults and is accompanied by fever, malaise, and enlarged lymph nodes. Ulcers develop in the interdental papillae. Then the destructive (necrotizing) process spreads along the gum margins, where a grayish pseudomembrane develops. The red, painful gums bleed easily; the breath is foul.

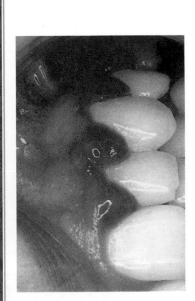

Chronic Gingivitis and Periodontitis

Chronic, untreated gingivitis may progress to periodontitis—inflammation of the deeper tissues, that normally hold the teeth in place. Attachments between gums and teeth are gradually destroyed, the gum margins recede, and the teeth eventually loosen. *Calculus* (calcified plaque), seen here as hard, cream-colored deposits on the teeth, contributes to the inflammation.

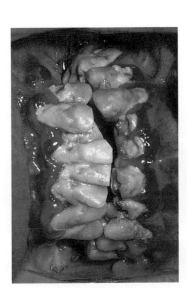

Gingival Hyperplasia

Gums enlarged by hyperplasia are swollen into heaped-up masses that may even cover the teeth. The redness of inflammation may coexist, as in this example. Causes include Dilantin therapy (as in this case), puberty, pregnancy, and leukemia.

(Sources of photos: *Marginal Gingivitis, Acute Necrotizing Ulcerative Gingivitis*—Tyldesley WR: A Colour Atlas of Orofacial Diseases, 2nd ed. London, Wolfe Medical Publications, 1991; *Chronic Gingivitis and Periodontitis* (Courtesy of Dr. Tom McDavid), *Gingival Hyperplasia* (Courtesy of Dr. James Cottone)—From Langlais RP, Miller CS: Color Atlas of Common Oral Diseases. Philadelphia, Lea & Febiger, 1992. Used with permission)

Continued

Table 7-20   *Findings in the Gums and Teeth*

TABLE 7-20 *(continued)*

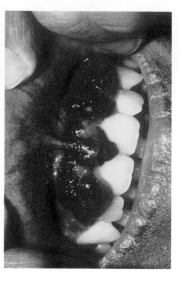

Pregnancy Tumor (Epulis, Pyogenic Granuloma)

Gingival enlargement may be localized, forming a tumorlike mass that usually originates in an interdental papilla. It is red and soft and usually bleeds easily. The estimated incidence of this lesion in pregnancy is about 1%. Note the accompanying gingivitis in this example.

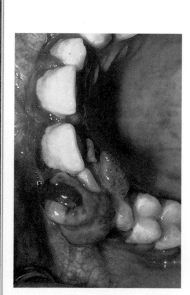

Lead Line

Now rare, a bluish black line on the gums may signal chronic lead poisoning. The line is about 1 mm from the gum margin, follows its contours, and is absent where there are no teeth. In this example, as is common, periodontitis coexists.

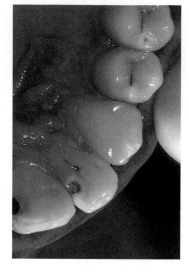

Kaposi's Sarcoma in AIDS

In people with AIDS, Kaposi's sarcoma may appear in the gums, as in other structures. The shape of the lesions in this advanced example might suggest hyperplasia, but the color suggests Kaposi's sarcoma. Be alert for less obvious lesions.

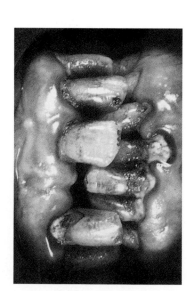

Dental Caries

Dental caries is first visible as a chalky white area in the enamel surface of a tooth. This area may then turn brown or black, become soft, and cavitate. Special dental techniques, including x-rays, are necessary for early detection.

(Sources of photos: *Pregnancy Tumor, Dental Caries*—From Langlais RP, Miller CS: Color Atlas of Common Oral Diseases. Philadelphia, Lea & Febiger 1992. Used with permission; *Kaposi's Sarcoma in AIDS*—Kelley WN (ed): Textbook of Internal Medicine, 2nd ed. Philadelphia, JB Lippincott, 1992; *Lead Line*—Courtesy of Dr. R. A. Cawson, from Cawson RA: Oral Pathology, 1st ed. London, UK, Gower Medical Publishing, 1987)

Table 7-20   Findings in the Gums and Teeth

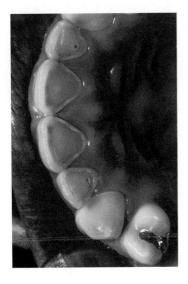

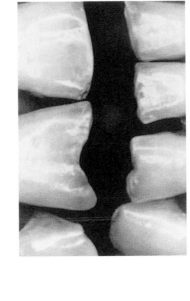

Erosion of Teeth

Teeth may be eroded by chemical action. Note here the erosion of the enamel from the lingual surfaces of the upper incisors, exposing the yellow-brown dentin. This results from recurrent regurgitation of stomach contents, as in bulimia.

Abrasion of Teeth With Notching

The biting surface of the teeth may become abraded or notched by recurrent trauma, such as holding nails or opening bobby pins between the teeth. Unlike Hutchinson's teeth, the sides of these teeth show normal contours; size and spacing of the teeth are unaffected.

Attrition of Teeth; Recession of Gums

In many elderly people, the chewing surfaces of the teeth have been worn down by repetitive use so that the yellow-brown dentin becomes exposed—a process called *attrition*. Note also the *recession of the gums*, which has exposed the roots of the teeth, giving a "long in the tooth" appearance.

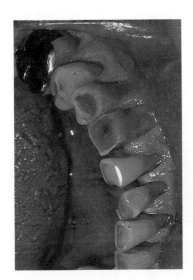

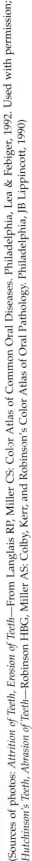

Hutchinson's Teeth

Hutchinson's teeth are smaller and more widely spaced than normal and are notched on their biting surfaces. The sides of the teeth taper toward the biting edges. The upper central incisors of the permanent (not the deciduous) teeth are most often affected. These teeth are a sign of congenital syphilis.

(Sources of photos: *Attrition of Teeth, Erosion of Teeth*—From Langlais RP, Miller CS: Color Atlas of Common Oral Diseases. Philadelphia, Lea & Febiger, 1992. Used with permission; *Hutchinson's Teeth, Abrasion of Teeth*—Robinson HBG, Miller AS: Colby, Kerr, and Robinson's Color Atlas of Oral Pathology. Philadelphia, JB Lippincott, 1990)

Table 7-21 Findings In or Under the Tongue

TABLE 7-21 Findings In or Under the Tongue

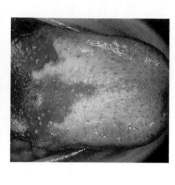

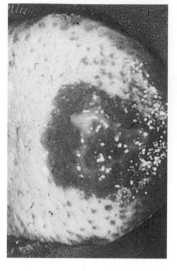

Geographic Tongue

The dorsum of a geographic tongue shows scattered smooth red areas that are denuded of papillae. Together with the normal rough and coated areas, they give a maplike pattern that changes over time. Of unknown cause, the condition is benign.

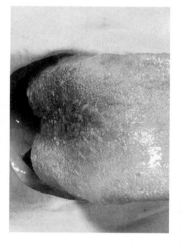

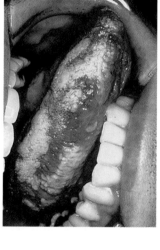

Hairy Tongue

The "hair" of hairy tongue consists of elongated papillae on the dorsum of the tongue, and is yellowish to brown or black. Hairy tongue may follow antibiotic therapy but may also occur spontaneously, without known cause. It is harmless.

Candidiasis

The thick white coat on this tongue is due to *Candida* infection. A raw red surface is left where the coat was scraped off. This infection may also cause redness of the tongue without the white coat. AIDS, among other factors, predisposes to this condition.

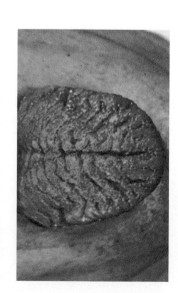

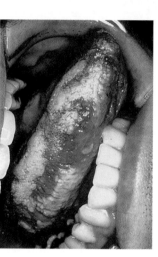

Fissured Tongue

Fissures may appear in the tongue with increasing age. Their appearance has led to the alternate term, *scrotal tongue.* Although food debris may accumulate in the crevices and become irritating, a fissured tongue usually has little significance.

Smooth Tongue *(Atrophic Glossitis)*

A smooth and often sore tongue that has lost its papillae suggests a deficiency in riboflavin, niacin, folic acid, vitamin B_{12}, pyridoxine, or iron. Specific diagnosis is often difficult. Anticancer drugs may also be responsible.

Hairy Leukoplakia

Whitish raised areas that have a feathery or corrugated pattern suggest hairy leukoplakia. Unlike candidiasis, these areas cannot be scraped off. The sides of the tongue are most often affected. This lesion is seen in HIV infection and AIDS.

(Sources of photos: *Fissured Tongue, Candidiasis*—Robinson HBG, Miller AS: Colby, Kerr, and Robinson's Color Atlas of Oral Pathology. Philadelphia, JB Lippincott, 1990; *Smooth Tongue*—Courtesy of Dr. R. A. Cawson, from Cawson RA: Oral Pathology. 1st ed. London, UK, Gower Medical Publishing, 1987; *Geographic Tongue*—The Wellcome Trust, National Medical Slide Bank, London, UK; *Hairy Leukoplakia*—Ioachim HL: Textbook and Atlas of Disease Associated With Acquired Immune Deficiency Syndrome. London, UK, Gower Medical Publishing, 1989)

Table 7-21   *Findings In or Under the Tongue*

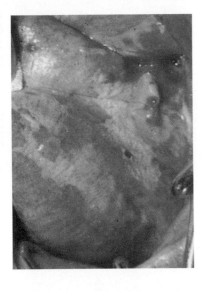

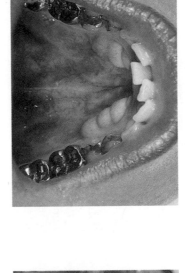

Leukoplakia

A persisting painless white patch in the oral mucosa is often called leukoplakia until biopsy reveals its nature. Here, the undersurface of the tongue looks as if it had been painted white. Mucous patches are more common. Leukoplakia of any size raises the possibility of malignant change.

Tori Mandibulares

Tori mandibulares are rounded bony protuberances that grow from the inner surfaces of the mandible. They are typically bilateral and asymptomatic. The overlying mucosa is normal in color. Like a torus palatinus (p. 237), these tori are harmless.

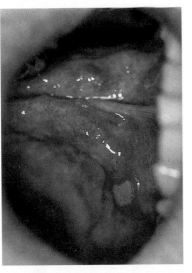

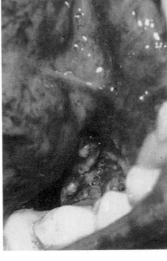

Aphthous Ulcer *(Canker Sore)*

A painful, small, round or oval ulcer that is white or yellowish gray and surrounded by a halo of reddened mucosa typifies the common aphthous ulcer. These ulcers may be single or multiple. They heal in 7 to 10 days, but may recur.

Carcinoma, Floor of the Mouth

This ulcerated lesion is in a common location for carcinoma, which also occurs on the side of the tongue. Medial to the carcinoma, note the reddened area of mucosa, called *erythroplakia*. Like leukoplakia, erythroplakia warns of possible malignancy.

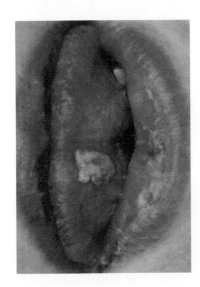

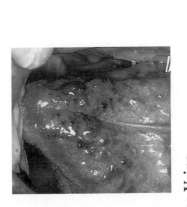

Mucous Patch of Syphilis

This painless lesion occurs in the secondary stage of syphilis and is highly infectious. It is slightly raised, oval, and covered by a grayish membrane. Mucous patches may be multiple and occur elsewhere in the mouth.

Varicose Veins

Small purplish or blue-black round swellings may appear under the tongue with age. They are dilatations of the lingual veins and have no clinical significance. Reassure a worried patient. These varicosities are also called *caviar lesions.*

(Sources of photos: *Mucous Patch, Leukoplakia, Carcinoma*—Robinson HBG, Miller AS: Colby, Kerr, and Robinson's Color Atlas of Oral Pathology. Philadelphia, JB Lippincott, 1990; *Varicose Veins*—From Neville B et al: Color Atlas of Clinical Oral Pathology. Philadelphia, Lea & Febiger, 1991. Used with permission)

Table 7-22 Thyroid Enlargement and Function

TABLE 7-22 Thyroid Enlargement and Function

Evaluation of the thyroid gland includes a description of the gland and a functional assessment.

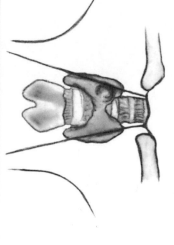

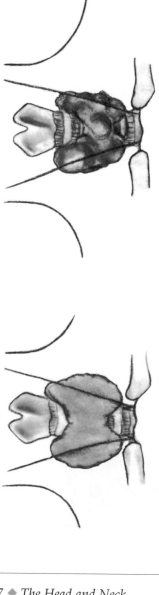

Diffuse Enlargement

A diffusely enlarged gland includes the isthmus and the lateral lobes, but there are no discretely palpable nodules. Causes include Graves' disease, Hashimoto's thyroiditis, and endemic goiter (related to iodine deficiency, now uncommon in the United States). Sporadic goiter refers to an enlarged gland with no apparent cause.

Multinodular Goiter

This term refers to an enlarged thyroid gland that contains two or more identifiable nodules. Multiple nodules suggest a metabolic rather than a neoplastic process, but irradiation during childhood, a positive family history, enlarged cervical nodes, or continuing enlargement of one of the nodules raises the suspicion of malignancy.

Single Nodule

A clinically single nodule may be a cyst, a benign tumor, or one nodule within a multinodular gland, but it also raises the question of a malignancy. Prior irradiation, hardness, rapid growth, fixation to surrounding tissues, enlarged cervical nodes, and occurrence in males increase the probability of malignancy.

Symptoms of Thyroid Dysfunction

Hyperthyroidism	Hypothyroidism
Nervousness	Fatigue, lethargy
Weight loss despite an increased appetite	Modest weight gain with anorexia
Excessive sweating and heat intolerance	Dry, coarse skin and cold intolerance
Palpitations	Swelling of face, hands, and legs
Frequent bowel movements	Constipation
Muscular weakness of the proximal type and tremor	Weakness, muscle cramps, arthralgias, paresthesias, impaired memory and hearing

Signs of Thyroid Dysfunction

Hyperthyroidism	Hypothyroidism
Tachycardia or atrial fibrillation	Bradycardia and, in late stages, hypothermia
Increased systolic and decreased diastolic blood pressures	Decreased systolic and increased diastolic blood pressures
Hyperdynamic cardiac pulsations with an accentuated S_1	Intensity of heart sounds sometimes decreased
Warm, smooth, moist skin	Dry, coarse, cool skin, sometimes yellowish from carotene, with nonpitting edema and loss of hair
Tremor and proximal muscle weakness	Impaired memory, mixed hearing loss, somnolence, peripheral neuropathy, carpal tunnel syndrome
With Graves' disease, eye signs such as stare, lid lag, and exophthalmos	Periorbital puffiness

The Thorax and Lungs

CHAPTER 8

Anatomy and Physiology

Review the *anatomy of the chest wall,* identifying the structures illustrated. Note that an interspace between two ribs is numbered by the rib above it.

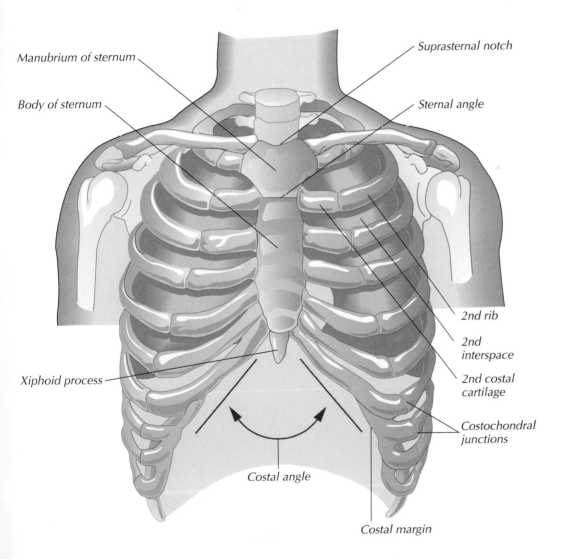

Manubrium of sternum

Body of sternum

Xiphoid process

Suprasternal notch

Sternal angle

2nd rib

2nd interspace

2nd costal cartilage

Costochondral junctions

Costal angle

Costal margin

Locating Findings on the Chest. To describe an abnormality on the chest, you need to locate it in two dimensions: along the vertical axis and around the circumference of the chest.

To locate vertically, you must be able to number the ribs and interspaces accurately. The *sternal angle* (angle of Louis) is the best guide. To find it, identify the suprasternal notch, and then move your finger down about 5 cm to find the horizontal bony ridge that joins the manubrium to the body of the sternum. Then move your finger laterally and find the adjacent 2nd rib and costal cartilage. From here, using two fingers, you can "walk down the interspaces," one space at a time, on an oblique line illustrated by the red numbers below. Do not try to count interspaces along the lower edge of the sternum; the ribs there are too close together. In a woman, to find the interspaces, either displace the breast laterally or palpate a little more medially than illustrated. Avoid pressing too hard on tender breast tissue.

Note that the costal cartilages of the first seven ribs articulate with the sternum. Those of the 8th, 9th, and 10th ribs articulate with the costal cartilages just above them. The 11th and 12th ribs, the so-called floating ribs, have no anterior attachments. The cartilaginous tip of the 11th rib can usually be felt laterally, and the 12th rib may be felt posteriorly. On palpation, costal cartilages cannot be distinguished from ribs.

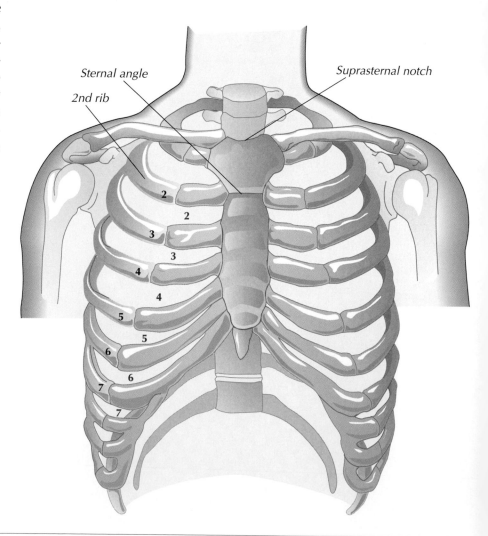

Sternal angle

Suprasternal notch

2nd rib

Posteriorly, the 12th rib gives you another possible starting point for counting ribs and interspaces. This is especially useful in locating findings on the lower posterior chest, and also helps when the anterior approach is unsatisfactory. With the fingers of one hand, press inward and up against the lower border of the 12th rib (see arrow). Then "walk" upward in the interspaces, numbered in red below, or obliquely upward and around to the front of the chest.

When estimating location, remember that the inferior angle of the scapula usually lies at the level of the 7th rib or interspace.

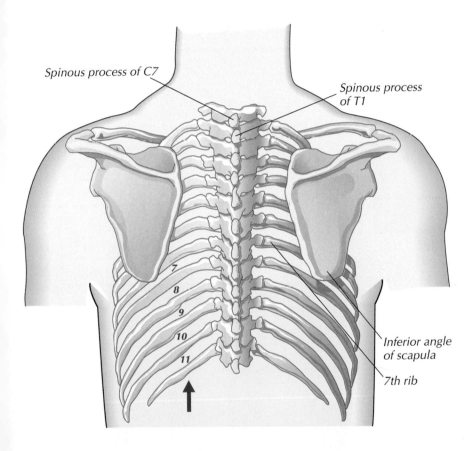

The spinous processes of the vertebrae can also help locate findings. When the neck is flexed forward, the most prominent process is usually that of C7. When two processes appear equally prominent, they are C7 and T1. The processes below them can often be felt and counted, especially when the spine is flexed.

To locate findings around the circumference of the chest, use a series of vertical lines, shown in the next three illustrations. The midsternal and vertebral lines are precise; the others are estimated. The midclavicular line drops vertically from the midpoint of the clavicle. To find it, you must identify both ends of the clavicle accurately (see p. 487). The anterior and posterior axillary lines drop vertically from the anterior and posterior axillary folds (the muscle masses that border the axilla). The midaxillary line drops from the apex of the axilla.

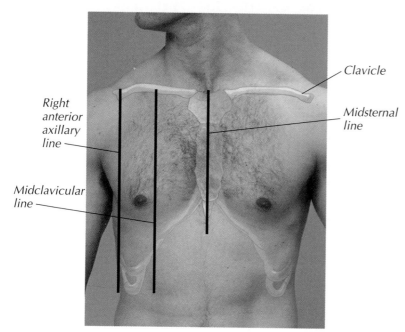

Right anterior axillary line

Midclavicular line

Clavicle

Midsternal line

ANTERIOR VIEW

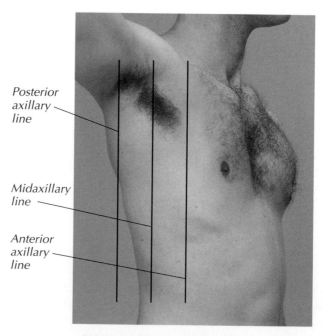

Posterior axillary line

Midaxillary line

Anterior axillary line

RIGHT ANTERIOR OBLIQUE VIEW

Posteriorly, the vertebral line follows the spinous processes of the vertebrae. Each scapular line drops from the inferior angle of the scapula.

Lungs, Fissures, and Lobes. The lungs and their fissures and lobes can be outlined mentally on the chest wall. Anteriorly, the apex of each lung rises about 2 cm to 4 cm above the inner third of the clavicle. The lower border of the lung crosses the 6th rib at the midclavicular line and the 8th rib at the midaxillary line. (Because ribs slant, a fairly horizontal line can drop a rib or more as it passes across the chest.) Posteriorly, the lower border of the lung lies at about the level of the T10 spinous process. On inspiration, it descends farther.

Each lung is divided about in half by an *oblique (major) fissure.* This fissure may be approximated by a string that runs from the T3 spinous process obliquely down and around the chest to the 6th rib at the midclavicular line. The right lung is further divided by the *horizontal (minor) fissure.* Anteriorly, this fissure runs close to the 4th rib and meets the oblique fissure in the midaxillary line near the 5th rib.

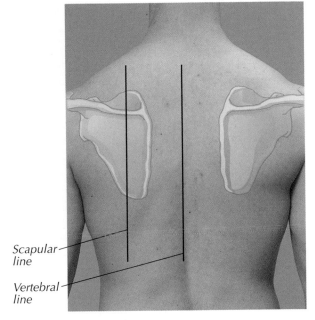

Scapular line

Vertebral line

POSTERIOR VIEW

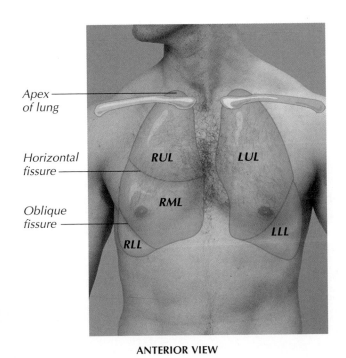

Apex of lung

Horizontal fissure

Oblique fissure

RUL

LUL

RML

LLL

RLL

ANTERIOR VIEW

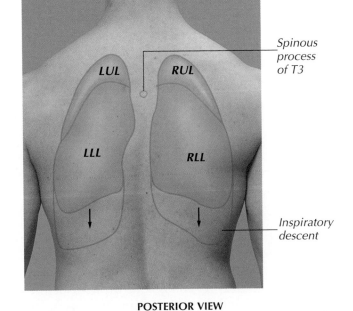

LUL

RUL

Spinous process of T3

LLL

RLL

Inspiratory descent

POSTERIOR VIEW

The right lung is thus divided into *upper, middle, and lower lobes.* The left lung has only two lobes, upper and lower.

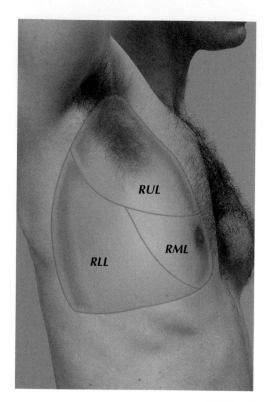 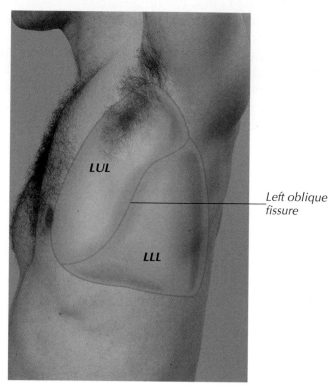

Left oblique fissure

RIGHT AND LEFT LATERAL VIEWS

Locations on the Chest. Be familiar with general anatomic terms used to locate chest findings, such as:

Supraclavicular—above the clavicles
Infraclavicular—below the clavicles
Interscapular—between the scapulae
Infrascapular—below the scapula
Bases of the lungs—the lowermost portions
Upper, middle, and lower lung fields

You may then infer what part(s) of the lung(s) are involved by an abnormal process. Signs in the right upper lung field, for example, almost certainly originate in the right upper lobe. Signs in the right middle lung field laterally, however, could come from any of three different lobes.

The Trachea and Major Bronchi. Breath sounds over the trachea and bronchi have a different quality than breath sounds over the lung parenchyma. Be sure you know the location of these structures. The trachea bifurcates into its mainstem bronchi at the levels of the sternal angle anteriorly and the T4 spinous process posteriorly.

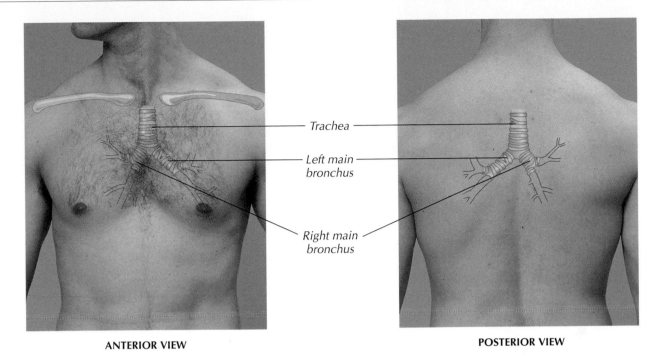

ANTERIOR VIEW　　　　　　　　　　　　　　**POSTERIOR VIEW**

The Pleurae. The pleurae are serous membranes that cover the outer surface of each lung (*visceral pleura*) and also line the inner rib cage and upper surface of the diaphragm (*parietal pleura*). Their smooth opposing surfaces, lubricated by pleural fluid, allow the lungs to move easily within the rib cage during inspiration and expiration. The *pleural space* is the potential space between visceral and parietal pleurae.

Breathing. Breathing is largely an automatic act, controlled in the brain-stem and mediated by the muscles of respiration. The dome-shaped *diaphragm* is the primary muscle of inspiration. When it contracts, it descends in the chest and enlarges the thoracic cavity. At the same time it compresses the abdominal contents, thus pushing the abdominal wall outward. Muscles in the rib cage and neck expand the thorax during inspiration. The major muscles here are the *parasternals,* which run obliquely from sternum to ribs, and the *scalenes,* which run from the cervical vertebrae to the first two ribs.

The thoracic enlargement caused by all these muscles during inspiration decreases intrathoracic pressure, draws air through the tracheobronchial tree into the alveoli (the distal air sacs), and expands the lungs. Oxygen diffuses into the blood of adjacent pulmonary capillaries, and carbon dioxide diffuses from the blood into the alveoli.

After the inspiratory effort stops, the chest wall and lungs recoil, the diaphragm rises passively, air flows outward, and the chest and abdomen return to their resting positions.

Normal breathing is quiet and easy—barely audible near the open mouth as a faint whish. When a healthy person lies supine, the breathing movements of the thorax are relatively slight. In contrast, the abdominal movements are usually easy to see. In the sitting position, movements of the thorax become more prominent.

During exercise and in certain diseases, extra work is required to breathe, and accessory muscles join the inspiratory effort. The sternomastoids are the most important of these, and the scalenes may become visible. Abdominal muscles assist in expiration.

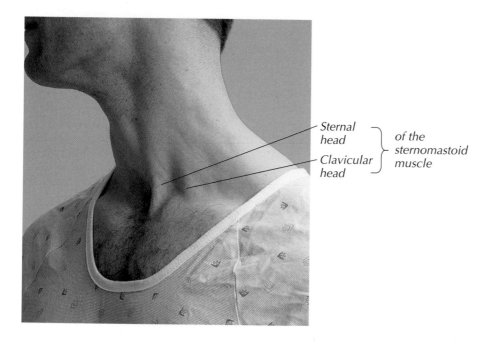

Sternal head
Clavicular head

} *of the sternomastoid muscle*

Changes With Age. As people age, their capacity for exercise decreases. The chest wall becomes stiffer and harder to move, respiratory muscles may weaken, and the lungs lose some of their elastic recoil. The speed of breathing out with maximal effort gradually diminishes. Skeletal changes associated with aging may accentuate the dorsal curve of the thoracic spine, producing kyphosis and increasing the anteroposterior diameter of the chest. The resulting "barrel chest," however, has little effect on function.

Techniques of Examination

General Approach

It is helpful to examine the posterior thorax and lungs while the patient is sitting, and the anterior thorax and lungs with the patient supine. Proceed in an orderly fashion: inspect, palpate, percuss, and auscultate. Try to visualize the underlying lobes, and compare one side with the other, so the patient serves as his or her own control. Arrange the patient's gown so that you can see the chest fully. For women, drape the gown over each half of the anterior chest as you examine the other half. Cover the woman's anterior chest when you examine the back.

With the patient sitting, examine the posterior thorax and lungs. The patient's arms should be folded across the chest with hands resting, if possible, on the opposite shoulders. This position moves the scapulae partly out of the way and increases your access to the lung fields. Then ask the patient to lie down.

With the patient supine, examine the anterior thorax and lungs. The supine position makes it easier to examine women because the breasts can be gently displaced. Furthermore, wheezes, if present, are more likely to be heard. (Some authorities, however, prefer to examine both the back and the front of the chest with the patient sitting. This technique is also satisfactory).

For patients unable to sit up without aid, try to get help so that you can examine the posterior chest in the sitting position. If this is impossible, roll the patient to one side and then to the other. Percuss the upper lung, and auscultate both lungs in each position. Because ventilation is relatively greater in the dependent lung, your chances of hearing wheezes or crackles are greater on the dependent side.

Survey of the Thorax and Respiration

Observe the rate, rhythm, depth, and effort of breathing. Note whether expiration lasts longer than usual. A normal resting adult breathes quietly and regularly about 14 to 20 times a minute. An occasional sigh is normal.

Prolonged expiration suggests narrowed lower airways. See Table 8-1, Abnormalities in Rate and Rhythm of Breathing (p. 269).

Check the patient's color for cyanosis.

Inspect the neck for supraclavicular retraction and for contraction of the sternomastoid or other accessory muscles during inspiration. Normally none of these signs is present.

Inspiratory subtraction of the sternomastoids during rest signals severe difficulty in breathing.

Listen to the patient's breathing. Are additional sounds such as wheezes audible? If so, where are they in the respiratory cycle?

Stridor, a chiefly inspiratory wheeze, suggests airway obstruction in the larynx or trachea.

Recall any relevant findings from earlier parts of your examination, such as:

- The shape of the fingernails

  Clubbing of the nails (p. 158)

- The position of the trachea, normally midline

  May be displaced laterally by a pleural effusion, pneumothorax, or atelectasis

Observe the shape of the chest. The anteroposterior diameter may increase with aging.

The anteroposterior diameter of the chest may increase in chronic obstructive pulmonary disease (COPD).

Examination of the Posterior Chest

Inspection

From a midline position behind the patient, note the *shape of the chest* and *the way in which it moves,* including:

- Deformities or asymmetry

  See Table 8-2, Deformities of the Thorax (p. 270).

- Abnormal retraction of the interspaces during inspiration. Retraction is most apparent in the lower interspaces. Supraclavicular retraction is often associated.

  Retraction in severe asthma, COPD, or upper airway obstruction.

- Impairment in respiratory movement on one or both sides or a unilateral lag (or delay) in that movement.

  Unilateral impairment or lagging of respiratory movement suggests disease of the underlying lung or pleura.

Palpation

As you palpate the chest, focus on areas of tenderness and abnormalities in the overlying skin, respiratory expansion, and fremitus.

Intercostal tenderness of an inflamed pleura

Identify tender areas. Carefully palpate any area where pain has been reported or where lesions are evident.

Assess any observed abnormalities such as masses or sinus tracts (blind, inflammatory, tubelike structures opening onto the skin)

Although rare, sinus tracts usually indicate infection of the underlying pleura and lung (e.g., tuberculosis, actinomycosis).

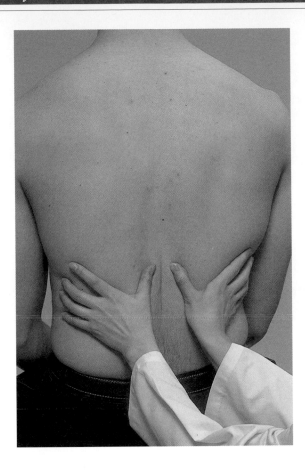

Test respiratory expansion. Place your thumbs about at the level of and parallel to the 10th ribs, your hands grasping the lateral rib cage. As you position your hands, slide them medially a bit in order to raise loose skin folds between your thumbs and the spine. Ask the patient to inhale deeply.

Watch the divergence of your thumbs during inspiration, and feel for the range and symmetry of respiratory movement.

Feel for tactile fremitus. Fremitus refers to the palpable vibrations transmitted through the bronchopulmonary tree to the chest wall when the patient speaks. To detect fremitus, use either the ball (the bony part of the palm at the base of the fingers) or the ulnar surface of your hand to optimize the vibratory sensitivity of the bones in your hand. Ask the patient to repeat the words "ninety-nine" or "one-one-one." If fremitus is faint, ask the patient to speak more loudly or in a deeper voice.

Use one hand until you have learned the feel of fremitus. Some clinicians find using one hand more accurate. The simultaneous use of both hands to compare sides, however, increases your speed and may facilitate detection of differences.

Causes of unilateral decrease or delay in chest expansion include chronic fibrotic disease of the underlying lung or pleura, pleural effusion, lobar pneumonia, pleural pain with associated splinting, and unilateral bronchial obstruction.

Fremitus is decreased or absent when the voice is soft or when the transmission of vibrations from the larynx to the surface of the chest is impeded. Causes include an obstructed bronchus; COPD; separation of the pleural surfaces by fluid (pleural effusion), fibrosis (pleural thickening), air (pneumothorax), or an infiltrating tumor; and also a very thick chest wall.

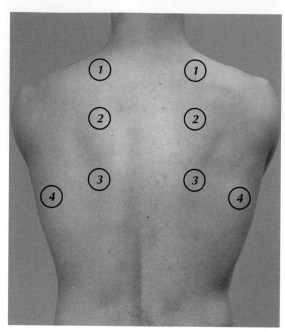

LOCATIONS FOR FEELING FREMITUS

Palpate and compare symmetrical areas of the lungs in the pattern shown above. Identify and locate any areas of increased, decreased, or absent fremitus. Fremitus is typically more prominent in the interscapular area than in the lower lung fields, and is often more prominent on the right side than on the left. It disappears below the diaphragm.

Fremitus is increased when transmission of sound is increased, as through the consolidated lung of lobar pneumonia.

Tactile fremitus is a relatively rough assessment tool, but as a scouting technique it directs your attention to possible abnormalities. Later in the examination you will check any hypotheses that it raises by listening for breath sounds, voice sounds, and whispered voice sounds. All these attributes tend to increase or decrease together.

See Table 8-3, Normal and Altered Breath and Voice Sounds (p. 271).

Percussion

Percussion of the chest sets the chest wall and underlying tissues into motion, producing audible sounds and palpable vibrations. Percussion helps to determine whether the underlying tissues are air-filled, fluid-filled, or solid. It penetrates only about 5 cm to 7 cm into the chest, however, and therefore will not help you to detect deep-seated lesions.

The *technique of percussion* can be practiced on any surface. The key points, described for a right-handed person, follow.

Hyperextend the middle finger of your left hand (the pleximeter finger). Press its distal interphalangeal joint *firmly* on the surface to be percussed. *Avoid surface contact by any other part of the hand,* because this would damp the vibrations.

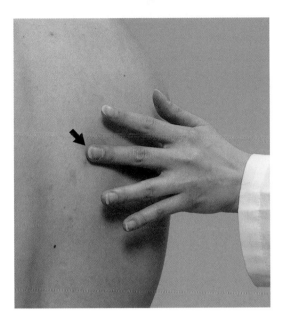

Position your right forearm quite close to the surface with the hand cocked upward. The right middle finger should be partially flexed, relaxed, and poised to strike.

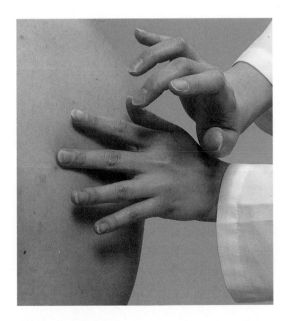

With a quick, sharp, but relaxed wrist motion, strike the pleximeter finger with the right middle finger (the plexor). Aim at your distal interphalangeal joint. You are trying to transmit vibrations through the bones of this joint to the underlying chest wall.

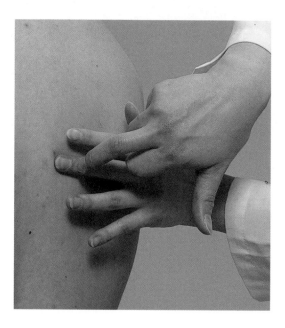

In making this strike, use the tip of your plexor finger, not the finger pad. Your finger should be almost at right angles to the pleximeter. To avoid self-injury, a short fingernail is advisable.

Withdraw your striking finger quickly to avoid damping the vibrations that you have created.

In summary, the movement is at the wrist. It is direct, brisk yet relaxed, and a bit bouncy.

Use the lightest percussion that produces a clear note. A thick chest wall requires heavier percussion than a thin one. In comparing two areas, however, keep your technique constant. Percuss about twice in one location and then move on. You will perceive the sounds better by comparing one area with another than by repetitive striking in one place. When percussing the lower posterior chest, stand somewhat to the side rather than directly behind the patient. Because your pleximeter finger then lies more firmly on the chest and your plexor is more effective, your percussion note is better.

Learn to identify five percussion notes. You can practice four of them on yourself. These notes can usually be distinguished by differences in their basic qualities of sound: intensity, pitch, and duration. Train your ear to detect these differences by concentrating on one quality at a time as you percuss first in one location, then in another.

Percussion Notes and Their Characteristics					Pathologic Examples
	Relative Intensity	Relative Pitch	Relative Duration	Example Location	
Flatness	Soft	High	Short	Thigh	Large pleural effusion
Dullness	Medium	Medium	Medium	Liver	Lobar pneumonia
Resonance	Loud	Low	Long	Normal lung	Simple chronic bronchitis
Hyperresonance	Very loud	Lower	Longer	None normally	Emphysema, pneumothorax
Tympany	Loud	High*	*	Gastric air bubble or puffed-out cheek	Large pneumothorax

* Distinguished mainly by its musical timbre.

While the patient keeps both arms crossed in front of the chest, *percuss the thorax* in symmetrical locations from the apices to the lung bases. Percuss one side of the chest and then the other at each level, as shown by the numbers below.

Dullness replaces resonance when fluid or solid tissue replaces air-containing lung or occupies the pleural space beneath your percussing fingers. Examples include: lobar pneumonia, in which the alveoli are filled with fluid and blood cells; and pleural accumulations of serous fluid (pleural effusion), blood (hemothorax), pus (empyema), fibrous tissue, or tumor.

Generalized hyperresonance may be heard over the hyperinflated lungs of emphysema or asthma, but it is not a reliable sign. Unilateral hyperresonance suggests a large pneumothorax or possibly a large air-filled bulla in the lung.

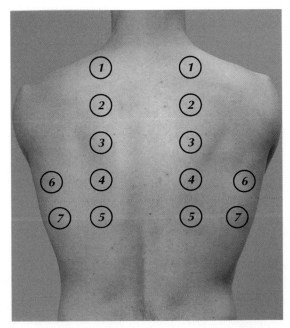

LOCATIONS FOR PERCUSSION AND AUSCULTATION

Omit the scapular areas; the thickness of muscle and bone there usually precludes worthwhile percussion.

Identify and locate any area of abnormal percussion note.

Identify the level of diaphragmatic dullness during quiet respiration. With the pleximeter finger held above and parallel to the expected level of dullness, percuss in progressive steps downward until dullness clearly replaces resonance. Check the level of this change near the middle of the hemithorax and also more laterally.

An abnormally high level suggests pleural effusion or a high diaphragm, as from atelectasis or diaphragmatic paralysis.

A typical left pleural effusion of moderate size is represented below.

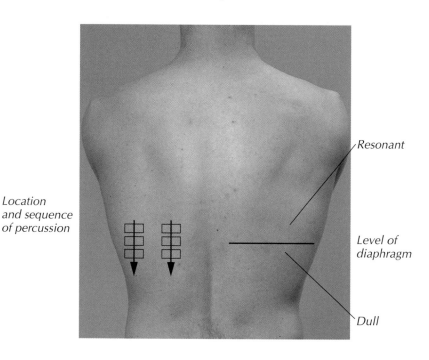

Location and sequence of percussion

Resonant

Level of diaphragm

Dull

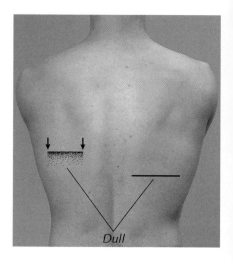

Dull

A paralyzed and therefore high left diaphragm causes similar dullness.

With this technique you are not percussing the diaphragm itself. If the boundary between the resonant lung tissue and the dull subdiaphragmatic tissue lies at a normal level, however, you can infer the probably normal location of the diaphragm.

Diaphragmatic excursion may be estimated by noting the distance between the levels of dullness on full expiration and full inspiration, normally around 5 cm or 6 cm. This estimate does not correlate well, however, with radiologic assessment of diaphragmatic movement.

Auscultation

Auscultation of the lungs is the most important examining technique for assessing air flow through the tracheobronchial tree. Together with percussion, it also helps the clinician to assess the condition of the sur-

Sounds from bedclothes, paper gowns, and the chest itself can generate confusion in ausculta-

rounding lungs and pleural space. Auscultation involves (1) listening to the sounds generated by breathing, (2) listening for any adventitious (added) sounds, and (3) if abnormalities are suspected, listening to the sounds of the patient's spoken or whispered voice as they are transmitted through the chest wall.

Breath Sounds (Lung Sounds). You will learn to identify patterns of breath sounds by their intensity, their pitch, and the relative duration of their inspiratory and expiratory phases. Normal breath sounds are:

- *Vesicular,* or soft and low pitched. They are heard through inspiration, continue without pause through expiration, and then fade away about one third of the way through expiration.

- *Bronchovesicular,* with inspiratory and expiratory sounds about equal in length, at times separated by a silent interval. Differences in pitch and intensity are often more easily detected during expiration.

- *Bronchial,* or louder and higher in pitch, with a short silence between inspiratory and expiratory sounds. Expiratory sounds last longer than inspiratory sounds.

The characteristics of these three kinds of breath sounds are summarized in the table below. Also shown are the *tracheal* breath sounds—very loud, harsh sounds that are heard by listening over the trachea in the neck.

tion. Hair on the chest may cause crackling sounds. Either press harder or wet the hair. If the patient is cold or tense, you may hear muscle contraction sounds—muffled, low-pitched rumbling or roaring noises. A change in the patient's position may eliminate this noise. You can reproduce this sound on yourself by doing a Valsalva maneuver (straining down) as you listen to your own chest.

Characteristics of Breath Sounds				
	Duration of Sounds	Intensity of Expiratory Sound	Pitch of Expiratory Sound	Locations Where Heard Normally
Vesicular*	Inspiratory sounds last longer than expiratory ones.	Soft	Relatively low	Over most of both lungs
Broncho-vesicular	Inspiratory and expiratory sounds are about equal.	Intermediate	Intermediate	Often in the 1st and 2nd interspaces anteriorly and between the scapulae
Bronchial	Expiratory sounds last longer than inspiratory ones.	Loud	Relatively high	Over the manubrium, if heard at all
Tracheal	Inspiratory and expiratory sounds are about equal.	Very loud	Relatively high	Over the trachea in the neck

If bronchovesicular or bronchial breath sounds are heard in locations distant from those listed, suspect that air-filled lung has been replaced by fluid-filled or solid lung tissue. See Table 8-3, Normal and Altered Breath and Voice Sounds (p. 271).

* The thickness of the bars indicates intensity; the steeper their incline, the higher the pitch.

Listen to the breath sounds with the diaphragm of a stethoscope after instructing the patient to breathe deeply through an open mouth. Use the pattern suggested for percussion, moving from one side to the other and comparing symmetrical areas of the lungs. If you hear or suspect abnormal sounds, auscultate adjacent areas so that you can fully describe the extent of any abnormality. Listen to at least one full breath in each location. Be alert for patient discomfort due to hyperventilation (e.g., lightheadedness, faintness), and allow the patient to rest as needed.

Note the *intensity* of the breath sounds. Breath sounds are usually louder in the lower posterior lung fields and may also vary a bit from area to area. If the breath sounds seem faint, ask the patient to breathe more deeply. You may then hear them easily. When patients do not breathe deeply enough or when they have a thick chest wall, as in obesity, breath sounds may remain diminished.

Breath sounds may be decreased when air flow is decreased (as by obstructive lung disease or muscular weakness) or when the transmission of sound is poor (as in pleural effusion, pneumothorax, or emphysema).

Is there a *silent gap* between the inspiratory and expiratory sounds?

A gap suggests bronchial breath sounds.

Listen for the *pitch, intensity, and duration of the expiratory and inspiratory sounds.* Are vesicular breath sounds distributed normally over the chest wall? Or are there bronchovesicular or bronchial breath sounds in unexpected places? If so, where are they?

Adventitious (Added) Sounds. Listen for any added, or adventitious, sounds that are superimposed on the usual breath sounds. Detection of adventitious sounds—crackles (sometimes called rales), wheezes, and rhonchi—is an important part of your examination, often leading to diagnosis of cardiac and pulmonary conditions. The most common kinds of these sounds are described below:

For further discussion and other added sounds, see Table 8-4, Adventitious (Added) Lung Sounds: Causes and Qualities (p. 272).

Adventitious Lung Sounds

DISCONTINUOUS SOUNDS (CRACKLES) are intermittent, nonmusical, and brief—like dots in time

  Fine crackles (· · · · ·) are soft, high pitched, and very brief (5–10 msec).

  Coarse crackles (• • • • •) are somewhat louder, lower in pitch, and not quite so brief (20–30 msec).

CONTINUOUS SOUNDS are > 250 msec, notably longer than crackles—like dashes in time—but do not necessarily persist throughout the respiratory cycle. Unlike crackles, they are musical.

  Wheezes (〰️) are relatively high pitched (around 400 Hz or higher) and have a hissing or shrill quality.

  Rhonchi (〰️) are relatively low pitched (around 200 Hz or lower) and have a snoring quality.

Crackles may be due to abnormalities of the lungs (pneumonia, fibrosis, early congestive heart failure) or of the airways (bronchitis, bronchiectasis).

Wheezes suggest narrowed airways, as in asthma, COPD, or bronchitis.

Rhonchi suggest secretions in large airways.

If you hear *crackles,* listen carefully for the following characteristics, which are clues to the underlying condition:

- Loudness, pitch, and duration (summarized as fine or coarse crackles)

- Number (few to many)

- Timing in the respiratory cycle

- Location on the chest wall

- Persistence of their pattern from breath to breath

- Any change after a cough or a change in the patient's position

Fine late inspiratory crackles that persist from breath to breath suggest abnormal lung tissue.

Clearing of crackles, wheezes, or rhonchi by cough suggests that secretions caused them, as in bronchitis or atelectasis.

In some normal people, crackles may be heard at the lung bases anteriorly after maximal expiration. Crackles in dependent portions of the lungs may also occur after prolonged recumbency.

If you hear *wheezes or rhonchi,* note their timing and location. Do they change with deep breathing or coughing?

Transmitted Voice Sounds. If you hear abnormally located bronchovesicular or bronchial breath sounds, continue on to assess transmitted voice sounds. With a stethoscope, listen in symmetrical areas over the chest wall as you:

Increased transmission of voice sounds suggests that air-filled lung has become airless. See Table 8-3, Normal and Altered Breath and Voice Sounds (p. 271).

- Ask the patient to say "ninety-nine." Normally the sounds transmitted through the chest wall are muffled and indistinct.

Louder, clearer voice sounds are called *bronchophony.*

- Ask the patient to say "ee." You will normally hear a muffled long E sound.

When "ee" is heard as "ay," an *E-to-A change (egophony)* is present. The quality sounds nasal.

- Ask the patient to whisper "ninety-nine" or "one-two-three." The whispered voice is normally heard faintly and indistinctly, if at all.

Louder, clearer whispered sounds are called *whispered pectoriloquy.*

Examination of the Anterior Chest

The patient, when examined in the supine position, should lie comfortably with arms somewhat abducted. A patient who is having difficulty in breathing should be examined in the sitting position or with the head of the bed elevated to a comfortable level.

Persons with severe COPD may prefer to sit leaning forward, with lips pursed during exhalation and arms supported on their knees or a table.

Inspection

Observe *the shape of the patient's chest* and *the movement of the chest wall.*
Note:

- Deformities or asymmetry

- Abnormal retraction of the lower interspaces during inspiration

- Local lag or impairment in respiratory movement

See Table 8-2, Deformities of
the Thorax (p. 270).

Severe asthma, COPD, or
upper airway obstruction

Underlying disease of lung or
pleura

Palpation

Palpation has four potential uses:

- *Identification of tender areas*

- *Assessment of observed abnormalities*

Tender pectoral muscles or
costal cartilages tend to corrob-
orate, but do not prove, that
chest pain has a musculoskeletal origin.

- *Further assessment of respiratory expansion.* Place your thumbs along
  each costal margin, your hands along the lateral rib cage. As you position your hands, slide them medially a bit to raise loose skin folds
  between your thumbs. Ask the patient to inhale deeply. Observe how
  far your thumbs diverge as the thorax expands, and feel for the extent
  and symmetry of respiratory movement.

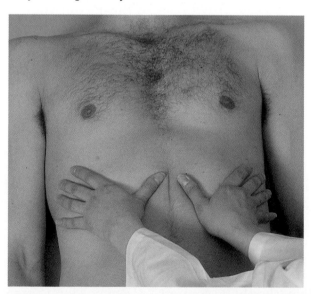

- *Assessment of tactile fremitus.* Compare both sides of the chest, using
  the ball or ulnar surface of your hand. Fremitus is usually decreased
  or absent over the precordium. When examining a woman, gently
  displace the breasts as necessary.

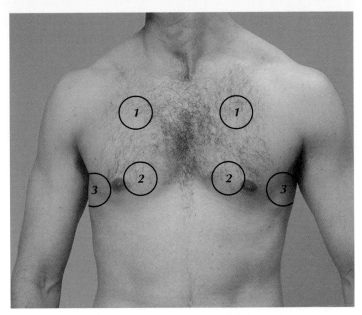

LOCATIONS FOR FEELING FREMITUS

Percussion

Percuss the anterior and lateral chest, again comparing both sides. The heart normally produces an area of dullness to the left of the sternum from the 3rd to the 5th interspaces. Percuss the left lung lateral to it.

Dullness replaces resonance when fluid or solid tissue replaces air-containing lung or occupies the pleural space. Because pleural fluid usually sinks to the lowest part of the pleural space (posteriorly in a supine patient), only a very large effusion can be detected anteriorly.

The hyperresonance of emphysema may totally replace cardiac dullness.

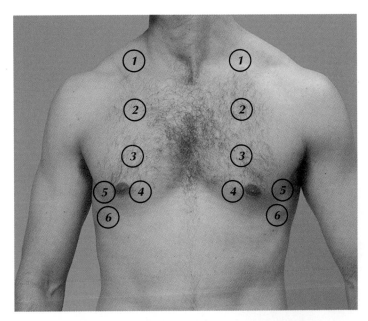

LOCATIONS FOR PERCUSSION AND AUSCULTATION

In a woman, to enhance percussion gently displace the breast with your left hand while percussing with the right.

The dullness of right middle lobe pneumonia typically occurs behind the right breast. Unless you displace the breast, you may miss the abnormal percussion note.

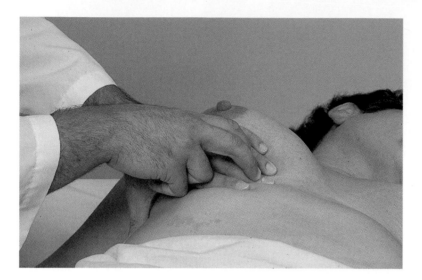

Alternatively, you may ask the patient to move her breast for you.

Identify and locate any area of abnormal percussion note.

With your pleximeter finger above and parallel to the expected upper border of liver dullness, percuss in progressive steps downward in the right midclavicular line. Identify the upper border of liver dullness. Later, during the abdominal examination, you will use this method to estimate the size of the liver. As you percuss down the chest on the left, the resonance of normal lung usually changes to the tympany of the gastric air bubble.

A lung affected by COPD often displaces the upper border of the liver downward. It also lowers the level of diaphragmatic dullness posteriorly.

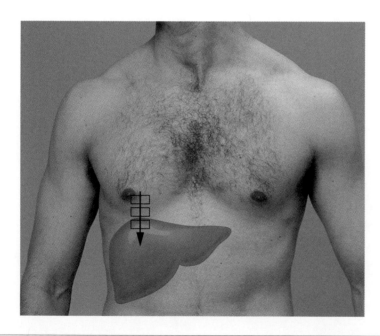

Auscultation

Listen to the chest, anteriorly and laterally, as the patient breathes with mouth open, somewhat more deeply than normal. Compare symmetrical areas of the lungs, using the pattern suggested for percussion and extending it to adjacent areas as indicated.

Listen to the breath sounds, noting their intensity and identifying any variations from normal vesicular breathing. Breath sounds are usually louder in the upper anterior lung fields. Bronchovesicular breath sounds may be heard over the large airways, especially on the right.

Identify any adventitious sounds, time them in the respiratory cycle, and locate them on the chest wall. Do they clear with deep breathing?

See Table 8-4, Adventitious (Added) Lung Sounds: Causes and Qualities (p. 272), and Table 8-5, Physical Signs in Selected Chest Disorders (pp. 274–275).

If indicated, *listen for transmitted voice sounds.*

Special Techniques

Clinical Assessment of Pulmonary Function. A simple but informative way to assess the complaint of breathlessness in an ambulatory patient is to walk with the patient down the hall or climb one flight of stairs. Observe the rate, effort, and sound of the patient's breathing.

Forced Expiratory Time. This test assesses the expiratory phase of breathing, which is typically slowed in obstructive pulmonary disease. Ask the patient to take a deep breath in and then breathe out as quickly and completely as possible, with mouth open. Listen over the trachea with the diaphragm of a stethoscope and time the audible expiration. Try to get three consistent readings, allowing a short rest between efforts if necessary.

If the patient understands and cooperates in performing the test, a forced expiration time of 6 or more seconds suggests obstructive pulmonary disease.

Identification of a Fractured Rib. Local pain and tenderness of one or more ribs raise the question of fracture. By anteroposterior compression of the chest, you can help to distinguish a fracture from soft-tissue injury. With one hand on the sternum and the other on the thoracic spine, squeeze the chest. Is this painful, and where?

An increase in the local pain (distant from your hands) suggests rib fracture rather than just soft-tissue injury.

Health Promotion and Counseling

Despite declines in smoking over the past several decades, 25% of U.S. adults still smoke.* All adults, pregnant women, parents, and adolescents who smoke should be counseled regularly to stop smoking. Smoking has been definitively linked to significant pulmonary, cardiovascular, and neoplastic disease, and accounts for one out of every five deaths in the United States.[†] It is considered the leading cause of preventable death. Nonsmokers exposed to smoke are also at increased risk for lung cancer, ear and respiratory infection, asthma, low birthweight, and residential fires. Smoking exposes patients not only to carcinogens, but also to nicotine, an addictive drug. Be especially alert to smoking by teenagers, the age group when tobacco use often begins, and by pregnant women, who often continue smoking during pregnancy.

The disease risks of smoking drop significantly within a year of smoking cessation. Effective interventions include targeted messages by clinicians, group counseling, and use of nicotine-replacement therapies. Clinicians are advised to adopt the four "As":

- **A**sk about smoking at each visit.
- **A**dvise patients regularly to stop smoking in a clear personalized message.
- **A**ssist patients to set stop dates and provide educational materials for self-help.
- **A**rrange for follow-up visits to monitor and support progress.

Combining clinician and group counseling with nicotine replacement therapy is especially effective for highly addicted patients.

Relapses are common and should be expected. Nicotine withdrawal, weight gain, stress, social pressure, and use of alcohol are often cited as explanations. Help patients to learn from these experiences: work with the patient to pinpoint the precipitating circumstances and develop strategies for alternative responses and health-promoting behaviors.

---

* Centers for Disease Control and Prevention. Cigarette Smoking Among Adults—United States. MMWR 43: 925–930, 1994.
[†] Centers for Disease Control and Prevention. Cigarette Smoking: Attributable Mortality and Years of Potential Life Cost—United States. MMWR 42: 645–649, 1993.

Table 8-1   Abnormalities in Rate and Rhythm of Breathing

TABLE 8-1   Abnormalities in Rate and Rhythm of Breathing

When observing respiratory patterns, think in terms of *rate, depth, and regularity* of the patient's breathing. Describe what you see in these terms. Traditional terms, such as tachypnea, are given below so that you will understand them, but simple descriptions are recommended for use.

Inspiration   Expiration

Normal

The respiratory rate is about 14–20 per min in normal adults and up to 44 per min in infants.

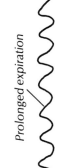

Rapid Shallow Breathing (*Tachypnea*)

Rapid shallow breathing has a number of causes, including restrictive lung disease, pleuritic chest pain, and an elevated diaphragm.

Rapid Deep Breathing (*Hyperpnea, Hyperventilation*)

Rapid deep breathing has several causes, including exercise, anxiety, and metabolic acidosis. In the comatose patient, consider infarction, hypoxia, or hypoglycemia affecting the midbrain or pons. *Kussmaul breathing* is deep breathing due to metabolic acidosis. It may be fast, normal in rate, or slow.

Slow Breathing (*Bradypnea*)

Slow breathing may be secondary to such causes as diabetic coma, drug-induced respiratory depression, and increased intracranial pressure.

Hyperpnea   Apnea

Cheyne–Stokes Breathing

Periods of deep breathing alternate with periods of apnea (no breathing). Children and aging people normally may show this pattern in sleep. Other causes include heart failure, uremia, drug-induced respiratory depression, and brain damage (typically on both sides of the cerebral hemispheres or diencephalon).

Ataxic Breathing (*Biot's Breathing*)

Ataxic breathing is characterized by unpredictable irregularity. Breaths may be shallow or deep, and stop for short periods. Causes include respiratory depression and brain damage, typically at the medullary level.

Sighs

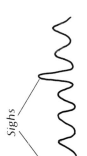

Sighing Respiration

Breathing punctuated by frequent sighs should alert you to the possibility of hyperventilation syndrome—a common cause of dyspnea and dizziness. Occasional sighs are normal.

Prolonged expiration

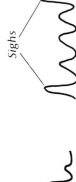

Obstructive Breathing

In obstructive lung disease, expiration is prolonged because narrowed airways increase the resistance to air flow. Causes include asthma, chronic bronchitis, and COPD.

Table 8-2   Deformities of the Thorax

TABLE 8-2   Deformities of the Thorax

Normal Adult

Cross Section of Thorax

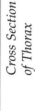

Clinical Appearance

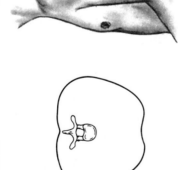

The thorax in the normal adult is wider than it is deep, i.e., its lateral diameter is larger than its anteroposterior diameter.

Barrel Chest

Cross Section of Thorax

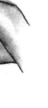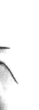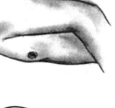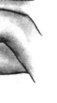

Clinical Appearance

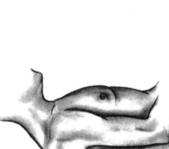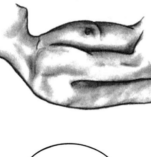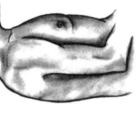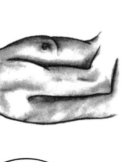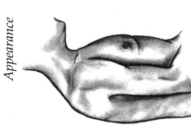

A barrel chest has an increased anteroposterior diameter. This shape is normal during infancy, and often accompanies normal aging and chronic obstructive pulmonary disease.

Traumatic Flail Chest

Cross Section of Thorax

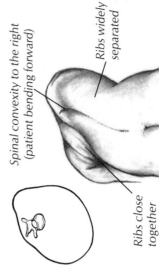

— Expiration
— Inspiration

If multiple ribs are fractured, paradoxical movements of the thorax may be seen. As descent of the diaphragm decreases intrathoracic pressure on inspiration, the injured area caves inward; on expiration, it moves outward.

Funnel Chest (*Pectus Excavatum*)

Cross Section of Thorax

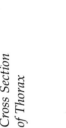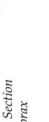

Clinical Appearance

A funnel chest is characterized by a depression in the lower portion of the sternum. Compression of the heart and great vessels may cause murmurs.

Pigeon Chest (*Pectus Carinatum*)

Cross Section of Thorax

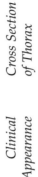

Depressed costal cartilages

Anteriorly displaced sternum

Clinical Appearance

In a pigeon chest, the sternum is displaced anteriorly, increasing the anteroposterior diameter. The costal cartilages adjacent to the protruding sternum are depressed.

Thoracic Kyphoscoliosis

Cross Section of Thorax

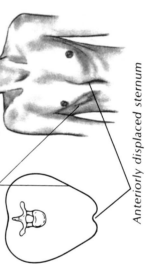

Spinal convexity to the right (patient bending forward)

Ribs widely separated

Ribs close together

Clinical Appearance

In thoracic kyphoscoliosis, abnormal spinal curvatures and vertebral rotation deform the chest. Distortion of the underlying lungs may make interpretation of lung findings very difficult.

Table 8-3   Normal and Altered Breath and Voice Sounds

TABLE 8-3   *Normal and Altered Breath and Voice Sounds*

The origins of breath sounds are still unclear. According to leading theories, turbulent air flow in the central airways produces the tracheal and bronchial breath sounds. As these sounds pass through the lungs to the periphery, lung tissue filters out their higher-pitched components and only the soft and lower-pitched components reach the chest wall. There they are heard as vesicular breath sounds. Normally, tracheal and bronchial sounds may be heard near their anatomic origins; vesicular breath sounds predominate elsewhere.

When lung tissue loses its air, it transmits high-pitched sounds much better. If the tracheobronchial tree is open, bronchial breath sounds may replace the normal vesicular sounds in areas that overlie airless lung. This change may be caused by lobar pneumonia, in which the alveoli fill with fluid, red cells, and white cells—a process called *consolidation*. Other causes include pulmonary edema or hemorrhage. The appearance of bronchial breath sounds usually correlates with an increase in tactile fremitus and transmitted voice sounds. These findings are summarized below.

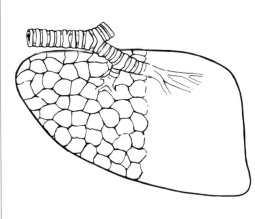

	Normally Air-Filled Lung	Airless Lung, as in Lobar Pneumonia
Breath Sounds	Predominantly vesicular	Bronchial or bronchovesicular over the involved area
Transmitted Voice Sounds	Spoken words muffled and indistinct	Spoken words louder, clearer (bronchophony)
	Spoken "ee" heard as "ee"	Spoken "ee" heard as "ay" (egophony)
	Whispered words faint and indistinct, if heard at all	Whispered words louder, clearer (whispered pectoriloquy)
Tactile Fremitus	Normal	Increased

Table 8-4   Adventitious (Added) Lung Sounds: Causes and Qualities

T A B L E   8 - 4   Adventitious (Added) Lung Sounds: Causes and Qualities

Crackles

Crackles have two leading explanations. (1) They result from a series of tiny explosions when small airways, deflated during expiration, pop open during inspiration. This mechanism probably explains the late inspiratory crackles of interstitial lung disease and early congestive heart failure. (2) Crackles result as air bubbles flow through secretions or lightly closed airways during respiration. This mechanism probably explains at least some coarse crackles.

Inspiration   Expiration

Late inspiratory crackles may begin in the first half of inspiration phase but must continue into late inspiration. They are usually fine and fairly profuse, and repeat themselves from breath to breath. These crackles appear first at the bases of the lungs, spread upward as the condition worsens, and shift to dependent regions with changes in posture. Causes include interstitial lung disease (such as fibrosis) and early congestive heart failure.

Early inspiratory crackles appear soon after the start of inspiration and do not continue into late inspiration. They are often but not always coarse and are relatively few in number. Expiratory crackles are sometimes associated. Causes include chronic bronchitis and asthma.

Midinspiratory and expiratory crackles are heard in bronchiectasis but are not specific for this diagnosis. Wheezes and rhonchi may be associated.

Wheezes and Rhonchi

Wheezes occur when air flows rapidly through bronchi that are narrowed nearly to the point of closure. They are often audible at the mouth as well as through the chest wall. Causes of wheezes that are generalized throughout the chest include asthma, chronic bronchitis, COPD, and congestive heart failure (cardiac asthma). In asthma, wheezes may be heard only in expiration or in both phases of the respiratory cycle. Rhonchi suggest secretions in the larger airways. In chronic bronchitis, wheezes and rhonchi often clear with coughing.

Occasionally in severe-obstructive pulmonary disease, the condition worsens to the point that the patient is no longer able to force enough air through the narrowed bronchi to produce wheezing. The resulting silent chest should raise concern and not be mistaken for improvement.

A persistent localized wheeze suggests a partial obstruction of a bronchus, as by a tumor or foreign body. It may be inspiratory, expiratory, or both.

Stridor

A wheeze that is entirely or predominantly inspiratory is called stridor. It is often louder in the neck than over the chest wall. It indicates a partial obstruction of the larynx or trachea, and demands immediate attention.

Pleural Rub

Inflamed and roughened pleural surfaces grate against each other as they are momentarily and repeatedly delayed by increased friction. These movements produce creaking sounds known as a pleural rub (or pleural friction rub).

Pleural rubs resemble crackles acoustically, although they are produced by different pathologic processes. The sounds may be heard as discrete, but sometimes are so numerous that they merge into an apparently continuous sound. A rub is usually confined to a relatively small area of the chest wall, and typically is heard in both phases of respiration. When inflamed pleural surfaces are separated by fluid, the rub often disappears.

Mediastinal Crunch
(Hamman's Sign)

A mediastinal crunch is a series of precordial crackles synchronous with the heart beat, not with respiration. Best heard in the left lateral position, it is due to mediastinal emphysema (pneumomediastinum).

Table 8-5   Physical Signs in Selected Chest Disorders

TABLE 8-5 Physical Signs in Selected Chest Disorders

The black boxes in this table suggest a framework for clinical assessment. Start with the three boxes under Percussion Note: resonant, dull, and hyperresonant. Then move from each of these to other boxes that emphasize some of the key differences among various conditions. The changes described vary with the extent and severity of the disorder. Abnormalities deep in the chest, moreover, usually produce fewer signs than do superficial ones, and may cause no signs at all. Use the table for the direction of typical changes, not for absolute distinctions.

Condition	Trachea	Percussion Note	Breath Sounds	Tactile Fremitus and Transmitted Voice Sounds	Adventitious Sounds
Normal The tracheobronchial tree and alveoli are clear; the pleurae are thin and close together; the mobility of the chest wall is unimpaired.	Midline	Resonant	Vesicular, except perhaps bronchovesicular and bronchial sounds over the large bronchi and trachea respectively	Normal	None, except perhaps a few transient inspiratory crackles at the bases of the lungs
Chronic Bronchitis The bronchi are chronically inflamed, and a productive cough is present. Airway obstruction may develop.	Midline	Resonant	Normal	Normal	None; or scattered coarse crackles in early inspiration and perhaps expiration; or wheezes or rhonchi
Left-Sided Heart Failure (Early) Increased pressure in the pulmonary veins causes congestion and interstitial edema (around the alveoli). The bronchial mucosa may become edematous.	Midline	Resonant	Normal	Normal	Late inspiratory crackles in the dependent portions of the lungs; possibly wheezes
Consolidation The alveoli fill with fluid or blood cells, as in pneumonia, pulmonary edema, or pulmonary hemorrhage.	Midline	Dull over the airless area	Bronchial over the involved area	Increased over the involved area, with bronchophony, egophony, and whispered pectoriloquy	Late inspiratory crackles over the involved area

Table 8-5   Physical Signs in Selected Chest Disorders

Condition	Trachea / Mediastinum	Percussion Note	Breath Sounds		Adventitious Sounds
Atelectasis *(Lobar Obstruction)* When a plug in a mainstem bronchus (as from mucus or a foreign object) obstructs air flow, the affected lung tissue collapses into an airless state.	May be shifted toward the involved side	Dull over the airless area	Usually absent when the bronchial plug persists. Exceptions include right upper lobe atelectasis, where adjacent tracheal sounds may be transmitted.	Usually absent when the bronchial plug persists. In exceptions, e.g., right upper lobe atelectasis, may be increased	None
Pleural Effusion When fluid accumulates in the pleural space, it separates the air-filled lung from the chest wall and blocks the transmission of sound.	Toward the opposite side in a large effusion	Dull to flat over the fluid	Decreased to absent, but bronchial breath sounds may be heard near the top of a large effusion.	Decreased to absent, but may be increased toward the top of a large effusion	None, except a possible pleural rub
Pneumothorax When air leaks into the pleural space, usually unilaterally, the lung recoils from the chest wall. Pleural air blocks the transmission of sound.	Toward the opposite side if much air	Hyperresonant or tympanitic over the pleural air	Decreased to absent over the pleural air	Decreased to absent over the pleural air	None, except a possible pleural rub
Emphysema This is a slowly progressive disorder in which the distal air spaces are enlarged and the lungs become hyperinflated. Chronic bronchitis is often associated.	Midline	Diffusely hyperresonant	Decreased to absent	Decreased	None, or the crackles, wheezes, and rhonchi of associated chronic bronchitis
Asthma Widespread narrowing of the tracheobronchial tree diminishes airflow to a fluctuating degree. During attacks, airflow decreases further and the lungs hyperinflate.	Midline	Normal to diffusely hyperresonant	Often obscured by wheezes	Decreased	Wheezes, possibly crackles

275

The Cardiovascular System

CHAPTER 9

Anatomy and Physiology

Surface Projections of the Heart and Great Vessels

It is helpful to visualize the underlying structures of the heart as you examine the anterior chest. The *right ventricle* occupies most of the anterior cardiac surface. This chamber and the pulmonary artery form a wedgelike structure behind and to the left of the sternum.

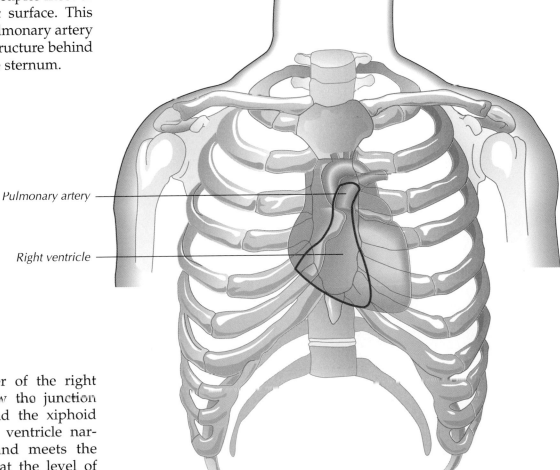

Pulmonary artery

Right ventricle

The inferior border of the right ventricle lies below the junction of the sternum and the xiphoid process. The right ventricle narrows superiorly and meets the pulmonary artery at the level of the 3rd left costal cartilage close to the sternum.

The *left ventricle,* behind the right ventricle and to the left, forms the lateral margin of the anterior cardiac surface. It is clinically important because it produces the *apical impulse.** This impulse locates the left border of the heart and is usually found in the 5th interspace, 7 cm to 9 cm from the midsternal line.

The right border of the heart is formed by the *right atrium,* a chamber not usually identifiable on physical examination. The *left atrium* is mostly posterior and cannot be examined directly, although its small atrial appendage may make up a segment of the left cardiac border between the pulmonary artery and the left ventricle.

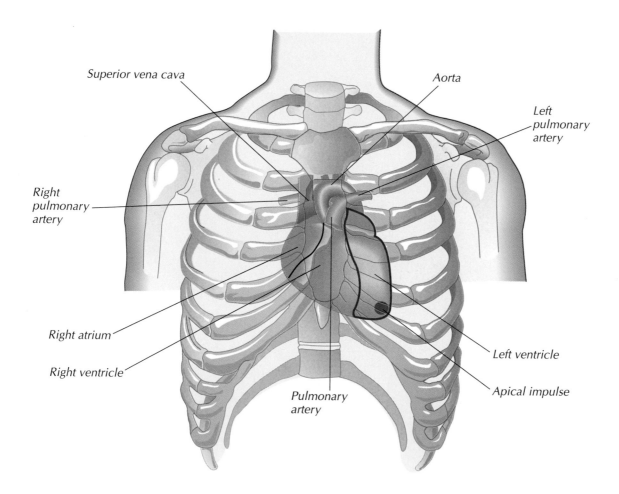

* The apical impulse is sometimes called the point of maximum impulse, or PMI. Because the most prominent cardiac impulse may not be apical, some authorities discourage use of this term.

Above the heart lie the great vessels. The pulmonary artery, already mentioned, bifurcates quickly into its left and right branches. The aorta curves upward from the left ventricle to the level of the sternal angle, where it arches backward to the left and then down. On the right, the superior vena cava empties into the right atrium.

Although not illustrated, the inferior vena cava also empties into the right atrium. The superior and inferior venae cavae carry venous blood from the upper and lower portions of the body, respectively.

Cardiac Chambers, Valves, and Circulation

Circulation through the heart is shown in the diagram below, which identifies the cardiac chambers, valves, and direction of blood flow. Because of their positions, the *tricuspid* and *mitral valves* are often called *atrioventricular valves.* The *aortic* and *pulmonic valves* are called *semilunar valves* because each of their leaflets is shaped like a half moon. Although this diagram shows all valves in an open position, they are not all open simultaneously in the living heart.

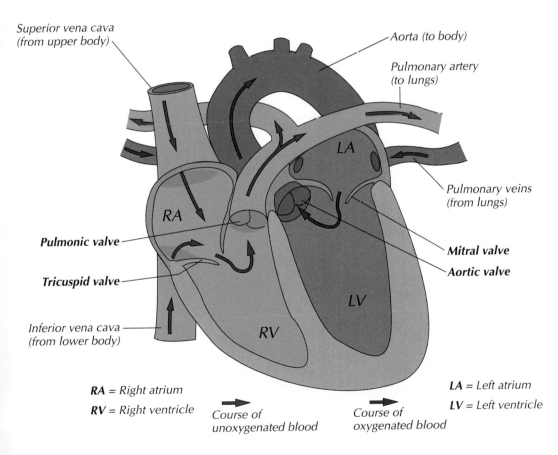

As the heart valves close, normal heart sounds arise from vibrations emanating from the leaflets, the adjacent cardiac structures, and the flow of blood. It is essential to understand the positions and movements of the valves in relation to events in the cardiac cycle.

Events in the Cardiac Cycle

The heart serves as a muscular pump that generates varying pressures as its chambers contract and relax. *Systole* is the period of ventricular contraction. In the diagram shown below, pressure in the left ventricle rises from less than 5 mm Hg in its resting state to a normal peak of 120 mm Hg. After the ventricle ejects much of its blood into the aorta, the pressure levels off and starts to fall. *Diastole* is the period of ventricular relaxation. Ventricular pressure falls further to below 5 mm Hg, and blood flows from atrium to ventricle. Late in diastole, ventricular pressure rises slightly during inflow of blood from atrial contraction.

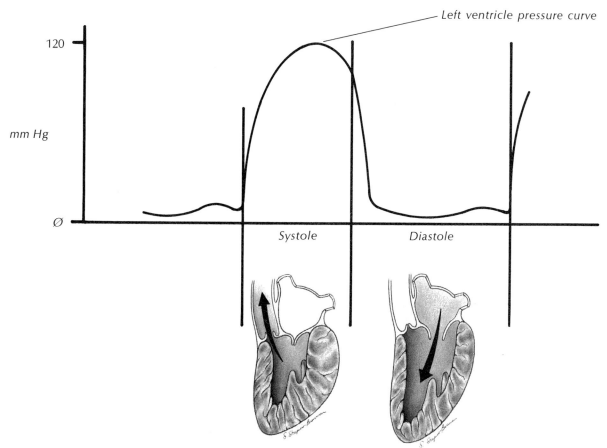

Note that during *systole* the aortic valve is open, allowing ejection of blood from the left ventricle into the aorta. The mitral valve is closed, preventing blood from regurgitating back into the left atrium. In contrast, during *diastole* the aortic valve is closed, preventing regurgitation of blood from the aorta back into the left ventricle. The mitral valve is open, allowing blood to flow from the left atrium into the relaxed left ventricle.

Understanding the interrelationships of the pressures in these three chambers—left atrium, left ventricle, and aorta—together with the position and movement of the valves is fundamental to the understanding of heart sounds. These changing pressures and the sounds that result are traced here through one cardiac cycle. Note that during auscultation the first and second heart sounds define the margins of *systole* and *diastole*.

During *diastole,* pressure in the blood-filled left atrium slightly exceeds that in the relaxed left ventricle, and blood flows from left atrium to left ventricle across the open mitral valve. Just before the onset of ventricular systole, atrial contraction produces a slight pressure rise in both chambers.

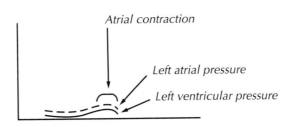

During *systole,* the left ventricle starts to contract and ventricular pressure rapidly exceeds left atrial pressure, thus shutting the mitral valve. Closure of the mitral valve produces the first heart sound (S$_1$).[†]

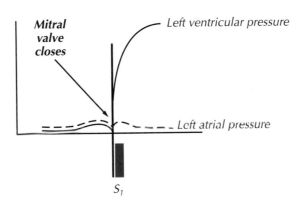

As left ventricular pressure continues to rise, it quickly exceeds the pressure in the aorta and forces the aortic valve open. In some pathologic conditions, opening of the aortic valve is accompanied by an early systolic ejection sound (Ej). Normally, maximal left ventricular pressure corresponds to systolic blood pressure.

As the left ventricle ejects most of its blood, ventricular pressure begins to fall. When left ventricular pressure drops below aortic pressure, the aortic valve shuts. Aortic valve closure produces the second heart sound (S$_2$) and another diastole begins.

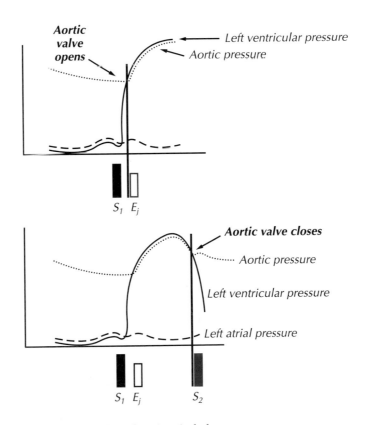

[†]An extensive literature deals with the exact causes of heart sounds. (Possible explanations include actual closure of valve leaflets, tensing of related structures, leaflet positions and pressure gradients at the time of atrial and ventricular systole, and the impact of columns of blood.) The explanations given here are oversimplified but retain clinical usefulness.

In diastole, left ventricular pressure continues to drop and falls below left atrial pressure. The mitral valve opens. This is usually a silent event, but may be audible as an opening snap (OS) if valve leaflet motion is restricted, as in mitral stenosis.

After the mitral valve opens, there is a period of rapid ventricular filling as blood flows early in diastole from left atrium to left ventricle. In children and young adults, a third heart sound (S_3) may arise from rapid deceleration of the column of blood against the ventricular wall.

Finally, although not often heard in normal adults, a fourth heart sound (S_4) marks atrial contraction. It immediately precedes S_1 of the next beat.

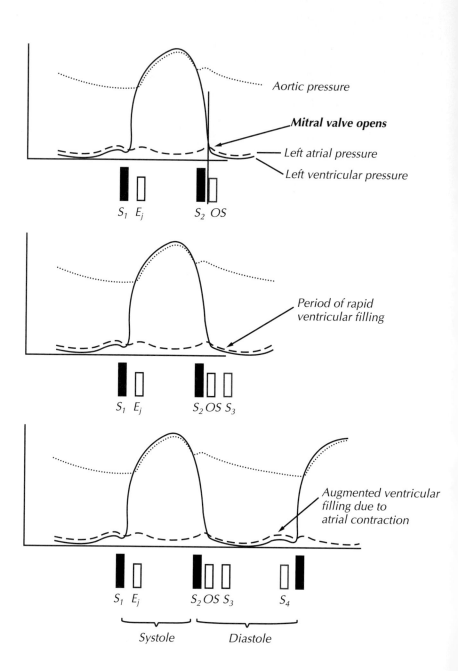

Aortic pressure

Mitral valve opens

Left atrial pressure

Left ventricular pressure

S_1 E_j S_2 OS

Period of rapid ventricular filling

S_1 E_j S_2 OS S_3

Augmented ventricular filling due to atrial contraction

S_1 E_j S_2 OS S_3 S_4

Systole   *Diastole*

The Splitting of Heart Sounds

While these events are occurring on the left side of the heart, similar changes are occurring on the right, involving the right atrium, right ventricle, tricuspid valve, pulmonic valve, and pulmonary artery. Right ventricular and pulmonary arterial pressures are significantly lower than corresponding levels on the left side. Furthermore, right-sided events usually occur slightly later than those on the left. Instead of a single heart sound, therefore, you may hear two discernible components, the first from left-sided valvular closure, the second from right-sided closure.

Consider the second heart sound and its two components, A_2 and P_2, which come from closure of the aortic and pulmonic valves, respectively. During expiration, these two components are fused into a single sound, S_2. During inspiration, however, A_2 and P_2 separate slightly, and S_2 splits into its two audible components.

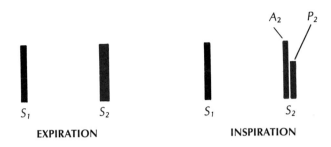

Current explanations of inspiratory splitting are technically complicated. In summary, inspiration prolongs ejection of blood from the right ventricle but shortens ejection from the left ventricle. P_2 is thus delayed, while A_2 comes slightly earlier.

Of the two components of the second heart sound, A_2 is normally the louder, reflecting the high pressure in the aorta. It is heard throughout the precordium. P_2, in contrast, is relatively soft, reflecting the lower pressure in the pulmonary artery. It is heard best in its own area—the 2nd and 3rd left interspaces close to the sternum. It is here that you should search for splitting of the second heart sound.

The first heart sound also has two components, an earlier mitral and a later tricuspid sound. The mitral sound, its principal component, is much louder, again reflecting the high pressures on the left side of the heart. It can be heard throughout the precordium and (like S_1 itself) is loudest at the cardiac apex. The softer tricuspid component is heard best at the lower left sternal border, and it is here that you may hear a split S_1. The earlier, louder mitral component may mask the tricuspid sound, however, and splitting is not always detectable. Splitting of the first heart sound does not vary with respiration.

Heart Murmurs

Heart murmurs are distinguishable from heart sounds by their longer duration. They are attributed to turbulent blood flow. Heart murmurs often have no pathologic significance, but they may indicate serious heart disease. A stenotic (abnormally narrowed) valvular orifice that partially obstructs the flow of blood, for example, causes a murmur. So does a valve that fails to close fully and allows blood to regurgitate (leak) back in a retrograde direction. To describe murmurs accurately, the clinician must be able to identify the location where they are best heard and to time them in the cardiac cycle.

Relation of Auscultatory Findings to the Chest Wall

The locations on the chest wall where you hear heart sounds and murmurs help to identify the valve or chamber where they originate. Sounds and murmurs arising from the mitral valve are usually heard best at and around the cardiac apex. Those originating in the tricuspid valve are heard best at or near the lower left sternal border. Murmurs arising from the pulmonic valve are usually heard best in the 2nd and 3rd left interspaces close to the sternum, but at times may also be heard at higher or lower levels, and those originating in the aortic valve may be heard anywhere from the right 2nd interspace to the apex. These areas overlap, as illustrated below, and you will need to correlate auscultatory findings with other portions of the cardiac examination to identify sounds and murmurs accurately.

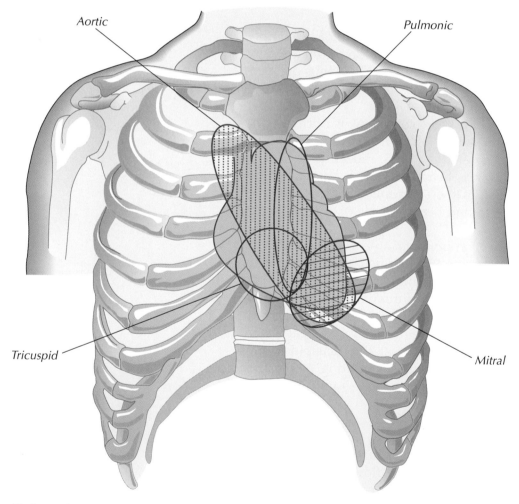

(Redrawn from Leatham A: Introduction to the Examination of the Cardiovascular System, 2nd ed. Oxford, Oxford University Press, 1979)

The "base of the heart"—a term often used clinically—refers to the right and left 2nd interspaces close to the sternum.

The Conduction System

An electrical conduction system stimulates and coordinates the contraction of cardiac muscle.

Each normal impulse is initiated in a group of cardiac cells known as the *sinus node.* Located in the right atrium near the junction of the vena cava, the sinus node acts as cardiac pacemaker and automatically discharges an impulse about 60 to 100 times a minute. This impulse travels through both atria to the *atrioventricular (AV) node,* a specialized group of cells located low in the atrial septum. Here the impulse is delayed before passing down the bundle of His and its branches to the ventricular myocardium. Muscular contraction follows: first the atria, then the ventricles. The normal conduction pathway is diagrammed in simplified form at the right.

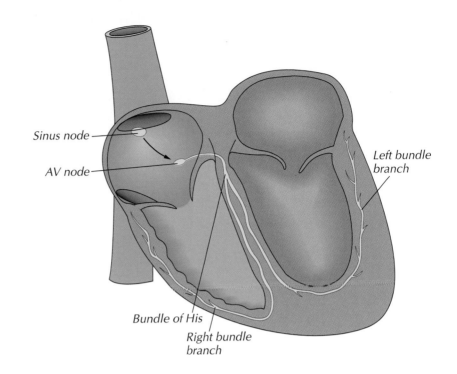

The electrocardiogram (ECG) records these events. Each normal impulse produces a series of waves:

1. A *small P wave* of atrial depolarization (electrical activation)
2. A *larger QRS complex* of ventricular depolarization. Each complex consists of one or more of the following:
   a. A *Q wave,* formed whenever the initial deflection is downward.
   b. An *R wave,* the upward deflection
   c. An *S wave,* a downward deflection following an R wave
3. A *T wave* of ventricular repolarization (recovery)

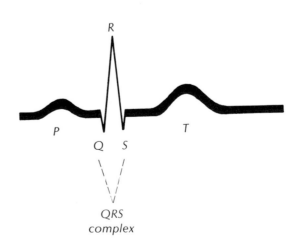

The electrical impulse slightly precedes the myocardial contraction that it stimulates. The relation of electrocardiographic waves to the cardiac cycle is shown below.

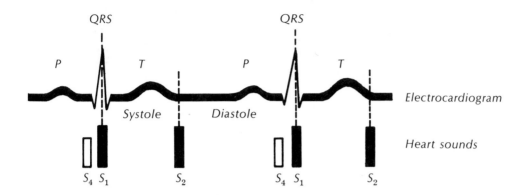

The Heart as a Pump

The left and right ventricles pump blood into the systemic and pulmonary arterial trees, respectively. *Cardiac output,* the volume of blood ejected from each ventricle during 1 minute, is the product of *heart rate* and *stroke volume.* Stroke volume (the volume of blood ejected with each heartbeat) depends in turn on preload, myocardial contractility, and afterload.

Preload refers to the load that stretches the cardiac muscle prior to contraction. The volume of blood in the right ventricle at the end of diastole, then, constitutes its preload for the next beat. Right ventricular preload is increased by increasing venous return to the right heart. Physiologic causes include inspiration and the increased volume of blood that flows from exercising muscles. The increased volume of blood in a dilated ventricle of congestive heart failure also increases preload. Causes of decreased right ventricular preload include exhalation, decreased left ventricular output, and pooling of blood in the capillary bed or the venous system.

Myocardial contractility refers to the ability of the cardiac muscle, when given a load, to shorten. Contractility increases when stimulated by action of the sympathetic nervous system, and decreases when blood flow or oxygen delivery to the myocardium is impaired.

Afterload refers to the vascular resistance against which the ventricle must contract. Sources of resistance to left ventricular contraction include the tone in the walls of the aorta, the large arteries, and the peripheral vascular tree (primarily the small arteries and arterioles), as well as the volume of blood already in the aorta.

Pathologic increases in preload and afterload, called *volume overload* and *pressure overload* respectively, produce changes in ventricular function that may be clinically detectable. These changes include alterations in ventricular impulses, detectable by palpation, and in normal heart sounds. Pathologic heart sounds and murmurs may also develop.

Arterial Pulses and Blood Pressure

With each contraction, the left ventricle ejects a volume of blood into the aorta and on into the arterial tree. The ensuing pressure wave moves rapidly through the arterial system, where it is felt as the *arterial pulse*. Although the pressure wave travels quickly—many times faster than the blood itself—a palpable delay between ventricular contraction and peripheral pulses makes the pulses in the arms and legs unsuitable for timing cardiac events.

Blood pressure in the arterial system varies with the cardiac cycle, reaching a systolic peak and a diastolic trough, levels that can be measured by sphygmomanometry. The difference between systolic and diastolic pressures is known as the *pulse pressure.*

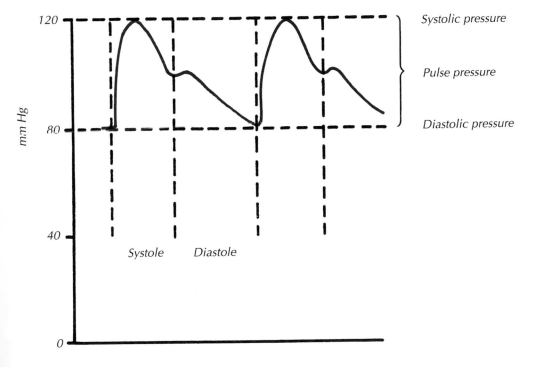

The principal factors influencing arterial pressure are:

1. Left ventricular stroke volume
2. The distensibility of the aorta and the large arteries
3. The peripheral vascular resistance, principally at the arteriolar level. This is controlled by the autonomic nervous system.
4. The volume of blood in the arterial system

Changes in any of these four factors alter systolic pressure, diastolic pressure, or both. Blood pressure levels fluctuate strikingly through any 24-hour period, varying, for example, with physical activity, emotional state, pain, noise, environmental temperature, the use of coffee, tobacco, and other drugs, and even the time of day.

Jugular Venous Pressure and Pulses

Jugular Venous Pressure. Systemic venous pressure is much lower than arterial pressure. Although venous pressure is ultimately dependent upon left ventricular contraction, much of this force is dissipated as the blood passes through the arterial tree and the capillary bed. Walls of veins contain less smooth muscle than do arterial walls, venous tone is less, and the veins are more distensible. Other important determinants of systemic venous pressure include blood volume and the capacity of the right heart to eject blood into the pulmonary arterial system. Cardiac disease may alter these variables, producing abnormalities in venous pressure. For example, venous pressure falls when left ventricular output or blood volume is significantly reduced; it rises when the right heart fails or when increased pressure in the pericardial sac impedes the return of blood to the right atrium.

It is important to assess pressure in the jugular veins, which reflects right atrial pressure. The best estimate is made from the internal jugular veins. If these are impossible to see, the external jugular veins can be used, but they are less reliable. To gauge the level of venous pressure, find the highest point of oscillation in the internal jugular veins or, if necessary, the point above which the external jugular veins appear collapsed.

The usual zero point for this estimate is the sternal angle, usually adjacent to the second rib, and venous pressure is always measured in vertical distance from it. Regardless of the patient's position—supine, sitting upright, or at any angle between these positions—the sternal angle remains roughly 5 cm above the right atrium.

The observer positions the patient to enhance detection of the jugular veins and their pulsations in the lower half of the neck. Elevating the head of the bed to about 15° to 30° from horizontal is usually sufficient. In the illustrations that follow, the pressure in the internal jugular vein is somewhat elevated. In *A*, the head of the bed is raised to about 30°. The venous pressure cannot be measured because the point that marks its level is above the jaw and therefore not visible. In *B*, the bed is raised to about 60°. The "top" of the jugular vein is now easily visible, and its vertical distance from the sternal angle can be measured. In *C*, the patient is upright and the veins are barely discernible above the clavicle. Note that the height of the venous pressure, measured from the sternal angle, is the same in all three positions, although the neck veins look much different.

Pressures measured as more than 3 cm or possibly 4 cm above the sternal angle are considered elevated.

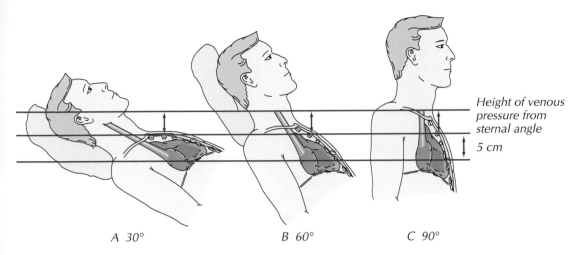

Height of venous pressure from sternal angle

↕ *5 cm*

A 30°   B 60°   C 90°

Jugular Venous Pulsations. The oscillations that you see in the internal jugular veins (and often in the externals as well) reflect changing pressures within the right atrium. The right internal jugular vein has the most direct channel to the right atrium and reflects these pressure changes best.

Careful observation reveals that the undulating pulsations of the internal jugular veins (and sometimes the externals) are composed of two quick elevations and two troughs.

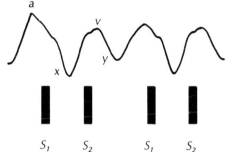

The first elevation, the *a wave*, reflects the slight rise in atrial pressure that accompanies atrial contraction. It occurs just before the first heart sound and before the carotid pulse. The following trough, the *x descent*, starts with atrial relaxation. It continues as the right ventricle, contracting during systole, pulls the floor of the atrium downward. During ventricular systole, blood continues to flow into the right atrium from the venae cavae. The tricuspid valve is closed, the chamber begins to fill, and right atrial pressure begins to rise again, creating the second elevation, the *v wave*. When the tricuspid valve opens early in diastole, blood in the right atrium flows passively into the right ventricle and right atrial pressure falls again, creating the second trough or *y descent*. To remember these four oscillations in a somewhat oversimplified way, think of the following sequence: atrial contraction, atrial relaxation, atrial filling, and atrial emptying. (You can think of the *a* wave as atrial contraction and the *v* wave as venous filling.)

To the naked eye, the two descents are the most obvious events in the normal jugular pulse. Of the two, the sudden collapse of the *x* descent late in systole is the more prominent, occurring just before the second heart sound. The *y* descent follows the second heart sound early in diastole.

Changes With Age

Cardiovascular findings vary importantly with age. Aging may affect the location of the apical impulse, the pitch of heart sounds and murmurs, the stiffness of the arteries, and blood pressure.

Changes in the Apical Impulse and Heart Sounds. The *apical impulse* is usually felt easily in children and young adults; as the chest deepens in its anteroposterior diameter, the impulse gets harder to find. For the same reason, *splitting of the second heart sound* may be harder to hear in older people as its pulmonic component becomes less audible. A physiologic *third heart sound,* commonly heard in children and young adults, may persist as late as the age of 40, especially in women. After approximately age 40, however, an S_3 strongly suggests either ventricular failure or volume overloading of the ventricle caused by valvular heart disease such as mitral regurgitation. In contrast, a *fourth heart sound* is seldom heard in young adults unless they are well conditioned athletes. An S_4 may be heard in apparently healthy older people, but is also frequently associated with heart disease. (See Table 9-8, Extra Heart Sounds in Diastole, p. 327).

Changes in Cardiac Murmurs. At some time over the life span, almost everyone has a *heart murmur.* Most murmurs occur without other evidence of cardiovascular abnormality, and may therefore be considered innocent normal variants. The nature of these common murmurs varies importantly with age, and familiarity with their patterns helps you to distinguish normal from abnormal.

Children, adolescents, and young adults frequently have an innocent systolic murmur, often called a *flow murmur,* that is felt to reflect pulmonic blood flow. It is usually heard best in the 2nd to 4th left interspaces (see p. 328).

Late in pregnancy and during lactation, many women have a so-called *mammary souffle*‡ secondary to increased blood flow in their breasts. Although this murmur may be noted anywhere in the breasts, it is often heard most easily in the 2nd or 3rd interspace on either side of the sternum. A mammary souffle is typically both systolic and diastolic, but sometimes only the louder systolic component is audible.

Middle-aged and older adults commonly have an *aortic systolic murmur.* This has been heard in about a third of people near the age of 60, and in well over half of those reaching 85. Aging thickens the bases of the aortic cusps with fibrous tissue, calcification follows, and audible vibrations result. Turbulence produced by blood flow into a dilated aorta may contribute to this murmur. In most people, this process of fibrosis and calcification—known as aortic sclerosis—does not impede blood flow. In some, however, the valve cusps become progressively calcified

‡ Souffle is pronounced soó-fl, not like cheese soufflé. Both words come from a French word meaning puff.

and immobile, and true aortic stenosis, or obstruction of flow, develops. A normal carotid upstroke may help distinguish aortic sclerosis from aortic stenosis (in which the carotid upstroke is delayed), but clinical differentiation between benign aortic sclerosis and pathologic aortic stenosis may be difficult.

A similar aging process affects the mitral valve, usually about a decade later than aortic sclerosis. Here degenerative changes with calcification of the mitral annulus, or valve ring, impair the ability of the mitral valve to close normally during systole, and cause the *systolic murmur of mitral regurgitation.* Because of the extra load placed on the heart by the leaking mitral valve, a murmur of mitral regurgitation cannot be considered innocent.

Murmurs may originate in large blood vessels as well as in the heart. The *jugular venous hum,* which is very common in children and may still be heard through young adulthood, illustrates this point (see p. 332). A second, more important example is the *cervical systolic murmur* or *bruit.* In older people, systolic bruits heard in the middle or upper portions of the carotid arteries suggest, but do not prove, a partial arterial obstruction secondary to atherosclerosis. In contrast, cervical bruits in younger people are usually innocent. In children and young adults, systolic murmurs (bruits) are frequently heard just above the clavicle. Studies have shown that, while cervical bruits can be heard in almost 9 out of 10 children under the age of 5, their prevalence falls steadily to about 1 out of 3 in adolescence and young adulthood and to less than 1 out of 10 in middle age.

Changes in Arteries and Blood Pressure. The aorta and large arteries stiffen with age as they become arteriosclerotic. As the aorta becomes less distensible, a given stroke volume causes a greater rise in systolic blood pressure; *systolic hypertension* with a *widened pulse pressure* often ensues. Peripheral arteries tend to lengthen, become tortuous, and feel harder and less resilient. These changes do not necessarily indicate atherosclerosis, however, and you can make no inferences from them as to disease in the coronary or cerebral vessels. Lengthening and tortuosity of the aorta and its branches occasionally result in kinking or buckling of the carotid artery low in the neck, especially on the right. The resulting pulsatile mass, which occurs chiefly in hypertensive women, may be mistaken for a carotid aneurysm—a true dilatation of the artery. A tortuous aorta occasionally raises the pressure in the jugular veins on the left side of the neck by impairing their drainage within the thorax.

In western societies, systolic blood pressure tends to rise from childhood through old age. Diastolic blood pressure stops rising, however, roughly around the sixth decade. On the other extreme, some elderly people develop an increased tendency toward *postural (orthostatic) hypotension*—a sudden drop in blood pressure when they rise to a sitting or standing position. Elderly people are also more likely to have abnormal heart rhythms. These arrhythmias, like postural hypotension, may cause *syncope* (temporary loss of consciousness).

Techniques of Examination

The cardiovascular examination usually begins with measuring the heart rate and blood pressure, although both may be taken along with other vital signs at the start of the physical examination. The clinician then examines the neck veins and carotid arteries, the radial pulses, and finally the heart itself. It is important to position yourself on the patient's right side whenever possible.

The Arterial Pulse

By examining arterial pulses you can count the rate of the heart and determine its rhythm, assess the amplitude and contour of the pulse wave, and sometimes detect obstructions to blood flow.

Heart Rate. The radial pulse is commonly used to assess the heart rate. With the pads of your index and middle fingers, compress the radial artery until a maximal pulsation is detected. If the rhythm is regular and the rate seems normal, count the rate for 15 seconds and multiply by 4. If the rate is unusually fast or slow, however, count it for 60 seconds.

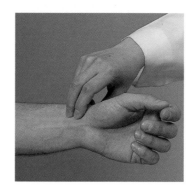

When the rhythm is irregular, the rate should be evaluated by cardiac auscultation, because beats that occur earlier than others may not be detected peripherally and the heart rate can thus be seriously underestimated.

Irregular rhythms include atrial fibrillation and atrial or ventricular premature contractions.

Rhythm. To begin your assessment of rhythm, feel the radial pulse. If there are any irregularities, check the rhythm again by listening with your stethoscope at the cardiac apex. Is the rhythm regular or irregular? If irregular, try to identify a pattern: (1) Do early beats appear in a basically regular rhythm? (2) Does the irregularity vary consistently with respiration? (3) Is the rhythm totally irregular?

Palpation of an irregularly irregular rhythm reliably indicates atrial fibrillation. For all other irregular patterns, an ECG is needed to identify the arrhythmia.

Amplitude and Contour. These are best assessed in the carotid or brachial arteries. The carotid reflects the aortic pulsation more accurately, but in patients with carotid obstruction, kinking, or thrills it is unsuitable. Although either of these arteries can be felt with the fingers, the thumb is convenient and can be positioned more comfortably.[§] The patient should be lying down and the head of the bed elevated to about 30°.

See Table 9-1, Selected Heart Rates and Rhythms (p. 320) and Table 9-2, Selected Irregular Rhythms (p. 321).

[§] Although there is a widespread prejudice against using thumbs to assess pulses, they are very useful for palpating large arteries.

When feeling the carotid artery, first inspect the neck for pulsations. Carotid pulsations may be visible just medial to the sternomastoid muscles. Then place your left thumb (or index and middle fingers) on the right carotid artery in the lower third of the neck, press posteriorly, and feel for the pulsations.

A tortuous and kinked carotid artery may produce a unilateral pulsatile bulge.

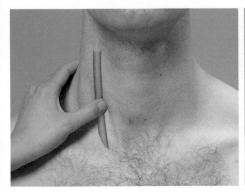
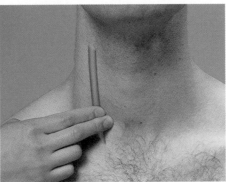

Decreased pulsations may be caused by decreased stroke volume, but may also be due to local factors in the artery such as atherosclerotic narrowing or occlusion.

Press just inside the medial border of a well relaxed sternomastoid muscle, roughly at the level of the cricoid cartilage. Avoid pressing on the carotid sinus, which lies at the level of the top of the thyroid cartilage. For the left carotid, use your right thumb or fingers. Never press both carotids at the same time. You might decrease the blood supply to the brain and cause syncope.

Pressure on the carotid sinus may cause a reflex drop in pulse rate or blood pressure.

When feeling the brachial artery, use the index and middle fingers or thumb of your opposite hand. Cup your hand under the patient's elbow

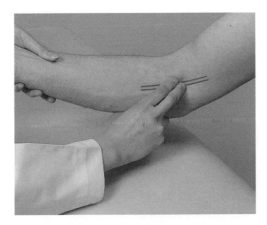

and feel for the pulse just medial to the biceps tendon. The patient's arm should rest with the elbow extended, palm up. With your free hand, you may need to flex the elbow to a varying degree to get optimal muscular relaxation.

Whichever artery you use, slowly increase the pressure until you feel a maximal pulsation, and then slowly decrease it until you can best sense the amplitude and contour. Try to assess:

See Table 9-3, Abnormalities of the Arterial Pulse and Pressure Waves (p. 322).

1. The amplitude of the pulse. This correlates reasonably well with the pulse pressure.

Small, weak pulses and large, bounding pulses (see p. 322)

2. The contour of the pulse wave (i.e., the speed of its upstroke, the duration of its summit, and the speed of its downstroke). The normal upstroke is smooth and rapid and follows the first heart sound almost immediately. The summit is smooth, rounded, and roughly midsystolic. The downstroke is less abrupt than the upstroke.

A delayed upstroke suggests aortic stenosis.

3. Any variations in amplitude
   a. From beat to beat

Pulsus alternans, bigeminal pulse (see p. 322)

   b. With respiration

Paradoxical pulse (see p. 322)

Bruits and Thrills. During palpation of the carotid artery, you may detect humming vibrations that feel like the throat of a purring cat. These are termed a *thrill.* If you feel them, listen over the area with the diaphragm of a stethoscope for a *bruit,* a murmurlike sound of vascular rather than cardiac origin.

You should also listen for bruits over the carotid arteries if the patient is middle-aged or elderly or if you suspect cerebrovascular disease. Ask the patient to hold breathing for a moment so that breath sounds do not obscure the vascular sound. Heart sounds alone do not constitute a bruit.

A carotid bruit with or without a thrill in a middle-aged or older person suggests but does not prove arterial narrowing. An aortic murmur may radiate to the carotid artery and sound like a bruit.

Further examination of arterial pulses is described in Chapter 16, The Peripheral Vascular System.

Blood Pressure

Choice of Sphygmomanometer. As many as 50 million Americans have elevated blood pressure. To measure blood pressure accurately, you must carefully choose a cuff of appropriate size. Proper size depends on the circumference of the limb you are evaluating. The inflatable bladder of the cuff should have a width of about 40% of the upper arm circumference—12 cm to 14 cm in an average adult. The length of the bladder should be about 80% of this circumference—almost long enough to encircle the arm. The sphygmomanometer may be either the aneroid or the mercury type. Because an aneroid instrument often becomes inaccurate with repeated use, it should be recalibrated periodically.

Cuffs that are too short or too narrow may give falsely high readings. Using a regular-size cuff on an obese arm may lead to a false diagnosis of hypertension.

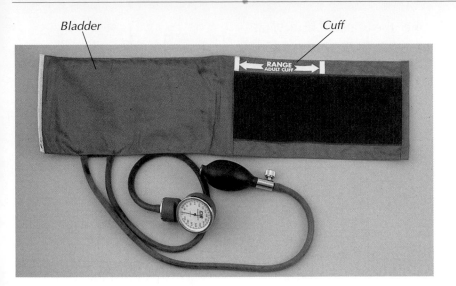

Bladder   Cuff

Technique. Ideally, before the blood pressure is recorded, the patient should avoid smoking or ingesting caffeine for 30 minutes and should rest for at least 5 minutes. The room should be quiet and comfortably warm. The arm selected should be resting and free of clothing. It should also be free of arteriovenous fistulas for dialysis, scarring from brachial artery cutdowns, and lymphedema, which may follow axillary node dissection and radiation therapy. If you have not already felt the brachial pulse, do so to make sure it is intact.

Position the arm so that the brachial artery (at the antecubital crease) is at heart level—roughly level with the 4th interspace at its junction with the sternum. When the patient is seated, rest the arm on a table a little above the patient's waist. When taking a standing blood pressure, try to support the arm at the midchest level.

Center the inflatable bladder over the brachial artery. The lower border of the cuff should be about 2.5 cm above the antecubital crease. Secure the cuff snugly. Position the patient's arm so that it is slightly flexed at the elbow.

To determine how high to raise the cuff pressure, first estimate the systolic pressure by palpation. As you feel the radial artery with the fingers of one hand, rapidly inflate the cuff until the radial pulse disappears. Read this pressure on the manometer and add 30 mm Hg to it. Use of this sum as the target for subsequent inflations prevents discomfort from unnecessarily high cuff pressures. It also avoids the occasional error caused by an auscultatory gap—a silent interval that may be present between the systolic and the diastolic pressures.

Deflate the cuff promptly and completely and wait 15 to 30 seconds.

If the brachial artery is much below heart level, blood pressure appears falsely high. The patient's own effort to support the arm may raise the blood pressure.

A loose cuff or a bladder that balloons outside the cuff leads to falsely high readings.

An unrecognized auscultatory gap may lead to serious underestimation of systolic pressure (e.g., 150/98 in the example on p. 296) or overestimation of diastolic pressure.

Now place the bell of a stethoscope lightly over the brachial artery, taking care to make an air seal with its full rim. Because the sounds to be heard (*Korotkoff sounds*) are relatively low in pitch, they are heard better with the bell.

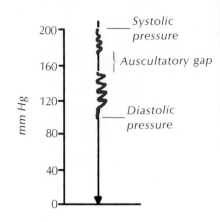

If you find an auscultatory gap, record your findings completely (e.g., 200/98 with an auscultatory gap from 170 to 150).

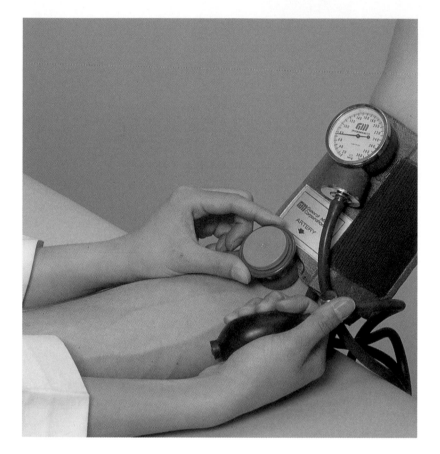

Inflate the cuff rapidly again to the level just determined, and then deflate it slowly at a rate of about 2 to 3 mm Hg per second. Note the level at which you hear the sounds of at least two consecutive beats. This is the systolic pressure.

Continue to lower the pressure slowly until the sounds become muffled and then disappear. To confirm the disappearance of sounds, listen as the pressure falls another 10 to 20 mm Hg. Then deflate the cuff rapidly to zero. The disappearance point, which is usually only a few mm Hg below the muffling point, enables the best estimate of true diastolic pressure in adults.

In some people, the muffling point and the disappearance point are farther apart. Occasionally, as in aortic regurgitation, the sounds never disappear. If there is more than 10 mm Hg difference, record both figures (e.g., 154/80/68).

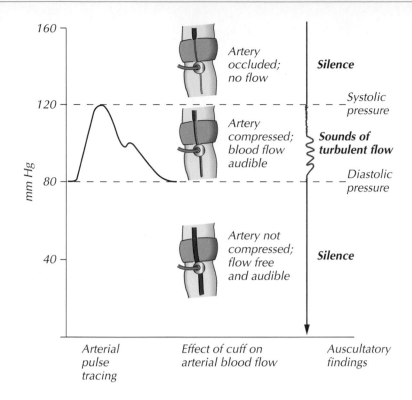

Read both the systolic and the diastolic levels to the nearest 2 mm Hg. Wait 2 or more minutes and repeat. Average your readings. If the first two readings differ by more than 5 mm Hg, take additional readings.

When using a mercury sphygmomanometer, keep the manometer vertical (unless you are using a tilted floor model) and make all readings at eye level with the meniscus. When using an aneroid instrument, hold the dial so that it faces you directly. Avoid slow or repetitive inflations of the cuff, because the resulting venous congestion can cause false readings.

By making the sounds less audible, venous congestion may produce artifactually low systolic and high diastolic pressures.

Blood pressure should be taken in both arms at least once. Normally, there may be a difference in pressure of 5 mm Hg and sometimes up to 10 mm Hg. Subsequent readings should be made on the arm with the higher pressure.

Pressure difference of more than 10–15 mm Hg suggests arterial compression or obstruction on the side with the lower pressure.

In patients taking antihypertensive medications or patients with a history of fainting, postural dizziness, or possible depletion of blood volume, take the blood pressure in three positions—supine, sitting, and standing (unless contraindicated). Normally, as the patient rises from the horizontal to a standing position, systolic pressure drops slightly or remains unchanged while diastolic pressure rises slightly. Another measurement after 1 to 5 minutes of standing may identify orthostatic hypotension missed by earlier readings. This repetition is especially useful in the elderly.

A fall in systolic pressure of 20 mm Hg or more, especially when accompanied by symptoms, indicates orthostatic (postural) hypotension. Causes include drugs, loss of blood, prolonged bed rest, and diseases of the autonomic nervous system.

Definitions of Normal and Abnormal Levels. In 1997, the Joint National Committee on Detection, Evaluation, and Treatment of High Blood Pressure recommended that hypertension should be diagnosed only when a higher than normal level has been found on at least two or more visits after initial screening. Either the diastolic blood pressure (DBP) or the systolic blood pressure (SBP) may be considered high. For adults (aged 18 or over), the Committee has categorized six levels of DBP and SBP:

Blood Pressure Classification (Adults)*		
Category	Systolic (mm Hg)	Diastolic (mm Hg)
Hypertension		
Stage 3 (severe)	≥180	≥110
Stage 2 (moderate)	160–179	100–109
Stage 1 (mild)	140–159	90–99
High Normal	130–139	85–89
Normal	<130	<85
Optimal	<120	<80

* When the systolic and diastolic levels indicate different categories, use the higher category. For example, 170/92 mm Hg is moderate hypertension and 170/120 mm Hg is severe hypertension.

In *isolated systolic hypertension,* systolic pressure is 140 mm Hg or more and diastolic pressure is less than 90 mm Hg.

Assessment of hypertension also includes its effects on target organs—the eyes, the heart, the brain, and the kidneys. Look for evidence of hypertensive retinopathy, left ventricular hypertrophy, and neurologic deficits suggesting a stroke. (Renal assessment requires urinalysis and blood tests.)

Relatively low levels of blood pressure should always be interpreted in the light of past readings and the patient's present clinical state.

A pressure of 110/70 would usually be normal, but could also indicate significant hypotension if past pressures have been high.

SPECIAL PROBLEMS

The Apprehensive Patient. Anxiety is a frequent cause of high blood pressure, especially during an initial visit. Try to get the patient relaxed. Repeat your measurements later in the encounter.

The Obese Arm. Use a wide cuff (15 cm). If the arm circumference exceeds 41 cm, use a thigh cuff (18 cm wide).

Leg Pulses and Pressures. To rule out coarctation of the aorta, two observations should be made at least once with every hypertensive patient:

• Compare the volume and timing of the radial and femoral pulses.
• Compare blood pressures in the arm and leg.

To determine blood pressure in the leg, use a wide, long thigh cuff that has a bladder size of 18 × 42 cm, and apply it to the midthigh. Center the bladder over the posterior surface, wrap it securely, and listen over the popliteal artery. If possible, the patient should be prone. Alternatively, ask the supine patient to flex one leg slightly, with the heel resting on the bed. When cuffs of the proper size are used for both the leg and the arm, blood pressures should be equal in the two areas. (The usual arm cuff, improperly used on the leg, gives a falsely high reading.) A systolic pressure lower in the legs than in the arms is abnormal.

A femoral pulse that is smaller and later than the radial pulse suggests coarctation of the aorta or occlusive aortic disease. Blood pressure is lower in the legs than in the arms in these conditions.

Weak or Inaudible Korotkoff Sounds. Consider technical problems such as erroneous placement of your stethoscope, failure to make full skin contact with the bell, and venous engorgement of the patient's arm from repeated inflations of the cuff. Consider also the possibility of shock.

When you cannot hear Korotkoff sounds at all, you may be able to estimate the systolic pressure by palpation. Alternative methods such as Doppler techniques or direct arterial pressure tracings may be necessary.

To intensify Korotkoff sounds, one of the following methods may be helpful:

* Raise the patient's arm before and while you inflate the cuff. Then lower the arm and determine the blood pressure.
* Inflate the cuff. Ask the patient to make a fist several times, and then determine the blood pressure.

Arrhythmias. Irregular rhythms produce variations in pressure and therefore unreliable measurements. Ignore the effects of an occasional premature contraction. With frequent premature contractions or atrial fibrillation, determine the average of several observations and note that your measurements are approximate.

Jugular Venous Pressure and Pulses

Jugular Venous Pressure (JVP). Examination of the jugular veins and their pulsations allows you to estimate the jugular venous pressure and the pressure in the right atrium (the central venous pressure). The internal jugular pulsations yield better estimates than external jugular pulsations. The jugular veins and pulses are difficult to see in children under 12 years of age, and are therefore of little use in evaluating the cardiovascular system in this age group.

Position the patient to promote comfort, with the head slightly elevated on a pillow and the sternomastoid muscles relaxed. Start with the head of the bed or table elevated about 30°; then adjust the angle so as to maximize visibility of the jugular venous pulsations in the lower half of the neck. Turn the patient's head slightly away from the side you are inspecting.

When the patient's venous pressure is increased, an elevation up to 60° or even 90° may be required. A hypovolemic patient, in contrast, may have to lie flat before you can see the veins. In all these positions the sternal angle usually remains about 5 cm above the right atrium, as diagrammed on p. 289.

Use *tangential (oblique) lighting* and *examine both sides of the neck.* Unilateral distention, especially of an external jugular vein, may be deceptive: it can be caused by local compression in the neck.

Identify the external jugular vein on each side. Then *find the pulsations of the internal jugular vein.* Because this vein lies deep to the sternomastoid muscle, you will not see the vein itself. Watch instead for the pulsations transmitted through the surrounding soft tissues. Look for them in the suprasternal notch, between the attachments of the sternomastoid muscle on the sternum and clavicle, or just posterior to the sternomastoid.

The following features help to distinguish jugular from carotid artery pulsations:

Internal Jugular Pulsations	Carotid Pulsations
Rarely palpable	Palpable
Soft, rapid, undulating quality, usually with two elevations and two troughs per heart beat	A more vigorous thrust with a single outward component
Pulsations eliminated by light pressure on the vein(s) just above the sternal end of the clavicle	Pulsations not eliminated by this pressure
Level of the pulsations changes with position, dropping as the patient becomes more upright.	Level of the pulsations unchanged by position
Level of the pulsations usually descends with inspiration.	Level of the pulsations not affected by inspiration

Identify the highest point of pulsation in the internal jugular vein. With a centimeter ruler, measure the vertical distance between this point and the sternal angle. Establishing true vertical and horizontal lines is difficult—much like the problem of hanging a picture straight when you are close to it. Place your ruler on the sternal angle and line it up with something in the room that you know to be vertical. Then place a long rectangular object such as a packaged tongue blade at an exact right angle to the ruler. This object constitutes your horizontal line. Move it up or down—still horizontal—so that its lower edge rests at the top of the jugular pulsations, and read the vertical distance on the ruler. Round your measurement off to the nearest centimeter.

Increased pressure suggests right-sided heart failure or, less commonly, constrictive pericarditis, tricuspid stenosis, or superior vena cava obstruction.

In patients with obstructive lung disease, venous pressure may appear elevated on expiration only; the veins collapse on inspiration. This finding does not indicate congestive heart failure.

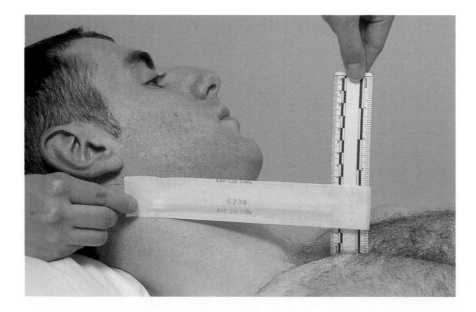

Venous pressure measured as greater than 3 cm or possibly 4 cm above the sternal angle is considered elevated.

The highest point of venous pulsations may lie below the level of the sternal angle. Under these circumstances, venous pressure is not elevated and seldom needs to be measured.

If you are unable to see pulsations in the internal jugular veins, look for them in the external jugulars, although they may not be visible here. If you see none, use *the point above which the external jugular veins appear to collapse.* Make this observation on each side of the neck. Measure the vertical distance of this point from the sternal angle.

Unilateral distention of the external jugular vein is usually due to local kinking or obstruction. Occasionally, even bilateral distention has a local cause.

Jugular Venous Pulsations. Observe the amplitude and timing of the jugular venous pulsations. In order to time these pulsations, feel the left carotid artery with your right thumb or listen to the heart simultaneously. The *a* wave just precedes S$_1$ and the carotid pulse, the *x* descent can be seen as a systolic collapse, the *v* wave almost coincides with S$_2$, and the *y* descent follows early in diastole. Look for absent or unusually prominent waves.

Prominent *a* waves indicate increased resistance to right atrial contraction. Causes include tricuspid stenosis or, more commonly, the decreased compliance of a hypertrophied right ventricle. The *a* waves disappear in atrial fibrillation. Larger *v* waves characterize tricuspid regurgitation.

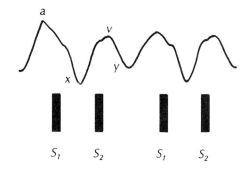

Considerable practice and experience are required to master jugular venous pulsations. A beginner is probably well advised to concentrate primarily on jugular venous pressure.

The Heart

General Approach

For most of the cardiac examination, the patient should be supine with the upper body raised by elevating the head of the bed or table to about 30°. Two other positions are also needed: (1) turning to the left side, and (2) leaning forward. The examiner should stand at the patient's right side.

The table below summarizes patient positions and a suggested sequence for the examination.

Sequence of the Cardiac Examination		Accentuated Findings
Patient Position	**Examination**	**Accentuated Findings**
Supine, with the head elevated 30°	Inspect and palpate the precordium: the 2nd interspaces; the right ventricle; and the left ventricle, including the apical impulse (diameter, location, amplitude, duration).	
Left lateral decubitus	Palpate the apical impulse if not previously detected. Listen at the apex with the bell of the stethoscope.	Low-pitched extra sounds (S_3, opening snap, diastolic rumble of mitral stenosis)
Supine, with the head elevated 30°	Listen at the tricuspid area with the bell. Listen at all the auscultatory areas with the diaphragm.	
Sitting, leaning forward, after full exhalation	Listen along the left sternal border and at the apex.	Soft decrescendo murmur of aortic insufficiency

During this examination, remember to correlate your cardiac findings with the patient's jugular venous pulsations and carotid pulse. It is important to identify both the anatomic location of your findings and their timing in the cardiac cycle.

Note the *anatomic location* of sounds in terms of interspaces and their distance from the midsternal, midclavicular, or axillary lines. The midsternal line offers the most reliable zero point for measurement, but the midclavicular line accommodates to the different sizes and shapes of patients.

Identify the *timing of impulses or sounds* in relation to the cardiac cycle. Timing of sounds is often possible through auscultation alone. In most people with normal or slow heart rates, it is easy to identify the paired heart sounds by listening through a stethoscope. S_1 is the first of these sounds, S_2 is the second, and the relatively long diastolic interval separates one pair from the next.

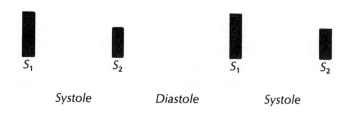

| S_1 | S_2 | S_1 | S_2 |

Systole   Diastole   Systole

The relative intensity of these sounds may also be helpful. S_1 is usually louder than S_2 at the apex; more reliably, S_2 is usually louder than S_1 at the base.

Even experienced clinicians are sometimes uncertain when timing what they hear, especially when they encounter extra heart sounds and murmurs. "Inching" can then be helpful. Return to a place on the chest—most often the base—where it is easy to identify S_1 and S_2. Get their rhythm clearly in mind. Then inch your stethoscope down the chest in steps until you hear the new sound.

Auscultation alone, however, can be a misleading tool for timing. The intensities of S_1 and S_2, for example, may be abnormal. At rapid heart rates, moreover, diastole shortens, and at about a rate of 120 the durations of systole and diastole become indistinguishable. *Palpation of either the carotid pulse or the apical impulse* must then guide the timing of observations. Both occur in early systole, right after the first heart sound.

For example, S_1 is decreased in first-degree heart block, and S_2 is decreased in aortic stenosis.

Inspection and Palpation

Careful inspection of the anterior chest may reveal the location of the apical impulse, or, less commonly, the ventricular movements of a left-sided S_3 or S_4.

Palpation yields further information. The characteristics of the apical impulse help you to determine the size of the left ventricle, and a left parasternal impulse may suggest enlargement of the right ventricle. Palpation may reveal an S_3 or an S_4, accentuated first and second heart sounds, and exaggerated pulsations of the aorta or pulmonary artery. In addition, a loud heart murmur may produce a palpable thrill.

The proper techniques facilitate these observations. Tangential light much improves your chances of seeing impulses. For feeling impulses, use your fingerpads, held flat or obliquely on the body surface: light pressure for the low-pitched S_3 and S_4 and firmer pressure for the relatively high-pitched S_1 and S_2. Thrills, like tactile fremitus, are felt best through bone—the ball of your hand pressed firmly on the chest. It is probably more efficient to feel for thrills after auscultation has revealed a loud murmur.

Thrills may accompany loud, harsh, or rumbling murmurs such as those of aortic stenosis, patent ductus arteriosus, ventricular septal defect, and, less commonly, mitral stenosis. They are palpated more easily in patient positions that accentuate the murmur.

From the patient's right side, systematically examine the anterior chest, paying special attention to each of the five areas illustrated below.

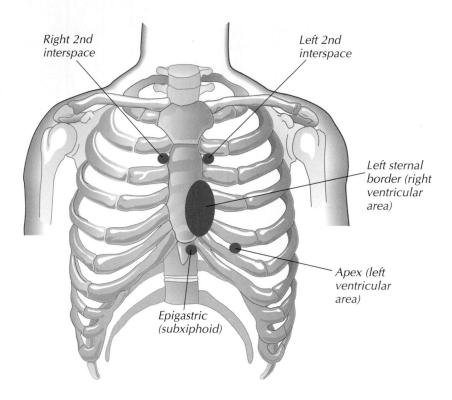

Right 2nd interspace

Left 2nd interspace

Left sternal border (right ventricular area)

Apex (left ventricular area)

Epigastric (subxiphoid)

The Cardiac Apex (Left Ventricular Area). This is normally at or medial to the midclavicular line in the 5th or possibly the 4th interspace. Here you can often see the apical impulse, the brief early systolic pulsation of the left ventricle as it moves anteriorly during contraction and touches the chest wall.

The apical impulse may not be visible in the supine patient, and often is most easily felt in the left lateral decubitus position. Ask the patient to roll partly onto the left side and look again. Then feel for the impulse. If inspection does not reveal its location, search for it first with the palmar surfaces of several fingers. If you cannot find it, ask the patient to exhale fully and stop breathing for a few seconds.

Cardiac impulses lateral to the midclavicular line suggest cardiac enlargement or displacement.

On rare occasions, a patient has *dextrocardia*—a heart situated on the right side. The apical impulse will then be found on the right. If you cannot find an apical impulse, percuss for the dullness of heart and liver and for the tympany of the stomach. In *situs inversus*, all three of these structures are on opposite sides from normal. A right-sided heart with a normally placed liver and stomach is usually associated with congenital heart disease.

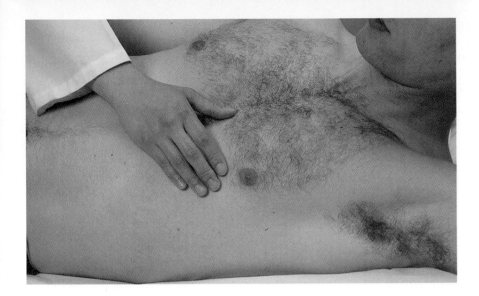

Once you have found the apical impulse, make finer assessments with your fingertips, and then with one finger.

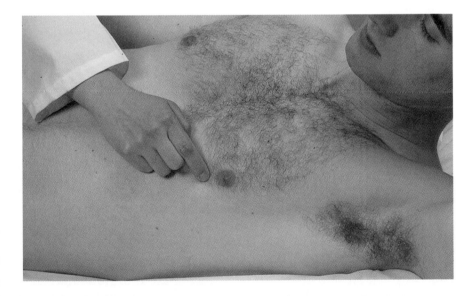

With experience, you will learn to feel the apical impulse in a high percentage of patients, but obesity, a very muscular chest wall, or an increased anteroposterior diameter of the chest may make it undetectable. Some apical impulses hide behind the rib cage, despite positioning.

When examining a woman with large breasts, gently displace the left breast upward or laterally as necessary. Alternatively, ask her to do this for you.

Assess the location, diameter, amplitude, and duration of the apical impulse. Having the patient breathe out and briefly stop breathing is helpful.

See Table 9-4, Variations and Abnormalities of the Ventricular Impulses (p. 323).

Location. If possible, assess the location of the apical impulse when the patient is supine. The left lateral decubitus position displaces this impulse to the left, though not normally beyond the midclavicular line. Note the interspace(s) that the impulse occupies, and measure its distance in centimeters from the midsternal or the midclavicular line.

The apical impulse may be displaced upward and to the left by pregnancy or a high left diaphragm. It may also be displaced by deformities of the thorax, by a mediastinal shift, or by enlargement of the heart.

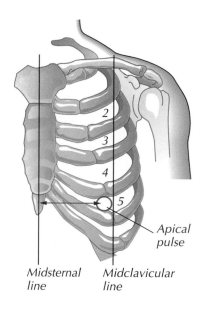

Diameter. Note the diameter of the apical impulse. In the supine patient, it usually measures less than 2.5 cm and occupies only one interspace. It may be larger in the left lateral decubitus position.

In the left lateral decubitus position, a diameter greater than 3 cm indicates left ventricular enlargement.

Amplitude. Estimate the amplitude of the impulse. It is usually small and feels like a gentle tap. An increased amplitude (hyperkinetic impulse) may be felt in some young persons, especially with excitement or after exercise. Duration, however, is normal.

Increased amplitude may also reflect hyperthyroidism, severe anemia, pressure overload of the left ventricle (e.g., aortic stenosis), or volume overload of the left ventricle (e.g., mitral regurgitation).

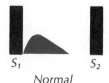

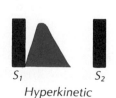

Duration. Of all the characteristics of the apical impulse, duration is the most useful in identifying hypertrophy of the left ventricle. To assess duration, listen to the heart sounds while you are feeling the apical impulse, or watch the movement of your stethoscope as you listen at the apex. Estimate the proportion of systole occupied by the apical impulse. The normal impulse may last through the first two thirds of systole, and often less, but does not continue to the second heart sound.

A sustained, high-amplitude impulse that is normally located suggests left ventricular hypertrophy from pressure overload (as in hypertension).

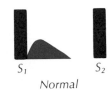

S_1 S_2

Normal

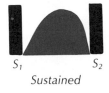

S_1 S_2

Sustained

If such an impulse is displaced laterally, consider volume overload.

A sustained low-amplitude (hypokinetic) impulse may be due to the dilated heart of cardiomyopathy.

S_3 and S_4. By inspection and palpation, you may also be able to detect the ventricular movements that are synchronous with pathologic third and fourth heart sounds. For the left ventricular impulses, feel the apical beat gently with one finger. The patient should lie partly on the left side, breathe out, and briefly stop breathing. By inking an X on the apex you may be able to see these movements.

A brief middiastolic impulse indicates an S_3; an impulse just before the systolic apical beat itself indicates an S_4.

The Left Sternal Border in the 3rd, 4th, and 5th Interspaces (Right Ventricular Area). The patient should rest supine at 30°. Place the tips of your curved fingers in the 3rd, 4th, and 5th interspaces and try to feel the systolic impulse of the right ventricle. Again, asking the patient to breathe out and then briefly stop breathing improves your observation.

If an impulse is palpable, assess its location, amplitude, and duration. A brief systolic tap of low or slightly increased amplitude is sometimes felt in thin or shallow-chested persons, especially when stroke volume is increased, as by anxiety.

A marked increased in amplitude with little or no change in duration occurs in chronic volume overload of the right ventricle, as from an atrial septal defect.

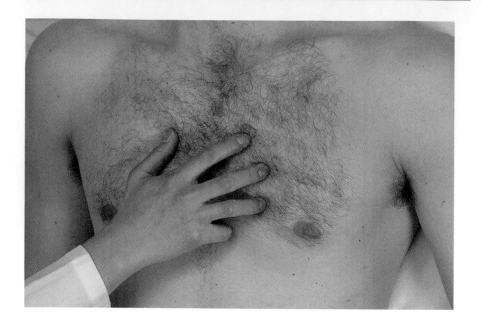

An impulse with increased amplitude and duration occurs with pressure overload of the right ventricle, as in pulmonic stenosis or pulmonary hypertension.

The diastolic movements of right-sided third and fourth heart sounds may be felt occasionally. Feel for them in the 4th and 5th left interspaces. Time them by auscultation or carotid palpation.

The Epigastric (Subxiphoid) Area. This location is especially useful when you are examining a person with an increased anteroposterior diameter of the chest. With your hand flattened, press your index finger just under the rib cage and up toward the left shoulder and try to feel right ventricular pulsations.

In pulmonary emphysema, hyperinflated lung may prevent palpation of an enlarged right ventricle in the left parasternal area. The impulse is felt easily, however, high in the epigastrium. In such patients, heart sounds are also often heard best here.

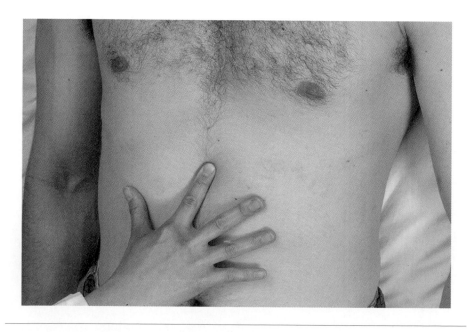

Asking the patient to inhale and briefly stop breathing is helpful. The inspiratory position moves your hand well away from the pulsations of the abdominal aorta, which might otherwise be confusing.

The diastolic movements of S_3 and S_4, if present, may also be felt here.

The Left 2nd Interspace, which overlies the *pulmonary artery.* During held expiration, look and feel for an impulse and feel for possible heart sounds. Firmer pressure is needed for the heart sounds. In thin or shallow-chested people, the pulsation of a pulmonary artery may sometimes be felt here, especially after exercise or with excitement.

A prominent pulsation here often accompanies dilatation or increased flow in the pulmonary artery. A palpable second heart sound suggests increased pressure in the pulmonary artery (pulmonary hypertension).

The Right 2nd Interspace. Again, search for pulsations and palpable heart sounds.

A palpable second heart sound suggests systemic hypertension. A pulsation here suggests a dilated or aneurysmal aorta.

Percussion

In most cases, palpation has replaced percussion in the estimation of cardiac size. When you cannot feel the apical impulse, however, percussion may suggest where to search for it. Occasionally, percussion may be your only tool. Under these circumstances, cardiac dullness often occupies a large area. Starting well to the left on the chest, percuss from resonance toward cardiac dullness in the 3rd, 4th, 5th, and possibly 6th interspaces.

A markedly dilated failing heart may have a hypokinetic apical impulse that is displaced far to the left. A large pericardial effusion may make the impulse undetectable.

Auscultation

Locations. Listen to the heart with your stethoscope in the right 2nd interspace close to the sternum, along the left sternal border in each interspace from the 2nd through the 5th, and at the apex.

In the past, most of these areas have had auscultatory names (shown in parentheses on p. 310 because they are still in common use). Because murmurs of more than one origin may occur in a given area these names may be misleading, and some authorities now discourage their use.

The areas designated on p. 310 should not limit your auscultation. If the heart is enlarged or displaced, you should alter your pattern accordingly. You should also listen in any area where you have observed an abnormality, and you should listen in areas adjacent to murmurs to determine where they are loudest and to trace their radiation. The room should be quiet.

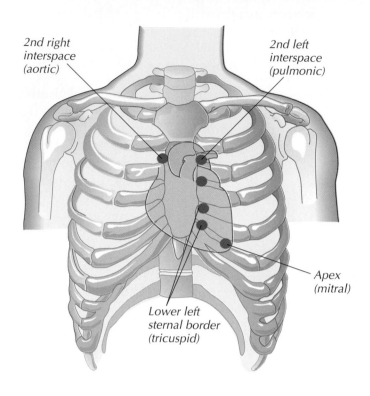

Heart sounds and murmurs that originate in the four valves are illustrated in the diagram below. Pulmonic sounds are usually heard best in the 2nd and 3rd left interspaces, but may extend further.

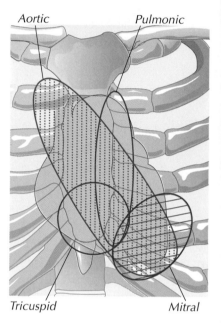

(Redrawm from Leatham A: Introduction to the Examination of the Cardiovascular System, 2nd ed. Oxford, Oxford University Press, 1979)

Sequence. Clinicians vary in their sequence of auscultation, some preferring to start at the apex, others preferring to start at the base. Either pattern is satisfactory.

Use of the Stethoscope. You should listen throughout the precordium with the diaphragm of your stethoscope, pressing it firmly on the chest. The diaphragm is better for picking up relatively high-pitched sounds such as S_1, S_2, the murmurs of aortic and mitral regurgitation, and pericardial friction rubs. The bell is more sensitive to low-pitched sounds such as S_3, S_4, and the murmur of mitral stenosis. Use the bell at the apex and more medially along the lower sternal border. Apply it lightly, with just enough pressure to produce an air seal with its full rim. Resting the heel of your hand on the chest, like a fulcrum, helps to maintain this light pressure.

Pressing the bell firmly on the chest stretches the underlying skin and makes the bell function more like a diaphragm. Low-pitched sounds such as S_3 and S_4 may disappear with this technique—an observation that helps to identify them. High-pitched sounds such as a midsystolic click, an ejection sound, or an opening snap, in contrast, persist or get louder.

Patient Positions. Listen to the entire precordium with the patient supine. In addition, use two other positions:

1. Ask the patient to *roll partly onto the left side,* thus bringing the left ventricle closer to the chest wall. Place the bell of your stethoscope lightly on the apical impulse.

This position accentuates or brings out a left-sided S_3 and S_4 and mitral murmurs, especially the murmur of mitral stenosis. You may otherwise miss these important findings.

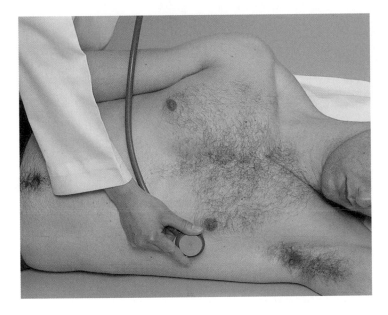

2. Ask the patient to *sit up, lean forward, exhale completely, and stop breathing* in expiration. With the diaphragm of your stethoscope pressed on the chest, listen along the left sternal border and at the apex, pausing periodically so the patient may breathe.

This position accentuates or brings out aortic murmurs. You may easily miss the murmur of aortic regurgitation unless you use this position.

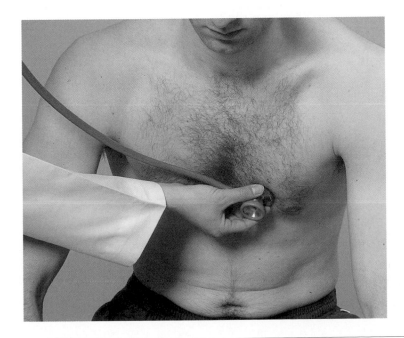

What to Listen for. Throughout your examination, take your time at each auscultatory area. Concentrate on each of the events in the cardiac cycle listed below and sounds you may hear in systole and diastole.

Auscultatory Sounds	
Heart Sounds	**Guides to Auscultation**
S_1	Note its intensity and any apparent splitting. Normal splitting is detectable along the lower left sternal border.
S_2	Note its intensity.
Split S_2	Listen for splitting of this sound in the 2nd and 3rd left interspaces. Ask the patient to breathe quietly, and then slightly more deeply than normal. Does S_2 split into its two components, as it normally does? If not, ask the patient to (1) breathe a little more deeply, or (2) sit up. Listen again. A thick chest wall may make the pulmonic component of S_1 inaudible.
	Width of split. How wide is the split? It is normally quite narrow.
	Timing of split. When in the respiratory cycle do you hear the split? It is normally heard late in inspiration.
	Does the split disappear as it should, during exhalation? If not, listen again with the patient sitting up.
	Intensity of A_2 and P_2. Compare the intensity of the two components, A_2 and P_2. A_2 is usually louder.
Extra Sounds in Systole	Such as ejection sounds or systolic clicks
	Note their location, timing, intensity, and pitch, and the effects of respiration on the sounds.
Extra Sounds in Diastole	Such as S_3, S_4, or an opening snap
	Note their location, timing, intensity, and pitch, and the effects of respiration on the sounds. (An S_3 or S_4 in athletes is a normal finding.)
Systolic and Diastolic Murmurs	Murmurs are differentiated from heart sounds by their longer duration.

See Table 9-5, Variations in the First Heart Sound (p. 324).

See Table 9-6, Variations in the Second Heart Sound (p. 325).

When either A_2 or P_2 is absent, as in disease of the respective valves, S_2 is persistently single.

Expiratory splitting suggests an abnormality (p. 325).

Persistent splitting results from delayed closure of the pulmonic valve or early closure of the aortic valve.

A loud P_2 suggests pulmonary hypertension.

The systolic click of mitral valve prolapse is the most common of these sounds. See Table 9-7, Extra Heart Sounds in Systole (p. 326)

See Table 9-8, Extra Heart Sounds in Diastole (p. 327)

See Table 9-9, Midsystolic Murmurs (pp. 328–329), Table 9-10, Pansystolic Murmurs (p. 330), and Table 9-11, Diastolic Murmurs (p. 331).

Attributes of Heart Murmurs. Any murmur should be described in terms of its timing, shape, location of maximal intensity, radiation or transmission from this location, intensity, pitch, and quality.

Timing. You must first be sure whether you are hearing a *systolic murmur,* which occurs between S_1 and S_2, or a *diastolic murmur,* which occurs between S_2 and S_1.

Diastolic murmurs usually indicate valvular heart disease. Systolic murmurs may indicate valvular disease, but often occur when the heart is entirely normal.

Systolic murmurs are usually *midsystolic* or *pansystolic.* Late systolic murmurs may also be heard.

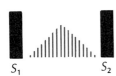

A *midsystolic murmur* begins after S_1 and stops before S_2. Brief gaps are audible between the murmur and the heart sounds. Listen carefully for the gap just before S_2. It is heard more easily and, if present, usually confirms the murmur as midsystolic, not pansystolic.

Midsystolic murmurs most often are related to blood flow across the semilunar (aortic and pulmonic) valves. See Table 9-9, Midsystolic Murmurs (pp. 328–329).

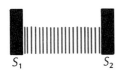

A *pansystolic (holosystolic) murmur,* in contrast, starts with S_1 and stops at S_2, without a gap between murmur and heart sounds.

Pansystolic murmurs often occur with regurgitant (backward) flow across the atrioventricular valves. See Table 9-10, Pansystolic (Holosystolic) Murmurs (p. 330).

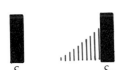

A *late systolic murmur* usually starts in mid- or late systole and persists up to S_2.

This is the murmur of mitral valve prolapse and is often, but not always, preceded by a systolic click (see p. 326).

Diastolic murmurs may be *early diastolic, middiastolic,* or *late diastolic.*

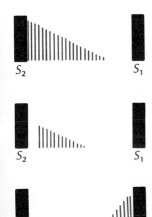

An *early diastolic murmur* starts right after S_2, without a discernible gap, and then usually fades into silence before the next S_1.

Early diastolic murmurs typically accompany regurgitant flow across incompetent semilunar valves.

A *middiastolic murmur* starts a short time after S_2. It may fade away, as illustrated, or merge into a late diastolic murmur.

Middiastolic and presystolic murmurs are related to turbulent flow across the atrioventricular valves. See Table 9-11, Diastolic Murmurs (p. 331).

A *late diastolic (presystolic) murmur* starts late in diastole and typically continues up to S_1.

An occasional murmur, such as that caused by a patent ductus arteriosus, starts in systole and continues without pause through S_2 into but not necessarily throughout diastole. It is then called a *continuous murmur*. Other cardiovascular sounds, such as pericardial friction rubs or venous hums, have *both systolic and diastolic components*. Observe and describe these sounds according to the characteristics used for systolic and diastolic murmurs.

The combination of systolic and diastolic murmurs, each with its own characteristics, may have similar timing. See Table 9-12, Cardiovascular Sounds With Both Systolic and Diastolic Components (p. 332).

Shape. The shape or configuration of a murmur is determined by its intensity over time.

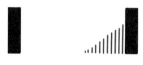

A *crescendo murmur* grows louder.

The presystolic murmur of mitral stenosis in normal sinus rhythm

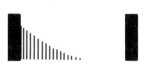

A *decrescendo murmur* grows softer.

The early diastolic murmur of aortic regurgitation

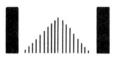

A *crescendo–descrescendo murmur* first rises in intensity, then falls.

The midsystolic murmur of aortic stenosis and innocent flow murmurs

A *plateau murmur* has the same intensity throughout.

The pansystolic murmur of mitral regurgitation

Location of Maximal Intensity. This is determined by the site where the murmur originates. Find the location by exploring the area in which you can hear the murmur, and describe where you hear it best in terms of the interspace and its relation to the sternum, the apex, or the midsternal, the midclavicular, or one of the axillary lines.

For example, a murmur best heard in the 2nd right interspace usually originates at or near the aortic valve.

Radiation or Transmission From the Point of Maximal Intensity. This reflects not only the site of origin but also the intensity of the murmur and the direction of blood flow. Explore the area around a murmur and determine where else you can hear it.

A loud murmur of aortic stenosis often radiates into the neck (in the direction of arterial flow).

Intensity. This is usually graded on a 6-point scale and expressed as a fraction. The numerator describes the intensity of the murmur wherever it is loudest, and the denominator indicates the scale you are using. Intensity is influenced by the thickness of the chest wall and the presence of intervening tissue.

An identical degree of turbulence would cause a louder murmur in a thin person than in a very muscular or obese one. Emphysematous lungs may diminish the intensity of murmurs.

You will learn to grade murmurs on the 6-point scale below:

Gradations of Murmurs	
Grade	**Description**
Grade 1	Very faint, heard only after listener has "tuned in"; may not be heard in all positions
Grade 2	Quiet, but heard immediately after placing the stethoscope on the chest
Grade 3	Moderately loud
Grade 4	Loud
Grade 5	Very loud. May be heard when the stethoscope is partly off the chest.
Grade 6	May be heard when stethoscope entirely off the chest.

Thrills are associated with murmurs of grades 4 through 6.

Pitch. This is categorized as high, medium, or low.

Quality. This is described in terms such as blowing, harsh, rumbling, and musical.

A fully described murmur might be: a "medium-pitched, grade 2/6, blowing decrescendo murmur, heard best in the 4th left interspace, with radiation to the apex" (aortic regurgitation).

Other useful characteristics of murmurs—and heart sounds too—include their variations, if any, with respiration, with the position of the patient, or with other special maneuvers.

Murmurs originating in the right side of the heart tend to change more with respiration than do left-sided murmurs.

A Note on Cardiovascular Assessment

A good cardiovascular examination requires more than observation. You need to think about the possible meanings of your individual observations, fit them together in a logical pattern, and correlate your cardiac findings with the patient's blood pressure, arterial pulses, venous pulsations, 2nd venous pressure, the remainder of your physical examination, and the patient's history.

Evaluating the common systolic murmur illustrates this point. In examining an asymptomatic teenager, for example, you might hear a grade 2/6 midsystolic murmur localized in the 2nd and 3rd left interspaces. Since this suggests a murmur of pulmonic origin, you should assess the size of the right ventricle by carefully palpating the left parasternal area. Because pulmonic stenosis and atrial septal defects can occasionally cause such murmurs, listen carefully to the splitting of the second heart sound and try to hear any ejection sounds. Listen to the murmur after the patient sits up. Look for evidence of anemia, hyperthyroidism, or pregnancy that

In a 60-year-old person with angina, you might hear a grade 3/6 harsh midsystolic murmur maximal in the right 2nd interspace radiating to the neck. You cannot feel a thrill. These findings suggest aortic stenosis, but could arise from a sclerotic valve without stenosis, a dilated aorta, or increased flow across a normal valve. Evaluate the apical impulse for evidence of left ventricular enlargement. Listen for the murmur of aortic regurgitation as the patient leans forward and exhales.

could produce such a murmur by increasing the flow across the aortic or the pulmonic valve. If all your findings are normal, your patient probably has an *innocent murmur*—one with no pathologic significance.

Special Techniques

Aids to Identify Systolic Murmurs. Elsewhere in this chapter you have learned how to improve your auscultation of heart sounds and murmurs by placing the patient in different positions. Two additional techniques will help you distinguish the murmurs of mitral valve prolapse and hypertrophic cardiomyopathy from aortic stenosis.

(1) Standing and Squatting. When a person stands, venous return to the heart decreases and so does peripheral vascular resistance. Arterial blood pressure, stroke volume, and the volume of blood in the left ventricle all decline. On squatting, changes occur in opposite directions. These changes help (1) to identify a prolapsed mitral valve, and (2) to distinguish hypertrophic cardiomyopathy from aortic stenosis.

Secure the patient's gown so that it will not interfere with your examination, and ready yourself for prompt auscultation. Instruct the patient in how to squat next to the examining table and how to hold on to it for balance. Listen to the heart with the patient in the squatting position and again in the standing position.

(2) Valsalva Maneuver. When a person strains down against a closed glottis, venous return to the right heart is decreased and after a few seconds left ventricular volume and arterial blood pressure both fall. Release of the effort has the opposite effects. These changes help to distinguish prolapse of the mitral valve and hypertrophic cardiomyopathy from aortic stenosis.

The patient should be lying down. Ask the patient to "bear down," or place one hand on the midabdomen and instruct the patient to strain against it. By adjusting your pressure you can alter the patient's effort to the desired level. Use your other hand to place your stethoscope on the patient's chest.

Pulsus Alternans. If you suspect left-sided heart failure, feel the pulse specifically for alternating amplitudes. These are usually felt best in the radial or the femoral arteries. A blood-pressure cuff gives you a more sensitive method. After raising the cuff pressure, lower it slowly to the systolic level and then below it. While you do this, the patient should breathe quietly or stop breathing in the respiratory midposition. If dyspnea prevents this, help the patient to sit up and dangle both legs over the side of the bed.

Alternately loud and soft Korotkoff sounds or a sudden doubling of the apparent heart rate as the cuff pressure declines indicates a pulsus alternans (see p. 322).

The upright position may accentuate the alternation.

Maneuvers to Identify Systolic Murmurs

Maneuver	Cardiovascular Effect	Effect on Systolic Sounds and Murmurs		
		Mitral Valve Prolapse	*Hypertrophic Cardiomyopathy*	*Aortic Stenosis*
Standing; Strain Phase of Valsalva	**Decreased left ventricular volume from** ↓ venous return to heart **Decreased vascular tone:** ↓ arterial blood pressure; ↓ peripheral vascular resistance	↑ prolapse of mitral valve Click moves earlier in systole and murmur lengthens	↑ outflow obstruction	↓ blood volume ejected into aorta
		↑ intensity of murmur	↑ intensity of murmur	↓ intensity of murmur
Squatting; Release of Valsalva	**Increased left ventricular volume:** ↑ venous return to heart ∴ ↑ left ventricular volume **Increased vascular tone:** ↑ arterial blood pressure; ↑ peripheral vascular resistance	↓ prolapse of mitral valve Delay of click and murmur shortens.	↓ outflow obstruction	↑ blood volume ejected into aorta
		↓ intensity of murmur	↓ intensity of murmur	↑ intensity of murmur

Paradoxical Pulse. If you have noted that the pulse varies in amplitude with respiration or if you suspect pericardial tamponade (because of increased jugular venous pressure, a rapid and diminished pulse, and dyspnea, for example), use a blood-pressure cuff to check for a paradoxical pulse. This is a greater than normal drop in systolic pressure during inspiration. As the patient breathes, quietly if possible, lower the cuff pressure slowly to the systolic level. Note the pressure level at which the first sounds can be heard. Then drop the pressure very slowly until sounds can be heard throughout the respiratory cycle. Again note the pressure level. The difference between these two levels is normally no greater than 3 or 4 mm Hg.

The level identified by first hearing Korotkoff sounds is the highest systolic pressure during the respiratory cycle. The level identified by hearing sounds throughout the cycle is the lowest systolic pressure. A difference between these levels of more than 10 mm Hg indicates a paradoxical pulse and suggests pericardial tamponade, possibly constrictive pericarditis, but most commonly obstructive airway disease (see p. 322).

Health Promotion and Counseling

Education and counseling will encourage your patients to maintain healthy levels of cholesterol, weight, and exercise. Screening for elevated cholesterol (≥200 mg/dL), even at age 20, establishes a baseline for education and diet modification. When total cholesterol is elevated, proceed to a lipid profile. Watch for three main patterns on the lipid profile: (1) normal to high levels of "the good cholesterol," namely high-density lipoprotein cholesterol (HDL)—associated with *low risk* of coronary heart disease (CHD); (2) low HDL levels—associated with *high risk* of CHD; and (3) high levels of low-density lipoprotein cholesterol (LDL) associated with *high risk* of CHD. Triglycerides may be elevated, but their role as a risk factor for CHD is still not clear.

For patients with low HDL and high LDL cholesterol, review the basic principles for *all* healthy diets: high intake of fruits, vegetables, and grains (such diets are naturally low in calories, saturated fat, cholesterol, salt, and sugar); use of lean meats, substituting chicken and fish when possible, and low-fat dairy products; and minimal intake of processed food and added salt and sugar in cooking and at the table. Eggs with yolks, the most concentrated source of dietary cholesterol, should be limited to two to four per week. Remember that LDL cholesterol levels are lowered most effectively by increasing intake of fiber, found in whole-grain breads, pasta, and oat, wheat, corn, or multigrain cereals. A rapid screen for dietary intake is shown below:

Rapid Screen for Dietary Intake		
	Portions Consumed	
	By Patient	*Recommended*
Grains, cereals, bread group	_____	6–11
Fruit group	_____	2–4
Vegetable group	_____	3–5
Meat and meat substitute group	_____	2–3
Dairy group	_____	2–3
Sugars, fats, snack foods	_____	—
Soft drinks	_____	—
Alcoholic beverages	_____	<2

Source: Nestle M: Chapter 8, Nutrition. In: Woolf SH, Jonas S, Lawrence RS (eds) Health Promotion and Disease Prevention in Clinical Practice. Baltimore, Williams & Wilkins, 1996.

Excess weight and sedentary lifestyle also increase risk of CHD. To initiate weight management, evaluate height, weight, and body fat. Determine if the patient is overweight. Patients whose body weight is 20% above the upper limit of normal by age, sex, and height are considered obese. Note that overly sedentary patients may have excess body fat (obesity) even at normal weights.

To maintain a desirable body weight, a person's energy expended must balance calories consumed. Excess calories are stored as fat. Metabolism of food fat, which contains 9 calories of potential energy per gram, uses up fewer calories than metabolism of foods high in carbohydrate or protein, which provide 4 calories of energy per gram. Patients with high fat intake are more likely to accumulate body fat than patients with increased protein and carbohydrate intake (and patients with low-fat diets may lose weight more quickly). Review the patient's eating habits and weight patterns in the family. Set realistic goals that will help the patient maintain healthy eating patterns *for life.*

Regular exercise is the number one recommendation of the U.S. Public Health Service's *Healthy People 2000.* To reduce risk for coronary artery disease, counsel patients to pursue *aerobic* exercise, or exercise that increases muscle oxygen uptake. (*Anaerobic* exercise relies on energy sources within contracting muscles rather than inhaled oxygen, and is usually nonsustained.) Deep breathing, sweating in cool temperatures, and pulse rates exceeding 60% of the maximum normal age-adjusted heart rate (220 minus the person's age) are markers of aerobic exercise. Since the cardiovascular benefits of exercise are long term, to help motivate patients be sure to emphasize that the patient will look and feel better as soon as exercise begins. Before selecting an exercise regimen, do a thorough evaluation of any cardiovascular, pulmonary, or musculoskeletal conditions presenting a risk for exercise. Guiding the patient to make time to exercise as a *regular activity* is often more important than the type of exercise chosen. For cardiovascular benefit, patients should exercise for 20 to 60 minutes at least 3 times a week. For patients losing weight, paradoxically, the metabolic rate may drop when caloric intake declines, known as the starvation response. Regular exercise will counteract this response.

During the physical examination, it is important to screen for hyper tension and for lipid-containing nodules on the skin, known as *xanthomas.* Hypertension (see p. 298) contributes significantly to death from CHD and stroke. Recommended blood pressure screening for healthy adults is generally once every 2 years. Search for xanthomas in patients with familial lipoprotein disorders. These may appear around the eyelids, over extensor tendons, and occasionally as small eruptive papules on the extremities, buttocks, and trunk.

Table 9-1 Selected Heart Rates and Rhythms

TABLE 9-1 Selected Heart Rates and Rhythms

Cardiac rhythms may be classified as regular or irregular. When rhythms are irregular or rates are fast or slow, an ECG is required to identify the origin of the beats (sinus node, AV node, atrium, or ventricle) and the pattern of conduction. Note that with AV (atrioventricular) block, arrhythmias may have a fast, normal, or slow ventricular rate.

IS THE RHYTHM REGULAR OR IRREGULAR?

REGULAR — WHAT IS THE RATE?

	ECG Pattern	Usual Resting Rate
FAST (>100)	Sinus tachycardia	100–180
	Supraventricular (atrial or nodal) tachycardia	150–250
	Atrial flutter with a regular ventricular response	100–175
	Ventricular tachycardia	110–250
NORMAL (60–100)	Normal sinus rhythm	60–100
	Second-degree AV block	60–100
	Atrial flutter with a regular ventricular response	75–100
SLOW (<60)	Sinus bradycardia	<60
	Second-degree AV block	30–60
	Complete heart block	<40

IRREGULAR — WHAT IS THE PATTERN OF IRREGULARITY?

	ECG Pattern	Usual Resting Rate
RHYTHMICALLY OR SPORADICALLY IRREGULAR	Early beats → Atrial or nodal (supraventricular) premature contractions; Ventricular premature contractions	See Table 9-2.
	Sinus arrhythmia	
TOTALLY IRREGULAR	Atrial fibrillation	
	Atrial flutter with varying block	

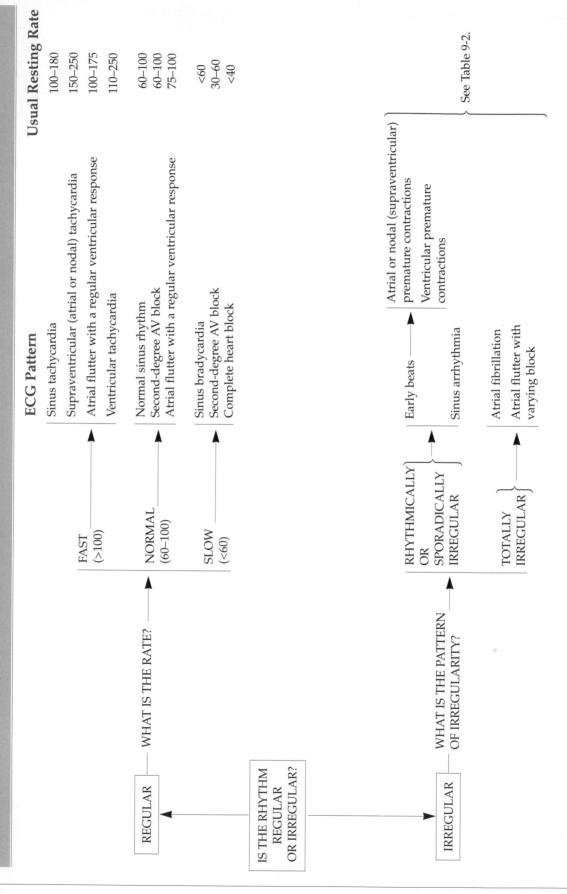

Table 9-2   Selected Irregular Rhythms

T A B L E 9 - 2   *Selected Irregular Rhythms*

Type of Rhythm	ECG Waves and Heart Sounds	Rhythm	Heart Sounds
Atrial or Nodal (*Supraventricular*) **Premature Contractions**		A beat of atrial or nodal origin comes earlier than the next expected normal beat. A pause follows and then the rhythm resumes.	S_1 may differ in intensity from the S_1 of normal beats, and S_2 may be decreased. Both sounds are otherwise similar to those of normal beats.
Ventricular Premature Contractions		A beat of ventricular origin comes earlier than the next expected normal beat. A pause follows and the rhythm resumes.	S_1 may differ in intensity from the S_1 of the normal beats, and S_2 may be decreased. Both sounds are likely to be split.
Sinus Arrhythmia		The heart varies cyclically, usually speeding up with inspiration and slowing down with expiration.	Normal, although S_1 may vary with the heart rate
Atrial Fibrillation and Atrial Flutter With Varying AV Block		The ventricular rhythm is totally irregular, although short runs of the irregular ventricular rhythm may seem regular.	S_1 varies in intensity.

Table 9-3 Abnormalities of the Arterial Pulse and Pressure Waves

TABLE 9 - 3 Abnormalities of the Arterial Pulse and Pressure Waves

Normal
mm Hg

The pulse pressure is about 30–40 mm Hg. The pulse contour is smooth and rounded. (The notch on the descending slope of the pulse wave is not palpable.)

Small, Weak Pulses

The pulse pressure is diminished, and the pulse feels weak and small. The upstroke may feel slowed, the peak prolonged. Causes include (1) decreased stroke volume, as in heart failure, hypovolemia, and severe aortic stenosis, and (2) increased peripheral resistance, as in exposure to cold and severe congestive heart failure.

Large, Bounding Pulses

The pulse pressure is increased and the pulse feels strong and bounding. The rise and fall may feel rapid, the peak brief. Causes include (1) an increased stroke volume, a decreased peripheral resistance, or both, as in fever, anemia, hyperthyroidism, aortic regurgitation, arteriovenous fistulas, and patent ductus arteriosus, (2) an increased stroke volume due to slow heart rates, as in bradycardia and complete heart block, and (3) decreased compliance (increased stiffness) of the aortic walls, as in aging or atherosclerosis.

Bisferiens Pulse

A bisferiens pulse is an increased arterial pulse with a double systolic peak. Causes include pure aortic regurgitation, combined aortic stenosis and regurgitation, and, though less commonly palpable, hypertrophic cardiomyopathy.

Pulsus Alternans

The pulse alternates in amplitude from beat to beat even though the rhythm is basically regular (and must be for you to make this judgment). When the difference between stronger and weaker beats is slight, it can be detected only by sphygmomanometry. Pulsus alternans indicates left ventricular failure and is usually accompanied by a left-sided S_3.

Bigeminal Pulse

This is a disorder of rhythm that may masquerade as pulsus alternans. A bigeminal pulse is caused by a normal beat alternating with a premature contraction. The stroke volume of the premature beat is diminished in relation to that of the normal beats, and the pulse varies in amplitude accordingly.

Premature contractions

Paradoxical Pulse

A paradoxical pulse may be detected by a palpable decrease in the pulse's amplitude on quiet inspiration. If the sign is less pronounced, a blood-pressure cuff is needed. Systolic pressure decreases by more than 10 mm Hg during inspiration. A paradoxical pulse is found in pericardial tamponade, constrictive pericarditis (though less commonly), and obstructive lung disease.

Inspiration *Expiration*

Table 9-4 Variations and Abnormalities of the Ventricular Impulses

TABLE 9-4 *Variations and Abnormalities of the Ventricular Impulses*

When a ventricle works under conditions of chronic pressure overload (increased afterload), its walls gradually thicken (hypertrophy). Volume overload (increased preload), in contrast, produces dilatation of the ventricle as well as thickening of its walls. A hyperkinetic impulse results from an increased stroke volume and does not necessarily signify heart disease. An impulse may feel hyperkinetic when the chest wall is unusually thin.

The Impulse	Left Ventricle				Right Ventricle			
	Normal	*Hyperkinetic*	*Pressure Overload*	*Volume Overload*	*Normal*	*Hyperkinetic*	*Pressure Overload*	*Volume Overload*
Location	5th or possibly 4th left interspace, medial to the midclavicular line	Normal	Normal	Displaced to the left and possibly downward	Indeterminate	3rd, 4th, or 5th left interspaces	3rd, 4th, or 5th left interspaces, also subxiphoid	Left sternal border, extending toward the left cardiac border, also subxiphoid
Diameter	Little more than 2 cm in adults (1 cm in children); 3 cm or less in left-sided position	Normal, though increased amplitude may make it seem larger	Increased	Increased	Indeterminate	Not useful	Not useful	Not useful
Amplitude	Small, gentle	Increased	Increased	Increased	Not palpable beyond infancy	Slightly increased	Increased	Slightly to markedly increased
Duration	Usually less than ⅔ of systole; the impulse stops before S_2	Normal	Prolonged, may be sustained up to S_2	Often slightly prolonged	Indeterminate	Normal	Prolonged	Normal to slightly prolonged
Examples of Causes		Anxiety, hyperthyroidism, severe anemia	Aortic stenosis, systemic hypertension	Aortic or mitral regurgitation		Anxiety, hyperthyroidism, severe anemia	Pulmonic stenosis, pulmonary hypertension	Atrial septal defect

Table 9-5 Variations in the First Heart Sound

TABLE 9-5 Variations in the First Heart Sound

Normal Variations	S_1 is softer than S_2 at the *base* (right and left 2nd interspaces). S_1 is often but not always louder than S_2 at the *apex*.
Accentuated S_1	S_1 is accentuated in (1) tachycardia, rhythms with a short PR interval, and high cardiac output states (e.g., exercise, anemia, hyperthyroidism), and (2) mitral stenosis. In these conditions, the mitral valve is still open wide at the onset of ventricular systole, and then closes quickly.
Diminished S_1	S_1 is diminished in first-degree heart block (delayed conduction from atria to ventricles). Here the mitral valve has had time after atrial contraction to float back into an almost closed position before ventricular contraction shuts it. It closes less loudly. S_1 is also diminished (1) when the mitral valve is calcified and relatively immobile, as in mitral regurgitation, and (2) when left ventricular contractility is markedly reduced, as in congestive heart failure or coronary heart disease.
Varying S_1	S_1 varies in intensity (1) in complete heart block, when atria and ventricles are beating independently of each other, and (2) in any totally irregular rhythm (e.g., atrial fibrillation). In these situations, the mitral valve is in varying positions before being shut by ventricular contraction. Its closure sound, therefore, varies in loudness.
Split S_1	S_1 may be split normally along the lower left sternal border where the tricuspid component, often too faint to be heard, becomes audible. This split may sometimes be heard at the apex, but consider also an S_4, an aortic ejection sound, and an early systolic click. Abnormal splitting of both heart sounds may be heard in right bundle branch block and in premature ventricular contractions.

Table 9-6   Variations in the Second Heart Sound

TABLE 9-6   *Variations in the Second Heart Sound*

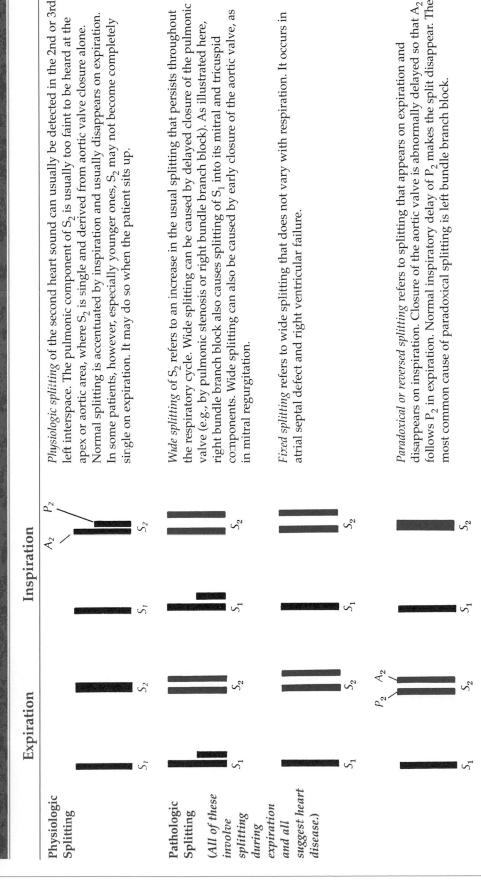

	Expiration	Inspiration	

Physiologic Splitting

Physiologic splitting of the second heart sound can usually be detected in the 2nd or 3rd left interspace. The pulmonic component of S_2 is usually too faint to be heard at the apex or aortic area, where S_2 is single and derived from aortic valve closure alone. Normal splitting is accentuated by inspiration and usually disappears on expiration. In some patients, however, especially younger ones, S_2 may not become completely single on expiration. It may do so when the patient sits up.

Pathologic Splitting

(All of these involve splitting during expiration and all suggest heart disease.)

Wide splitting of S_2 refers to an increase in the usual splitting that persists throughout the respiratory cycle. Wide splitting can be caused by delayed closure of the pulmonic valve (e.g., by pulmonic stenosis or right bundle branch block). As illustrated here, right bundle branch block also causes splitting of S_1 into its mitral and tricuspid components. Wide splitting can also be caused by early closure of the aortic valve, as in mitral regurgitation.

Fixed splitting refers to wide splitting that does not vary with respiration. It occurs in atrial septal defect and right ventricular failure.

Paradoxical or reversed splitting refers to splitting that appears on expiration and disappears on inspiration. Closure of the aortic valve is abnormally delayed so that A_2 follows P_2 in expiration. Normal inspiratory delay of P_2 makes the split disappear. The most common cause of paradoxical splitting is left bundle branch block.

Increased Intensity of A_2 in the Right Second Interspace (where only A_2 can usually be heard) occurs in systemic hypertension because of the increased pressure. It also occurs when the aortic root is dilated, probably because the aortic valve is then closer to the chest wall.

A Decreased or Absent A_2 in the Right Second Interspace is noted in calcific aortic stenosis because of immobility of the valve. If A_2 is inaudible, no splitting is heard.

Increased Intensity of P_2. When P_2 is equal to or louder than A_2, pulmonary hypertension may be suspected. Other causes include a dilated pulmonary artery and an atrial septal defect. Splitting of the second heart sound that is heard widely, even at the apex and the right base, indicates an accentuated P_2.

A Decreased or Absent P_2 is most commonly due to the increased anteroposterior diameter of the chest associated with aging. It can also result from pulmonic stenosis. If P_2 is inaudible, no splitting is heard.

Table 9-7   *Extra Heart Sounds in Systole*

TABLE 9-7   *Extra Heart Sounds in Systole*

Extra heart sounds in systole are of two kinds: (1) early ejection sounds, and (2) clicks, most commonly heard in mid- and late systole.

Early Systolic Ejection Sounds

Early systolic ejection sounds occur shortly after the first heart sound, coincident with the opening of the aortic and pulmonic valves. They are relatively high in pitch, have a sharp, clicking quality, and are heard better with the diaphragm of the stethoscope. An ejection sound indicates cardiovascular disease.

An *aortic ejection sound* is heard at both base and apex and may be louder at the apex. It does not usually vary with respiration. An aortic ejection sound may accompany a dilated aorta or aortic valve disease, such as congenital stenosis or a bicuspid valve.

A *pulmonic ejection sound* is heard best in the 2nd and 3rd left interspaces. When the first heart sound, usually relatively soft in this area, appears to be loud, you may instead be hearing a pulmonic ejection sound. Its intensity often decreases with inspiration. Causes include dilatation of the pulmonary artery, pulmonary hypertension, and pulmonic stenosis.

S_1 E_j S_2

Systolic Clicks

Systolic clicks are usually due to *mitral valve prolapse*—an abnormal systolic ballooning of part of the mitral valve into the left atrium. The clicks are usually mid- or late systolic. Prolapse of the mitral valve is a common cardiac condition, affecting about 5% of the general population. It is now felt to have equal prevalence in men and women. The click is usually single, but more than one may be heard. A click is heard best at or medial to the apex but may also be heard at the lower left sternal border. It is high-pitched and clicking in quality and is heard better with the diaphragm. The click is often followed by a late systolic murmur, which usually represents mitral regurgitation—a flow of blood from left ventricle to left atrium. The murmur usually crescendos up to S_2. Systolic clicks may also be of extracardial or mediastinal origin.

Auscultatory findings are notably variable. Most patients have only a click, some have only a murmur, and some have both. Findings vary from time to time and often change with body position. Several positions are recommended to identify the syndrome: supine, seated, squatting, and standing. Squatting delays the click and murmur; standing moves them closer to S_1.

S_1 C_I S_2

Squatting

S_1 C_I S_2

Standing

S_1 C_I S_2

Table 9-8   Extra Heart Sounds in Diastole

TABLE 9-8   Extra Heart Sounds in Diastole

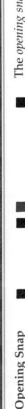

Opening Snap

The *opening snap* is a very early diastolic sound usually produced by the opening of a stenotic mitral valve. It is heard best just medial to the apex and along the lower left sternal border. When it is loud, an opening snap radiates to the apex and to the pulmonic area, where it may be mistaken for the pulmonic component of a split S_2. Its high pitch and snapping quality help to distinguish it from an S_2. It is heard better with the diaphragm.

S_3

A *physiologic third heart sound* is heard frequently in children. It may persist in young adults to the age of 35 or 40. It is common during the last trimester of pregnancy. Occurring early in diastole during rapid ventricular filling, it is later than an opening snap, dull and low in pitch, and heard best at the apex in the left lateral decubitus position. The bell of the stethoscope should be used with very light pressure.

A *pathologic S_3* or *ventricular gallop* sounds just like a physiologic S_3. An S_3 in a person over age 40 (possibly a little older in women) is almost certainly pathologic. Causes include decreased myocardial contractility, myocardial failure, and volume overloading of a ventricle, as from mitral or tricuspid regurgitation. A left-sided S_3 is heard typically at the apex in the left lateral position. A right-sided S_3 is usually heard along the lower left sternal border or below the xiphoid with the patient supine. It is louder on inspiration. The term gallop comes from the cadence of three heart sounds, especially at rapid heart rates.

S_4

An S_4 (*atrial sound* or *atrial gallop*) occurs just before S_1. It is dull, low in pitch, and heard better with the bell. An S_4 is heard occasionally in an apparently normal person, especially in trained athletes and also in older age groups. More commonly, it is due to increased resistance to ventricular filling following atrial contraction. This increased resistance is related to decreased compliance (increased stiffness) of the ventricular myocardium. Causes of a left-sided S_4 include hypertensive heart disease, coronary artery disease, aortic stenosis, and cardiomyopathy. A left-sided S_4 is heard best at the apex in the left lateral position. The less common right-sided S_4 is heard along the lower left sternal border or below the xiphoid. It often gets louder with inspiration. Causes of a right-sided S_4 include pulmonary hypertension and pulmonic stenosis.

An S_4 may also be associated with delayed conduction between atria and ventricles. This delay separates the normally faint atrial sound from the louder S_1 and makes it audible. An S_4 is never heard in the absence of atrial contraction, as occurs with atrial fibrillation.

Occasionally, a patient has both an S_3 and an S_4, producing a *quadruple rhythm* of four heart sounds. At rapid heart rates the S_3 and S_4 may merge into one loud extra heart sound, called a *summation gallop.*

S_1 S_2 OS

S_1 S_2 S_3

S_4 S_1 S_2

Table 9-9 Midsystolic Murmurs

TABLE 9-9 Midsystolic Murmurs

Midsystolic (ejection) murmurs—the most common kind of heart murmur—may be (1) *pathologic* (secondary to structural cardiovascular abnormality), (2) *physiologic* (secondary to physiologic alteration in the body), and (3) *innocent* (not associated with any detectable physiologic or structural abnormality). Midsystolic murmurs tend to peak near midsystole, and usually stop before S_2. The crescendo-decrescendo shape is not always obvious to the ear, but the gap between the murmur and S_2 helps to distinguish midsystolic from pansystolic murmurs.

	Mechanism	The Murmur	Associated Findings
Innocent Murmurs	Innocent murmurs result from turbulent blood flow, probably generated by left ventricular ejection of blood into the aorta. Occasionally, turbulence from right ventricular ejection may also cause them. There is no evidence of cardiovascular disease. Innocent murmurs—very common in children and young adults—may also be heard in older people.	*Location.* 2nd to 4th left interspaces between the left sternal border and the apex *Radiation.* Little *Intensity.* Grade 1 to 2, possibly 3 *Pitch.* Medium *Quality.* Variable *Aids.* Usually decreases or disappears on sitting	None: normal splitting, no ejection sounds, no diastolic murmurs, and no palpable evidence of ventricular enlargement. Occasionally, a patient has both an innocent murmur and another kind of murmur.
Physiologic Murmurs	Turbulence due to a temporary increase in blood flow causes this murmur. Predisposing conditions include anemia, pregnancy, fever, and hyperthyroidism.	Similar to innocent murmurs	Possible signs of a likely cause
Pathologic Murmurs *Pulmonic Stenosis*	Stenosis of the pulmonic valve impairs flow across the valve, and increases the afterload on the right ventricle. It is congenital and most often found in children. *Pathologically increased flow across the pulmonic valve* may mimic the murmur of pulmonic stenosis. The systolic murmur associated with an atrial septal defect originates from this flow, not from the defect itself.	*Location.* 2nd and 3rd left interspaces *Radiation.* If loud, toward the left shoulder and neck, especially on the left *Intensity.* Soft to loud; if loud, associated with a thrill *Pitch.* Medium *Quality.* Often harsh	In severe stenosis, S_2 is widely split and P_2 is diminished. When P_2 is inaudible, no splitting is heard. An early pulmonic ejection sound is common. A right-sided S_4 may be present. The right ventricular impulse is often increased in amplitude and may be prolonged.

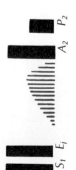

Table 9-9   Midsystolic Murmurs

Aortic Stenosis

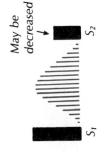

Significant stenosis of the aortic valve impairs blood flow across the valve, causing turbulence, and increases the afterload on the left ventricle. Causes are congenital, rheumatic, and degenerative, and findings may differ with each cause.

Other conditions may mimic the murmur of aortic stenosis without obstructing flow:

- *Aortic sclerosis*, a stiffening of aortic valve leaflets associated with aging
- A *bicuspid aortic valve*, a congenital condition, which may not be recognized until adulthood
- A *dilated aorta*, as from arteriosclerosis, syphilis, or Marfan's syndrome
- *A pathologically increased flow across the aortic valve during systole, as in aortic regurgitation*

Location. Right 2nd interspace

Radiation. Often to the neck and down the left sternal border, even to the apex

Intensity. Sometimes soft but often loud, with a thrill

Pitch. Medium; at the apex, it may be higher

Quality. Often harsh; at the apex it may be more musical

Aids. Heard best with the patient sitting and leaning forward

A_2 decreases as the stenosis worsens. A_2 may be delayed, merging with P_2 to form a single sound or causing paradoxical splitting. An S_4, reflecting the decreased compliance of the hypertrophied left ventricle, may be present at the apex. An aortic ejection sound, if present, suggests a congenital cause. A sustained apical impulse often reveals left ventricular hypertrophy. The carotid artery impulse may rise slowly and feel small in amplitude.

Hypertrophic Cardiomyopathy

Massive hypertrophy of ventricular muscle is associated with unusually rapid ejection of blood from the left ventricle during systole. Obstruction to flow may coexist. Accompanying distortion of the mitral valve may cause mitral regurgitation.

Location. 3rd and 4th left interspaces

Radiation. Down the left sternal border to the apex, possibly to the base, but not to the neck

Intensity. Variable

Pitch. Medium

Quality. Harsh

Aids. Decreases with squatting, increases with straining down

An S_3 may be present.

An S_4 is often present at the apex (unlike in mitral regurgitation).

The apical impulse may be sustained and have two palpable components.

The carotid pulse rises quickly (unlike the pulse in aortic stenosis).

Table 9-10 Pansystolic (Holosystolic) Murmurs

TABLE 9-10   *Pansystolic (Holosystolic) Murmurs*

Pansystolic (holosystolic) murmurs are pathologic. They are heard when blood flows from a chamber of high pressure to one of lower pressure through a valve or other structure that should be closed. The murmur begins immediately with S_1 and continues up to S_2.

	Mechanism	The Murmur	Associated Findings
Mitral Regurgitation 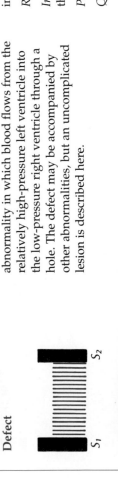	When the mitral valve fails to close fully in systole, blood regurgitates from left ventricle to left atrium, causing a murmur. This leakage creates a volume overload on the left ventricle, with subsequent dilatation and hypertrophy. Several structural abnormalities cause this condition, and findings may vary accordingly.	*Location.* Apex *Radiation.* To the left axilla, less often to the left sternal border *Intensity.* Soft to loud; if loud, associated with an apical thrill *Pitch.* Medium to high *Quality.* Blowing *Aids.* Unlike the murmur of tricuspid regurgitation, it does not become louder in inspiration.	S_1 is often decreased. An apical S_3 reflects the volume overload on the left ventricle. The apical impulse is increased in amplitude and may be prolonged.
Tricuspid Regurgitation	When the tricuspid valve fails to close fully in systole, blood regurgitates from right ventricle to right atrium, producing a murmur. The most common cause is right ventricular failure and dilatation, with resulting enlargement of the tricuspid orifice. Either pulmonary hypertension or left ventricular failure is the usual initiating cause.	*Location.* Lower left sternal border *Radiation.* To the right of the sternum, to the xiphoid area, and perhaps to the left midclavicular line, but not into the axilla *Intensity.* Variable *Pitch.* Medium *Quality.* Blowing *Aids.* Unlike in the murmur of mitral regurgitation, the intensity may increase slightly with inspiration.	The right ventricular impulse is increased in amplitude and may be prolonged. An S_3 may be audible along the lower left sternal border. The jugular venous pressure is often elevated, and large v waves may be seen in the jugular veins.
Ventricular Septal Defect	A ventricular septal defect is a congenital abnormality in which blood flows from the relatively high-pressure left ventricle into the low-pressure right ventricle through a hole. The defect may be accompanied by other abnormalities, but an uncomplicated lesion is described here.	*Location.* 3rd, 4th, and 5th left interspaces *Radiation.* Often wide *Intensity.* Often very loud, with a thrill *Pitch.* High *Quality.* Often harsh	A_2 may be obscured by the loud murmur. Findings vary with the severity of the defect and with associated lesions.

Table 9-11   Diastolic Murmurs

TABLE 9-11   Diastolic Murmurs

Diastolic murmurs almost always indicate heart disease. There are two basic types. *Early decrescendo diastolic murmurs* signify regurgitant flow through an incompetent semilunar valve, more commonly the aortic. *Rumbling diastolic murmurs in mid- or late diastole suggest stenosis of an atrioventricular valve*, more often the mitral.

	Mechanism	The Murmur	Associated Findings
Aortic Regurgitation	The leaflets of the aortic valve fail to close completely during diastole, and blood regurgitates from the aorta back into the left ventricle. A volume overload on the left ventricle results. Two other murmurs may be associated: (1) a midsystolic murmur from the resulting increased forward flow across the aortic valve, and (2) a mitral diastolic (*Austin Flint*) murmur. The latter is attributed to diastolic impingement of the regurgitant flow on the anterior leaflet of the mitral valve.	*Location.* 2nd to 4th left interspaces *Radiation.* If loud, to the apex, perhaps to the right sternal border *Intensity.* Grade 1 to 3 *Pitch.* High. Use a diaphragm. *Quality.* Blowing; may be mistaken for breath sounds *Aids.* The murmur is heard best with the patient sitting, leaning forward, with breath held in exhalation.	An ejection sound may be present. An S_3 or S_4 if present, suggests severe regurgitation. Progressive changes in the apical impulse include increased amplitude, displacement laterally and downward, widened diameter, and increased duration. The pulse pressure increases, and arterial pulses are often large and bounding. Either a midsystolic flow murmur or an Austin Flint murmur suggests a large regurgitant flow.
Mitral Stenosis	When the leaflets of the mitral valve thicken, stiffen, and become distorted from the effects of rheumatic fever, the valve fails to open sufficiently in diastole. The resulting murmur has two components: (1) middiastolic (during rapid ventricular filling), and (2) presystolic (during atrial contraction). The latter disappears if atrial fibrillation develops, leaving only a middiastolic rumble.	*Location.* Usually limited to the apex *Radiation.* Little or none *Intensity.* Grade 1 to 4 *Pitch.* Low. Use a bell. *Aids.* Placing the bell exactly on the apical impulse, turning the patient into a left lateral position, and mild exercise all help to make the murmur audible. It is heard better in exhalation.	S_1 is accentuated and may be palpable at the apex. An opening snap (OS) often follows S_2 and initiates the murmur. If pulmonary hypertension develops, P_2 is accentuated and the right ventricular impulse becomes palpable. Mitral regurgitation and aortic valve disease may be associated with mitral stenosis.

Table 9-12 Cardiovascular Sounds With Both Systolic and Diastolic Components

Some cardiovascular sounds are not confined to one portion of the cardiac cycle. Three examples are: (1) a pericardial friction rub, produced by inflammation of the pericardial sac, (2) patent ductus arteriosus, a congenital abnormality in which an open channel persists between aorta and pulmonary artery, and (3) a venous hum, a benign sound produced by turbulence of blood in the jugular veins (common in children). Their characteristics are contrasted below. The term *continuous murmur* is defined as one that begins in systole and continues through the second sound into all or part of diastole. It need not continue through diastole. The murmur of patent ductus arteriosus, therefore, may be classified as continuous.

	Pericardial Friction Rub	Patent Ductus Arteriosus	Venous Hum
Timing	May have three short components, each associated with cardiac movement: (1) atrial systole, (2) ventricular systole, and (3) ventricular diastole. Usually the first two components are present; all three make diagnosis easy; only one (usually the systolic) invites confusion with a murmur.	Continuous murmur in both systole and diastole, often with a silent interval late in diastole. Is loudest in late systole, obscures S_2, and fades in diastole	Continuous murmur without a silent interval. Loudest in diastole
Location	Variable, but usually heard best in the 3rd interspace to the left of the sternum	Left 2nd interspace	Above the medial third of the clavicles, especially on the right
Radiation	Little	Toward the left clavicle	1st and 2nd interspaces
Intensity	Variable. May increase when the patient leans forward and exhales	Usually loud, sometimes associated with a thrill	Soft to moderate. Can be obliterated by pressure on the jugular veins
Quality	Scratchy, scraping	Harsh, machinerylike	Humming, roaring
Pitch	High (heard better with a diaphragm)	Medium	Low (heard better with a bell)

The Breasts and Axillae

CHAPTER 10

Anatomy and Physiology

The female breast lies against the anterior thoracic wall, extending from the 2nd to the 6th ribs, and from the sternal edge to the midaxillary line. The posterior surface overlies the pectoralis major and, inferiorly, the serratus anterior.

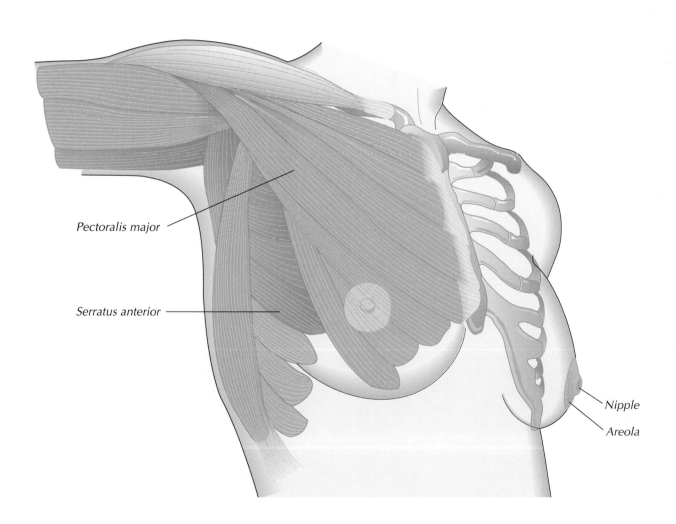

Pectoralis major

Serratus anterior

Nipple

Areola

To describe clinical findings, the breast is often divided into four quadrants based on horizontal and vertical lines crossing at the nipple. An axillary tail of breast tissue extends toward the anterior axillary fold. Alternatively, findings can be localized as the "time" on the face of a clock (e.g., 3 o'-clock) and the distance in centimeters from the nipple.

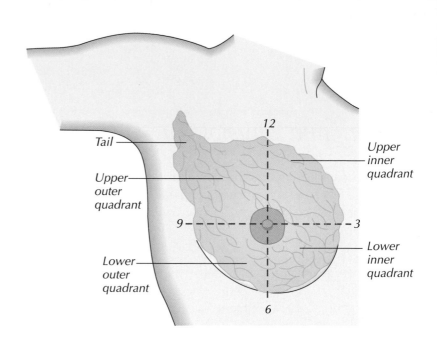

The breast is hormonally sensitive tissue that changes with monthly cycling and aging. *Glandular tissue*, namely secretory tubuloalveolar glands and ducts, forms 15 to 20 septated lobes radiating around the nipple, each draining into a lactiferous duct and dilated sinus opening onto the nipple surface. *Fibrous connective tissue* provides structural support in the form of fibrous bands or suspensory ligaments connected to both the skin and the fascia underlying the breast. *Adipose tissue*, or fat, surrounds the breast and predominates superficially and peripherally. The proportions of these components vary with age, the general state of nutrition, pregnancy, and other factors.

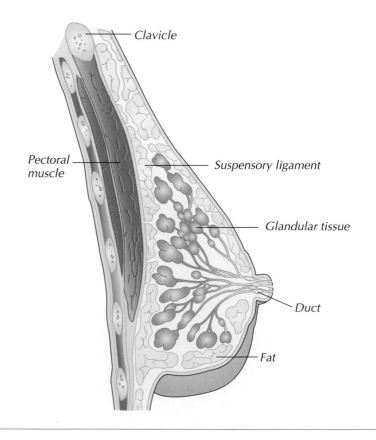

The surface of the areola has small, rounded elevations formed by sebaceous glands, sweat glands, and accessory areolar glands. A few hairs are often seen on the areola.

Both the nipple and the areola are well supplied with smooth muscle that contracts to express milk from the ductal system when the mother is nursing an infant. Rich sensory innervation, especially in the nipple, triggers "milk letdown" following neurohormonal stimulation from infant sucking. Tactile stimulation of the area, including the breast examination, makes the nipple smaller, firmer, and more erect, while the areola puckers and wrinkles. These normal smooth muscle reflexes should not be mistaken for signs of breast disease.

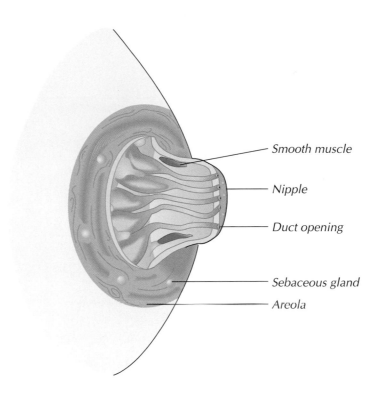

Smooth muscle

Nipple

Duct opening

Sebaceous gland

Areola

Occasionally, one or more extra (supernumerary) breasts are located along the "milk line," illustrated on the right. They are found most commonly in the axilla or just below the normal breast. Only a small nipple and areola are usually present, often mistaken for a common mole. Glandular tissue may be present. An extra breast has no pathologic significance.

The male breast consists chiefly of a small nipple and areola. These overlie a thin disc of undeveloped breast tissue that may not be distinguishable clinically from the surrounding tissues. A firm button of breast tissue 2 cm or more in diameter has been described in roughly one out of three adult men. The limits of normal have not yet been clearly established.

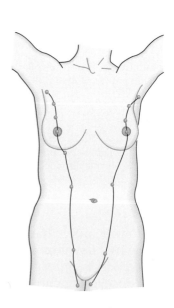

Changes With Age

Adolescence. Development of a woman's breasts begins during puberty. The preadolescent breast consists of a small elevated nipple, with no elevation of underlying breast tissue. Between the ages of 8 and 13 (average around 11), secondary sex characteristics become apparent. Breast buds appear, and further enlargement of breasts and areolae follows.

The five stages of breast development as defined by Tanner's sex maturity ratings (SMR) are shown below.

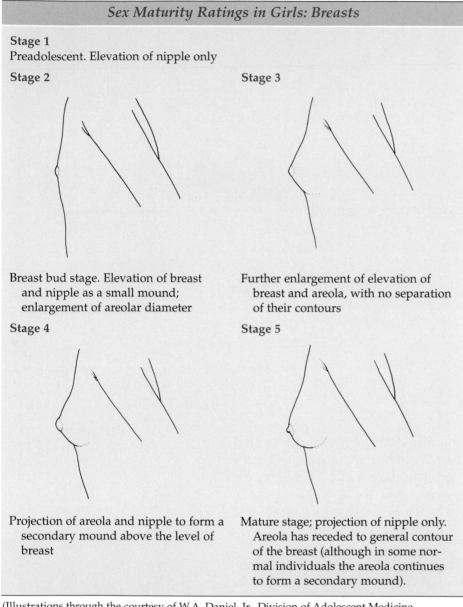

Sex Maturity Ratings in Girls: Breasts

Stage 1
Preadolescent. Elevation of nipple only

Stage 2

Stage 3

Breast bud stage. Elevation of breast and nipple as a small mound; enlargement of areolar diameter

Further enlargement of elevation of breast and areola, with no separation of their contours

Stage 4

Stage 5

Projection of areola and nipple to form a secondary mound above the level of breast

Mature stage; projection of nipple only. Areola has receded to general contour of the breast (although in some normal individuals the areola continues to form a secondary mound).

(Illustrations through the courtesy of W.A. Daniel, Jr., Division of Adolescent Medicine, University of Alabama, Birmingham)

Concomitantly, pubic hair appears and spreads, as illustrated on page 408. These two developmental changes—in breasts and pubic hair—are useful in assessing growth and maturation, although they do not necessarily proceed synchronously. The sequence from SMR 2 to SMR 5 takes about 3 years on the average, with a range of 1.5 to 6 years. Axillary hair usually appears about 2 years after pubic hair.

Menarche usually occurs when a girl is in breast stage 3 or 4. By then, she has characteristically reached the peak of her adolescent growth spurt; further growth will be slower. The relationships of menarche to breast development and to growth are useful in counseling a girl who is worried that she may grow too tall or that her menarche is too late. The usual sequence of these changes is summarized in the diagram below.

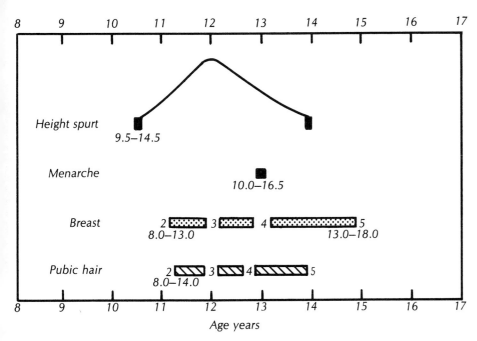

Numbers below the bars indicate the ranges in age within which certain changes occur. (Redrawn from Marshall WA, Tanner JM: Variations in the pattern of pubertal changes in boys. Arch Dis Child 45:22, 1970)

Tanner's figures are based on studies of white English girls. An American survey indicates that African American girls tend to be more advanced in their secondary sex characteristics than are whites of the same age. African American girls, too, develop axillary hair earlier than do their Caucasian counterparts, sometimes before their pubic hair appears. These differences, together with the relatively fine, sparse pubic hair described in Asian women, illustrate the caution required in applying group norms.

In about 1 out of 12 girls, breasts develop at different rates, and considerable asymmetry may result. This is usually temporary and, unless it is very marked, reassurance is indicated.

Adulthood. The normal adult breast may be soft, but it often feels granular, nodular, or lumpy. This uneven texture is normal and may be termed *physiologic nodularity.* It is often bilateral. It may be evident throughout the breast or only in parts of it. The nodularity may increase premenstrually—a time when breasts often enlarge and become tender or even painful. For breast changes during pregnancy, see pp. 431–432.

Aging. The breasts of an aging woman tend to diminish in size as glandular tissue atrophies and is replaced by fat. Although the proportion of fat increases, its total amount may also decrease. The breasts often become flaccid and more pendulous, as shown on p. 139. The ducts surrounding the nipple may become more easily palpable as firm, stringy strands. Axillary hair diminishes.

The Adolescent Male. Approximately 2 out of 3 adolescent boys develop *gynecomastia*—breast enlargement on one or both sides. This is usually slight, but obvious enlargement may be embarrassing. Pubertal gynecomastia usually resolves spontaneously within a year or two.

Lymphatics

Lymphatics from most of the breast drain toward the axilla. Of the axillary lymph nodes, the *central nodes* are palpable most frequently. They lie along the chest wall, usually high in the axilla and midway between the anterior and posterior axillary folds. Into them drain channels from three other groups of lymph nodes, which are seldom palpable:

1. The *pectoral (anterior) nodes* are located along the lower border of the pectoralis major inside the anterior axillary fold. These nodes drain the anterior chest wall and much of the breast.
2. The *subscapular (posterior) nodes* lie along the lateral border of the scapula and are felt deep in the posterior axillary fold. They drain the posterior chest wall and a portion of the arm.
3. The *lateral nodes* lie along the upper humerus and drain most of the arm.

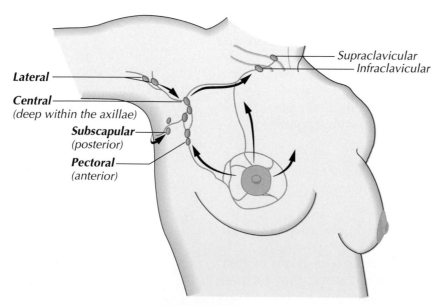

ARROWS INDICATE DIRECTION OF LYMPH FLOW

Lymph drains from the central axillary nodes to the infraclavicular and supraclavicular nodes.

Not all the lymphatics of the breast drain into the axilla. Malignant cells from a breast cancer may spread directly to the infraclavicular nodes or into deep channels within the chest.

Techniques of Examination

The Female Breast

General Approach

Women and girls may be apprehensive about having their breasts examined, and fearful about what the clinician may discover. Reassure the patient and adopt a courteous and gentle approach. Tell the patient that you are going to examine her breasts. This may be a good time to ask if she has noted any lumps or other problems and whether she does monthly self-examinations. If she is unfamiliar with self-examination, you should teach her good technique for examining her breasts and help her to repeat maneuvers after you.

An adequate inspection requires full exposure of the chest, but later in the examination you may find it helpful to cover one breast while you are palpating the other. Because breasts tend to swell and become more nodular premenstrually, the best time to examine them is a week after onset of the menstrual period. If you find suspicious nodules during the premenstrual phase, arrange to reevaluate them later.

Risk factors for breast cancer include increasing age, prior cancer in the opposite breast, a mother or sister who has had it, early menarche, late or no pregnancies, late menopause, and exposure to ionizing radiation.

Inspection

Inspect the breasts and nipples with the patient in the sitting position and disrobed to the waist. A thorough examination of the breast includes careful inspection for skin changes, symmetry, contours, and retraction in four views—arms at sides, arms over head, arms pressed against hips, and leaning forward.

Arms at sides. Note the clinical features listed below.

• The *appearance of the skin,* including

  Color

Redness from local infection or inflammatory carcinoma

  Thickening of the skin and unusually prominent pores, which may accompany lymphatic obstruction

Thickening and prominent pores suggest a breast cancer.

• The *size and symmetry of the breasts.* Some difference in the size of the breasts, including the areolae, is common and is usually normal, as shown in the photograph on page 341.

• The *contour of the breasts.* Look for changes such as masses, dimpling, or flattening. Compare one side with the other.

Flattening of the normally convex breast suggests cancer. See Table 10-1, Visible Signs of Breast Cancer (p. 352).

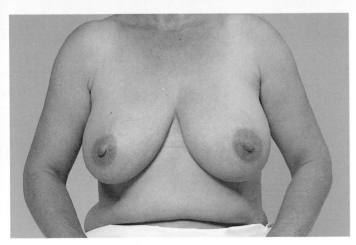

ARMS AT SIDES

- The *characteristics of the nipple*:

    Their *size and shape*. Occasionally, a nipple is inverted—depressed below the areolar surface and sometimes enveloped by folds of areolar skin, as illustrated. Longstanding inversion is usually a normal variant; except for possible difficulty in nursing an infant, it is of no clinical consequence.

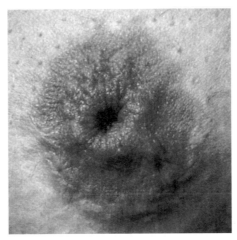

INVERTED NIPPLE

Recent or fixed flattening or depression of the nipple suggests nipple retraction. A retracted nipple may also be broadened and thickened. It suggests an underlying cancer.

The direction in which they point (normally outward and often downward)

Asymmetry of the directions in which nipples point suggests an underlying cancer.

Any rashes or ulcerations

Paget's disease of the breast (see p. 352).

Any discharge

When examining an adolescent girl, assess her breast development according to Tanner's sex maturity ratings (SMR) described on page 336. Because an adolescent girl is often concerned about her breasts, it may be helpful to tell her that she is developing normally (if she is) and, using the diagrams, to review with her the usual developmental sequence. You will rate pubic hair development separately, later in the examination.

Arms Over Head; Hands Pressed Against Hips. In order to bring out dimpling or retraction that may otherwise be invisible, ask the patient to raise her arms over her head, and then to press her hands against her hips to contract the pectoral muscles. Inspect the breast contour carefully in each position.

Dimpling or retraction of the breasts with either of these positions suggests an underlying cancer. When a cancer or its associated fibrous strands are

341

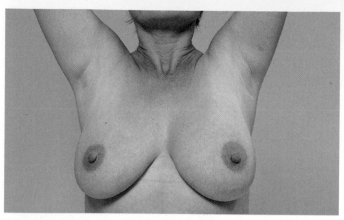

ARMS OVER HEAD

attached to both the skin and the fascia overlying the pectoral muscles, pectoral contraction can draw the skin inward, causing dimpling.

Occasionally, these signs may be associated with benign lesions such as posttraumatic fat necrosis or mammary duct ectasia, but they must always be evaluated with great care.

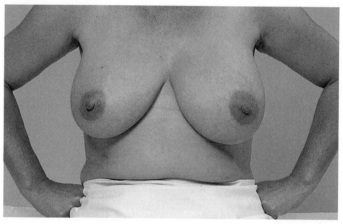

HANDS PRESSED AGAINST HIPS

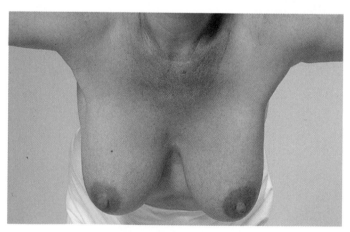

LEANING FORWARD

Leaning Forward. If the breasts are large or pendulous, a fourth position may be useful. Ask the patient to stand and lean forward, supported by the back of a chair or the examiner's hands.

This position may reveal an asymmetry of the breast or nipple not otherwise visible. Retraction of the nipple and areola suggests an underlying cancer. See Table 10-1, Visible Signs of Breast Cancer (p. 352).

Palpation

The Breast. Ask the patient to lie down. Unless the breasts are small, place a small pillow under the patient's shoulder on the side you are examining and ask her to rest her arm over her head. These maneuvers help to spread the breast more evenly across the chest and make it easier to find nodules.

With your fingers flat on the breast, compress the tissues gently in a rotary motion against the chest wall. You will need to press more firmly to reach the deeper tissues of a large breast. Proceed systematically, examining the entire breast including the periphery, tail, and areola.

When pressing deeply on the breast, you may mistake a normal rib for a hard breast mass.

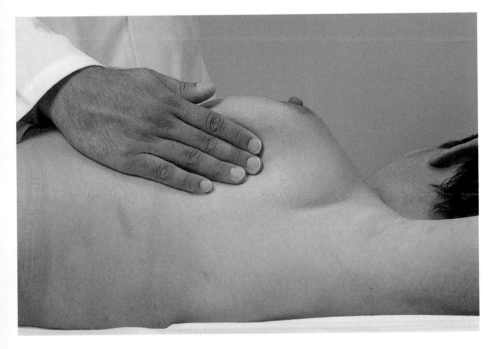

Nodules in the tail of the breast are sometimes mistaken for enlarged axillary lymph nodes (and vice versa).

Using a pattern such as concentric circles, parallel lines, or consecutive clock times, palpate the entire breast from clavicle to inframammary fold, from midsternal line to posterior axillary line, and well into the axilla for the tail of the breast. Check carefully for:

- The *consistency of the tissues.* Normal consistency varies widely, depending in part on the relative proportions of soft fat and firmer glandular tissue. Physiologic nodularity may be present and may increase premenstrually. Especially in large breasts, a firm transverse ridge of compressed tissue may be present along the lower edge of the breast. This is the normal inframammary ridge, not a tumor.
- *Tenderness,* as in premenstrual fullness

Tender cords suggest *mammary duct ectasia,* a benign but sometimes painful condition with dilatation of the ducts and inflammation around them. Masses may be associated.

- *Nodules.* Feel carefully for any lump or mass that is larger than or qualitatively different from the rest of the breast tissue. This is sometimes called a dominant mass and, if persistent, suggests a pathologic change that may require evaluation by mammogram, aspiration, or biopsy. Describe the characteristics of any nodules:

Location, by quadrant or clock, with centimeters from the nipple
Size in centimeters
Shape (e.g., round or disclike, regular or irregular)
Consistency (e.g., soft, firm, or hard)
Delimitation (i.e., well circumscribed or not)

Mobility, in relation to the skin, pectoral fascia, and chest wall. Gently move the breast near the mass and watch for dimpling.

See Table 10-2, Differentiation of Common Breast Nodules (p. 353).

Hard, irregular, poorly circumscribed nodules, fixed to the skin or underlying tissues, strongly suggest cancer.

Dimpling suggests an underlying cancer.

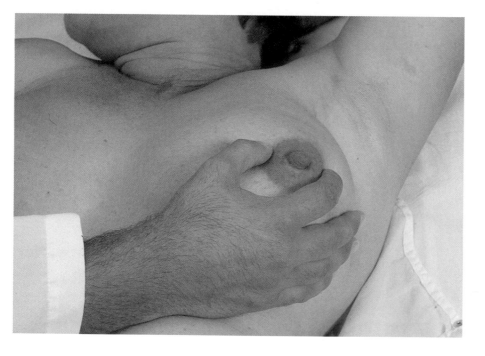

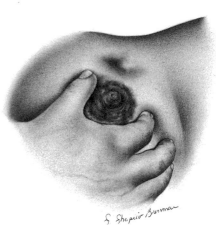

Next, try to move the mass itself while the patient relaxes her arm and then while she presses her hand against her hip.

If a mobile mass becomes fixed when the patient presses her hand against her hip, the mass is attached to the pectoral fascia. If it is immobile with the patient relaxed, it is attached to the ribs and intercostal muscles.

Tenderness

Cysts, inflamed areas, and sometimes cancer may be tender.

The Nipple. Palpate each nipple, noting its elasticity.

Thickening of the nipple and loss of elasticity suggest an underlying cancer.

The Male Breast

Examination of the male breast may be brief but is sometimes important.

Inspect the nipple and areola for nodules, swelling, or ulceration.

Palpate the areola for nodules. If the breast appears enlarged, distinguish between the soft fatty enlargement that may accompany obesity and the firm disc of glandular enlargement, called gynecomastia.

Gynecomastia is attributed to an imbalance of estrogens and androgens, sometimes drug-related. A hard, irregular, eccentric, or ulcerating nodule is not gynecomastia and suggests breast cancer.

The Axillae

Although the axillae may be examined with the patient lying down, a sitting position is preferable.

Inspection

Inspect the skin of each axilla, noting evidence of:

- Rash

- Infection

- Unusual pigmentation

Deodorant and other rashes

Sweat gland infection (*hidradenitis suppurativa*)

Deeply pigmented, velvety axillary skin suggests *acanthosis nigricans,* one form of which is associated with internal malignancy.

Palpation

To examine the left axilla, ask the patient to relax with the left arm down. Help by supporting the left wrist or hand with your left hand. Cup together the fingers of your right hand and reach as high as you can toward the apex of the axilla. Warn the patient that this may feel uncomfortable. Your fingers should lie directly behind the pectoral muscles, pointing toward the midclavicle. Now press your fingers in toward the chest wall and slide them downward, trying to feel the central nodes against the chest wall. Of the axillary nodes, these are the most often palpable. One or more soft, small (<1 cm), nontender nodes are frequently felt.

Enlarged axillary nodes are most commonly due to infection of the hand or arm or to recent immunizations or skin tests in the arm. They may also be part of a generalized lymphadenopathy. Check the epitrochlear nodes and other groups of lymph nodes.

Nodes that are large (≥ 1 cm) and firm or hard, matted together, or fixed to the skin or to underlying tissues suggest malignant involvement.

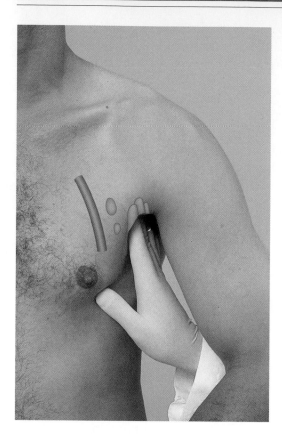

Use your left hand to examine the right axilla.

If the central nodes feel large, hard, or tender, or if there is a suspicious lesion in the drainage areas for the axillary nodes, feel for the other groups of axillary lymph nodes:

- Pectoral nodes: grasp the anterior axillary fold between your thumb and fingers, and with your fingers palpate inside the border of the pectoral muscle.
- Lateral nodes: from high in the axilla, feel along the upper humerus.
- Subscapular nodes: step behind the patient and with your fingers feel inside the muscle of the posterior axillary fold.

Also, feel for infraclavicular nodes and reexamine the supraclavicular nodes.

Special Techniques

Assessment of Spontaneous Nipple Discharge. If there is a history of spontaneous nipple discharge, try to determine its origin by compressing the areola with your index finger, placed in radial positions around the nipple. Watch for discharge appearing through one of the duct openings on the nipple's surface. Note the color, consistency, and quantity of any discharge and the exact location where it appears.

Milky discharge unrelated to a prior pregnancy and lactation is called *nonpuerperal galactorrhea.* Leading causes are hormonal and pharmacologic.

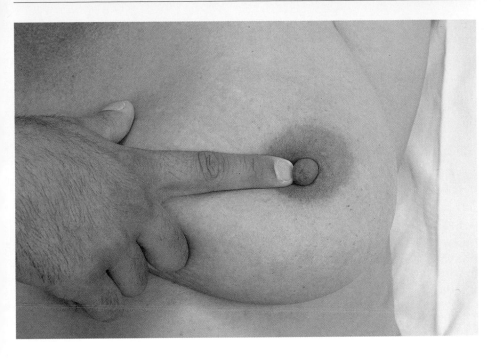

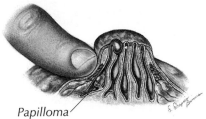

Papilloma

A nonmilky unilateral discharge suggests local breast disease. The causative lesion is usually benign, but may be malignant, especially in elderly women. A benign intraductal papilloma is shown above in its usual subareolar location. Note the drop of blood exuding from a duct opening.

Examination of The Mastectomy Patient. The woman with a mastectomy warrants special care on examination. Inspect the mastectomy scar and axilla carefully for any masses or unusual nodularity. Note any change in color or signs of inflammation. Lymphedema may be present in the axilla and upper arm from impaired lymph drainage after surgery. Palpate gently along the scar—these tissues may be unusually sensitive. Use a circular motion with two or three fingers. Pay special attention to the upper outer quadrant and axilla. Note any enlargement of the lymph nodes or signs of inflammation or infection.

It is especially important to palpate carefully the breast tissue and incision lines of women with breast augmentation or reconstruction.

Instructions for The Breast Self-Examination. The office or hospital visit is an important time to teach the patient how to perform the breast self-examination (BSE). A high proportion of breast masses are detected by women examining their own breasts. Although BSE has not been shown to reduce breast cancer mortality, monthly BSE is inexpensive and may promote stronger health awareness and more active self-care. For early detection of breast cancer, the BSE is most useful when coupled with regular breast examination by an experienced clinician and mammography. The BSE is best timed just after menses, when hormonal stimulation of breast tissue is low.

Patient Instructions for the Self-Examination (BSE)

Lying Supine

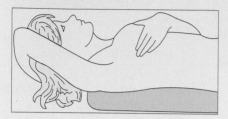

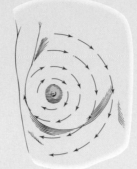

1. Lie down with a pillow under your right shoulder. Place your right arm behind your head.
2. Use the finger pads of the three middle fingers on your left hand to feel for lumps in the right breast. The finger pads are the top third of each finger.
3. Press firmly enough to know how your breast feels. A firm ridge in the lower curve of each breast is normal. If you're not sure how hard to press, talk with your health care provider, or try to copy the way the doctor or nurse does it.

4. Move around the breast in a set way. You can choose the circle, the up and down line, or the wedge, but be sure to do it the same way every time. Go over the entire breast area, and remember how your breast feels from month to month.
5. Repeat the exam on your left breast, using the finger pads of the right hand.
6. If you find any changes, see your doctor right away.

Standing

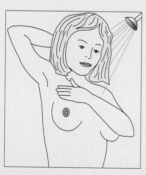

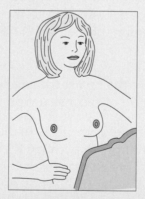

1. Repeat the examination of both breasts while standing, with one arm behind your head. The upright position makes it easier to check the upper, outer part of the breasts (toward your armpit). This is where about half of breast cancers are found. You may want to do the upright part of the BSE while you are in the shower. Your soapy hands will make it easy to check how your breasts feel as they glide over the wet skin.

2. For added safety, you might want to check your breasts by standing in front of a mirror right after your BSE each month. See if there are any changes in the way your breasts look, such as dimpling of the skin, changes in the nipple, redness, or swelling.

Source: American Cancer Society, 1997

Health Promotion and Counseling

Women may experience a wide range of changes in breast tissue and sensation, from cyclic swelling and nodularity to a distinct lump or mass. The examination of the breast provides a meaningful opportunity for the clinician and the woman patient to explore concerns important to women's health—what to do if a lump or mass is detected, risk factors for breast cancer, and screening measures such as breast self-examination, the clinical breast examination (CBE) by a skilled clinician, and mammography.

Breast masses show marked variation in etiology, from fibroadenomas and cysts seen in younger women, to abscess or mastitis, to primary breast cancer. All breast masses warrant careful evaluation. On initial assessment, the woman's age and physical characteristics of the mass provide clues to its origin, but definitive diagnostic measures should be pursued.

Palpable Masses of the Breast		
Age	Common Lesion	Characteristics
15–25	Fibroadenoma	Usually fine, round, mobile, nontender
25–50	Cysts	Usually soft to firm, round, mobile; often tender
	Fibrocystic changes	Nodular, ropelike
	Cancer	Irregular, stellate, firm, not clearly delineated from surrounding tissue
Over 50	Cancer until proven otherwise	As above
Pregnancy/lactation	Lactating adenomas, cysts, mastitis, and cancer	As above

Adapted from Schultz MZ, Ward BA, Reiss M: Ch. 149. Breast Diseases. In Noble J, Greene HL, Levinson W, Modest GA, Young MJ (eds): Primary Care Medicine, 2nd ed. St. Louis, Mosby, 1996.

Risk Factors for Breast Cancer. A woman in the United States has a 12% lifetime risk of developing breast cancer and 23.5% risk of dying from the disease.* Although 70% of affected women have no known predisposition, definite risk factors are well established. The clinician and the inquiring patient should understand and review such factors as age, family history, reproductive history, and prior history of benign breast disease.

Age. Although one in nine women will eventually develop breast cancer, it is important to note that this is a cumulative risk estimate—more than half of a woman's risk occurs over the age of 65. For women between the ages of 35 and 55 without major risk factors, the chance of developing breast cancer is only 2.5%.

*Harris JR, Morrow M, Bonadonna G: Cancer of the breast. In DeVita VT, Hellman S, Rosenberg SA (eds): Cancer Principles & Practice of Oncology, 5th ed. Philadelphia, Lippincott-Raven, 1997.

Family History. The relative risk (or risk relative to an individual without a given risk factor) of breast cancer associated with menstrual history, pregnancy, and breast conditions and diseases is summarized in the table below. Risk from familial breast cancer falls into two patterns: family history of breast cancer and genetic predisposition. First-degree relatives, namely a mother or sister with breast cancer, establish a "positive family history." Within this group, menopausal status and extent of disease play a key role. Having first-degree relatives with breast cancer who are premenopausal with bilateral disease confers the highest risk. Even when a mother and a sister have bilateral breast cancer, however, the probability of breast cancer is only 25%.

Inherited disease in women carrying mutations in breast cancer susceptibility genes accounts for only 5% to 10% of breast cancers. However, these genes confer a 50% risk of the disease in women under 50, and an 80% risk by age 65. Red flags for possible inherited disease include multiple relatives (maternal or paternal) with breast cancer, a family history of combined breast cancer and ovarian cancer, and a family history of bilateral and/or early onset of breast cancer.

Menstrual History and Pregnancy. Late menarche, delayed menopause, and first live birth after age 35 or no pregnancy all raise the risk of breast cancer two- to three-fold.

Summary of Breast Cancer Risk Factors	
Factor	Relative Risk
Family History	
First-degree relative with breast cancer	1.2–3.0
Premenopausal	3.1
Premenopausal and bilateral	8.5–9.0
Postmenopausal	1.5
Postmenopausal and bilateral	4.0–5.4
Menstrual History	
Age at menarche <12	1.3
Age at menopause >55	1.5–2.0
Pregnancy	
First live birth from ages 25–29	1.5
First live birth after age 30	1.9
First live birth after age 35	2.0–3.0
Nulliparous	3.0
Breast Conditions and Diseases	
Nonproliferative disease	1.0
Proliferative disease	1.9
Proliferative with atypical hyperplasia	4.4
Lobular carcinoma in situ	6.9–12.0

Adapted from Bilmoria MM and Morrow M: The woman at increased risk for breast cancer: evaluation and management strategies. Ca 45(5):263, 1995.

Breast Conditions and Diseases. Benign breast disease with biopsy findings of atypical hyperplasia or lobular carcinoma in situ carry significantly increased relative risks—4.4 and 6.9 to 12.0, respectively.

Breast Cancer Screening. Screening with clinical breast examination (CBE) and/or mammography is universally recommended, depending on the patient's age. All women aged 40 or older are generally advised to undergo annual CBE, and women with increased risk factors may benefit from CBE even earlier. The guidelines for mammography continue to change as more facts are established. Currently, for women aged 50 to 69, performing mammograms alone or with CBE is advised every 1 to 2 years. In women aged 40 to 50, the benefits of screening mammography remain controversial, since before menopause breast tissue is generally more glandular and mammography appears to be less sensitive. Clinicians often recommend a baseline mammogram at age 40. In women aged 70 and older, the benefits of screening mammograms are also less clear and testing should be considered on an individual basis.

Table 10-1   Visible Signs of Breast Cancer

TABLE 10-1 *Visible Signs of Breast Cancer*

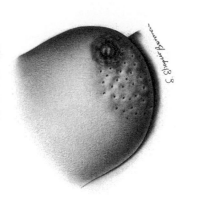

Retraction Signs

Mechanism

As breast cancer advances, it causes fibrosis (scar tissue). Shortening of this fibrotic tissue produces retraction signs, including dimpling, changes in contour, and retraction or deviation of the nipple. Other causes of retraction signs include fat necrosis and mammary duct ectasia.

Retracted nipple

Dimpling

Cancer

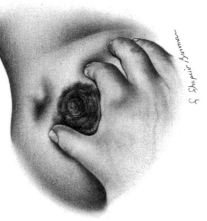

Skin Dimpling

Look for this sign with the patient's arm at rest, during special positioning, and on moving or compressing the breast, as illustrated here.

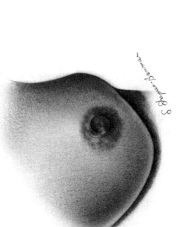

Dermatitis of areola

Erosion of nipple

Edema of the Skin

Edema of the skin is produced by lymphatic blockade. It appears as thickened skin with enlarged pores—the so-called *peau d'orange* (orange peel) *sign*. It is often seen first in the lower portion of the breast or areola.

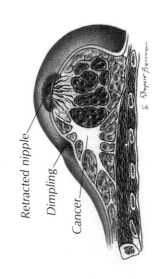

Abnormal Contours

Look for any variation in the normal convexity of each breast, and compare one side with the other. Special positioning may again be useful. Shown here is marked flattening of the lower outer quadrant of the left breast.

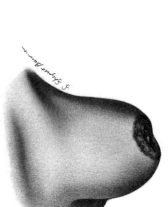

Nipple Retraction and Deviation

A retracted nipple is flattened or pulled inward, as illustrated here. It may also be broadened, and feels thickened. When involvement is radially asymmetrical, the nipple may deviate, i.e., point in a different direction from its normal counterpart, typically toward the underlying cancer.

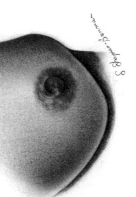

Paget's Disease of the Nipple

This is an uncommon form of breast cancer that usually starts as a scaly, eczemalike lesion. The skin may also weep, crust, or erode. A breast mass may be present. Suspect Paget's disease in any persisting dermatitis of the nipple and areola.

Table 10-2   Differentiation of Common Breast Nodules

TABLE 10-2   Differentiation of Common Breast Nodules

The three most common kinds of breast nodules are gross cysts, fibroadenoma (a benign tumor), and breast cancer. The classic clinical characteristics of these three conditions, outlined below, are not always predictive of the final diagnosis. The nodules illustrated are rather large for illustrative purposes. Identification of a breast cancer is made ideally when it is small. *Fibrocystic changes*, not illustrated, are also commonly palpable in women 25–50 as nodular rope-like densities, at times tender or painful. Such changes are considered benign.

	Fibroadenoma	Gross Cysts	Cancer
Usual Age	15–25, usually puberty and young adulthood, but up to age 55	30–50, regress after menopause except with estrogen therapy	30–90, most common over 50 in middle-aged and elderly women
Number	Usually single, may be multiple	Single or multiple	Usually single, although may coexist with other nodules
Shape	Round, disclike, or lobular	Round	Irregular or stellate
Consistency	May be soft, usually firm	Soft to firm, usually elastic	Firm or hard
Delimitation	Well delineated	Well delineated	Not clearly delineated from surrounding tissues
Mobility	Very mobile	Mobile	May be fixed to skin or underlying tissues
Tenderness	Usually nontender	Often tender	Usually nontender
Retraction Signs	Absent	Absent	May be present

The Abdomen

CHAPTER 11

Anatomy and Physiology

Review the anatomy of the abdominal wall and pelvis, identifying the landmarks illustrated. The rectus abdominis muscles can be identified when a person raises the head and shoulders from the supine position.

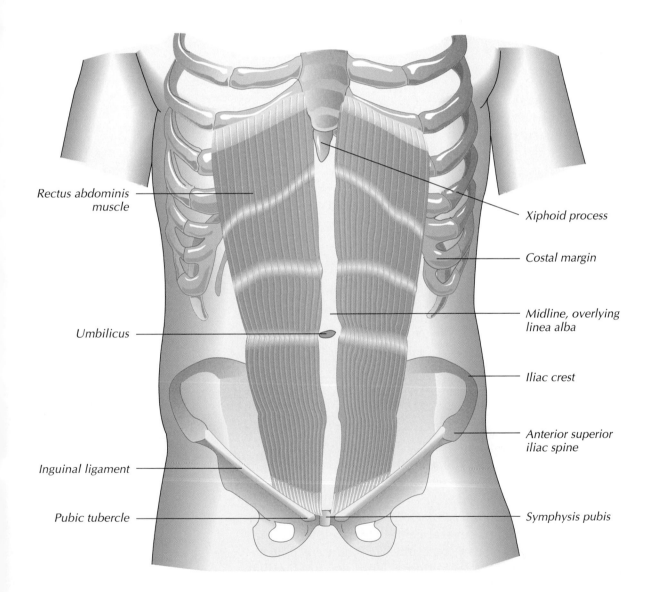

Rectus abdominis muscle

Xiphoid process

Costal margin

Midline, overlying linea alba

Umbilicus

Iliac crest

Anterior superior iliac spine

Inguinal ligament

Pubic tubercle

Symphysis pubis

Anatomy and Physiology

For descriptive purposes, the abdomen is often divided into four quadrants by imaginary lines crossing at the umbilicus: right upper, right lower, left upper, and left lower quadrants. Another system divides the abdomen into nine sections. Terms for three of them are commonly used: epigastric, umbilical, and hypogastric or suprapubic.

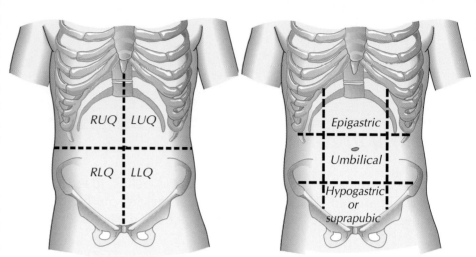

When examining the abdomen, you may be able to feel several normal structures. The sigmoid *colon* is frequently palpable as a firm, narrow tube in the left lower quadrant, while the cecum and part of the ascending colon form a softer, wider tube in the right lower quadrant. Portions of the transverse and descending colon may also be palpable. None of these structures should be mistaken for a tumor. Although the normal *liver* often extends down just below the right costal margin, its soft consistency makes it difficult to feel through the abdominal wall. The lower margin of the liver, the liver edge, is often palpable. Also in the right upper quadrant, but usually at a deeper level, lies the lower pole of the right kidney. It is occasionally palpable, especially in thin individuals with relaxed abdominal muscles. Pulsations of the *abdominal aorta* are frequently visible and usually palpable in the upper abdomen, while the pulsations of the *iliac arteries* may sometimes be felt in the lower quadrants.

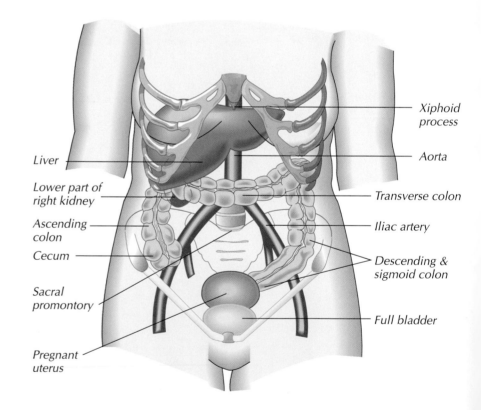

A distended *bladder* and a pregnant *uterus* each may rise above the symphysis pubis. With deep palpation several centimeters below the umbilicus in thin relaxed persons, you can sometimes feel the *sacral promontory,* the anterior edge of the first sacral vertebra. Until you are familiar with this normal structure, you may mistake its stony hard outlines for a tumor. Another stony hard lump that can sometimes mislead you, and occasionally also alarms a patient who discovers it first, is a normal *xiphoid process*.

The abdominal cavity extends up under the rib cage to the dome of the diaphragm. In this protected location, beyond the reach of the palpating hand, are much of the liver and *stomach* and all of the usual normal spleen. The *spleen* lies against the diaphragm at the level of the 9th, 10th, and 11th ribs, mostly posterior to the left midaxillary line. It is lateral to and behind the stomach, and just above the left kidney. The tip of a normal spleen is palpable below the left costal margin in a small percentage of adults.

Most of the normal *gallbladder* lies deep to the liver, from which it cannot be distinguished clinically. The *duodenum* and *pancreas* lie deep in the upper abdomen, where they are not normally palpable.

The *kidneys* are posterior organs, the upper portions of which are protected by the ribs. The costovertebral angle—the angle formed by the lower border of the 12th rib and the transverse processes of the upper lumbar vertebrae—defines the region to assess for kidney tenderness.

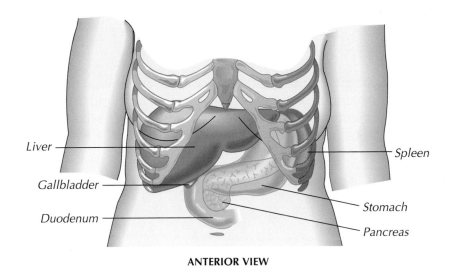

ANTERIOR VIEW

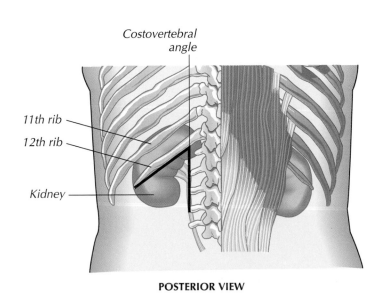

POSTERIOR VIEW

Changes With Age

During the middle and later years, fat tends to accumulate in the lower abdomen and near the hips, even when total body weight is stable. This accumulation, together with weakening of the abdominal muscles, often produces a potbelly. Occasionally a person notes this change with alarm and interprets it as fluid or evidence of disease.

Old age may blunt the manifestations of acute abdominal disease. Pain may be less severe, fever is often less pronounced, and signs of peritoneal inflammation, such as muscular guarding and rebound tenderness (pp. 363–364) may be diminished or even absent.

Techniques of Examination

General Approach

For a good abdominal examination you need (1) good light, (2) a relaxed patient, and (3) full exposure of the abdomen from above the xiphoid process to the symphysis pubis. The groins should be visible, although the genitalia should be kept draped. To encourage relaxation:

- The patient should *not* have a full bladder.

- Make the patient comfortable in a supine position, with a pillow for the head and perhaps another under the knees. Check to see if the patient is relaxed and flat on the table by trying to insert you hand underneath the low back.

An arched back thrusts the abdomen forward, thus tightening the abdominal muscles.

- Have the patient keep arms at the sides or folded across the chest. Although patients commonly put their arms over their heads, this move should be discouraged because it stretches and tightens the abdominal wall and makes palpation difficult.

- Before palpation, ask the patient to point to any areas of pain, and examine painful or tender areas last.

- Monitor your examination by watching the patient's face for signs of discomfort.

- Have warm hands, a warm stethoscope, and short fingernails. Rubbing your hands together or running hot water over them may help to warm them. If necessary, you may start your palpation through the patient's gown. This contact with the patient's body usually warms your hand, and you can then expose the abdomen properly. Anxious examiners often have cold hands. This problem decreases over time.

- Approach slowly and avoid quick, unexpected movements.

- Distract the patient if necessary with conversation or questions.

- If the patient is very frightened or very ticklish, begin palpation with the patient's hand beneath yours. In a few moments you can slip your hand underneath to palpate directly.

Make a habit of visualizing each organ in the region you are examining. From the patient's right side, proceed in an orderly fashion: inspection, auscultation, percussion, and palpation of the abdomen, and assessment of the liver, spleen, kidneys, and aorta.

The Abdomen

Inspection

Starting from your usual standing position at the right side of the bed, inspect the abdomen. When looking at the contour of the abdomen and watching for peristalsis, it is helpful to sit or bend down so that you can view the abdomen tangentially.

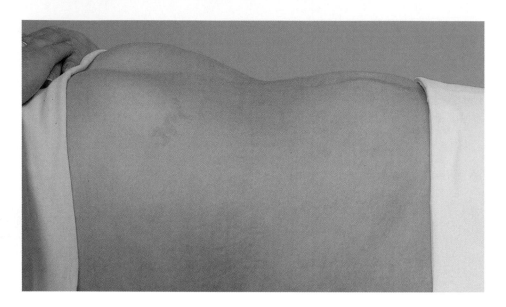

Note:

- *The skin,* including:

    Scars. Describe or diagram their location.

    Striae. Old silver striae or stretch marks, as illustrated above, are normal.

    Pink purple striae of Cushing's syndrome

    Dilated veins. A few small veins may be visible normally.

    Dilated veins of hepatic cirrhosis or of inferior vena cava obstruction

    Rashes and lesions

- *The umbilicus*—its contour and location, and any signs of inflammation or hernia

    See Table 11-1, Localized Bulges in the Abdominal Wall (p. 380).

- *The contour of the abdomen.*

    Is it flat, rounded, protuberant, or scaphoid (markedly concave or hollowed)?

    See Table 11-2, Protuberant Abdomens (p. 381).

    Do the flanks bulge or are there any local bulges? Include in this survey the inguinal and femoral areas.

    Bulging flanks of ascites; suprapubic bulge of a distended bladder or pregnant uterus; hernias

Is the abdomen symmetrical?	Asymmetry due to an enlarged organ or mass
Are there visible organs or masses? Look for an enlarged liver or spleen that has descended below the rib cage.	Lower abdominal mass of an ovarian or a uterine tumor
• *Peristalsis.* Observe for several minutes if you suspect intestinal obstruction. Peristalsis may be visible normally in very thin people.	Increased peristaltic waves of intestinal obstruction
• *Pulsations.* The normal aortic pulsation is frequently visible in the epigastrium.	Increased pulsation of an aortic aneurysm or of increased pulse pressure

Auscultation

Auscultation of the abdomen is useful in assessing bowel motility and abdominal complaints, in searching for renal artery stenosis as a cause of hypertension, and in exploring for other vascular obstructions. You should practice the technique until you become thoroughly familiar with normal variations and can listen intelligently when you need to.

Listen to the abdomen before percussing and feeling it, because the latter maneuvers may alter the frequency of bowel sounds. Place the diaphragm of your stethoscope gently on the abdomen.

Listen for *bowel sounds* and note their frequency and character. Normal sounds consist of clicks and gurgles, occurring at an estimated frequency of 5 to 34 per minute. Occasionally you may hear *borborygmi*—long prolonged gurgles of hyperperistalsis—the familiar "stomach growling." Because bowel sounds are widely transmitted through the abdomen, listening in one spot, such as the right lower quadrant, is usually sufficient.	Bowel sounds may be altered in diarrhea, intestinal obstruction, paralytic ileus, and peritonitis. See Table 11-3, Sounds in the Abdomen (p. 382).
If the patient has high blood pressure, listen in the epigastrium and in each upper quadrant for *bruits*—vascular sounds resembling heart murmurs. Later in the examination, when the patient sits up, listen also in the costovertebral angles. Epigastric bruits confined to systole may be heard in normal persons.	A bruit in one of these areas that has both systolic and diastolic components strongly suggests renal artery stenosis as the cause of hypertension.
If you suspect arterial insufficiency in the legs, listen for bruits over the aorta, the iliac arteries, and the femoral arteries. Bruits confined to systole are relatively common, however, and do not necessarily signify occlusive disease.	Bruits with both systolic and diastolic components suggest the turbulent blood flow of partial arterial occlusion. See Table 11-3, Sounds in the Abdomen (p. 382).

Listening points for bruits in these vessels are illustrated on p. 362.

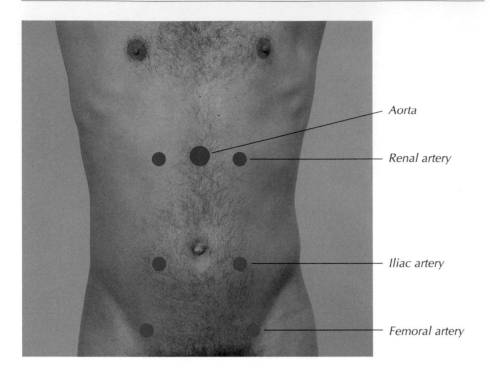

Aorta

Renal artery

Iliac artery

Femoral artery

If you suspect a liver tumor, gonococcal infection around the liver, or splenic infarction, listen over the liver and spleen for *friction rubs*.

See Table 11-3, Sounds in the Abdomen (p. 382).

Percussion

Percussion helps you to assess the amount and distribution of gas in the abdomen and to identify possible masses that are solid or fluid filled. Its use in estimating the size of the liver and spleen will be described in later sections.

Percuss the abdomen lightly in all four quadrants to assess the distribution of tympany and dullness. Tympany usually predominates because of gas in the gastrointestinal tract, but scattered areas of dullness due to fluid and feces there are also typical.

A protuberant abdomen that is tympanitic throughout suggests intestinal obstruction. See Table 11-2, Protuberant Abdomens (p. 381).

• Note any large dull areas that might indicate an underlying mass or enlarged organ. This observation will guide your palpation.

Pregnant uterus, ovarian tumor, distended bladder, large liver or spleen

• On each side of a protuberant abdomen, note where abdominal tympany changes to the dullness of solid posterior structures.

Dullness in both flanks indicates further assessment for ascites (see pp. 374–375).

Briefly percuss the lower anterior chest, between lungs above and costal margins below. On the right, you will usually find the dullness of liver; on the left, the tympany that overlies the gastric air bubble and the splenic flexure of the colon.

In situs inversus (rare), organs are reversed: air bubble on the right, liver dullness on the left.

Palpation

Light Palpation. Feeling the abdomen gently is especially helpful in identifying abdominal tenderness, muscular resistance, and some superficial organs and masses. It also serves to reassure and relax the patient.

Keeping your hand and forearm on a horizontal plane, with fingers together and flat on the abdominal surface, palpate the abdomen with a light, gentle, dipping motion. When moving your hand from place to place, raise it just off the skin. Moving smoothly, feel in all quadrants.

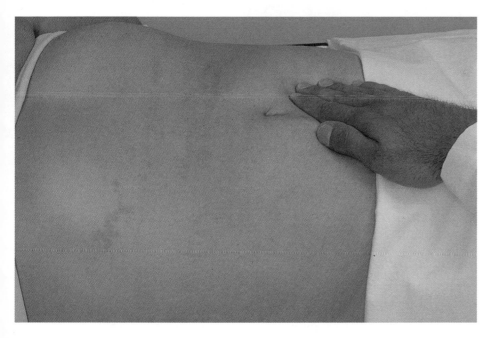

Identify any superficial organs or masses and any area of tenderness or increased resistance to your hand. If resistance is present, try to distinguish voluntary guarding from involuntary muscular spasm. To do this:

- Try all the relaxing methods you know (see p. 359).

- Feel for the relaxation of abdominal muscles that normally accompanies exhalation.

- Ask the patient to mouth-breathe with jaw dropped open.

Voluntary guarding usually decreases with these maneuvers.

Deep palpation. This is usually required to delineate abdominal masses. Again using the palmar surfaces of your fingers, feel in all four quadrants. Identify any masses and note their location, size, shape, consistency, tenderness, pulsations, and mobility (e.g., with respiration or with the examining hand). Correlate your palpable findings with your percussion note.

Involuntary rigidity (muscular spasm) typically persists despite these maneuvers. It indicates peritoneal inflammation.

Abdominal masses may be categorized in several ways: physiologic (pregnant uterus), inflammatory (diverticulitis of the colon), vascular (an aneurysm of the abdominal

When deep palpation is difficult—as in obesity—use two hands, one on top of the other. Exert pressure with the outside hand while concentrating on feeling with the inside hand.

aorta), neoplastic (carcinoma of the colon), or obstructive (a distended bladder or dilated loop of bowel).

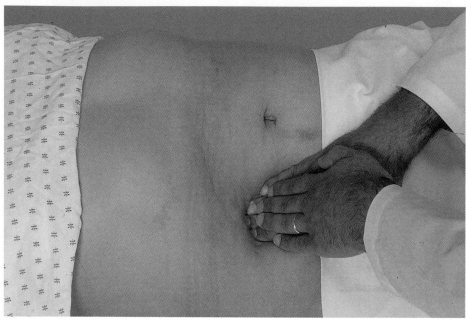

TWO-HANDED DEEP PALPATION

Assessment for Peritoneal Inflammation. Abdominal pain and tenderness, especially when associated with muscular spasm, suggest inflammation of the parietal peritoneum. Localize the pain as accurately as possible. First, even before palpation, *ask the patient to cough* and determine where the cough produced pain. Thus guided, *palpate gently with one finger* to map the tender area. Pain produced by light percussion has similar localizing value. These gentle maneuvers may be all you need to establish an area of peritoneal inflammation.

Abdominal pain on coughing or with light percussion suggests peritoneal inflammation. See Table 11-4, Tender Abdomens (pp. 383–384).

If not, *look for rebound tenderness.* Press your fingers in firmly and slowly, and then quickly withdraw them. Watch and listen to the patient for signs of pain. Ask the patient (1) to compare which hurt more, the pressing or the letting go, and (2) to show you exactly where it hurt. Pain induced or increased by quick withdrawal constitutes rebound tenderness. It results from the rapid movement of inflamed peritoneum.

Rebound tenderness suggests peritoneal inflammation. If tenderness is felt elsewhere than where you were trying to elicit rebound, that area may be the real source of the problem.

The Liver

Because most of the liver is sheltered by the rib cage, assessing it is difficult. Its size and shape can be estimated by percussion and perhaps palpation, however, and the palpating hand may enable you to evaluate its surface, consistency, and tenderness.

Percussion

Measure the vertical span of liver dullness in the right midclavicular line. Starting at a level below the umbilicus (in an area of tympany, not dullness), lightly percuss upward toward the liver. Ascertain the lower border of liver dullness in the midclavicular line.

Next, identify the upper border of liver dullness in the midclavicular line. Lightly percuss from lung resonance down toward liver dullness. Gently displace a woman's breast as necessary to be sure that you start in a resonant area. The course of percussion is shown below.

The span of liver dullness is increased when the liver is enlarged.

The span of liver dullness is decreased when the liver is small. It may also be decreased when free air is present below the diaphragm, as from a perforated hollow viscus. Serial observations may show a decreasing span of dullness with resolution of hepatitis or congestive heart failure or, less commonly, with progression of fulminant hepatitis.

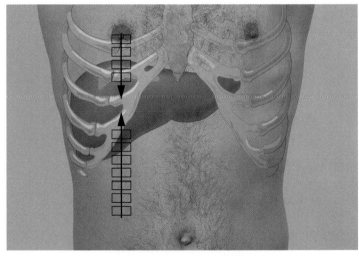

PERCUSSING LIVER SPAN

Liver dullness may be displaced downward by the low diaphragm of chronic obstructive lung disease. Span, however, remains normal.

Now measure in centimeters the distance between your two points—the vertical span of liver dullness. Normal liver spans are shown at the top of p. 366. They are generally greater in men than in women, in tall people than in short. If the liver seems to be enlarged, outline the lower edge by percussing in other areas.

Although percussion is probably the most accurate clinical method for estimating the vertical size of the liver, it typically leads to underestimation.

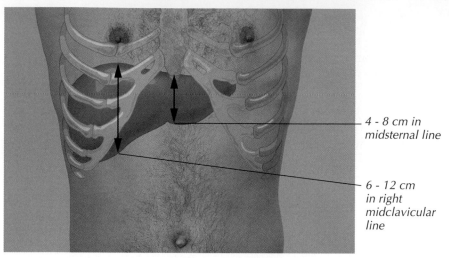

4 - 8 cm in
midsternal line

6 - 12 cm
in right
midclavicular
line

NORMAL LIVER SPANS

Dullness of a right pleural effusion or consolidated lung, if adjacent to liver dullness, may falsely increase the estimate of liver size.

Gas in the colon may produce tympany in the right upper quadrant, obscure liver dullness, and falsely decrease the estimate of liver size.

Palpation

Place your left hand behind the patient, parallel to and supporting the right 11th and 12th ribs and adjacent soft tissues below. Remind the patient to relax on your hand if necessary. By pressing your left hand forward, the patient's liver may be felt more easily by your other hand.

Place your right hand on the patient's right abdomen lateral to the rectus muscle, with your fingertips well below the lower border of liver dullness.

Some examiners like to point their fingers up toward the patient's head, while others prefer a somewhat more oblique position, as shown in the two photos on the following page. In either case, press gently in and up. Then ask the patient to take a deep breath.

Try to feel the liver edge as it comes down to meet your fingertips. If you feel it, lighten the pressure of your palpating hand slightly so that the liver can slip under your finger pads and you can feel its anterior surface. Note any tenderness. If palpable at all, the edge of a normal liver is soft, sharp, and regular, its surface smooth. The normal liver may be slightly tender.

Firmness or hardness of the liver, bluntness or rounding of its edge, and irregularity of its contour suggest an abnormality of the liver.

On inspiration, the liver below is palpable about 4 cm below the right costal margin in the mid-clavicular line.

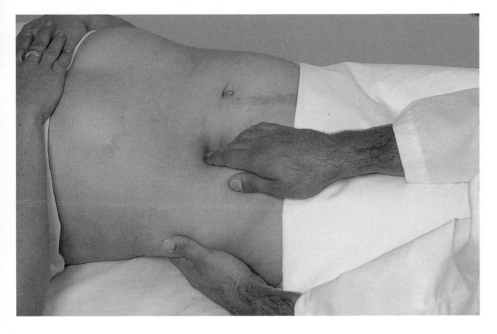

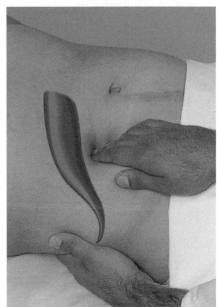

The edge of an enlarged liver may be missed by starting palpation too high in the abdomen, as shown below.

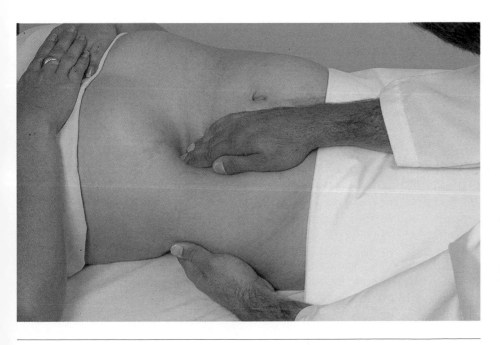

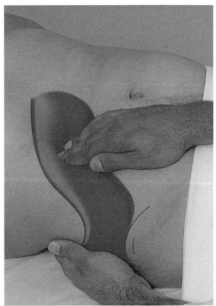

Try to trace the liver edge both laterally and medially. Palpation through the rectus muscles, however, is especially difficult. Describe or sketch the liver edge, and measure its distance from the right costal margin in the midclavicular line.

In order to feel the liver, you may have to alter your pressure according to the thickness and resistance of the abdominal wall. If you cannot feel it, move your palpating hand closer to the costal margin and try again.

The "hooking technique" may be helpful, especially when the patient is obese. Stand to the right of the patient's chest. Place both hands, side by side, on the right abdomen below the border of liver dullness. Press in with your fingers and up toward the costal margin. Ask the patient to take a deep breath.

See Table 11-5, Liver Enlargement: Apparent and Real (pp. 385–386). An obstructed, distended gallbladder may form an oval mass below the edge of the liver and merging with it. It is dull to percussion.

The liver edge shown below is palpable with the fingerpads of both hands.

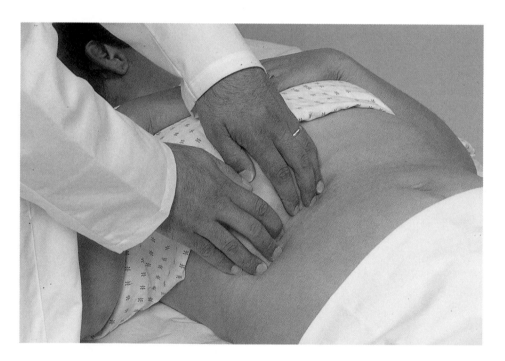

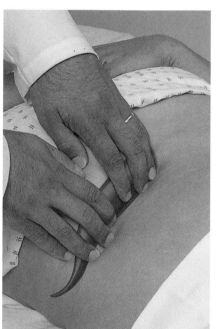

Some people breathe more with their chests than with their diaphragms. It may be helpful to train such a patient to "breathe with the abdomen," thus bringing the liver, as well as the spleen and kidneys, into a palpable position during inspiration.

Assessing Tenderness of a Nonpalpable Liver. Place your left hand flat on the lower right rib cage and then gently strike your hand with the ulnar surface of your right fist. Ask the patient to compare the sensation with that produced by a similar strike on the left side.

Tenderness over the liver suggests inflammation, as in hepatitis, or congestion, as in heart failure.

The Spleen

When a spleen enlarges, it does so anteriorly, downward, and medially, often replacing the tympany of stomach and colon with the dullness of a solid organ. It then becomes palpable below the costal margin. Percussion cannot confirm splenic enlargement but can raise your suspicions of it. Palpation can confirm the enlargement, but often misses large spleens that do not descend below the costal margin.

Percussion

Two techniques may help you to detect *splenomegaly*, an enlarged spleen:

• *Percuss the left lower anterior chest wall* between lung resonance above and the costal margin below (an area termed *Traube's space*). As you percuss along the routes suggested by the arrow below, note the lateral extent of tympany.

Dullness, as shown below, raises the question of splenomegaly.

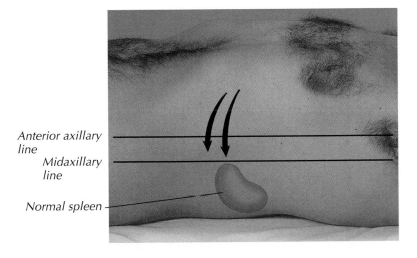

Anterior axillary line
Midaxillary line
Normal spleen

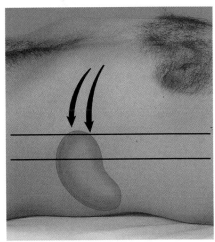

This is variable, but if tympany is prominent, especially laterally, splenomegaly is not likely. The dullness of a normal spleen is usually hidden within the dullness of other posterior tissues.

Fluid or solids in the stomach or colon may also cause dullness in Traube's space.

• *Check for a splenic percussion sign.* Percuss the lowest interspace in the left anterior axillary line, as shown on the following page. This area is usually tympanitic. Then ask the patient to take a deep breath, and percuss again. When spleen size is normal, the percussion note usually remains tympanitic.

If either or both of these tests is positive, pay extra attention to palpating the spleen.

A change in percussion note from tympany to dullness on inspiration suggests splenic enlargement. This is a *positive splenic percussion sign.*

The splenic percussion sign may also be positive when spleen size is normal.

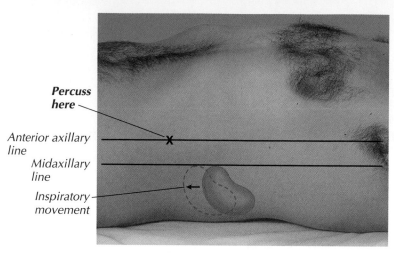

Percuss here

Anterior axillary line

Midaxillary line

Inspiratory movement

NEGATIVE SPLENIC PERCUSSION SIGN

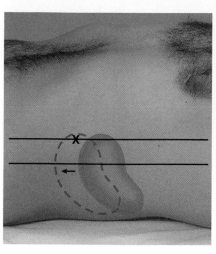

POSITIVE SPLENIC PERCUSSION SIGN

Palpation

With your left hand, reach over and around the patient to support and press forward the lower left rib cage and adjacent soft tissue. With your right hand below the left costal margin, press in toward the spleen. Begin palpation low enough so that you are below a possibly enlarged spleen. (If your hand is close to the costal margin, moreover, it is not sufficiently mobile to reach up under the rib cage.) Ask the patient to take a deep breath. Try to feel the tip or edge of the spleen as it comes down to meet your fingertips. Note any tenderness, assess the splenic contour, and measure the distance between the spleen's lowest point and the left costal margin. In a small percentage of normal adults, the tip of the spleen is palpable. Causes include a low, flat diaphragm, as in chronic obstructive pulmonary disease, and a deep inspiratory descent of the diaphragm.

An enlarged spleen may be missed if the examiner starts too high in the abdomen to feel the lower edge.

A palpable spleen tip, though not necessarily abnormal, may indicate splenic enlargement. The spleen tip below is just palpable deep to the left costal margin.

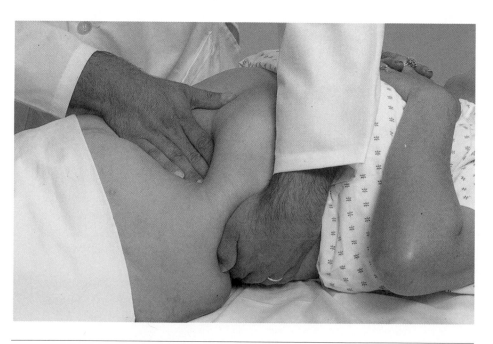

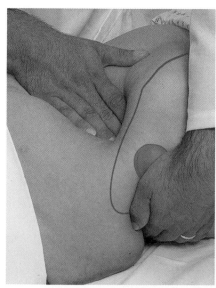

Repeat with the patient lying on the right side with legs somewhat flexed at hips and knees. In this position, gravity may bring the spleen forward and to the right into a palpable location.

The enlarged spleen below is palpable about 2 cm below the left costal margin on deep inspiration.

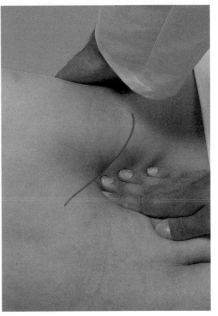

Marked and massive splenomegaly are shown below.

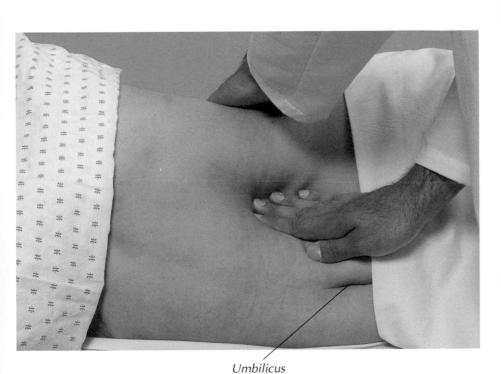

Umbilicus

**PALPATING SPLEEN—
ANTERIOR VIEW WITH PATIENT LYING ON RIGHT SIDE**

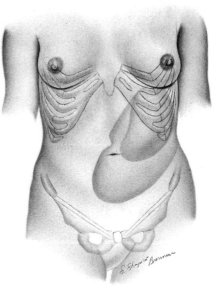

In assessment of a mass in the left flank, attributes that favor an enlarged spleen over an

The Kidneys

Palpation of the Right Kidney

Although kidneys are not usually palpable, you should learn and practice the techniques. Detecting an enlarged kidney may prove to be very important.

Place your left hand behind the patient just below and parallel to the 12th rib, with your fingertips just reaching the costovertebral angle. Lift, trying to displace the kidney anteriorly. Place your right hand gently in the right upper quadrant, lateral and parallel to the rectus muscle. Ask the patient to take a deep breath. At the peak of inspiration, press your right hand firmly and deeply into the right upper quadrant, just below the costal margin, and try to "capture" the kidney between your two hands. Ask the patient to breathe out and then to stop breathing briefly. Slowly release the pressure of your right hand, feeling at the same time for the kidney to slide back into its expiratory position. If the kidney is palpable, describe its size, contour, and tenderness.

enlarged left kidney are a notch on the medial border, extension beyond the midline, dullness to percussion, and the ability to get your fingers deep to its medial and lower borders but not between the mass and the costal margin. Definitive differentiation, however, cannot usually be made on clinical criteria alone.

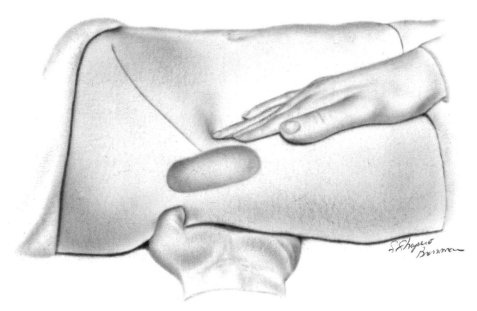

A normal right kidney may be palpable, especially in thin, well relaxed women. It may or may not be slightly tender. The patient is usually aware of a capture and release. Occasionally, a right kidney is located more anteriorly than usual and then must be distinguished from the liver. The edge of the liver, if palpable, tends to be sharper and to extend farther medially and laterally. It cannot be captured. The lower pole of the kidney is rounded.

Causes of kidney enlargement include hydronephrosis, cysts, and tumors. Bilateral enlargement suggests polycystic disease.

Palpation of the Left Kidney

To capture the left kidney, move to the patient's left side. Use your right hand to lift from in back, and your left hand to feel deep in the left upper quadrant. Proceed as before.

In assessment of a mass in the left flank, attributes that favor an enlarged kidney over an

Alternatively, try to feel for the left kidney by a method somewhat similar to feeling for the spleen. With your left hand, reach over and around the patient to lift the left loin, and with your right hand feel deep in the left upper quadrant. Ask the patient to take a deep breath, and feel for a mass. A normal left kidney is rarely palpable.

enlarged spleen are the preservation of normal tympany in the left upper quadrant, and the ability to get your fingers between the mass and the costal margin but not deep to its medial and lower borders.

Assessing Kidney Tenderness

Tenderness may be noted during abdominal palpation, but search for it also in each costovertebral angle. Pressure from your fingertips may be enough to reveal tenderness here; if not, use fist percussion. Place the ball of one hand in the costovertebral angle and strike it with the ulnar surface of your fist. Use force sufficient to cause a perceptible but painless jar or thud in a normal person.

Pain with pressure or with fist percussion in the costovertebral angle suggests kidney infection, but it may also have a musculoskeletal cause.

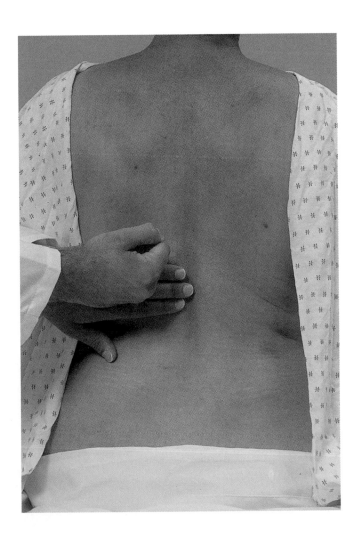

To save the patient needless exertion, integrate this assessment with your examination of the back (see p. 133).

The Aorta

Press firmly deep in the upper abdomen, slightly to the left of the midline, and identify the aortic pulsations. In persons over age 50, try to assess the width of the aorta by pressing deeply in the upper abdomen with one hand on each side of the aorta, as illustrated. In this age group, a normal aorta is not more than 3.0 cm wide (average 2.5 cm). This measurement does not include the thickness of the abdominal wall. The ease with which you can feel aortic pulsations varies greatly with the thickness of the abdominal wall and with the anteroposterior diameter of the abdomen.

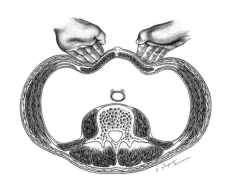

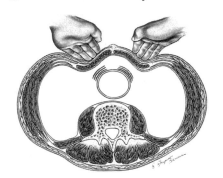

In an older person, a periumbilical or upper abdominal mass with expansile pulsations suggests an aortic aneurysm.

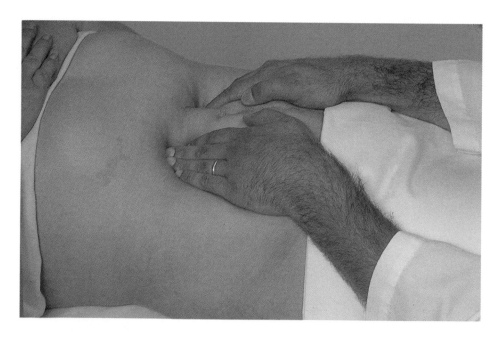

This is a pathologic dilatation of the aorta, usually due to arteriosclerosis. A merely tortuous abdominal aorta, however, may be difficult to distinguish from an aneurysm on clinical grounds.

Although an aneurysm is usually painless, pain may herald its most dreaded and frequent complication—rupture of the aorta.

Apparent enlargement of the aorta indicates assessment by ultrasound.

Special Techniques

To Assess Possible Ascites. A protuberant abdomen with bulging flanks suggests the possibility of ascitic fluid. Because ascitic fluid characteristically sinks with gravity while gas-filled loops of bowel float to the top, percussion gives a dull note in dependent areas of the abdomen. Look for such a pattern by percussing outward in several directions from the central area of tympany. Map the border between tympany and dullness.

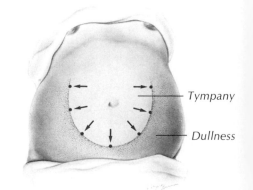

Tympany

Dullness

Two further techniques help to confirm the presence of ascites, although both signs may be misleading.

1. *Test for shifting dullness.* After mapping the borders of tympany and dullness, ask the patient to turn onto one side. Percuss and mark the borders again. In a person without ascites, the borders between tympany and dullness usually stay relatively constant.

In ascites, dullness shifts to the more dependent side, while tympany shifts to the top.

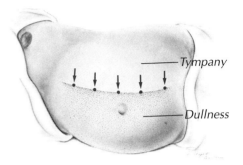

2. *Test for a fluid wave.* Ask the patient or an assistant to press the edges of both hands firmly down the midline of the abdomen. This pressure helps to stop the transmission of a wave through fat. While you tap one flank sharply with your fingertips, feel on the opposite flank for an impulse transmitted through the fluid. Unfortunately, this sign is often negative until ascites is obvious, and it is sometimes positive in people without ascites.

An easily palpable impulse suggests ascites.

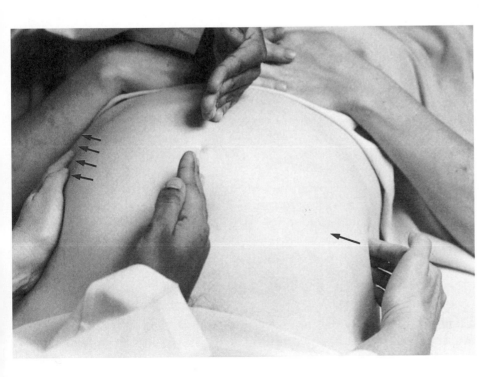

To Identify an Organ or a Mass in an Ascitic Abdomen. Try to *ballotte* the organ or mass, exemplified here by an enlarged liver. Straighten and stiffen the fingers of one hand together, place them on the abdominal surface, and make a brief jabbing movement directly toward the anticipated structure. This quick movement often displaces the fluid so that your fingertips can briefly touch the surface of the structure through the abdominal wall.

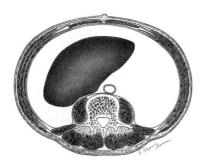 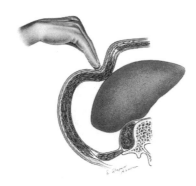

To Assess Possible Appendicitis

- Ask the patient to point to where the pain began and where it is now. Ask the patient to cough. Determine whether and where pain results.

  The pain of appendicitis classically begins near the umbilicus and then shifts to the right lower quadrant, where coughing increases it. Elderly patients report this pattern less frequently than younger ones.

- Search carefully for an area of local tenderness.

  Localized tenderness anywhere in the right lower quadrant, even in the right flank, may indicate appendicitis.

- Feel for muscular rigidity.

  Early voluntary guarding may be replaced by involuntary muscular rigidity.

- Perform a rectal examination and, in women, a pelvic examination. These maneuvers may not help you to discriminate well between a normal and an inflamed appendix, but they may help to identify an inflamed appendix atypically located within the pelvic cavity. They may also suggest other causes of the abdominal pain.

  Right-sided rectal tenderness may be caused by, for example, inflamed adnexa or an inflamed seminal vesicle, as well as by an inflamed appendix.

Some additional techniques are sometimes helpful.

- Check the tender area for rebound tenderness. (If other signs are typically positive, you can save the patient unnecessary pain by omitting this test.)

  Rebound tenderness suggests peritoneal inflammation, as from appendicitis.

- Check for *Rovsing's sign* and for referred rebound tenderness. Press deeply and evenly in the *left* lower quadrant. Then quickly withdraw your fingers.

    Pain in the *right* lower quadrant during *left*-sided pressure suggests appendicitis (a positive Rovsing's sign). So does right lower quadrant pain on quick withdrawal (referred rebound tenderness).

- Look for a *psoas sign.* Place your hand just above the patient's right knee and ask the patient to raise that thigh against your hand. Alternatively, ask the patient to turn onto the left side. Then extend the patient's right leg at the hip. Flexion of the leg at the hip makes the psoas muscle contract; extension stretches it.

    Increased abdominal pain on either maneuver constitutes a positive psoas sign, suggesting irritation of the psoas muscle by an inflamed appendix.

- Look for an *obturator sign.* Flex the patient's right thigh at the hip, with the knee bent, and rotate the leg internally at the hip. This maneuver stretches the internal obturator muscle. (Internal rotation of the hip is described on p. 530.)

    Right hypogastric pain constitutes a positive obturator sign, suggesting irritation of the obturator muscle by an inflamed appendix.

- Test or *cutaneous hyperesthesia.* At a series of points down the abdominal wall, gently pick up a fold of skin between your thumb and index finger, without pinching it. This maneuver should not normally be painful.

    Localized pain with this maneuver, in all or part of the right lower quadrant, may accompany appendicitis.

To Assess Possible Acute Cholecystitis. When right upper quadrant pain and tenderness suggest acute cholecystitis, look for *Murphy's sign.* Hook your left thumb or the fingers of your right hand under the costal margin at the point where the lateral border of the rectus muscle intersects with the costal margin. Alternatively, if the liver is enlarged, hook your thumb or fingers under the liver edge at a comparable point below. Ask the patient to take a deep breath. Watch the patient's breathing and note the degree of tenderness.

A sharp increase in tenderness with a sudden stop in inspiratory effort constitutes a positive Murphy's sign of acute cholecystitis. Hepatic tenderness may also increase with this maneuver, but is usually less well localized.

To Assess Ventral Hernias (hernias in the abdominal wall exclusive of groin hernias). If you suspect but do not see an umbilical or incisional hernia, ask the patient to raise both head and shoulders off the table.

The bulge of a hernia will usually appear with this action (see p. 378).

Inguinal and femoral hernias are discussed in the next chapter. They can give rise to important abdominal problems and must not be overlooked.

The cause of intestinal obstruction or peritonitis may be missed by overlooking a strangulated femoral hernia.

To Distinguish an Abdominal Mass From a Mass in the Abdominal Wall. An occasional mass is in the abdominal wall rather than inside the abdominal cavity. Ask the patient either to raise the head and shoulders or to strain down, thus tightening the abdominal muscles. Feel for the mass again.

A mass in the abdominal wall remains palpable; an intraabdominal mass is obscured by muscular contraction.

Health Promotion and Counseling

Health promotion and counseling relevant to the abdomen include screening for alcoholism, risk of infectious hepatitis, and risk of colon cancer. Clues from social patterns and behavioral problems in the history and findings of liver enlargement or tenderness on physical examination often alert the clinician to possible alcoholism or risk of infectious hepatitis. Past medical history and family history are important when assessing risk of colon cancer.

The impact of alcohol and substance abuse on public health may be even greater than that of illicit drugs. Assessing patients for use of alcohol and other substances is a primary responsibility of all clinicians. The clinician should focus on detection, counseling, and, for significant impairment, specific recommendations for treatment. These interventions need not be time-consuming. Use the four CAGE questions, validated across many studies, to screen for alcohol dependence or abuse in all adolescents and adults, including pregnant women (see p. 18). Brief counseling interventions have been shown to reduce alcohol consumption by up to 25%.* Focus on (1) sharing concern about the adverse effects of alcohol and education about harmful consequences, and (2) setting goals for behavioral change and follow-up. Tailor recommendations for treatment to the severity of the problem, ranging from support groups to inpatient detoxification to more extended rehabilitation.

Protective measures against infectious hepatitis include counseling about how the viruses are spread and the need for immunization. Transmission of Hepatitis A is fecal–oral: fecal shedding in food handlers leads to contamination of water and foods. Illness occurs approximately 30 days after exposure. Hepatitis A vaccine is recommended for travelers to endemic areas, food handlers, military personnel, selected health-care and laboratory workers, and caretakers of children. For immediate protection and prophylaxis for household contacts and travelers, consider the administration of immunoglobulin.

Hepatitis B poses more serious threats to patients' health, including risk of fulminant hepatitis as well as chronic infection and subsequent cirrhosis and hepatocellular carcinoma. Transmission occurs during contact with infected body fluids, such as blood, semen, saliva, and vaginal secretions. Adults between the ages of 20 and 39 are most affected, especially injection drug users and sex workers. Up to a tenth of infected adults become chronically infected asymptomatic carriers. Behavioral counseling and serologic screening are advised for patients at risk. Because up to 30% of patients have no identifiable risk factors, hepatitis B vaccine is recommended for all young adults not previously immunized, injection drug users and their sexual partners, persons at risk for sexually transmitted disease, travelers to endemic areas, recipients of

---

* U.S. Preventive Services Task Force: Guide to Clinical Preventive Services, 2nd ed. Baltimore, Williams & Wilkins, 1996, p. 572.

blood products as in hemodialysis, and health-care workers with frequent exposure to blood products. Many of these groups should also be screened for HIV infection.

It is also important to screen patients for colorectal cancer, second highest of the malignancies in both prevalence and mortality. Risk factors include family history of colonic polyps, history of colorectal cancer or adenoma in a first-degree relative, and a personal history of ulcerative colitis, adenomatous polyps, or prior diagnosis of endometrial, ovarian, or breast cancer. The U.S. Preventive Services Task Force recommends annual testing of all persons over age 50 with the fecal occult blood test (FOBT), sigmoidoscopy, or both, but details several caveats.** The FOBT has a highly variable sensitivity (26%–92%), but good specificity (90%–99%). It produces many false positives related to diet, selected medications, and gastrointestinal conditions such as ulcer disease, diverticulosis, and hemorrhoids. The benefits of sigmoidoscopy are linked to the length of the sigmoidoscope and its depth of insertion. Detection rates for colorectal cancer and insertion depths are roughly as follows: 25%–30% at 20 cm; 50%–55% at 35 cm; 40%–65% at 40–50 cm. Full colonoscopy or air contrast barium enema detects 80%–95% of colorectal cancers, but these procedures are more uncomfortable and colonoscopy is more expensive. When counseling patients about prevention, there is preliminary but inconsistent evidence that diets high in fiber may reduce risk of colorectal malignancy.

** U.S. Preventive Services Task Force: Guide to Clinical Preventive Services, 2nd ed. Baltimore, Williams & Wilkins, 1996, pp. 89–103.

Table 11-1   Localized Bulges in the Abdominal Wall

TABLE 11-1   Localized Bulges in the Abdominal Wall

Localized bulges in the abdominal wall include ventral hernias (defects in the wall through which tissue protrudes) and subcutaneous tumors such as lipomas. The more common ventral hernias are umbilical, incisional, and epigastric. Rectus diastasis is also sometimes so classified. Hernias and a rectus diastasis usually become more evident when the patient raises head and shoulders from a supine position.

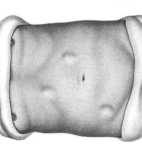

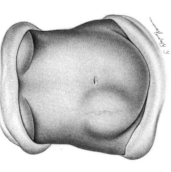

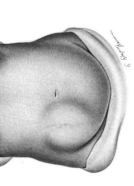

INFANT

Umbilical Hernia

Umbilical hernias protrude through a defective umbilical ring. They are most common in infants but also occur in adults. In infants, but not in adults, they usually close spontaneously within a year or two.

Incisional Hernia

An incisional hernia protrudes through an operative scar. By palpation, note the length and width of the defect in the abdominal wall. A small defect, through which a large hernia has passed, has a greater risk of complications than a large defect.

Epigastric Hernia

An epigastric hernia is a small midline protrusion through a defect in the linea alba, somewhere between the xiphoid process and the umbilicus. With the patient's head and shoulders raised (or with the patient standing), look for it, and run your fingerpad down the linea alba to feel it.

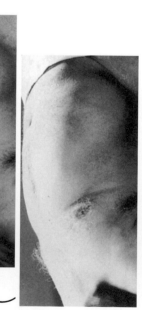
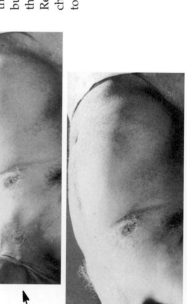

Lipoma

Lipomas are common, benign, fatty tumors usually located in the subcutaneous tissues almost anywhere in the body, including the abdominal wall. Small or large, they are usually soft and often lobulated. When your finger presses down on the edge of a lipoma, the tumor typically slips out from under it.

Diastasis Recti

A rectus diastasis is a separation of the two rectus abdominis muscles, through which abdominal contents bulge to form a midline ridge when the patient raises head and shoulders. Repeated pregnancies, obesity, and chronic lung disease may predispose to it. It has no clinical consequences.

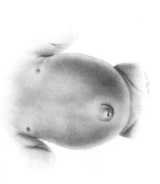

Ridge

Table 11-2   Protuberant Abdomens

TABLE 11-2   Protuberant Abdomens

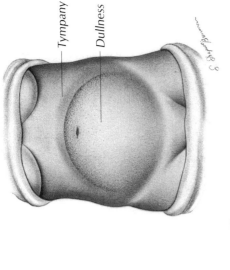

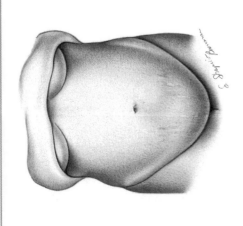

Fat

Fat is the most common cause of a protuberant abdomen and is associated with generalized obesity. The abdominal wall is thick. Fat in the mesentery and omentum also contributes to abdominal size. The umbilicus may appear sunken. The percussion note is normal. An apron of fatty tissue may extend below the inguinal ligaments. Lift it to look for inflammation in the skin fold or even for a hidden hernia.

Gas

Gaseous distention may be localized, as shown, or generalized. It causes a tympanitic percussion note. Increased intestinal gas production due to certain foods may cause mild distention. More serious are intestinal obstruction and adynamic (paralytic) ileus. Note the location of the distention. Distention becomes more marked in colonic than in small bowel obstruction.

Tumor

A large, solid tumor, usually rising out of the pelvis, is dull to percussion. Air-filled bowel is displaced to the periphery. Causes include ovarian tumors and uterine myomata. Occasionally, a markedly distended bladder may be mistaken for such a tumor.

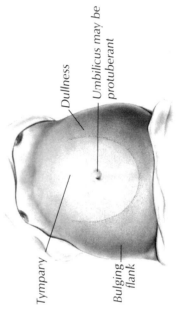

Tympany

Dullness

Pregnancy

Pregnancy is a common cause of a pelvic "tumor." Listen for the fetal heart (see pp. 441–442).

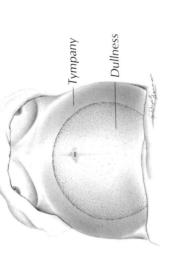

Tympany

Dullness

Ascitic Fluid

Ascitic fluid seeks the lowest point in the abdomen, producing bulging flanks that are dull to percussion. The umbilicus may protrude. Turn the patient onto one side to detect the shift in position of the fluid level (shifting dullness). (See pp. 374–375 for the assessment of ascites.)

Table 11-3 Sounds in the Abdomen

TABLE 11-3 Sounds in the Abdomen

Bowel Sounds

Bowel sounds may be:

- Increased, as from diarrhea or early intestinal obstruction.
- Decreased, then absent, as in adynamic ileus and peritonitis. Before deciding that bowel sounds are absent, sit down and listen where shown for 2 min or even longer.

High-pitched tinkling sounds suggest intestinal fluid and air under tension in a dilated bowel. Rushes of high-pitched sounds coinciding with an abdominal cramp indicate intestinal obstruction.

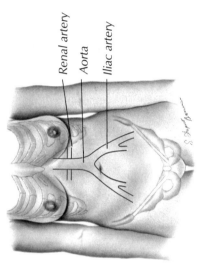

Bruits

A *hepatic bruit* suggests carcinoma of the liver or alcoholic hepatitis. *Arterial bruits* with both systolic and diastolic components suggest partial occlusion of the aorta or large arteries. Partial occlusion of a renal artery may cause and explain hypertension.

Renal artery
Aorta
Iliac artery

Venous Hum

A venous hum is rare. It is a soft humming noise with both systolic and diastolic components. It indicates increased collateral circulation between portal and systemic venous systems, as in hepatic cirrhosis.

Epigastric and umbilical

Friction Rubs

Friction rubs are rare. They are grating sounds with respiratory variation. They indicate inflammation of the peritoneal surface of an organ, as from a liver tumor, chlamydial or gonococcal perihepatitis, recent liver biopsy, or splenic infarct. When a systolic bruit accompanies a hepatic friction rub, suspect carcinoma of the liver.

Hepatic
Splenic

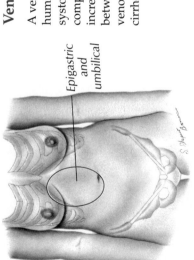

Table 11-4   Tender Abdomens

T A B L E   1 1 - 4   *Tender Abdomens*

Abdominal Wall Tenderness

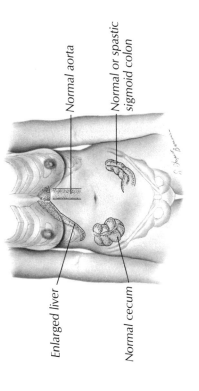

Superficial tender area

Deep tender areas

Tenderness may originate in the abdominal wall. When the patient raises head and shoulders, this tenderness persists, whereas tenderness from a deeper lesion (protected by the tightened muscles) decreases.

Visceral Tenderness

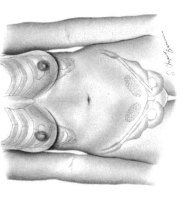

Normal aorta

Normal or spastic sigmoid colon

Enlarged liver

Normal cecum

The structures shown may be tender to deep palpation. Usually the discomfort is dull and there is no muscular ridigity or rebound tenderness. A reassuring explanation to the patient may prove quite helpful.

Tenderness From Disease in the Chest and Pelvis

Acute Pleurisy

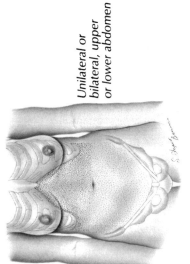

Unilateral or bilateral, upper or lower abdomen

Abdominal pain and tenderness may be due to acute pleural inflammation. When unilateral, it may mimic acute cholecystitis or appendicitis. Rebound tenderness and rigidity are less common; chest signs are usually present.

Acute Salpingitis

Frequently bilateral, the tenderness of acute salpingitis (inflammation of the fallopian tubes) is usually maximal just above the inguinal ligaments. Rebound tenderness and rigidity may be present. On pelvic examination, motion of the uterus causes pain.

Continued

Table 11-4   Tender Abdomens

TABLE 11-4 (continued)

Tenderness of Peritoneal Inflammation

Tenderness associated with peritoneal inflammation is usually more severe than visceral tenderness. Muscular rigidity and rebound tenderness are frequently but not necessarily present. Generalized peritonitis causes exquisite tenderness throughout the abdomen, together with boardlike muscular rigidity. Local causes of peritoneal inflammation include:

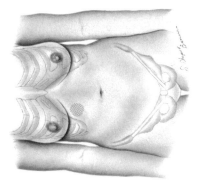

Acute Cholecystitis

Signs are maximal in the right upper quadrant. Check for Murphy's sign (see p. 377).

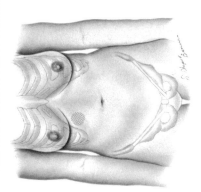

Just below the middle of a line joining the umbilicus and the anterior superior iliac spine

Right rectal tenderness

Acute Appendicitis

Right lower quadrant signs are typical of acute appendicitis, but may be absent early in the course. The typical area of tenderness is illustrated. Explore other portions of the right lower quadrant as well as the right flank.

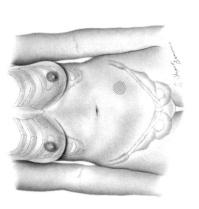

Acute Pancreatitis

In acute pancreatitis, epigastric tenderness and rebound tenderness are usually present, but the abdominal wall may be soft.

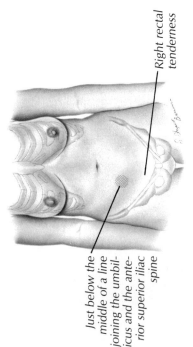

Acute Diverticulitis

Acute diverticulitis most often involves the sigmoid colon and then resembles a left-sided appendicitis.

Table 11-5   Liver Enlargement: Apparent and Real

TABLE 11-5   Liver Enlargement: Apparent and Real

A palpable liver does not necessarily indicate hepatomegaly (an enlarged liver), but more often results from a change in consistency—from the normal softness to an abnormal firmness or hardness, as in cirrhosis. Clinical estimates of liver size should be based on both percussion and palpation, although even then they are far from perfect.

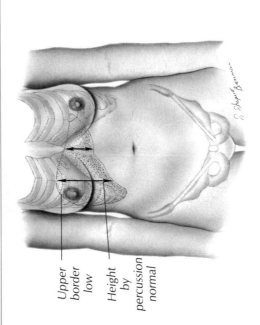

Downward Displacement of the Liver by a Low Diaphragm

This is a common finding (e.g., in emphysema) when the diaphragm is low. The liver edge may be readily palpable well below the costal margin. Percussion, however, reveals a low upper edge also, and the vertical span of the liver is normal.

Upper border low

Height by percussion normal

Elongated right lobe

Normal Variations in Liver Shape

In some persons, especially those with a lanky build, the liver tends to be somewhat elongated so that its right lobe is easily palpable as it projects downward toward the iliac crest. Such an elongation, sometimes called *Riedel's* lobe, represents a variation in shape, not an increase in liver volume or size. This variant illustrates the basic limitations of assessing liver size. We can only estimate the upper and lower borders of an organ that has three dimensions and differing shapes. Some error is unavoidable.

Continued

Table 11-5   *Liver Enlargement: Apparent and Real*

T A B L E   1 1 - 5   *(continued)*

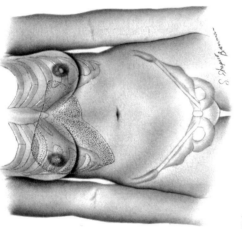

Smooth Large Nontender Liver

Cirrhosis may produce an enlarged liver with a firm nontender edge. The liver is not always enlarged in this condition, however, and many other diseases may produce similar findings.

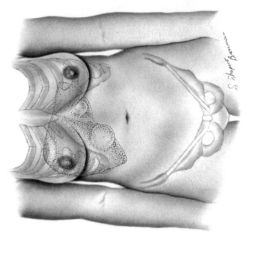

Large Irregular Liver

An enlarged liver that is firm or hard and has an irregular edge or surface suggests malignancy. There may be one or more nodules. The liver may or may not be tender.

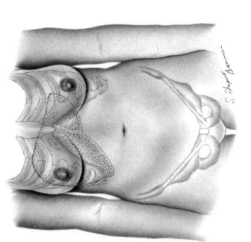

Smooth Large Tender Liver

An enlarged liver with a smooth tender edge suggests inflammation, as in hepatitis, or venous congestion, as in right-sided heart failure.

Male Genitalia and Hernias

CHAPTER 12

Anatomy and Physiology

Review the anatomy of the male genitalia.

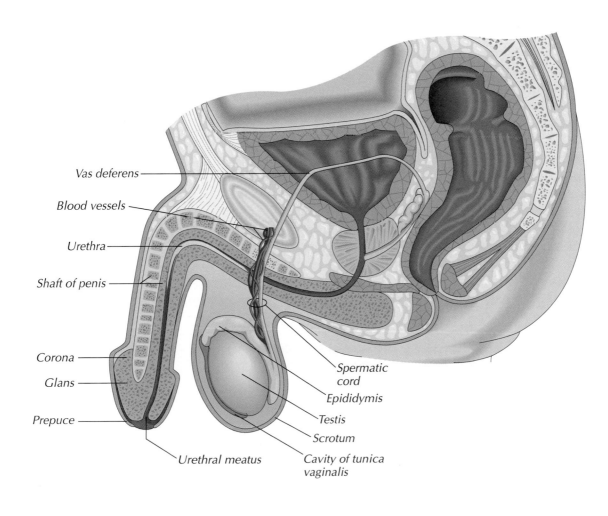

Vas deferens

Blood vessels

Urethra

Shaft of penis

Corona

Glans

Prepuce

Urethral meatus

Spermatic cord

Epididymis

Testis

Scrotum

Cavity of tunica vaginalis

The *shaft of the penis* is formed by three columns of vascular erectile tissue bound together by fibrous tissue. At the end of the penis is the cone-shaped *glans* with its expanded base, or *corona.* Unless the person has been circumcised, the glans is covered by a loose, hoodlike fold of skin called the *prepuce* or *foreskin.* The urethra is located ventrally in the shaft of the penis, within one of the vascular columns, and urethral abnormalities may sometimes be felt here. The urethra opens into the vertical, slit-like *urethral meatus,* located somewhat ventrally at the tip of the glans.

The *scrotum* is a loose, wrinkled pouch divided into two compartments, each of which contains a testis (testicle). The *testes* are ovoid, somewhat rubbery structures, about 4.5 cm long in the adult, with a range from 3.5 cm to 5.5 cm. The left usually lies somewhat lower than the right. On the posterolateral surface of each testis is the softer, comma-shaped *epididymis.* It is most prominent along the superior margin of the testis. (The epididymis may be located anteriorly in 6% to 7% of males.) Surrounding the testis, except posteriorly, is the *tunica vaginalis,* a serous membrane enclosing a potential cavity.

The testes produce spermatozoa and testosterone. Testosterone stimulates the pubertal growth of the male genitalia, prostate, and seminal vesicles. It also stimulates the development of masculine secondary sex characteristics, including the beard, body hair, musculoskeletal development, and enlarged larynx with its male voice.

The *vas deferens,* a cordlike structure, begins at the tail of the epididymis, ascends within the scrotal sac, and passes through the external inguinal ring on its way to the abdomen and pelvis. Behind the bladder it is joined by the duct from the seminal vesicle and enters the urethra within the prostate gland. Sperm thus pass from the testis and the epididymis through the vas deferens into the urethra. Secretions from the vasa deferentia, the seminal vesicles, and the prostate all contribute to the semen. Within the scrotum each vas is closely associated with blood vessels, nerves, and muscle fibers. These structures make up the *spermatic cord.*

Lymphatics. Lymphatics from the penile and scrotal surfaces drain into the inguinal nodes. When you find an inflammatory or possibly malignant lesion on these surfaces, assess the inguinal nodes especially carefully for enlargement or tenderness. The lymphatics of the testes, however, drain into the abdomen, where enlarged nodes are clinically undetectable. See page 468 for further discussion of the inguinal nodes.

Anatomy of the Groin. Because hernias are relatively common, it is important to understand the anatomy of the groin. The basic landmarks are the anterior superior iliac spine, the pubic tubercle, and the inguinal ligament which runs between them. Find these on yourself or a colleague.

The *inguinal canal,* which lies above and approximately parallel to the inguinal ligament, forms a tunnel for the vas deferens as it passes through the abdominal muscles. The exterior opening of the tunnel—the *external inguinal ring*—is a triangular slitlike structure palpable just above and lateral to the pubic tubercle. The internal opening of the canal—or internal inguinal ring—is about 1 cm above the midpoint of the inguinal ligament. Neither canal nor internal ring is palpable through the abdominal wall. When loops of bowel force their way through weak areas of the inguinal canal they produce inguinal hernias, as illustrated on pp. 402 and 403.

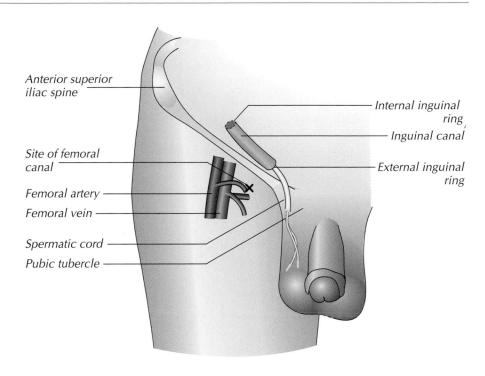

Anterior superior iliac spine

Site of femoral canal

Femoral artery

Femoral vein

Spermatic cord

Pubic tubercle

Internal inguinal ring

Inguinal canal

External inguinal ring

Another potential route for a herniating mass is the *femoral canal.* This lies below the inguinal ligament. Although you cannot see it, you can estimate its location by placing your right index finger, from below, on the right femoral artery. Your middle finger will then overlie the femoral vein; your ring finger, the femoral canal. Femoral hernias protrude here.

Changes With Age

Adolescence. Important anatomic changes in the male genitalia accompany puberty and help to define its progress. A noticeable increase in the size of the testes constitutes the first reliable sign and usually begins between the ages of 9.5 years and 13.5 years. Next, pubic hair appears and the penis begins to grow. The complete change from preadolescent to adult form requires about 3 years, with a range from less than 2 years to almost 5 years.

By observing the pubic hair and the development of the penis, testes, and scrotum, you can assess sexual development according to the five stages described by Tanner. These are outlined and illustrated on the next page.

In about 80% of men, pubic hair spreads farther up the abdomen in a triangular pattern pointing toward the umbilicus. Because this kind of spread, known as stage 6, is not completed until the mid-20s or later, it is not considered a pubertal change.

		Genital	
	Pubic Hair	*Penis*	*Testes and Scrotum*
Stage 1	Preadolescent—no pubic hair except for the fine body hair (vellus hair) similar to that on the abdomen	Preadolescent—same size and proportions as in childhood	Preadolescent—same size and proportions as in childhood
Stage 2	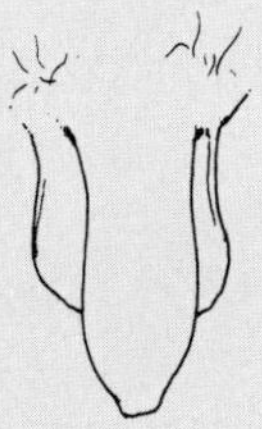 Sparse growth of long, slightly pigmented, downy hair, straight or only slightly curled, chiefly at the base of the penis	Slight or no enlargement	Testes larger; scrotum larger, somewhat reddened, and altered in texture
Stage 3	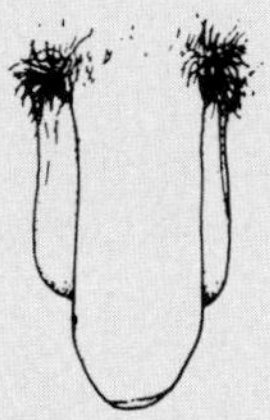 Darker, coarser, curlier hair spreading sparsely over the pubic symphysis	Larger, especially in length	Further enlarged
Stage 4	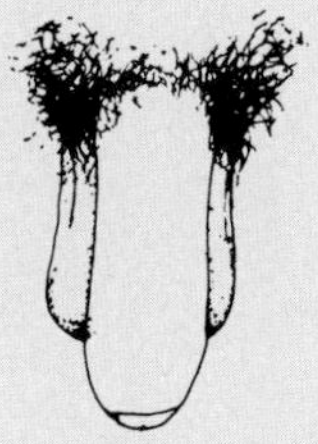 Coarse and curly hair, as in the adult; area covered greater than in stage 3 but not as great as in the adult and not yet including the thighs	Further enlarged in length and breadth, with development of the glans	Further enlarged; scrotal skin darkened
Stage 5	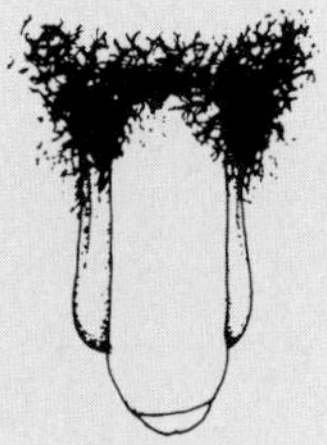 Hair adult in quantity and quality, spread to the medial surfaces of the thighs but not up over the abdomen	Adult in size and shape	Adult in size and shape

Sex Maturity Ratings in Boys

In assigning SMRs in boys, observe each of the three characteristics separately because they may develop at different rates. Record two separate ratings: pubic hair and genital. If the penis and testes differ in their stages, average the two into a single figure for the genital rating.

(Illustrations through the courtesy of W.A. Daniel, Jr., Division of Adolescent Medicine, University of Alabama, Birmingham)

An average developmental sequence is diagrammed below. Note the rather wide age ranges for the start and completion of pubertal changes. Some normal boys may have completed their genital development while others of the same age have not yet begun. Boys often begin to experience ejaculation as they approach SMR 3, and sometimes mistake nocturnal emissions for urine or the discharge of sexually transmitted disease. Discussion and explanation are indicated.

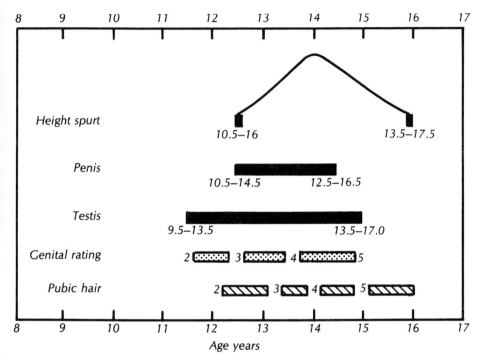

Numbers below the bars indicate the ranges in age within which certain changes occur. (Redrawn from Marshall WA, Tanner JM: Variations in the patterns of pubertal changes in boys. Arch Dis Child 45:22, 1970)

Aging. In elderly patients, pubic hair may decrease and become gray. The penis decreases in size and the testicles hang lower in the scrotum. Although the testes often decrease in size with protracted, debilitating illnesses, they do not necessarily decrease with aging *per se*.

Techniques of Examination

General Approach

Many students feel anxious about examining a man's genitalia. "How will the patient react?" "Will he have an erection?" "Will he let me examine him?" It may be reassuring to explain each step of the examination so the patient knows what to expect. A male patient may occasionally have an erection. If so, you should explain that this is a normal response, finish your examination, and proceed with an unruffled demeanor. If the man refuses to be examined, you should respect his wishes.

A good genital examination can be done with the patient either standing or supine. To check for hernias or varicoceles, however, the patient should stand, and you should sit comfortably on a chair or stool. A gown conveniently covers the patient's chest and abdomen. Wear gloves throughout the examination. Expose the genitalia and inguinal areas.

Assessment of Sexual Development

Assess sexual maturation by noting the size and shape of the penis and testes, the color and texture of the scrotal skin, and the character and distribution of the pubic hair. Assessment of testicular size requires palpation (see p. 394).

In adolescents, make two separate sex maturity ratings according to Tanner's stages: one for pubic hair, the other for genital development. If a boy's testes have increased in size to 2.5 cm or more, or if his pubic hair has reached stage 2, you can tell him that his sexual development has started. You may also use Tanner's diagrams to show your patient how he is developing, to review the wide range of normals for his age, and to answer any questions he may have.

Delayed puberty is often familial or related to chronic illness. It may also be due to abnormalities in the hypothalamus, anterior pituitary gland, or testes.

The Penis

Inspection

Inspect the penis, including:

- The skin

- The prepuce (foreskin). If it is present, retract it or ask the patient to retract it. This step is essential for the detection of many chancres and carcinomas. A cheesy, whitish material called smegma may accumulate normally under the foreskin.

See Table 12-1, Abnormalities of the Penis (p. 399).

Phimosis is a tight prepuce that cannot be retracted over the glans. *Paraphimosis* is a tight prepuce that, once retracted, cannot be returned. Edema ensues.

- The glans. Look for any ulcers, scars, nodules, or signs of inflammation.

Balanitis (inflammation of the glans); *balanoposthitis* (inflammation of the glans and prepuce)

Check the skin around the base of the penis for excoriations or inflammation. Look for nits or lice at the bases of the pubic hairs.

Pubic or genital excoriations suggest the possibility of lice (crabs) or sometimes scabies.

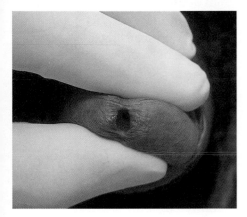

Note the location of the urethral meatus.

Hypospadias is a congenital, ventral displacement of the meatus on the penis (p. 398).

Compress the glans gently between your index finger above and your thumb below. This maneuver should open the urethral meatus and allow you to inspect it for discharge. Normally there is none.

The discharge of gonococcal urethritis tends to be profuse and yellow, while that of nongonococcal urethritis tends to be scanty and white or clear. Definitive diagnosis, however, requires a Gram stain and culture.

If the patient has reported a discharge but you do not see any, ask him to strip, or milk, the shaft of the penis from its base to the glans. Alternatively, do it yourself. This maneuver may bring some discharge out of the urethral meatus for appropriate examination. Have a glass slide and culture materials ready.

Palpation

Palpate any abnormality of the penis, noting any tenderness or induration. Palpate the shaft of the penis between your thumb and first two fingers, noting any induration. Palpation of the shaft may be omitted in a young, asymptomatic male patient.

Induration along the ventral surface of the penis suggests a urethral stricture or possibly a carcinoma. Tenderness of such an indurated area suggests periurethral inflammation secondary to a urethral stricture.

If you retract the foreskin, replace it before proceeding on to examine the scrotum.

The Scrotum and Its Contents

Inspection

See Table 12-2, Abnormalities of the Scrotum (pp. 400–401).

Inspect the scrotum, including:

- The skin. Lift up the scrotum so that you can see its posterior surface.

Rashes, epidermoid cysts, rarely skin cancer

- The scrotal contours. Note any swelling, lumps, or veins.

A poorly developed scrotum on one or both sides suggests *cryptorchidism* (an undescended testicle). Common scrotal swellings include indirect inguinal hernias, hydroceles, and scrotal edema. A tender, painful scrotal swelling occurs in acute epididymitis, acute orchitis, torsion of the spermatic cord, and a strangulated inguinal hernia.

Palpation

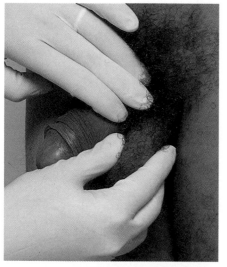

Palpate each testis and epididymis between your thumb and first two fingers.

Note their size, shape, consistency, and tenderness; feel for any nodules. Pressure on the testis normally produces a deep visceral pain.

Any painless nodule in the testis must raise the possibility of testicular cancer, a potentially curable cancer with a peak incidence between the ages of 20 and 35 years.

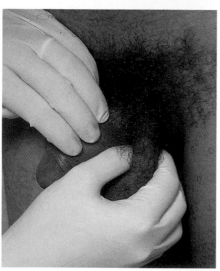

Palpate each spermatic cord, including the vas deferens, between your thumb and fingers from the epididymis to the superficial inguinal ring.

Note any nodules or swellings.

Multiple tortuous veins in this area, usually on the left, may be palpable and even visible. They indicate a varicocele (p. 400).

The vas deferens, if chronically infected, may feel thickened or beaded. A cystic structure in the spermatic cord suggests a hydrocele of the cord.

Any swelling in the scrotum other than the testicles should be evaluated by transillumination. After darkening the room, shine the beam of a strong flashlight from behind the scrotum through the mass. Look for transmission of the light as a red glow.

Swellings that contain serous fluid, such as a hydrocele, transilluminate: they light up with a red glow. Those that contain blood or tissue, such as a normal testis, a tumor, and most hernias, do not.

Hernias

Inspection

Inspect the inguinal and femoral areas carefully for bulges. While you continue your observation, ask the patient to strain down.

A bulge that appears on straining suggests a hernia.

Palpation

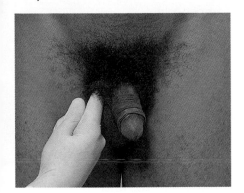

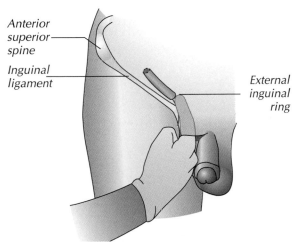

Anterior superior spine

Inguinal ligament

External inguinal ring

Palpate for an inguinal hernia. Using in turn your right hand for the patient's right side and your left hand for the patient's left side, invaginate loose scrotal skin with your index finger. Start at a point low enough to be sure that your finger will have enough mobility to reach as far as the internal inguinal ring if this proves possible. Follow the spermatic cord upward to above the inguinal ligament and find the triangular slitlike opening of the external inguinal ring. This is just above and lateral to the pubic tubercle. If the ring is somewhat enlarged, it may admit your index finger. If possible, gently follow the inguinal canal laterally in its oblique course. With your finger located either at the external ring or within the canal, ask the patient to strain down or cough. Note any palpable herniating mass as it touches your finger.

See Table 12-3, Course and Presentation of Hernias in the Groin (p. 402).

See Table 12-4, Differentiation of Hernias in the Groin (p. 403).

Palpate for a femoral hernia by placing your fingers on the anterior thigh in the region of the femoral canal. Ask the patient to strain down again or cough. Note any swelling or tenderness.

Evaluating a Possible Scrotal Hernia. If you find a large scrotal mass and suspect that it may be a hernia, ask the patient to lie down. The mass may return to the abdomen by itself. If so, it is a hernia. If not:

- Can you get your fingers above the mass in the scrotum?

- Listen to the mass with a stethoscope for bowel sounds.

If the findings suggest a hernia, gently try to reduce it (return it to the abdominal cavity) by sustained pressure with your fingers. Do not attempt this maneuver if the mass is tender or the patient reports nausea and vomiting.

History may be helpful here. The patient can usually tell you what happens to his swelling on lying down and may be able to demonstrate how he reduces it himself. Remember to ask him.

If you can, suspect a hydrocele.

Bowel sounds may be heard over a hernia, but not over a hydrocele.

A hernia is *incarcerated* when its contents cannot be returned to the abdominal cavity. A hernia is *strangulated* when the blood supply to the entrapped contents is compromised. Suspect strangulation in the presence of tenderness, nausea, and vomiting, and consider surgical intervention.

Special Techniques

The Testicular Self-Examination

The incidence of testicular cancer is low, about 4 per 100,000 men, but it is the most common cancer of young men between ages 20 and 35. Although the testicular self-examination (TSE) has not been formally endorsed as a screen for testicular carcinoma, you may wish to teach your patient the TSE to enhance health awareness and self-care. When detected early, testicular carcinoma has an excellent prognosis. Risk factors include cryptorchidism, which confers a high risk of testicular carcinoma in the undescended testicle, a history of carcinoma in the contralateral testicle, mumps orchitis, inguinal hernia, and hydrocele in childhood.

Instructions for Testicular Self-Examination

1. Check your testicles once a month.
2. Roll each testicle between your thumb and finger. Feel for hard lumps or bumps.
3. If you notice a change or have aches or lumps, tell your doctor right away so something can be done about it.

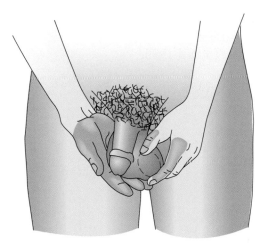

Encourage men to perform the TSE at regular intervals and seek evaluation of any masses promptly.

Health Promotion and Counseling

Health promotion and counseling should address patient education about sexually transmitted diseases (STDs) and the human immunodeficiency virus (HIV), early detection of infection during history taking and physical examination, and identification and treatment of infected partners. Discussion of risk factors for STDs and HIV is especially important for adolescents and younger patients, the age groups that are most adversely affected. Clinicians must be comfortable with eliciting the sexual history and with asking frank but tactful questions about sexual practices. A minimal history includes identifying the patient's sexual orientation, the number of sexual partners in the past month, and any history of STDs (see Chap. 1, p. 19). Questions should be clear and nonjudgmental. You should also identify use of alcohol and drugs, particularly injection drugs. Counsel patients at risk about limiting the number of partners, using condoms, and establishing regular medical care for treatment of STDs and HIV. It is important for men to seek prompt attention for any genital lesions or penile discharge.

The U.S. Preventive Services Task Force recommends counseling and testing for HIV infection in the following groups: all persons at increased risk for infection with HIV and/or STDs; men with male partners; past or present injection drug users; any past or present partners of individuals with HIV infection, bisexual practices, or injection drug use; and patients with a history of transfusion between 1978 and 1985.

In addition, encourage men, especially those between the ages of 20 and 35, to perform the TSE at regular intervals.

Table 12-1   Abnormalities of the Penis

TABLE 12-1   *Abnormalities of the Penis*

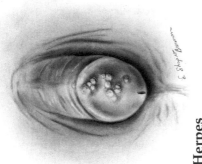

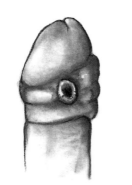

Hypospadias

Hypospadias is a congenital displacement of the urethral meatus to the inferior surface of the penis. A groove extends from the actual urethral meatus to its normal location on the tip of the glans.

Syphilitic Chancre

A syphilitic chancre usually appears as an oval or round, dark red, painless erosion or ulcer with an indurated base. Nontender enlarged inguinal lymph nodes are typically associated. Chancres may be multiple, and when secondarily infected may be painful. They may then be mistaken for the lesions of herpes. Chancres are infectious.

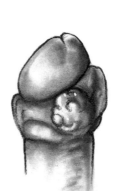

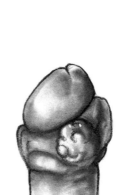

Genital Herpes

A cluster of small vesicles, followed by shallow, painful, nonindurated ulcers on red bases, suggests a herpes simplex infection. The lesions may occur anywhere on the penis. Usually there are fewer lesions when the infection recurs.

Peyronie's Disease

In Peyronie's disease, there are palpable nontender hard plaques just beneath the skin, usually along the dorsum of the penis. The patient complains of crooked, painful erections.

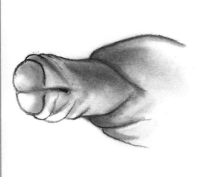

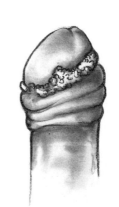

Venereal Wart *(Condyloma acuminatum)*

Venereal warts are rapidly growing excrescences that are moist and often malodorous. They result from infection by human papillomavirus.

Carcinoma of the Penis

Carcinoma may appear as an indurated nodule or ulcer that is usually nontender. Limited almost completely to men who are not circumcised in childhood, it may be masked by the prepuce. Any persistent penile sore must be considered suspicious.

Table 12-2   Abnormalities of the Scrotum

TABLE 12-2   *Abnormalities of the Scrotum*

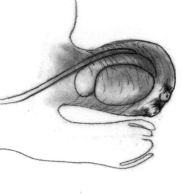

Late

As a testicular neoplasm grows and spreads, it may seem to replace the entire organ. The testicle characteristically feels heavier than normal.

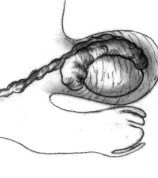

Early

Tumor of the Testis

A tumor of the testis usually appears as a painless nodule. It does not transilluminate. Any nodule within the testis must raise the suspicion of malignancy.

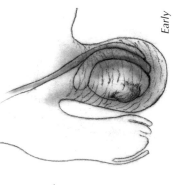

Fingers cannot get above mass

Scrotal Hernia

A hernia located within the scrotum is usually an indirect inguinal hernia. Since it comes through the external inguinal ring, the examining fingers cannot get above it in the scrotum.

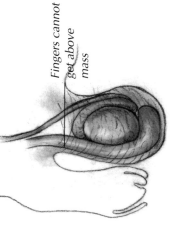

Fingers can get above mass

Hydrocele

A hydrocele is a nontender, fluid-filled mass that occupies the space within the tunica vaginalis. The examining fingers can get above the mass within the scrotum. The mass transilluminates.

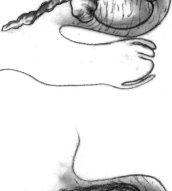

Epidermoid Cysts

These are firm, yellowish, nontender, cutaneous cysts up to about 1 cm in diameter. They are common and frequently multiple.

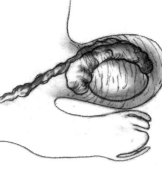

Tuberculous Epididymitis

The chronic inflammation of tuberculosis produces a firm enlargement of the epididymis, which is sometimes tender, with thickening or beading of the vas deferens.

Varicocele

Varicocele refers to varicose veins of the spermatic cord, usually found on the left. It feels like a soft "bag of worms" separate from the testis, and slowly collapses when the scrotum is elevated in the supine patient. Infertility may be associated.

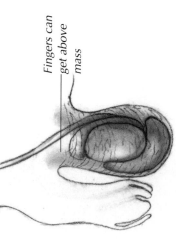

Spermatocele and Cyst of the Epididymis

A painless, movable cystic mass just above the testis suggests a spermatocele or an epididymal cyst. Both transilluminate. The former contains sperm and the latter does not, but they are clinically indistinguishable.

Table 12-2   Abnormalities of the Scrotum

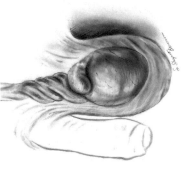

Acute Orchitis

An acutely inflamed testis is painful, tender, and swollen. The testis may be difficult to distinguish from the epididymis. The scrotum may be reddened. Look for evidence of postpubertal mumps, such as parotid swelling, or other less common infectious causes.

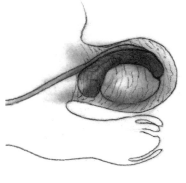

Acute Epididymitis

An acutely inflamed epididymis is tender and swollen and may be difficult to distinguish from the testis. The scrotum may be reddened, and the vas deferens may also be inflamed. Epididymitis occurs chiefly in adults. Coexisting urinary tract infection or prostatitis supports the diagnosis.

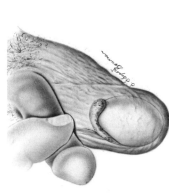

Torsion of the Spermatic Cord

Torsion, or twisting, of the testicle on its spermatic cord produces an acutely painful, tender, and swollen organ that is retracted upward in the scrotum. The scrotum becomes red and edematous. There is no associated urinary infection. Torsion, most common in adolescents, is a surgical emergency because of obstructed circulation.

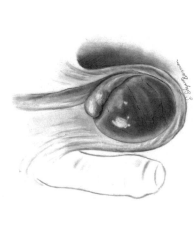

Small Testis

Adult testes are considered small when they are less than 3.5 cm long. Small, firm testes (usually less than 2 cm long) suggest *Klinefelter's syndrome.* Small, soft testes suggest atrophy, associated with several conditions (e.g., cirrhosis, myotonic dystrophy, administration of estrogens, and hypopituitarism). Atrophy may also follow orchitis (e.g., from mumps).

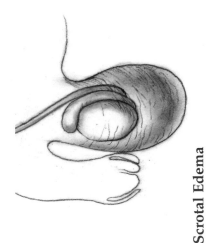

Cryptorchidism

An undeveloped scrotum suggests cryptorchidism, as shown here on the patient's left. No left testis or epididymis is palpable in this scrotal sac. They may lie in the inguinal canal or abdomen. Cryptorchidism leads to testicular atrophy on the involved side(s) and markedly increases the risk of testicular cancer.

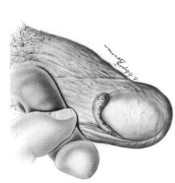

Scrotal Edema

The scrotal skin may become taut with pitting edema. Scrotal edema is usually associated with generalized edema, as in chronic congestive heart failure or the nephrotic syndrome.

Table 12-3   Course and Presentation of Hernias in the Groin

TABLE 12-3   *Course and Presentation of Hernias in the Groin*

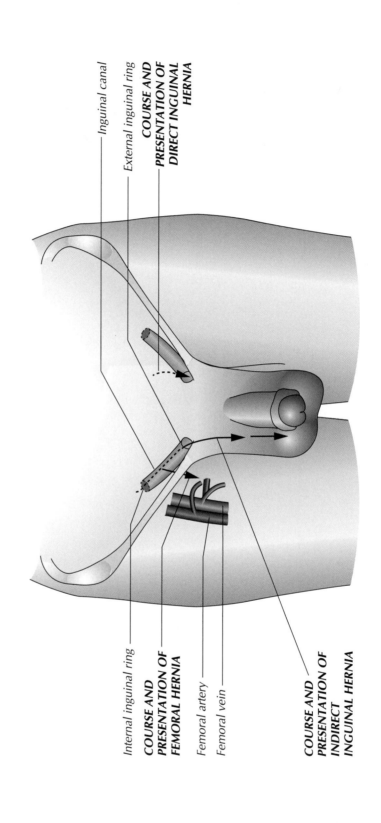

Inguinal canal

External inguinal ring

COURSE AND PRESENTATION OF DIRECT INGUINAL HERNIA

Internal inguinal ring

COURSE AND PRESENTATION OF FEMORAL HERNIA

Femoral artery

Femoral vein

COURSE AND PRESENTATION OF INDIRECT INGUINAL HERNIA

Table 12-4 Differentiation of Hernias in the Groin

TABLE 12-4 Differentiation of Hernias in the Groin

Differentiation among these hernias is not always clinically possible. Understanding their features, however, improves your observation.

	Inguinal		Femoral
	Indirect	Direct	
Frequency	Most common, all ages, both sexes	Less common	Least common
Age and Sex	Often in children, may be in adults	Usually in men over age 40, rare in women	More common in women than in men
Point of Origin	Above inguinal ligament, near its midpoint (the internal inguinal ring)	Above inguinal ligament, close to the pubic tubercle (near the external inguinal ring)	Below the inguinal ligament; appears more lateral than an inguinal hernia and may be hard to differentiate from lymph nodes
Course	Often into the scrotum	Rarely into the scrotum	Never into the scrotum
With the examining finger in the inguinal canal during straining or cough	The hernia comes down the inguinal canal and touches the fingertip.	The hernia bulges anteriorly and pushes the side of the finger forward.	The inguinal canal is empty.

Female Genitalia

CHAPTER 13

Anatomy and Physiology

Review the anatomy of the external female genitalia (vulva), including the *mons pubis,* a hair-covered fat pad overlying the symphysis pubis; the *labia majora,* rounded folds of adipose tissue; the *labia minora,* thinner pinkish red folds that extend anteriorly to form the *prepuce;* and the *clitoris.* The *vestibule* is the boat-shaped fossa between the labia minora. In its posterior portion lies the vaginal opening (*introitus*), which in virgins may be hidden by the *hymen.* The term *perineum,* as commonly used clinically, refers to the tissues between the introitus and the anus.

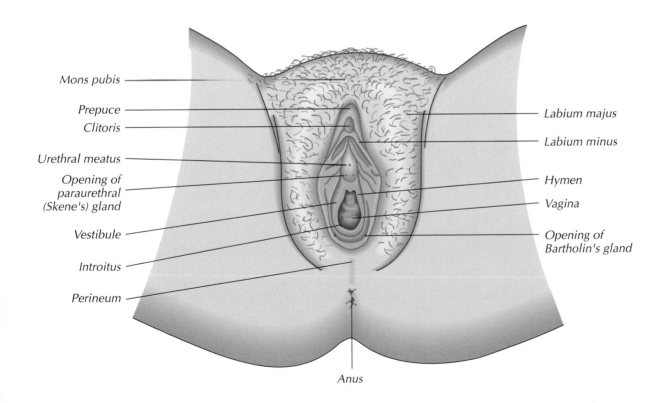

Mons pubis

Prepuce

Clitoris

Urethral meatus

Opening of paraurethral (Skene's) gland

Vestibule

Introitus

Perineum

Labium majus

Labium minus

Hymen

Vagina

Opening of Bartholin's gland

Anus

The *urethral meatus* opens into the vestibule between the clitoris and the vagina. Just posterior to it on either side lie the openings of the *paraurethral (Skene's) glands.*

The openings of *Bartholin's glands* are located posteriorly on either side of the vaginal opening, but are not usually visible. Bartholin's glands themselves are situated more deeply.

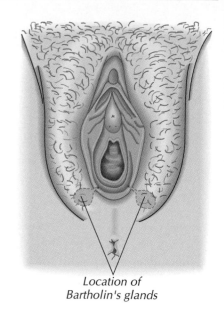

Location of Bartholin's glands

The *vagina* is a hollow tube extending upward and posteriorly between urethra and rectum. It terminates in the cup-shaped fornix. The vaginal mucosa lies in transverse folds, or rugae.

At almost right angles to the vagina sits the *uterus,* a flattened fibro-muscular structure shaped like an inverted pear. The uterus has two parts: the body (corpus) and the cervix, which are joined together by the isthmus. The convex upper surface of the body is called the *fundus* of the uterus. The lower part of the uterus, the *cervix,* protrudes into the vagina, dividing the fornix into anterior, posterior, and lateral fornices.

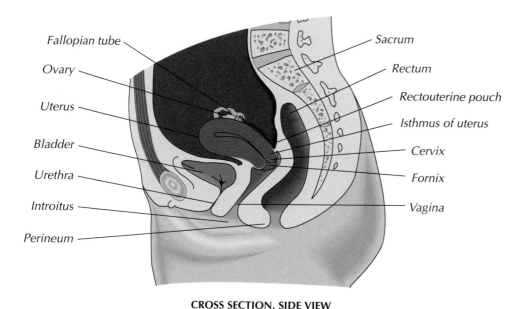

Fallopian tube
Ovary
Uterus
Bladder
Urethra
Introitus
Perineum

Sacrum
Rectum
Rectouterine pouch
Isthmus of uterus
Cervix
Fornix
Vagina

CROSS SECTION, SIDE VIEW

The vaginal surface of the cervix, the *ectocervix,* is seen easily with the help of a speculum. At its center is a round, oval, or slitlike depression, the *external os* of the cervix, that marks the opening into the endocervical canal. The ectocervix is covered by epithelium of two possible types: a shiny pink squamous epithelium, contiguous with the vaginal lining, and a deep red columnar epithelium resembling the lining of the endocervical canal. The columnar epithelium is often visible around the os. The *squamocolumnar junction* marks the boundary between the two types of epithelium.

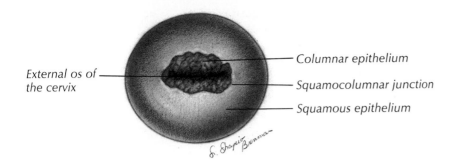

External os of the cervix

Columnar epithelium

Squamocolumnar junction

Squamous epithelium

A *fallopian tube* with a fanlike tip extends from each side of the uterus toward the ovary. The two ovaries are almond-shaped structures that vary considerably in size but average about 3.5 × 2 × 1.5 cm from adulthood through menopause. The ovaries are often palpable on pelvic examination during a woman's reproductive years, but normally fallopian tubes cannot be felt. The term *adnexa* (a plural Latin word meaning appendages) refers to the ovaries, tubes, and supporting tissues.

The ovaries have two primary functions: the production of ova and the secretion of hormones, including estrogen, progesterone, and testosterone. Increased hormonal secretions during puberty stimulate the growth of the uterus and its endometrial lining. They enlarge the vagina and thicken its epithelium. They also stimulate the development of secondary sex characteristics, including the breasts and pubic hair.

The parietal peritoneum extends downward behind the uterus into a cul de sac called the *rectouterine pouch* (pouch of Douglas). You can just reach this area on rectal examination.

The pelvic organs are supported by a sling of tissues composed of muscle, ligaments, and fascia, through which the urethra, vagina, and rectum all pass.

Lymphatics. Lymph from the vulva and the lower vagina drains into the inguinal nodes. Lymph from the internal genitalia, including the upper vagina, flows into the pelvic and abdominal lymph nodes, which are not palpable clinically.

Changes With Age

Adolescence. During the pubertal years, the vulva and the internal genitalia grow and change to their adult proportions. Assessment of sexual maturity in girls, as classified by Tanner, depends not on internal examination, however, but on the growth of pubic hair and the development of breasts. Tanner's stages, or sex maturity ratings, as they relate to pubic hair are shown below; those relating to breasts are shown on p. 336.

Sex Maturity Ratings in Girls: Pubic Hair

Stage 1
Preadolescent—no pubic hair except for the fine body hair (vellus hair) similar to that on the abdomen

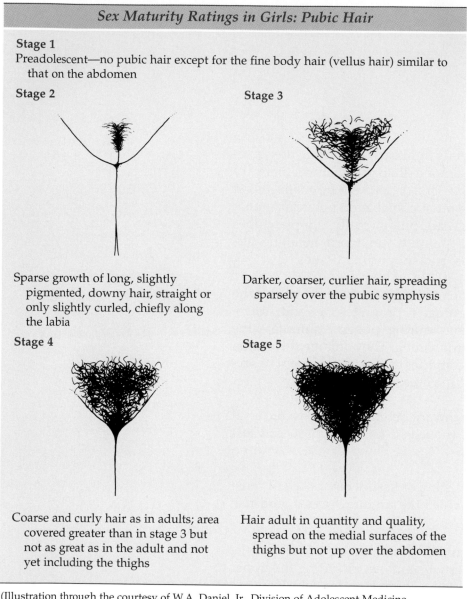

Stage 2

Sparse growth of long, slightly pigmented, downy hair, straight or only slightly curled, chiefly along the labia

Stage 3

Darker, coarser, curlier hair, spreading sparsely over the pubic symphysis

Stage 4

Coarse and curly hair as in adults; area covered greater than in stage 3 but not as great as in the adult and not yet including the thighs

Stage 5

Hair adult in quantity and quality, spread on the medial surfaces of the thighs but not up over the abdomen

(Illustration through the courtesy of W.A. Daniel, Jr., Division of Adolescent Medicine, University of Alabama, Birmingham)

A girl's first sign of puberty is usually the appearance of breast buds. Sometimes, however, pubic hair appears first. On average, these changes start at around 11 years of age, with a range from 8 to 13 years for breast buds, 8 to 14 years for pubic hair. The transformation from preadolescent to adult form takes about 3 years, with a range of 1.5 to 6 years. Menarche tends to occur during breast stage 3 or 4, at ages ranging from 10 to 16.5 years according to Tanner's studies in England, which are summarized graphically on p. 409. The age of menarche in the United States is a little earlier, roughly from 9 to 16 years.

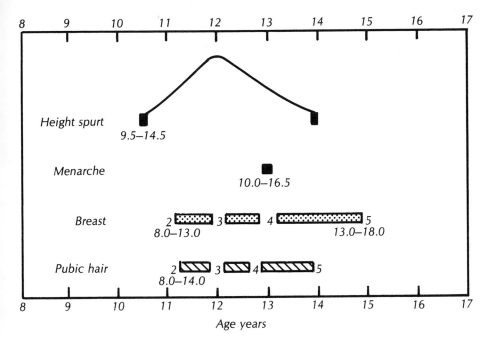

Numbers below the bars indicate the ranges in age within which certain changes occur. (Redrawn from Marshall WA, Tanner JM: Variations in the pattern of pubertal changes in boys. Arch Dis Child 45:22, 1970)

As in boys, there is a wide range of normal in pubertal development. Some girls may have completed the development of their secondary sex characteristics while others of the same age have not yet begun.

In 10% or more of women, pubic hair spreads further up the abdomen in a triangular pattern, pointing toward the umbilicus. This spread can be classified as stage 6; because it is usually not completed until the mid-20s or later, however, it is not considered a pubertal change.

Just before menarche there is a physiologic increase in vaginal secretions—a normal change that sometimes worries a girl or her mother. As menses become established, increased secretions (*leukorrhea*) coincide with ovulation. They also accompany sexual arousal. These normal kinds of discharges must be differentiated from those of infectious processes.

Aging. Ovarian function usually starts to diminish during a woman's 40s, and menstrual periods cease on the average between the ages of 45 and 52, sometimes earlier and sometimes later. Pubic hair becomes sparse as well as gray. As estrogen stimulation falls, the labia and the clitoris become smaller. The vagina narrows and shortens and its mucosa becomes thin, pale, and dry. The uterus and ovaries diminish in size.

Techniques of Examination

General Approach

Many students feel anxious or uncomfortable when first examining the genitalia of another person. At the same time, patients have their own concerns. Some women have had painful, embarrassing, or even demeaning experiences during previous pelvic examinations, while others may be facing their first examination. Patients may fear what the clinician will find and how these findings may affect their lives.

A patient's reactions and behavior may give you important clues to such feelings and to her attitudes toward sexuality. If she adducts her thighs, pulls away, or expresses negative feelings during the examination, you can gently confront her as you would during the interview. "I notice you are having some trouble relaxing. Is it just being here, or are you troubled by the examination?. . . is anything worrying you?" Behavior that seems to present an obstacle to your examination may become the key to understanding your patient's concerns.

A patient who has never had a pelvic examination is often fearful, embarrassed, and unsure of what to expect. Try to shape the experience so that she learns about both her body and the examination itself and becomes more comfortable with them. Before she undresses, explain the relevant anatomy with the help of three-dimensional models. Show her the speculum and other equipment and encourage her to handle them during the examination so that she can better understand your explanations and procedures. It is especially important to avoid hurting the patient during her first encounter.

Indications for a pelvic examination during adolescence include menstrual abnormalities such as amenorrhea, excessive bleeding, or dysmenorrhea, unexplained abdominal pain, vaginal discharge, the prescription of contraceptives, bacteriologic and cytologic studies in a sexually active girl, and the patient's own desire for assessment.

Regardless of age, rape merits special evaluation, usually requiring gynecologic consultation and documentation.

Getting a patient to relax is essential for an adequate examination. Be sensitive to her feelings. In addition:

- Ask the patient to empty her bladder before the examination.
- Position and drape her appropriately. Elevating her head and shoulders slightly helps the patient to relax her abdominal muscles and to see what is going on. The drape should cover the area from the midabdomen to the knees. Depressing it in the midline enables both patient and examiner to see each other's face. A girl or woman may wish to use a mirror to see her genitalia during the examination. When possible, offer her this opportunity.

- The patient's arms should be at her sides or folded across her chest—not over her head, a position that may cause tightening of the abdominal muscles.
- Explain in advance each step of the examination and tell the patient what she may feel. Avoid any sudden or unexpected movements. When beginning palpation or using a speculum, it may be helpful to make initial contact not on the genitalia themselves but on the upper inner thigh.
- Your hands and the speculum should be warm.
- Monitor your examination when possible by watching the patient's face.
- Finally, of course, be as gentle as possible.

Wear gloves throughout the examination and afterward when handling equipment used.

Equipment. You should have within reach a good light, a vaginal speculum of appropriate size, water-soluble lubricant, and equipment for taking Papanicolaou smears, bacteriologic cultures, or other diagnostic tests. Review the supplies and procedures of your own facility before taking cultures and other samples.

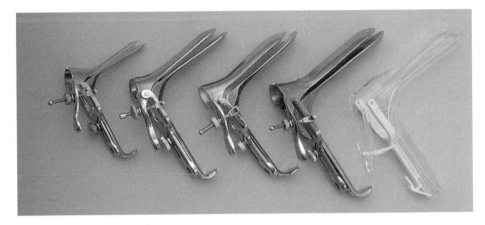

Specula are made of metal or plastic and come in two basic shapes. Graves specula are usually best for sexually active women. They are available in small, medium, and large sizes. The narrow-bladed Pedersen speculum is useful for a patient with a relatively small introitus, such as a virgin or an elderly woman, and is often more comfortable for other patients as well.

Before using a speculum, become thoroughly familiar with how to open and close its blades, lock the blades in an open position, and release them again. Although the instructions in this chapter refer to a metal speculum, you can easily adapt them to a plastic one by handling the speculum before using it.

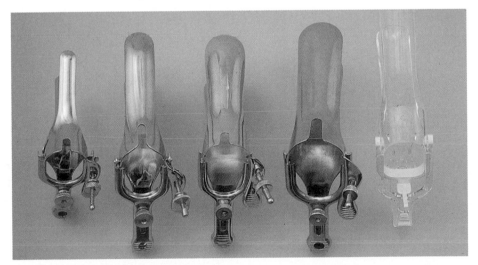

Speculae, from left to right: small metal Pedersen, medium metal Pedersen, medium metal Graves, large metal Graves, and large plastic Pedersen

Plastic specula typically make a loud click when locked or released. Forewarning the patient about this click helps to avoid unnecessary surprise.

Male examiners are customarily attended by female assistants. Female examiners may or may not prefer to work alone, but should also be assisted if the patient is physically disabled or emotionally disturbed.

Position. Drape the patient appropriately and then assist her into the lithotomy position. Help her to place first one heel and then the other into the stirrups. She may be more comfortable with shoes on than with bare feet. Then ask her to move toward the end of the examining table until her buttocks extend slightly beyond the edge. Her thighs should be flexed, abducted, and externally rotated at the hips. A pillow should support her head.

External Examination

Assess the Sexual Maturity of an Adolescent Patient. You can assess pubic hair during either the abdominal or the pelvic examination. Note its character and distribution, and rate it according to Tanner's stages described on p. 408.

Delayed puberty is often familial or related to chronic illness. It may also be due to abnormalities in the hypothalamus, anterior pituitary gland, or ovaries.

Inspect the Patient's External Genitalia. Seat yourself comfortably and inspect the mons pubis, labia, and perineum. Separate the labia and inspect:

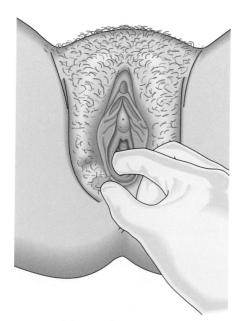

PALPATING BARTHOLIN'S GLAND

- The labia minora

- The clitoris

- The urethral meatus

- The vaginal opening or introitus

Note any inflammation, ulceration, discharge, swelling, or nodules. If there are any lesions, palpate them.

If there is a history or an appearance of labial swelling, check Bartholin's glands. Insert your index finger into the vagina near the posterior end of the introitus. Place your thumb outside the pos-

Excoriations or itchy, small, red maculopapules suggest pediculosis pubis (lice or "crabs"). Look for nits or lice at the bases of the pubic hairs.

Enlarged clitoris in masculinizing conditions

Urethral caruncle, prolapse of the urethral mucosa (p. 424)

Syphilitic chancre, epidermoid cyst. See Table 13-1, Lesions of the Vulva (p. 423).

A Bartholin's gland may become acutely or chronically infected and then produce a swelling. See Table 13-2, Bulges and Swelling of Vulva, Vagina, and Urethra (p. 424).

terior part of the labium majus. On each side in turn, palpate between your finger and thumb for swelling or tenderness. Note any discharge exuding from the duct opening of the gland. If any is present, culture it.

If you suspect urethritis or inflammation of the paraurethral glands, insert your index finger into the vagina and milk the urethra gently from inside outward. Note any discharge from or about the urethral meatus. If present, culture it.

Urethritis may arise from infection with *Chlamydia trachomatis* or *Neisseria gonorrhoeae*.

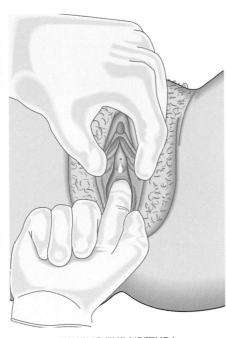

MILKING THE URETHRA

Internal Examination

Locate the Cervix. Insert your index finger into the vagina and identify the firm, rounded surface of the cervix. Locating the cervix manually will help you to angle the speculum more accurately. This technique also helps you to assess the size of the introitus and guides your choice of speculum. You may need to lubricate your finger with water, but do not use other lubricants.

Assess the Support of the Vaginal Walls. With the labia separated by your middle and index fingers, ask the patient to strain down. Note any bulging of the vaginal walls.

Cystocele and rectocele. See Table 13-2, Bulges and Swelling of Vulva, Vagina, and Urethra (p. 424).

Insert the Speculum. Select a speculum of appropriate size and shape, and lubricate it with warm water. (Other lubricants may interfere with cytologic studies and bacterial or viral cultures.) You can enlarge the vaginal introitus by applying downward pressure with two fingers at its lower margin. This greatly eases insertion of the speculum and the patient's comfort. With your other hand (usually the left), introduce the closed speculum past your fingers at a somewhat downward slope. Be careful not to pull on the pubic hair or pinch the labia with the speculum.

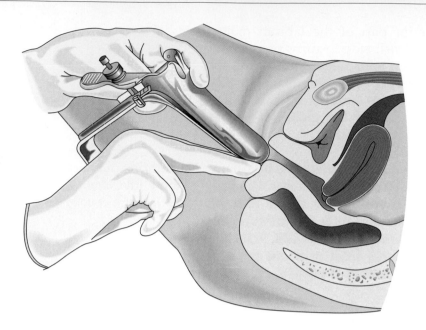

Two methods avoid the discomfort caused by pressure on the sensitive urethra. (1) When inserting the speculum, hold it at an angle (shown below on the left), and then (2) slide the speculum inward along the posterior wall of the vagina.

After the speculum has entered the vagina, remove your fingers from the introitus. You may wish to switch the speculum to the right hand to enhance maneuverability of the speculum and subsequent collection of specimens. Rotate the speculum into a horizontal position, maintaining the pressure posteriorly, and insert it to its full length.

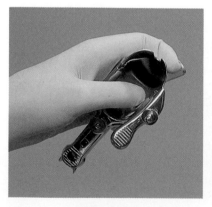

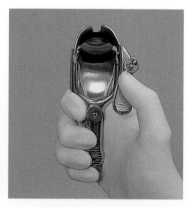

ENTRY ANGLE   **ANGLE AT FULL INSERTION**

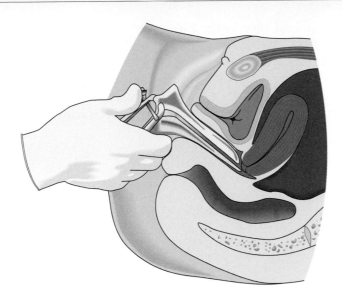

Inspect the Cervix. Open the speculum and adjust it until it cups the cervix and brings it into full view. Position the light to see well. When the uterus is retroverted, the cervix points more anteriorly than illustrated. If you have difficulty in finding the cervix, withdraw the speculum slightly and reposition it on a different slope. If discharge obscures your view, wipe it away gently with a large cotton swab.

See retroversion of the uterus, p. 429.

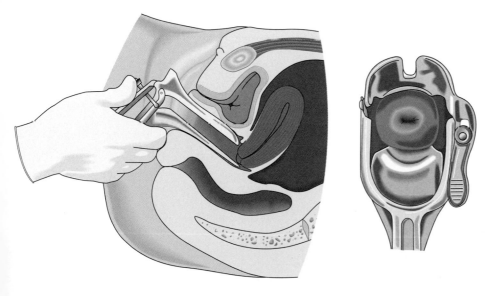

Inspect the cervix and its os. Note the color of the cervix, its position, the characteristics of its surface, and any ulcerations, nodules, masses, bleeding, or discharge.

See Table 13-3, Variations in the Cervix (p. 425), and Table 13-4, Abnormalities of the Cervix (p. 426).

Maintain the open position of the speculum by tightening the thumb screw.

Obtain Specimens for Cervical Cytology (Papanicolaou Smears): One from the endocervix and another from the ectocervix, or a combination specimen using the cervical brush ("broom"). For best results the patient should not be menstruating. She should have avoided sexual intercourse, douching, or using vaginal suppositories during the prior 24 to 48 hours.

Endocervical Swab. Moisten the end of a cotton applicator stick with saline and insert it into the cervical os. Roll it between your thumb and index finger, clockwise and counterclockwise. Remove it. Smear a glass slide with the cotton swab, gently, in a painting motion. (Rubbing hard on the slide will destroy the cells.) Either place the slide into an ether–alcohol fixative at once, or spray it promptly with a special fixative.

A yellowish discharge on the endocervical swab suggests a mucopurulent cervicitis, commonly caused by *Chlamydia trachomatis, Neisseria gonorrhoeae,* or herpes simplex (p. 426).

Cervical Scrape. Place the longer end of the scraper into the os of the cervix. Press, turn, and scrape in a full circle, making sure to include the squamocolumnar junction. Prepare a second slide as before.

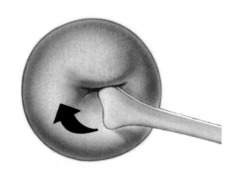

Cervical Brush (Broom). In women who are not pregnant, many clinicians use a plastic brush with a fringed broomlike tip for collection of a single specimen combining squamous and columnar epithelial cells. Rotate the tip of the brush in the cervical os, and then stroke each side of the brush on the glass slide. Use fixative promptly as described above.

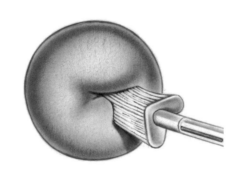

Inspect the Vagina. Withdraw the speculum slowly while observing the vagina. As the speculum clears the cervix, release the thumb screw and maintain the open position of the speculum with your thumb. Close the speculum as it emerges from the introitus, avoiding both excessive stretching and pinching of the mucosa. During withdrawal inspect the vaginal mucosa, noting its color and any inflammation, discharge, ulcers, or masses.

See Table 13-5, Vaginitis (p. 427).

Cancer of the vagina

Perform a Bimanual Examination. Lubricate the index and middle fingers of one of your gloved hands, and *from a standing position* insert them into the vagina, again exerting pressure primarily posteriorly. Your thumb should be abducted, your ring and little fingers flexed into your palm. Pressing inward on the perineum with your flexed fingers causes little if any discomfort and allows you to position your palpating fingers correctly. Note any nodularity or tenderness in the vaginal wall, including the region of the urethra and the bladder anteriorly.

Stool in the rectum may simulate a rectovaginal mass, but unlike a tumor mass can usually be dented by digital pressure. Rectovaginal examination confirms the distinction.

Palpate the cervix, noting its position, shape, consistency, regularity, mobility, and tenderness. Normally the cervix can be moved somewhat without pain. Feel the fornices around the cervix.

Palpate the uterus. Place your other hand on the abdomen about midway between the umbilicus and the symphysis pubis. While you elevate the cervix and uterus with your pelvic hand, press your abdominal hand in and down, trying to grasp the uterus between your two hands. Note its size, shape, consistency, and mobility, and identify any tenderness or masses.

Pain on movement of the cervix, together with adnexal tenderness, suggests pelvic inflammatory disease.

See Table 13-6, Abnormalities and Positions of the Uterus (pp. 428–429).

Uterine enlargement suggests pregnancy or benign or malignant tumors.

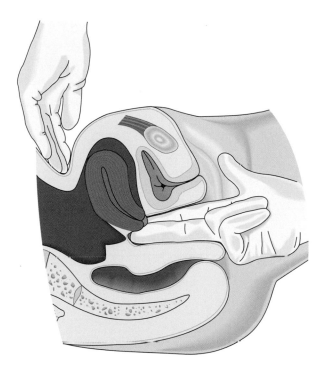

Now slide the fingers of your pelvic hand into the anterior fornix and palpate the body of the uterus between your hands. In this position your pelvic fingers can feel the anterior surface of the uterus, and your abdominal hand can feel part of the posterior surface.

Nodules on the uterine surfaces suggest myomas (see p. 428).

If you cannot feel the uterus with either of these maneuvers, it may be tipped posteriorly (retrodisplaced). Slide your pelvic fingers into the posterior formix and feel for the uterus butting against your fingertips. An obese or poorly relaxed abdominal wall may also prevent you from feeling the uterus even when it is located anteriorly.

See retroversion and retroflexion of the uterus (p. 429).

Palpate each ovary. Place your abdominal hand on the right lower quadrant, your pelvic hand in the right lateral formix. Press your abdominal hand in and down, trying to push the adnexal structures toward your pelvic hand. Try to identify the right ovary or any adjacent adnexal masses. By moving your hands slightly, slide the adnexal structures be-

Three to five years after menopause, the ovaries have usually atrophied and are no longer palpable. If you can feel an ovary in a postmenopausal

tween your fingers, if possible, and note their size, shape, consistency, mobility, and tenderness. Repeat the procedure on the left side.

woman, consider an abnormality such as a cyst or a tumor.

Adnexal masses include ovarian cysts and tumors, the swollen fallopian tube(s) of pelvic inflammatory disease, and a tubal pregnancy. A uterine myoma may simulate an adnexal mass. See Table 13-7, Adnexal Masses (p. 430).

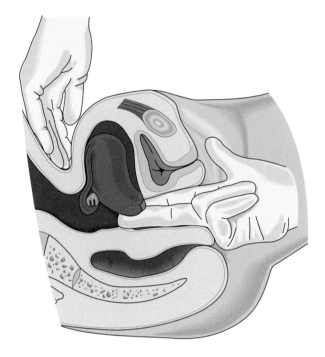

Normal ovaries are somewhat tender. They are usually palpable in slender, relaxed women but are difficult or impossible to feel in others who are obese or poorly relaxed.

Assess the Strength of the Pelvic Muscles. Withdraw your two fingers slightly, just clear of the cervix, and spread them to touch the sides of the vaginal walls. Ask the patient to squeeze her muscles around them as hard and long as she can. A squeeze that compresses your fingers snugly, moves them upward and inward, and lasts 3 seconds or more is full strength.

Impaired strength may be due to age, vaginal deliveries, or neurologic deficits. Weakness may be associated with urinary stress incontinence.

Do a Rectovaginal Examination. Withdraw your fingers. Lubricate your gloves again if necessary. (See note on using lubricant p. 419.) Then slowly reintroduce your index finger into the vagina, your middle finger into the rectum. Ask the patient to strain down as you do this so that her anal sphincter will relax. Tell her that this examination may make her feel as if she has to move her bowels but that she will not do so. Repeat the maneuvers of the bimanual examination, giving special attention to the region behind the cervix that may be accessible only to the rectal finger.

Rectovaginal palpation is especially valuable in assessing a retrodisplaced uterus, as illustrated.

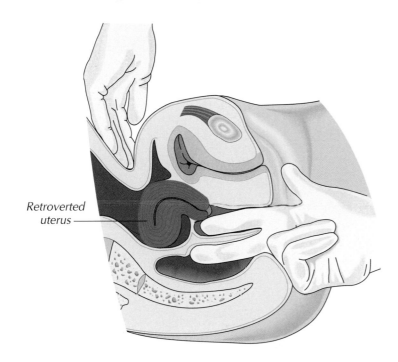

Retroverted uterus

Proceed to the rectal examination (see Chap. 15). After your examination, wipe off the external genitalia and anus or offer the patient some tissue so she can do it herself.

A Note on the Small Introitus. Many virginal vaginal orifices will readily admit a single examining finger. Modify your technique so as to use your index finger only. A small Pedersen speculum may make inspection possible. When the vaginal orifice is even smaller, a fairly good bimanual examination can be performed by placing one finger in the rectum rather than in the vagina.

An imperforate hymen occasionally delays menarche. Be sure to check for this possibility when menarche seems unduly late in relation to the development of a girl's breasts and pubic hair.

Similar techniques may be indicated in elderly women in whom the introitus has become atrophied and tight.

A Note on Using Lubricant. If you use a large tube of lubricant during a pelvic or rectal examination, you may inadvertently contaminate it by touching the tube with your gloved fingers after touching the patient. To avoid this problem, let the lubricant drop onto your gloved fingers without allowing contact between the tube and the gloves. If you or your assistant should inadvertently contaminate the tube, discard it. Small disposable tubes for use with one patient circumvent this problem.

Hernias

Hernias of the groin occur in women as well as in men, but they are much less common. Search for one if symptoms suggest the possibility. The examination techniques (see p. 395) are basically the same as for men, and a woman too should stand up to be examined. To feel an indirect inguinal hernia, however, palpate in the labia majora and upward to just lateral to the pubic tubercles.

An indirect inguinal hernia is the most common hernia that occurs in the female groin. A femoral hernia ranks next in frequency.

Health Promotion and Counseling

To promote health for women, direct attention to the importance of screening for cervical cancer with the Papanicolaou (Pap) smear, options for family planning, and risk factors for infection from sexually transmitted diseases (STDs) and the human immunodeficiency virus (HIV).

Widespread testing by Pap smear has contributed to a significant drop in the incidence of invasive cervical cancer. Careful technique to ensure sampling of endocervical cells at the squamocolumnar junction and use of accredited laboratories to interpret smears improve accuracy of the test. Screening should begin at age 18 or with onset of sexual activity. Recommendations about frequency of testing are undergoing revision. Annual testing until age 65 has been common, but does not appear to improve detection compared to longer intervals. A number of professional organizations recommend annual Pap smears for 3 years and then, if these are normal, less frequent testing based on clinician discretion. The U.S. Preventive Health Services Task Force recommends a 3-year interval beginning with onset of sexual activity. More frequent testing is warranted for women at increased risk—those with early onset of sexual activity, multiple partners, infection with human papillomavirus or HIV, or limited access to regular medical care. The upper age limit for the Pap smear testing is not well established. For women over 65, continued testing is indicated if recent tests have been abnormal or screening over the prior 10 years has been incomplete. Women who have never had sexual intercourse or with complete hysterectomies (cervix removed) do not require screening.

It is important to counsel women, particularly adolescents, about the timing of ovulation in the menstrual cycle and how to plan or prevent pregnancy. Survey data indicate that more than half of U.S. pregnancies are unintended, with this number rising to 80% of the one million teen pregnancies each year.* Clinicians should be familiar with the numerous options for family planning and their effectiveness. These include: natural methods (periodic abstinence, withdrawal, lactation); barrier methods (condom, diaphragm, cervical cap); implantable methods (intrauterine device, subdermal implant); pharmacologic interventions (spermicide, birth control pill, subdermal implant of levonorgestrel, injection of depo-medroxyprogesterone acetate); and surgery (tubal ligation). The clinician must take the time to understand the patient or couple's concerns and preferences and respect these preferences whenever possible. Continued use of a preferred method is superior to a more effective method that is abandoned. For teenagers, providing a confidential setting eases discussion of topics that may seem private and difficult to explore.

As with men, the clinician should assess risk factors for infection with STDs and HIV by taking a careful sexual history and counseling patients

* U.S. Preventive Health Services Task Force: Guide to Clinical Preventive Services, 2nd ed. Philadelphia, Williams & Wilkins, 1996, pp. 739–740.

about spread of disease and ways to reduce high-risk practices (see Chap. 1, p. 19 and Chap. 12, p. 398). Women with STDs are at higher risk for asymptomatic infection and loss of fertility. Learn to assess women for genital and pelvic infections through careful examination and collection of appropriate cultures and to apply recommended guidelines for serologic testing for infection with HIV (see Chap. 12, p. 398).

For middle age and older women, the clinician should be familiar with the psychological and physiological changes of menopause—mood shifts and changes in self-concept, vasomotor changes ("hot flashes"), accelerated bone loss, increases in total and LDL cholesterol, and vulvo-vaginal atrophy leading to symptoms of vaginal drying, dysuria, and sometimes dyspareunia. The clinician must be knowledgeable about estrogen and progesterone replacement therapy and help the patient to weigh the benefits and risks of treatment, taking into account the personal and family history of cardiovascular disease and osteoporosis (risk of developing these conditions decreases with hormone treatment) and breast cancer and endometrial cancer (treatment increases risk). Counseling patients about these decisions may extend over several visits.

Table 13-1   Lesions of the Vulva

TABLE 13-1   Lesions of the Vulva

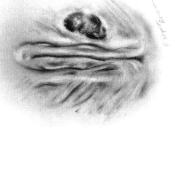

Flat, gray papules

Secondary Syphilis
(Condyloma Latum)

Slightly raised, flat, round or oval papules covered by a gray exudate suggest condylomata lata. These constitute one manifestation of secondary syphilis and are contagious.

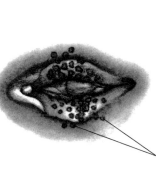

Carcinoma of the Vulva

An ulcerated or raised red vulvar lesion in an elderly woman may indicate vulvar carcinoma.

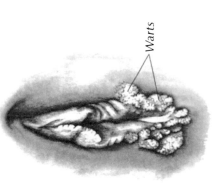

Warts

Venereal Wart
(Condyloma Acuminatum)

Warty lesions on the labia and within the vestibule suggest condylomata acuminata. They are due to infection with human papillomavirus.

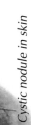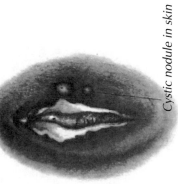

Shallow ulcers on red bases

Genital Herpes

Shallow, small, painful ulcers on red bases suggest a herpes infection. Initial infection may be extensive, as illustrated here. Recurrent infections are usually confined to a small local patch.

Cystic nodule in skin

Epidermoid Cyst

Small, firm, round cystic nodules in the labia suggest epidermoid cysts. They are sometimes yellowish in color. Look for the dark punctum marking the blocked opening of the gland.

Syphilitic Chancre

A firm, painless ulcer suggests the chancre of primary syphilis. Since most chancres in women develop internally, they often go undetected.

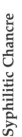

Table 13-2   Bulges and Swelling of Vulva, Vagina, and Urethra

TABLE 13-2   Bulges and Swelling of Vulva, Vagina, and Urethra

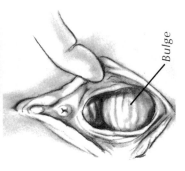

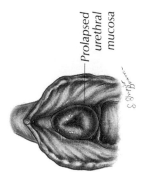

Bulge

Cystocele

A cystocele is a bulge of the anterior vaginal wall, together with the bladder above it, that results from weakened supporting tissues. The upper two thirds of the vaginal wall are involved.

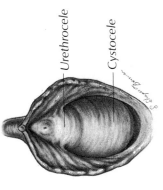

Urethrocele

Cystocele

Cystourethrocele

When the entire anterior vaginal wall, together with the bladder and the urethra, is involved in the bulge, a cystourethrocele is present. A groove sometimes defines the border between urethrocele and cystocele, but is not always present.

Rectocele

A rectocele is a bulging of the posterior wall of the vagina, together with the rectal wall behind it. Weakened supporting structures are the cause.

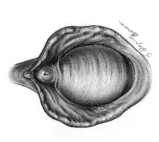

Labial swelling

Bartholin's Gland Infection

Causes of a Bartholin's gland infection include gonococci, *Chlamydia trachomatis*, and other organisms. Acutely, it appears as a tense, hot, very tender abscess. Look for pus coming out of the duct or erythema around the duct opening. Chronically, a nontender cyst is felt. It may be large or small.

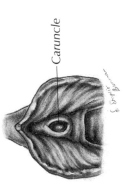

Caruncle

Urethral Caruncle

A urethral caruncle is a small, red, benign tumor visible at the posterior part of the urethral meatus. It occurs chiefly in postmenopausal women, and usually causes no symptoms. Occasionally, a carcinoma of the urethra is mistaken for a caruncle. To check for this, palpate the urethra through the vagina for thickening, nodularity, or tenderness, and feel for inguinal lymphadenopathy.

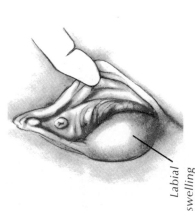

Prolapsed urethral mucosa

Prolapse of the Urethral Mucosa

Prolapsed urethral mucosa forms a swollen red ring around the urethral meatus. It usually occurs before menarche or after menopause. Identify the urethral meatus at the center of the swelling to make this diagnosis

Table 13-3   Variations in the Cervix

TABLE 13-3   *Variations in the Cervix*

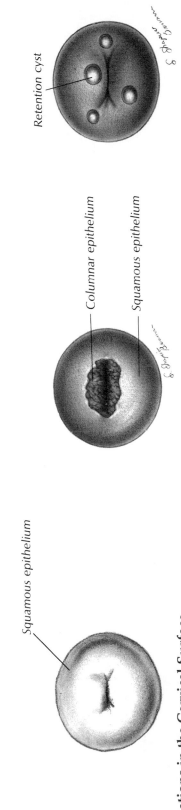

Squamous epithelium

Columnar epithelium

Squamous epithelium

Retention cyst

Shapes of the Cervical Os

The normal cervical os may be round, oval, or slitlike. The trauma of one or more vaginal deliveries may tear the cervix, producing lacerations. Illustrated here, from left to right, are an oval os, a slitlike os, and lacerations described as unilateral transverse, bilateral transverse, and stellate.

Variations in the Cervical Surface

Two kinds of epithelia may cover the cervix: (1) shiny pink *squamous epithelium,* which resembles the vaginal epithelium, and (2) deep red, plushy, *columnar epithelium,* which is continuous with the endocervical lining. These two meet at the squamocolumnar junction. When this junction is at or inside the cervical os, only squamous epithelium is seen. A ring of columnar epithelium is often visible to a varying extent around the os—the result of a normal process that accompanies fetal development, menarche, and the first pregnancy.*

By another process termed *metaplasia,* all or part of this columnar epithelium is transformed into squamous epithelium again. This change may block the secretions of columnar epithelium and thus cause retention cysts (*nabothian cysts*). These appear as one or more translucent nodules on the cervical surface, and have no pathologic significance.

*Terminology is in flux. Other terms for the columnar epithelium that is visible on the ectocervix are ectropion, ectopy, and eversion.

Table 13-4   *Abnormalities of the Cervix*

TABLE 13-4   *Abnormalities of the Cervix*

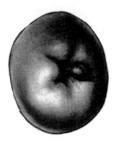

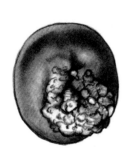

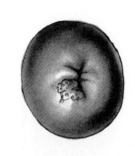

Carcinoma of the Cervix

Carcinoma of the cervix begins in an area of metaplasia. In its earliest stages, it cannot be distinguished from a normal cervix. In a late stage, an extensive, irregular, cauliflowerlike growth may develop. Early frequent intercourse, multiple partners, and infection with human papillomavirus increase the risk for cervical cancer.

Cervical Polyp

A cervical polyp usually arises from the endocervical canal, becoming visible when it protrudes through the cervical os. It is bright red, soft, and rather fragile. When only the tip is seen, it cannot be differentiated clinically from a polyp originating in the endometrium. Polyps are benign but may bleed.

Mucopurulent Cervicitis

Mucopurulent cervicitis produces purulent yellow drainage from the cervical os, usually due to infection from *Chlamydia trachomatis, Neisseria gonorrhoeae,* or herpes. These infections are sexually transmitted, and may occur without symptoms or signs.

Vaginal adenosis

Columnar epithelium

Collar

Fetal Exposure to Diethylstilbestrol (DES)*

Daughters of women who took DES during pregnancy are at much higher risk for a number of abnormalities, including (1) columnar epithelium that covers most or all of the cervix, (2) vaginal adenosis, i.e., extension of this epithelium to the vaginal wall, and (3) a circular collar or ridge of tissue, of varying shapes, between cervix and vagina. Much less common is an otherwise rare carcinoma of the upper vagina.

* In the United States, exposure to DES diminished in the late 1960s and stopped in 1971 when the drug was banned.

Table 13-5   Vaginitis

TABLE 13-5   *Vaginitis*

The vaginal discharge that often accompanies vaginitis must be distinguished from a physiologic discharge. The latter is clear or white and may contain white clumps of epithelial cells; it is not malodorous. It is also important to distinguish vaginal from cervical discharges. Use a large cotton swab to wipe off the cervix. If no cervical discharge is present in the os, suspect a vaginal origin and consider the causes below. Remember that diagnosis of cervicitis or vaginitis hinges on careful collection and analysis of the appropriate laboratory specimens.

	Trichomonas Vaginitis	Candida Vaginitis (*Monilia*)	Bacterial Vaginosis	Atrophic Vaginitis
Cause	*Trichomonas vaginalis*, a protozoa. Often but not always acquired sexually.	*Candida albicans*, a yeast (a normal vaginal inhabitant). Many factors predispose.	Unknown; probably anaerobic bacteria. May be transmitted sexually	Decreased estrogen production after menopause
Discharge	Yellowish green or gray, possibly frothy; often profuse and pooled in the vaginal fornix; may be malodorous	White and curdy; may be thin but typically thick; not as profuse as in *Trichomonas* infection; not malodorous	Gray or white, thin, homogeneous, malodorous; coats the vaginal walls. Usually not profuse, may be minimal	Variable in color, consistency, and amount; may be blood-tinged; rarely profuse
Other Symptoms	Pruritus (though not usually as severe as with *Candida* infection), pain on urination from skin inflammation or possibly urethritis), and dyspareunia	Pruritus, vaginal soreness, pain on urination (from skin inflammation), and dyspareunia	Unpleasant fishy or musty genital odor	Pruritus, vaginal soreness, or burning and dyspareunia
Vulva	The vestibule and labia minora may be reddened.	The vulva and even the surrounding skin are often inflamed and sometimes swollen to a variable extent.	Usually normal	Atrophic
Vaginal Mucosa	May be diffusively reddened, with small red granular spots or petechiae in the posterior fornix. In mild cases, the mucosa looks normal.	Often reddened, with white, often tenacious patches of discharge. The mucosa may bleed when these patches are scraped off. In mild cases, the mucosa looks normal.	Usually normal	Atrophic, dry, pale; may be red, petechial, or ecchymotic; bleeds easily; may show erosions or filmy adhesions
Laboratory Evaluation	Scan saline wet mount for trichomonads.	Scan potassium hydroxide (KOH) preparation for branching hyphae of *Candida*.	Scan saline wet mount for clue cells (epithelial cells with stippled borders); sniff for fishy odor after applying KOH ("whiff test").	

* Previously termed *Gardnerella* vaginitis.

Table 13-6   Abnormalities and Positions of the Uterus

TABLE 13-6   *Abnormalities and Positions of the Uterus*

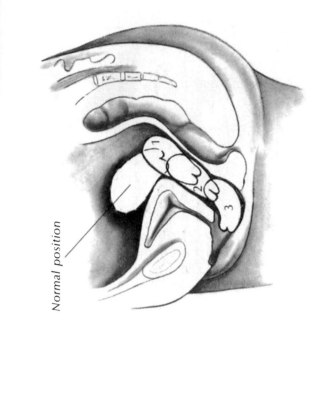

Normal position

Myomas

Myomas of the Uterus (Fibroids)

Myomas are very common benign uterine tumors. They may be single or multiple and vary greatly in size, occasionally reaching massive proportions. They feel like firm, irregular nodules in continuity with the uterine surface. Occasionally, a myoma projecting laterally can be confused with an ovarian mass; a nodule projecting posteriorly can be mistaken for a retroflexed uterus. Submucous myomas project toward the endometrial cavity and are not themselves palpable, although they may be suspected because of an enlarged uterus.

Prolapse of the Uterus

Prolapse of the uterus results from weakness of the supporting structures of the pelvic floor, and is often associated with a cystocele and rectocele. In progressive stages, the uterus becomes retroverted and descends down the vaginal canal to the outside. In first-degree prolapse, the cervix is still well within the vagina. In second-degree prolapse, it is at the introitus. In third-degree prolapse (procidentia), the cervix and vagina are outside the introitus.

Table 13-6   Abnormalities and Positions of the Uterus

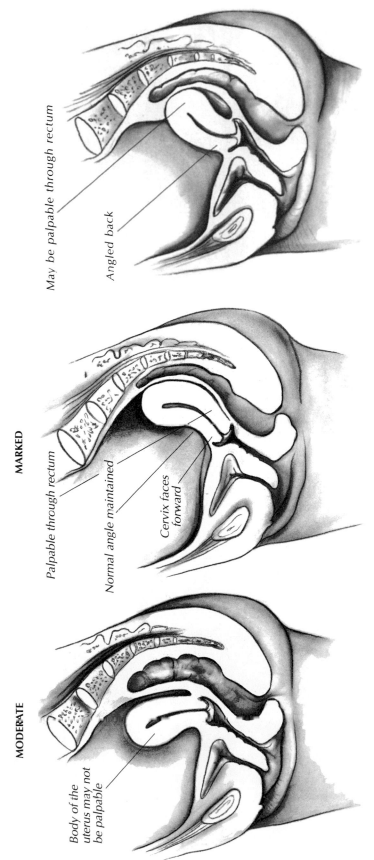

MODERATE

Body of the uterus may not be palpable

MARKED

Palpable through rectum

Normal angle maintained

Cervix faces forward

May be palpable through rectum

Angled back

Retroversion of the Uterus

Retroversion of the uterus refers to a tilting backward of the entire uterus, including both body and cervix. It is a common variant occurring in about 1 out of 5 women. Early clues on pelvic examination are a cervix that faces forward and a uterine body that cannot be felt by the abdominal hand. In moderate retroversion, shown on the left, the body may not be palpable with either hand. In marked retroversion, shown on the right, the body can be felt posteriorly, either through the posterior fornix or through the rectum. A retroverted uterus is usually both mobile and asymptomatic. Occasionally, such a uterus is fixed and immobile, held in place by conditions such as endometriosis or pelvic inflammatory disease.

Retroflexion of the Uterus

Retroflexion of the uterus refers to a backward angulation of the body of the uterus in relation to the cervix. The cervix maintains its usual position. The body of the uterus is often palpable through the posterior fornix or through the rectum.

Both retroversion and retroflexion are usually normal variants.

429

Table 13-7   Adnexal Masses

TABLE 13-7   *Adnexal Masses*

Adnexal masses most commonly result from disorders of the fallopian tubes or ovaries. Three examples—often hard to differentiate—are described. In addition, inflammatory disease of the bowel (such as diverticulitis), carcinoma of the colon, and a pedunculated myoma of the uterus may simulate an adnexal mass.

Ovarian Cysts and Tumors

Ovarian cysts and tumors may be detected as adnexal masses on one or both sides. Later, they may extend out of the pelvis. Cysts tend to be smooth and compressible, tumors more solid and often nodular. Uncomplicated cysts and tumors are not usually tender.

Small (≤6 cm in diameter), mobile, cystic masses in a young woman are usually benign and often disappear after the next menstrual period.

Ruptured Tubal Pregnancy

A ruptured tubal pregnancy spills blood into the peritoneal cavity, causing severe abdominal pain and tenderness. Guarding and rebound tenderness are sometimes associated. A unilateral adnexal mass may be palpable, but tenderness often prevents its detection. Faintness, syncope, nausea, vomiting, tachycardia, and shock may be present, reflecting the hemorrhage. There may be a prior history of amenorrhea or other symptoms of a pregnancy.

Pelvic Inflammatory Disease

Pelvic inflammatory disease (PID) is most often a result of sexually transmitted infection of the fallopian tubes (salpingitis) or of the tubes and ovaries (salpingo-oophoritis). It is caused by *Neisseria gonorrhoeae*, *Chlamydia trachomatis*, and other organisms. *Acute* disease is associated with very tender, bilateral adnexal masses, although pain and muscle spasm usually make it impossible to delineate them. Movement of the cervix produces pain. If not treated, a tuboovarian abscess or infertility may ensue.

Infection of the fallopian tubes and ovaries may also follow delivery of a baby or gynecologic surgery.

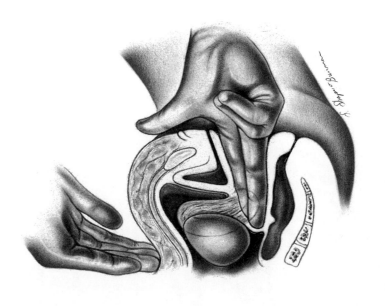

The Pregnant Woman

CHAPTER 14

Joyce E. (Beebe) Thompson

This chapter focuses on the evaluation of the healthy adult woman who is pregnant. Overall assessment of the pregnant woman is similar to that of nonpregnant women. However, changes in anatomy and physiology during pregnancy result in symptoms and physical signs that are important to recognize as pregnancy related rather than abnormal. Common variations of normal findings are presented, and easily identified problems or danger signs are discussed briefly.

The chapter highlights the initial assessment of the pregnant woman, including the history and physical examination used to diagnose or confirm pregnancy. This assessment ideally takes place within 6 to 8 weeks of conception, although some women do not come for their first pregnancy visit until much later. If a woman appears late in pregnancy for her first visit, additional techniques such as modified Leopold's maneuvers for abdominal palpation are needed. Because normal pregnancy lasts 38 to 42 weeks and changes in the organs of reproduction that begin with conception continue throughout, these changes will be outlined briefly. Also included are health promotion recommendations on nutrition and exercise for the pregnant woman, as well as information on screening for domestic violence.

Anatomy and Physiology

In preparation for physical examination of the pregnant woman, you may wish to review the anatomy in Chapter 10, The Breasts and Axillae, and Chapter 13, Female Genitalia. The major anatomical changes related to pregnancy occur in the thyroid gland, breasts, abdomen, and pelvis. Minor skin changes, including the mask of pregnancy and abdominal striae, may be noted in some women.

During pregnancy, the thyroid gland enlarges moderately due to hyperplasia of the glandular tissue and increased vascularity. The breasts also enlarge for the same reasons, and become nodular by the third month of gestation as the mammary tissue hypertrophies. The nipples enlarge, darken, and become more erectile. From mid- to late pregnancy a normal thick, yellowish discharge called *colostrum* may be expressed from the nipple. The areolae darken, and Montgomery's glands appear prominent around the nipples. The venous pattern over the breasts becomes increasingly visible as pregnancy progresses.

The abdomen's most notable anatomical change is distention, primarily related to the increasing size of the growing uterus and fetus. Early distention from fluid retention and from the relaxation of abdominal muscles may be noted before the uterus becomes an abdominal organ (12–14 weeks of gestation). The expected growth patterns of the normal uterus and fetus are illustrated on the right, and the standing contours of the primigravid abdomen in each trimester of pregnancy are illustrated below.

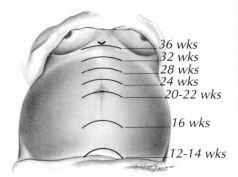

**EXPECTED HEIGHT OF THE UTERINE
FUNDUS BY MONTH OF PREGNANCY**

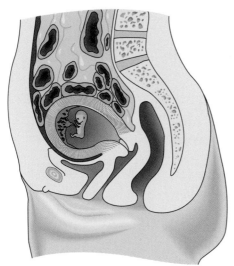

First Trimester

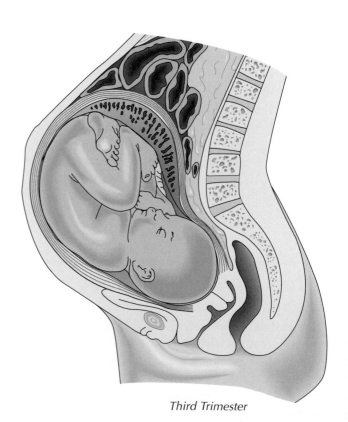

Third Trimester

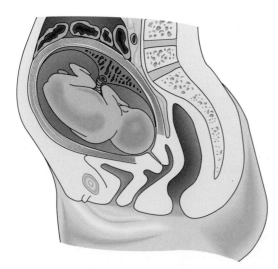

Second Trimester

CHANGING CONTOURS OF THE PRIMIGRAVID ABDOMEN

As the skin stretches to accommodate the growth of the fetus, purplish striae may appear. *Linea nigra,* a brownish black pigmented line following the midline of the abdomen, may become evident. Muscle tone is diminished as pregnancy advances, and *diastasis recti* (separation of the rectus muscles at the midline of the abdomen) may be noticeable in the latter trimesters of pregnancy. If diastasis is severe (as it may be in multiparous women), only a layer of skin, fascia, and peritoneum covers most of the anterior uterine wall. The fetus is felt easily through this muscular gap.

Many anatomical changes take place in the pelvis through the course of pregnancy. The early diagnosis of pregnancy is based in part on the changes in the vagina and the uterus. With the increased vascularity throughout the pelvic region, the vagina takes on a bluish or violet color. The vaginal walls appear thicker and deeply rugated because of an increased thickness of the mucosa, loosening of the connective tissue, and hypertrophy of smooth muscle cells. Vaginal secretions are considerably increased, thick, and white. The pH becomes more acidic as a result of increased lactic acid from the action of *Lactobacillus acidophilus* on the increased levels of glycogen stored in the vaginal epithelium. This changing pH protects the pregnant woman from some vaginal infections, but the increased glycogen may contribute to higher rates of *Candida* (yeast) infection during pregnancy (see Table 13-5).

The uterus is clearly the organ most affected. Early in pregnancy, it loses the firmness and resistance of the nonpregnant organ. The palpable softening at the isthmus (*Hegar's sign*) is an early diagnostic sign of pregnancy, and is illustrated on the right.

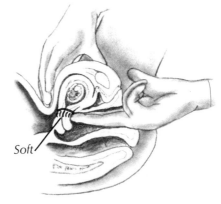

Soft

HEGAR'S SIGN

Over the course of 9 months, the uterus increases in weight from 2 ounces to 2 pounds, largely because of increased size of muscle cells, an accumulation of fibrous tissue, a considerable increase in elastic tissue, and a great increase in the size and number of blood vessels and lymphatics. There is a 500- to 1000-fold increase in size, so that by the end of pregnancy the uterus has a capacity of approximately 10 liters.

As the uterus grows, it changes shape and position. Prior to 12 weeks of gestation, it is a pelvic organ. As it enlarges, the anteverted uterus quickly takes up space normally occupied by the bladder, thus creating a need for frequent voiding. Irrespective of uterine position (anteverted, retroverted, or retroflexed), the uterus straightens and rises out of the pelvis by the end of 12 weeks' gestation, then becoming palpable abdominally.

As it grows, it displaces the intestinal contents laterally and superiorly and also stretches the ligaments that support it, sometimes resulting in lower quadrant pain. The usually pear-shaped organ is altered by fetal growth and positions, and as the uterus grows it tends to rotate to the right to accommodate the rectosigmoid in the left side of the pelvis.

The cervix also looks and feels quite different. Pronounced softening and cyanosis appear very early after conception and continue throughout pregnancy (*Chadwick's sign*). The cervical canal is filled with a tenacious mucus (*mucous plug*) that protects the developing fetus from infection. Red, velvety mucosa around the os is common on the cervix during pregnancy and is considered normal.

Common Concerns During Pregnancy and Their Explanation

Common Concerns	Time in Pregnancy	Explanation and Effects on Woman's Body
No menses (*amenorrhea*)	Throughout	Continued high levels of estrogen, progesterone, and human chorionic gonadotropin following fertilization of the ovum allow the uterine endometrium to build up and support the developing pregnancy rather than to slough as menses.
Nausea with or without vomiting	1st trimester	Possible causes include hormonal changes of pregnancy leading to slowed peristalsis throughout the GI tract, changes in taste and smell, the growing uterus, or emotional factors. Women may have a modest (2–5 lb) weight loss in the first trimester.
Breast tenderness, tingling	1st trimester	The hormones of pregnancy stimulate the growth of breast tissue. As the breasts enlarge throughout pregnancy, women may experience upper backache from their increased weight. There is also increased blood flow throughout the breasts, increasing pressure on the tissue.
Urinary frequency (nonpathologic)	1st/3rd trimesters	There is increased blood volume and increased filtration rate in the kidneys with increased urine production. Due to less space for the bladder from pressure from the growing uterus (1st trimester) or from the descent of the fetal head (3rd trimester), the woman needs to empty her bladder more frequently.
Fatigue	1st/3rd trimesters	Rapid change in energy requirements; hormonal changes (progesterone has a sedative effect); in 3rd trimester, weight gain, changes in mechanics of movement, and sleep disturbances contribute.
Heartburn Constipation	Throughout	Relaxation of the lower esophageal sphincter allows stomach contents to back up into the lower esophagus. The decreased GI motility caused by pregnancy hormones slows peristalsis and causes constipation. Constipation may cause or aggravate existing hemorrhoids.
Leukorrhea	Throughout	Increased secretions from the cervix and the vaginal epithelium, due to the hormones and vasocongestion of pregnancy, result in an asymptomatic milky white vaginal discharge.
Weight loss	1st trimester	If a woman experiences nausea and vomiting, she may not be eating normally in early pregnancy, see nausea above.
Backache (nonpathologic)	Throughout	Hormonally induced relaxation of joints and ligaments and the minor lordosis required to balance the growing uterus sometimes result in a lower backache. Pathologic causes must be ruled out.
Edema	3rd trimester	There is increased venous pressure in the legs, obstruction of lymphatic flow, and reduced plasma colloid osmotic pressure.

The ovaries and fallopian tubes undergo changes as well, but few are noticeable during physical examination. Early in pregnancy, the *corpus luteum* (the ovarian follicle that has discharged its ovum) may be sufficiently prominent to be felt on the affected ovary as a small nodule, but it disappears by midpregnancy. The major reason for thorough examination of the fallopian tubes is the need to rule out a tubal pregnancy (see p. 430).

Reproductive physiology is reviewed briefly in the table on p. 434. Physiological alterations during pregnancy affect anatomical changes that explain many of the normal symptoms and physical findings. One example is what happens to a woman's breasts in early pregnancy. Hormonal influences (estrogen, progesterone, and prolactin) lead to vasodilation and growth and proliferation of ducts and glands. These changes, in turn, result in tenderness, fullness, and tingling of the breasts and can make breast examination difficult as well as uncomfortable for the newly pregnant woman. Care is needed during palpation to avoid undue discomfort while distinguishing between normal nodular changes of pregnancy and other breast masses.

The Pregnancy History

Accurate historical details are essential for directing both the order and the content of the physical examination. This examination is usually targeted to confirming the woman's suspicion of pregnancy, and the woman is most interested in pregnancy-related information and symptoms. The examiner, however, should also ascertain the general health of the woman. Details of the medical and psychosocial history related to pregnancy can be found in texts of nurse-midwifery and obstetrics noted in the bibliography.

In large measure, the history is directed toward risk factors known or suspected to diminish the health of either the woman or her developing fetus. The sociodemographic history includes age, income, adequacy of the social support network, and the woman's attitude toward this pregnancy, including whether she plans to keep it. Personal and family history of chronic diseases such as hypertension, diabetes, and cardiac conditions are important, along with family history of genetic disease. Past obstetrical history is particularly significant if the woman has had any major complication of pregnancy, labor, or birth or has given birth to a premature or growth-retarded infant. These conditions tend to repeat in subsequent pregnancies.

Exposure to teratogenic drugs, toxic substances in the workplace, or high levels of stress needs to be known early in pregnancy, though prevention is done better before the woman conceives. Personal behaviors known to have adverse effects on the health of the pregnant woman and fetus include over- or undernutrition, cigarette smoking, and use of alcohol and illicit drugs. Knowledge of these behaviors should prompt appropriate counseling during this first pregnancy assessment.

In addition, the clinician should get the history necessary to calculate the *expected weeks of gestation by dates.* This is currently counted in weeks from either (1) the first day of the last menstrual period (*LMP*), known as *menstrual age,* or (2) the date of conception, if this is known (*conception age*). Menstrual age is used most frequently to express the weeks of gestation calculated by dates. The first day of the LMP is also used to calculate the *expected date of confinement (EDC)* or projected time of term labor and birth for women with regular 28- to 30-day cycles. The EDC can be determined by adding 7 days to the first day of the LMP, subtracting 3 months, and adding one year (*Naegele's rule*). This information is often one of the first questions the pregnant woman asks when seeking confirmation of pregnancy.

The weeks of gestation at the time of examination tell you the expected size of the uterus if the LMP was normal, the dates were remembered accurately, and conception actually occurred. You should ascertain this size before examining the woman. You can then compare the expected size by dates with what you actually palpate during the bimanual examination (or abdominally, if pregnancy is beyond 14 weeks of gestation). Uterine size is measured by the palpable size of the uterus if still within the pelvic cavity, or by the height of the fundus if above the symphysis pubis. If there is a discrepancy, you need to look for the causes. Accurately dating the pregnancy is best done early, and contributes to good decision-making later in pregnancy if the fetus is not growing well, if preterm labor is suspected, or if the pregnancy goes beyond 42 weeks of gestation. If the woman does not remember her LMP or has irregular menstrual cycles, dating the pregnancy is done by palpation and subsequent monitoring of the growth curve (see p. 432) along with the time of first fetal movements. In some cases, ultrasound is an appropriate adjunct in dating an early pregnancy.

Other historical data needed prior to examination include the symptoms of pregnancy, such as breast tenderness, nausea or vomiting, urinary frequency, change in bowel habits, and fatigue (see table on p. 434). It is also important to ask whether the woman has ever had a complete pelvic examination. If not, time will be needed to explain its details and seek her cooperation throughout. Explaining what you do and what you find is important if you are to maintain rapport and educate the woman about her body, its response to pregnancy, and how she can maintain her health.

Techniques of Examination

General Approach

As with all patients, as you begin your examination of the pregnant woman show consideration for her comfort and sense of privacy, as well as for her individual needs and sensitivities. Have the needed equipment readily at hand. If the examiner has not met the woman before, taking the history before asking her to gown shows respect for her right to be treated with dignity. Ask the woman to put on the gown with the opening in front to ease the examination of both the breasts and the pregnant abdomen. Draping for the abdominal and pelvic examinations is similar to that discussed in earlier chapters.

Positioning. Positioning is important when examining the abdomen of a pregnant woman given the added time and attention needed to palpate the uterus and listen to the fetal heart. The semi-sitting position with the knees bent, as shown below, affords the greatest comfort, as well as protection from the negative effects of the weight of the gravid uterus on abdominal organs and vessels.

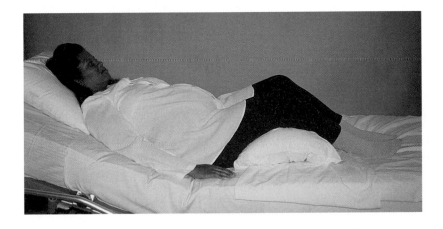

This position is especially important when examining a woman with an advanced pregnancy. Prolonged periods of lying on the back should be avoided because the uterus then lies directly on the woman's vertebral column and may compress the descending aorta and inferior vena cava, interfering with return of venous blood from the lower extremities and the pelvic vessels. Therefore, abdominal palpation should be efficient in time and results.

Encourage the woman to sit again briefly before proceeding to the pelvic evaluation. This pause also provides time for the woman to empty her bladder again. Make sure, however, that she is acclimated to sitting before allowing her to stand up. The pelvic examination should likewise be relatively quick. All other examination procedures should be done in sitting or left-side–lying position.

Supine hypotension is a severe form of this diminished circulation and may lead the woman to experience dizziness and feel faint, especially when lying down.

Equipment. The examiner's hands are the primary equipment for examination of the pregnant woman; they should be warm, and firm yet gentle in palpation. Whenever possible the fingers should be together and flat against the abdominal or pelvic tissue to minimize discomfort. Likewise, all touching and palpation should be done with smooth continuous contact against the skin rather than kneading or abrupt motion. The more sensitive palmar surfaces of the ends of the fingers will attain the greatest amount of information. Avoid tender areas on the woman's body until the end of the examination.

The gynecologic speculum is used for inspecting the cervix and the vagina and for taking specimens for cytologic or bacteriologic study. Because the vaginal walls are relaxed during pregnancy and may fall medially, obscuring your view, a speculum of larger than expected size may be needed. The relaxation of perineal and vulvar structures allows its use with minimal discomfort for the woman. Because of the increased vascularity of the vaginal and cervical structures, insert and open the speculum gently. You will thus avoid tissue trauma and bleeding. (Bleeding interferes with the interpretation of Pap smears.)

The cervical brush is not recommended for Pap smears in pregnant women because it often causes bleeding. The Ayre wooden spatula and/or cotton-tipped applicator is appropriate.

Review Chapter 13 for instruments and techniques used to take cervical smears.

General Inspection

Inspect the overall health, nutritional status, neuromuscular coordination, and emotional state as the woman walks into the exam room and climbs on the examination table. Discussion of the woman's priorities for the examination, her responses to pregnancy, and her general health provide useful information and help to put the woman at ease.

Vital Signs and Weight

Take the blood pressure. A baseline reading helps to determine the woman's usual range. In early and midpregnancy, blood pressure is normally lower than in the nonpregnant state.

High blood pressure prior to 24 weeks indicates chronic hypertension. After 24 weeks, further evaluation is required to diagnose and treat *pregnancy-induced hypertension (PIH)*.

Weigh the woman. First trimester weight loss related to nausea and vomiting is common but should not exceed 5 pounds.

Weight loss of more than 5 pounds during the first trimester may be due to excessive vomiting (*hyperemesis*).

Head and Neck

Stand facing the seated woman and observe the head and neck, including the:

- *Face.* The mask of pregnancy (*chloasma*) is normal. It consists of irregular brownish patches around the eyes or across the bridge of the nose.

- *Hair,* including texture, moisture, and distribution. Dryness, oiliness, and sometimes minor generalized hair loss may be noted.

- *Eyes.* Note the conjunctival color.

- *Nose,* including the mucous membranes and the septum. Nasal congestion is common during pregnancy.

- *Mouth,* especially the gums and teeth.

- *Thyroid gland.* Inspect and palpate the gland. Symmetrical enlargement is expected.

Facial edema after 24 weeks of gestation suggests PIH.

Localized patches of hair loss should not be attributed to pregnancy.

Anemia of pregnancy may cause pallor.

Nosebleeds are more common during pregnancy. Signs of cocaine use may be present.

Gingival enlargement with bleeding (p. 239) is common during pregnancy.

Marked or asymmetrical enlargement is not due to pregnancy.

Thorax and Lungs

Inspect the thorax for the pattern of breathing. Although women late in pregnancy sometimes report difficulty in breathing, there are usually no abnormal physical signs.

If signs of respiratory distress are noted, examine the lungs thoroughly.

Heart

Palpate for the apical impulse (PMI). In advanced pregnancy, it may be slightly higher than normal because of dextrorotation of the heart due to the higher diaphragm.

Auscultate the heart. Soft, blowing murmurs are common during pregnancy, reflecting increased blood flow in normal vessels.

These murmurs may also accompany anemia.

Breasts

Inspect the breasts and nipples for symmetry and color. The venous pattern may be marked, the nipples and areolae are dark, and Montgomery's glands are prominent.

An inverted nipple needs attention if breastfeeding is planned.

Palpate for masses. During pregnancy, breasts are tender and nodular.

A pathologic mass may be difficult to isolate.

Compress each nipple between your index finger and thumb. This maneuver may express colostrum from the nipples.

A bloody or purulent discharge should not be attributed to pregnancy.

Abdomen

Position the pregnant woman in a semi-sitting position with her knees flexed (see p. 437).

Inspect for scars, striae, the shape and contour of the abdomen, and the fundal height. Purplish striae and linea nigra are normal in pregnancy. The shape and contour may indicate pregnancy size (see figures on p. 432).

Scars may confirm the type of prior surgery, especially cesarean section.

Palpate the abdomen for:

- *Organs or masses.* The mass of pregnancy is expected.

- *Fetal movements.* These can usually be felt by the examiner after 24 weeks (and by the mother at 18–20 weeks).

If movements cannot be felt after 24 weeks, consider error in calculating gestation, fetal death or morbidity, or false pregnancy.

- *Uterine contractility.* The uterus contracts irregularly after 12 weeks and often in response to palpation during the third trimester. The abdomen then feels tense or firm to the examiner, and it is difficult to feel fetal parts. If the hand is left resting on the fundal portion of the uterus, the fingers will sense the relaxation of the uterine muscle.

Prior to 37 weeks, regular uterine contractions with or without pain or bleeding are abnormal, suggesting preterm labor.

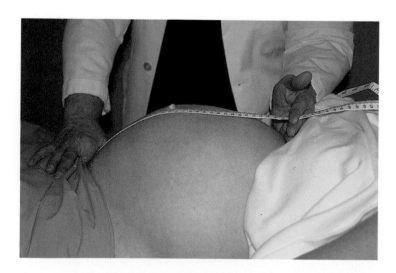

Measure the fundal height with a tape measure if the woman is more than 20 weeks pregnant. Holding the tape as illustrated and following the

If fundal height is more than 2 cm higher than expected, con-

midline of the abdomen, measure from the top of the symphysis pubis to the top of the uterine fundus. After 20 weeks, measurement in centimeters should roughly equal the weeks of gestation. For estimating fetal height between 12 and 20 weeks, see p. 432.

Auscultate the fetal heart, noting its rate (FHR), location, and rhythm. Use either:

- Doptone, with which the FHR is audible after 12 weeks, or

- A fetoscope, with which it is audible after 18 weeks.

sider multiple gestation, a big baby, extra amniotic fluid, or uterine myomata. If it is lower than expected by more than 2 cm, consider missed abortion, transverse lie, growth retardation, or false pregnancy.

Lack of an audible fetal heart may indicate pregnancy of fewer weeks than expected, fetal demise, or false pregnancy.

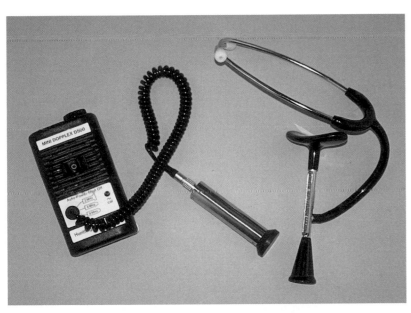

DOPTONE (LEFT) AND FETOSCOPE (RIGHT)

The *rate* is usually in the 160s during early pregnancy, and then slows to the 120s to 140s near term. After 32 to 34 weeks, the FHR should increase with fetal movement.

An FHR that near term drops noticeably with fetal movement could indicate poor placental circulation.

The *location* of the audible FHR is in the midline of the lower abdomen from 12 to 18 weeks of gestation. After 28 weeks, the fetal heart is heard best over the fetal back or chest. The location of the FHR then depends on how the fetus is positioned. Palpating the fetal head and back helps you identify where to listen. (See Modified Leopold's Maneuvers, pp. 444–445.) If the fetus is head down with the back on the woman's left side, the FHR is heard best in the lower left quadrant. If the fetal head is under the xiphoid process (*breech presentation*) with the back on the right, the FHR is heard in the upper right quadrant.

After 24 weeks, auscultation of more than one FHR (with varying rate) in different locations suggests more than one fetus.

Rhythm becomes important in the third trimester. Expect a variance of 10 to 15 beats per minute (BPM) over 1 to 2 minutes.

Lack of beat-to-beat variability late in pregnancy suggests fetal compromise.

Genitalia, Anus, and Rectum

Inspect the *external genitalia,* noting the hair distribution, the color, and any scars. Parous relaxation of the introitus and noticeable enlargement of the labia and clitoris are normal. Scars from an *episiotomy* (a perineal incision to facilitate delivery of an infant) or from perineal lacerations may be present in multiparous women.

Some women have labial varicosities that become tortuous and painful.

Inspect the *anus* for varicosities (*hemorrhoids*). If these are present, note their size and location.

Varicosities often engorge later in pregnancy. They may be painful and bleed.

Palpate *Bartholin's and Skene's glands.* No discharge or tenderness should be present.

Check for a *cystocele or rectocele.*

May be pronounced due to the muscle relaxation of pregnancy

Speculum Examination. Take *Pap smears* and, if indicated, other vaginal or cervical specimens. The cervix may bleed more easily when touched due to the vasocongestion of pregnancy.

Vaginal infections are more common during pregnancy, and specimens may be needed for diagnosis.

Inspect the *vaginal walls* for color, discharge, rugae, and relaxation. A bluish or violet color, deep rugae, and an increased milky white discharge (*leukorrhea*) are normal.

A pink vagina suggests a non-pregnant state. Vaginal irritation and itching with discharge suggest infection.

Inspect the *cervix* for color, shape, and healed lacerations. A parous cervix may look irregular because of lacerations (see p. 425).

A pink cervix suggests a non-pregnant state.

Bimanual Examination. Insert two lubricated fingers into the introitus, palmar side down, with slight pressure downward on the perineum. Slide the fingers into the posterior vaginal vault. Maintaining downward pressure, gently turn the fingers palmar side up. Avoid the sensitive urethral structures at all times. With the relaxation of pregnancy, the bimanual examination is usually accomplished more easily. Tissues are soft and the vaginal walls usually close in on the examining fingers, giving the sensation of being immersed in a bowl of oatmeal. It may be difficult to distinguish the cervix at first because of its softer texture.

Place your finger gently in the os, then sweep it around the *surface of the cervix.* A nulliparous cervix should be closed, while a multiparous cervix may admit a fingertip through the external os. The internal os—the narrow passage between the endocervical canal and the uterine cavity—should be closed in both situations. The surface of a normal multiparous cervix may feel irregular due to the healed lacerations from a previous birth.

A shortened (effaced) cervix prior to 32 weeks may indicate preterm labor.

Estimate the *length of the cervix* by palpating the lateral surface of the cervix from the cervical tip to the lateral fornix. Prior to 34 to 36 weeks, the cervix should retain its normal length of about 1.5 to 2 cm.

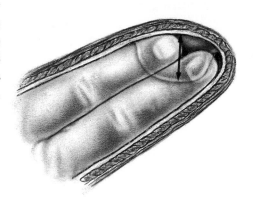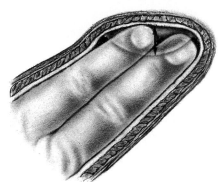

Palpate the *uterus* for size, shape, consistency, and position. These depend on the weeks of gestation. Early softening of the isthmus (Hegar's sign) is characteristic of pregnancy. The uterus is shaped like an inverted pear until 8 weeks, with slight enlargement in the fundal portion. The uterus becomes globular by 10 to 12 weeks. Anteflexion or retroflexion is lost by 12 weeks, with the fundal portion measuring about 8 cm in diameter.

With your internal fingers placed at either side of the cervix, palmar surfaces upward, gently lift the uterus toward the abdominal hand. Capture the fundal portion of the uterus between your two hands and gently estimate uterine size.

An irregularly shaped uterus suggests uterine myomata or a *bicornuate uterus* (two distinct uterine cavities separated by a septum).

Palpate the *left and right adnexa.* The corpus luteum may feel like a small nodule on the affected ovary during the first few weeks after conception. Late in pregnancy, adnexal masses may be difficult to feel.

Early in pregnancy, it is important to rule out a tubal (*ectopic*) pregnancy. See Table 13-7, Adnexal Masses, p. 430.

Palpate for *pelvic muscle strength* as you withdraw your examining fingers.

A *rectovaginal examination* may be done if you need to confirm uterine size or the integrity of the rectovaginal septum. A pregnancy of less than 10 weeks in a retroverted and retroflexed uterus lies totally in the posterior pelvis. Its size can be confirmed only by this examination.

Extremities

General inspection may be done with the woman seated or lying on her left side.

Inspect the legs for *varicose veins*.

Inspect the hands and legs for *edema*. Palpate for pretibial, ankle, and pedal edema. Edema is rated on a 0 to 4+ scale. Physiologic edema is more common in advanced pregnancy, during hot weather, and in women who stand a lot.

Obtain knee and ankle *reflexes*.

Special Techniques

Modified Leopold's Maneuvers. These maneuvers are important adjuncts to palpation of the pregnant abdomen beginning at 28 weeks of gestation. They help determine where the fetus is lying in relation to the woman's back (longitudinal or transverse), what end of the fetus is presenting at the pelvic inlet (head or buttocks), where the fetal back is located, how far the presenting part of the fetus has descended into the maternal pelvis, and the estimated weight of the fetus. This information is necessary to assess the adequacy of fetal growth and the probability of successful vaginal birth.

First Maneuver (Upper Pole). Stand at the woman's side facing her head. Keeping the fingers of both examining hands together, palpate gently with the fingertips to determine what part of the fetus is in the upper pole of the uterine fundus.

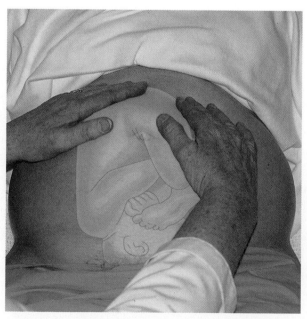

Varicose veins may begin or worsen during pregnancy.

Pathologic edema associated with PIH is often 3+ or more pretibially; it also affects the hands and face.

After 24 weeks, reflexes greater than 2+ may indicate PIH.

Interpretation
Common deviations include breech presentation (the fetal buttocks presenting at the outlet of the maternal pelvis) and absence of the presenting part well down into the maternal pelvis at term. Neither situation necessarily precludes vaginal birth. The most serious findings are a transverse lie close to term and slowed fetal growth that could represent *intrauterine growth retardation (IUGR)*.

Most commonly, the fetal buttocks are at the upper pole. They feel firm but irregular, and less globular than the head. The fetal head feels firm, round, and smooth.

Second Maneuver (Sides of the Maternal Abdomen). Place one hand on each side of the woman's abdomen, aiming to capture the body of the fetus between them. Use one hand to steady the uterus and the other to palpate the fetus.

The hand on the fetal back feels a smooth, firm surface the length of the hand (or longer) by 32 weeks of gestation. The hand on the fetal arms and legs feels irregular bumps, and also perhaps kicking if the fetus is awake and active.

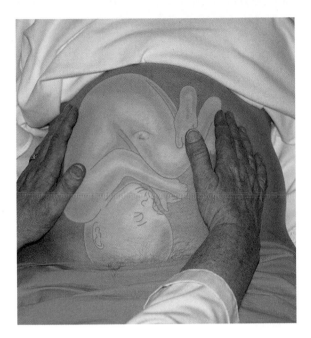

Third Maneuver (Lower Pole). Turn and face the woman's feet. Using the flat palmar surfaces of the fingers of both hands and, at the start, touching the fingertips together, palpate the area just above the symphysis pubis. Note whether the hands diverge with downward pressure or stay together. This tells you whether or not the presenting part of the fetus (head or buttocks) is descending into the pelvic inlet.

If the fetal head is presenting, the fingers feel a smooth, firm, rounded surface on both sides.

If the hands diverge, the presenting part is descending into the pelvic inlet, as illustrated.

If the hands stay together and you can gently depress the tissue over the bladder without touching the fetus, the presenting part is above your hands.

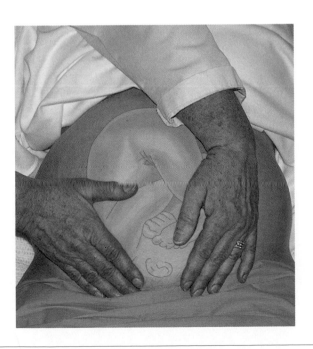

If the presenting fetal part is descending, palpate its texture and firmness. If not, gently move your hands up the lower abdomen and capture the presenting part between your hands.

Fourth Maneuver (Confirmation of the Presenting Part). With your dominant hand grasp the part of the fetus in the lower pole, and with your nondominant hand the part of the fetus in the upper pole. With this maneuver, you may be able to distinguish between the head and the buttocks.

The fetal head feels smooth, firm, and rounded; the buttocks, firm but irregular.

Most commonly, the head is in the lower pole and the fetal buttocks are in the upper pole. If the head is above the pelvic inlet, it moves somewhat independently of the rest of the fetal body.

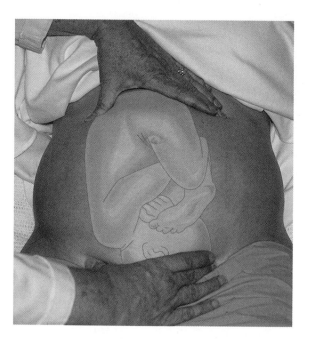

Concluding the Visit

Once the examination is completed and the woman is dressed, review the findings with her. If further data are necessary to confirm pregnancy, discuss how these may be obtained. Reinforce the importance of regular prenatal care. Record all the findings on the prenatal record.

Health Promotion and Counseling

Counseling about nutrition and exercise is important for the health of the pregnant woman and baby. Evaluate the nutritional status of the woman at the first prenatal visit, including a diet history, measurement of height and weight, and screening for anemia by checking the hematocrit. Be sure to explore the woman's habits and attitudes about eating and weight gain, as well as her use of needed vitamin and mineral supplements. Develop a nutrition plan that is appropriate to the woman's cultural preferences. Be sure there is a balanced increase in calories and protein, since protein will be used for energy, rather than growth, unless sufficient calories are consumed. Women with low incomes should be helped to obtain additional food. At each visit, monitor weight gain and review nutritional goals for women at risk.

Ideal weight gain during pregnancy follows a pattern: very little gain the first trimester, rapid increase in the second, and a mild slowing of the increase in the third trimester. Women should be weighed at each visit, with the results plotted on a graph for the woman and health-care provider to review and discuss.

Recommended Total Weight Gain Ranges for Pregnant Women

Prepregnancy Weight-for-Height Category	Recommended Total Gain	
	lb	kg
Low (BMI <19.8)	28–40	12.5–18
Normal (BMI 19.8 to 26.0)	25–35	11.5–16
High (BMI 26.0 to 29.0)	15–25	7.0–11.5
Obese (BMI >29.0)	≥15	≥7.0

Figures are for single pregnancies. The range for women carrying twins is 35 to 45 lb (16 to 20 kg). Young adolescents (<2 years after menarche) and African American women should strive for gains at the upper end of the range. Short women (<62 in. or <157 cm) should strive for gains at the lower end of the range.

Institute of Medicine. Nutrition During Pregnancy. Part I, Weight Gain. Committee on Nutritional Status During Pregnancy and Lactation, Food and Nutrition Board, National Academy Press, Washington, DC, 1990.

Exercise is an important part of the lifestyle of many women. Guidelines are contradictory, but the recommendations of the American College of Obstetrics and Gynecology (1994) suggest that, in the absence of either obstetric or medical complications, most women can perform moderate exercise to maintain cardiorespiratory and muscular fitness throughout pregnancy and the postpartum period. Women exercising regularly prior to pregnancy can continue mild to moderate exercise, preferably for short periods three times per week. Women initiating exercise during pregnancy should be more cautious, and consider programs developed specifically for pregnant women. After the first trimester, women should avoid exercise in the supine position, which can compress the inferior vena cava and decrease blood flow to the placenta. The pregnant woman should stop exercise when she feels fatigued or uncomfortable and avoid overheating and dehydration. Since the center of gravity shifts in the third trimester, advise her that exercises that could cause loss of balance are unwise.

Pregnancy may be a time when women are more likely to be abused by an intimate partner, increasing risk of miscarriage and low birthweight babies. Abuse in pregnancy occurs more often than any other major antepartum complication.* Because victims of violence are often likely to disclose their experiences to their health-care provider before confiding in their family, clergy, or friends, many experts consider universal screening an ethical imperative. Ask pregnant women about domestic violence at least three times during pregnancy. Often a woman will be too ashamed to acknowledge domestic violence initially, but will feel more trusting at future visits and more willing to share her situation. Clues to physical violence may also arise from behavior during the interview or from frequent changes in appointments at the last minute to avoid detection of bruises.

* Centers for Disease Control and Prevention. MMWR 43:132, 1994.

The Anus, Rectum, and Prostate

CHAPTER 15

Anatomy and Physiology

The gastrointestinal tract terminates in a short segment, the anal canal. Its external margin is poorly demarcated, but the skin of the anal canal can usually be distinguished from the surrounding perianal skin by its moist, hairless appearance. The anal canal is normally held in a closed position by action of the voluntary external muscular sphincter and the involuntary internal sphincter, the latter an extension of the muscular coat of the rectal wall.

The direction of the anal canal on a line roughly between anus and umbilicus should be noted carefully. Unlike the rectum above it, the canal is liberally supplied by somatic sensory nerves, and a poorly directed finger or instrument will produce pain.

The anal canal is demarcated from the rectum superiorly by a serrated line marking the change from skin to mucous membrane. This anorectal

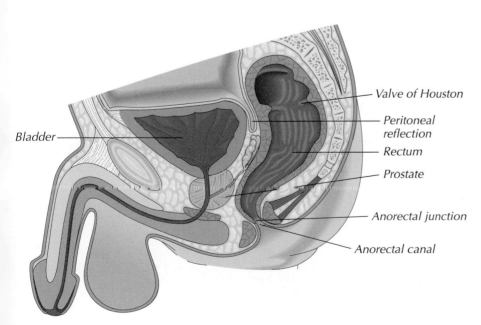

Bladder

Valve of Houston

Peritoneal reflection

Rectum

Prostate

Anorectal junction

Anorectal canal

MEDIAN SECTION—VIEW FROM THE LEFT SIDE

junction (often called the *pectinate* or *dentate line*) also denotes the boundary between somatic and visceral nerve supplies. It is readily visible on proctoscopic examination, but is not palpable.

Above the anorectal junction, the rectum balloons out and turns posteriorly into the hollow of the coccyx and the sacrum. In the male, the prostate gland is palpable anteriorly as a rounded, heart-shaped structure about 2.5 cm in length. Its two lateral lobes are separated by a shallow median sulcus or groove. The seminal vesicles, shaped like rabbit ears above the prostate, are not normally palpable.

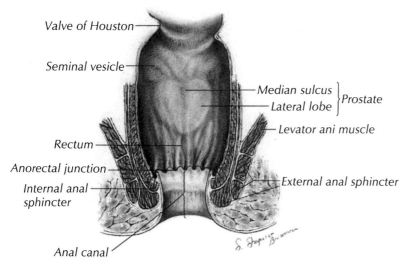

CORONAL SECTION OF THE ANUS AND RECTUM. VIEW FROM BEHIND, SHOWING THE ANTERIOR WALL

Through the anterior wall of the female rectum, the uterine cervix can usually be felt.

The rectal wall contains three inward foldings, called *valves of Houston.* The lowest of these can sometimes be felt, usually on the patient's left.

Most of the rectum that is accessible to digital examination does not have a peritoneal surface. The anterior rectum usually does, however, and you may reach it with the tip of your examining finger. You may thus be able to identify the tenderness of peritoneal inflammation or the nodularity of peritoneal metastases.

Changes With Age

The prostate gland is small during boyhood, but between puberty and the age of about 20 years it increases roughly five-fold in size. Starting in about the fifth decade, further enlargement is increasingly common as the gland becomes hyperplastic (see p. 459).

Techniques of Examination

For most patients, the rectal examination is probably the least popular segment of the entire physical examination. It may cause discomfort for the patient, perhaps embarrassment, but, if skillfully done, should not be truly painful in most circumstances. Although you may choose to omit a rectal examination in adolescents who have no relevant complaints, you should do one in adult patients. In middle-aged and older persons, omission risks missing an asymptomatic carcinoma. A successful examination requires gentleness, slow movement of your finger, a calm demeanor, and an explanation to the patient of what he or she may feel.

Male

The anus and rectum may be examined with the patient in one of several positions. For most purposes, the side-lying position is satisfactory and allows good views of the perianal and sacrococcygeal areas. This is the position described below. The lithotomy position may help you to reach a cancer high in the rectum. It also permits a bimanual examination, enabling you to delineate a pelvic mass. Some clinicians prefer to examine a patient while he stands with his hips flexed and his upper body resting across the examining table.

Ask the patient to lie on his left side with his buttocks close to the edge of the examining table near you. Flexing the patient's hips and knees, especially in the top leg, stabilizes his position and improves visibility. Drape the patient appropriately and adjust the light for the best view. Glove your hands and spread the buttocks apart.

No matter how you position the patient, your examining finger cannot reach the full length of the rectum. If a rectosigmoid cancer is suspected or screening is warranted, inspection by sigmoidoscopy is necessary.

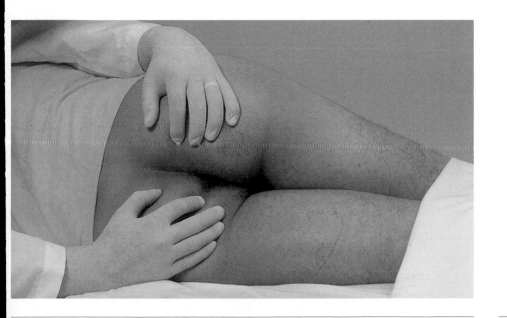

Inspect the sacrococcygeal and perianal areas for lumps, ulcers, inflammation, rashes, or excoriations. Adult perianal skin is normally more pigmented and somewhat coarser than the skin over the buttocks. Palpate any abnormal areas, noting lumps or tenderness.

Examine the anus and rectum. Lubricate your gloved index finger, explain to the patient what you are going to do, and tell him that the examination may make him feel as if he were moving his bowels but that he will not do so. Ask him to strain down. Inspect the anus, noting any lesions.

As the patient strains, place the pad of your lubricated and gloved index finger over the anus. As the sphincter relaxes, gently insert your fingertip into the anal canal, in a direction pointing toward the umbilicus.

Anal and perianal lesions include hemorrhoids, venereal warts, herpes, syphilitic chancre, and carcinoma. A perianal abscess produces a painful, tender, indurated, and reddened mass. Pruritus ani causes swollen, thickened, fissured skin with excoriations.

Soft, pliable tags of redundant skin at the anal margin are common. Though sometimes due to past anal surgery or previously thrombosed hemorrhoids, they are often unexplained.

See Table 15-1, Abnormalities of the Anus, Surrounding Skin, and Rectum (pp. 457–458).

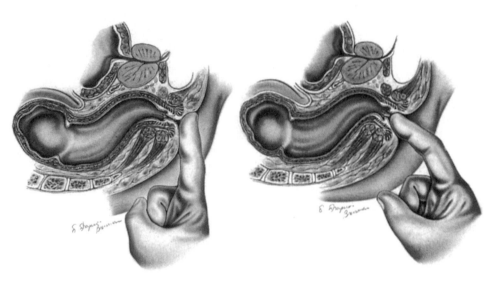

MEDIAN SECTIONS—VIEW FROM THE PATIENT'S RIGHT SIDE. PATIENT LYING ON HIS LEFT SIDE

If you feel the sphincter tighten, pause and reassure the patient. When in a moment the sphincter relaxes, proceed. Occasionally, severe tenderness prevents you from examining the anus. Do not try to force it. Instead, place your fingers on both sides of the anus, gently spread the orifice, and ask the patient to strain down. Look for a lesion, such as an anal fissure, that might explain the tenderness.

If you can proceed without undue discomfort, note:

• The sphincter tone of the anus. Normally, the muscles of the anal sphincter close snugly around your finger.

• Tenderness, if any

Sphincter tightness in anxiety, inflammation, or scarring; laxity in some neurologic diseases

- Induration

Induration may be due to inflammation, scarring, or malignancy.

- Irregularities or nodules

Insert your finger into the rectum as far as possible. Rotate your hand clockwise to palpate as much of the rectal surface as possible on the patient's right side, then counterclockwise to palpate the surface posteriorly and on the patient's left side.

Note any nodules, irregularities, or induration. To bring a possible lesion into reach, take your finger off the rectal surface, ask the patient to strain down, and palpate again.

The irregular border of a rectal cancer is shown below.

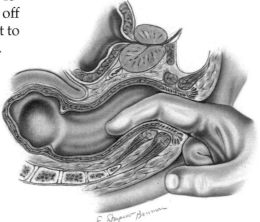

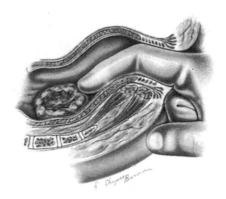

Then rotate your hand further counterclockwise so that your finger can *examine the posterior surface of the prostate gland.* By turning your body somewhat away from the patient, you can feel this area more easily. Tell the patient that you are going to feel his prostate gland, and that it may make him want to urinate but he will not do so.

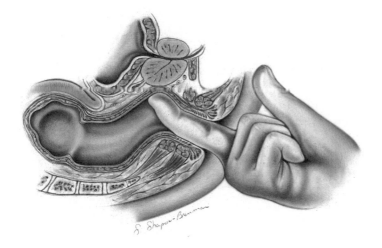

Sweep your finger carefully over the prostate gland, identifying its lateral lobes and the median sulcus between them. Note the size, shape, and consistency of the prostate, and identify any nodules or tenderness. The normal prostate is rubbery and nontender.

See Table 15-2, Abnormalities of the Prostate (p. 459).

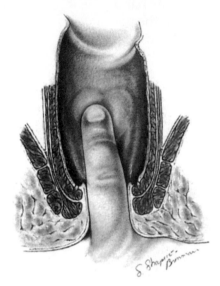

PALPATING THE PROSTATE—VIEW FROM BELOW

If possible, *extend your finger above the prostate* to the region of the seminal vesicles and the peritoneal cavity. Note nodules or tenderness.

A rectal "shelf" of peritoneal metastases (see p. 458) or the tenderness of peritoneal inflammation

Gently withdraw your finger, and wipe the patient's anus or give him tissues to do it himself. Note the color of any fecal matter on your glove, and test it for occult blood.

Female

The rectum is usually examined after the female genitalia, while the patient is in the lithotomy position. If a rectal examination alone is indicated, the lateral position offers a satisfactory alternative. It affords a much better view of the perianal and sacrococcygeal areas.

The technique is basically similar to that described for males. The cervix is usually felt readily through the anterior rectal wall. Sometimes, a retroverted uterus is also palpable. Neither of these, nor a vaginal tampon, should be mistaken for a tumor.

Health Promotion and Counseling

Clinicians should discuss screening issues related to prostate cancer to promote health for men, and provide screening recommendations to both men and women for detection of colorectal cancer and adenomatous colonic polyps.

Prostate cancer is the second leading cause of death in North American men. Groups at increased risk are men over 50, African American men, and men with a family history of prostate cancer. To educate patients about prostate cancer, clinicians must be knowledgeable about a number of issues related to general screening of patients *without symptoms*. Prognosis is most favorable when the cancer is confined to the prostate, and worsens with extracapsular or metastatic spread. Autopsy studies show that many men over 50, and even some who are younger, have nests of cancerous prostate cells that have never caused disease. Since many of these tumors are quiescent, early detection may increase unnecessary testing and treatment without affecting survival. A further complication in decisions about screening is that currently available screening tests are not highly accurate, which heightens patient concern and leads to additional noninvasive and invasive testing.

The two principal screening tests for prostate cancer are the digital rectal examination (DRE) and the prostate specific antigen test (PSA). Each of these tests has distinct limitations that warrant careful review with the patient.* The DRE reaches only the posterior and lateral surfaces of the prostate, missing 25% to 35% of tumors in other areas. Sensitivity of the DRE for prostate cancer is low, ranging from 20% to 68%. In addition, because the DRE has a high rate of false positives, further testing by transrectal ultrasound or even biopsy is common. Many professional societies recommend annual DRE between the ages of 40 or 50 and 70. In contrast, the U.S. Preventive Health Services Task Force currently recommends against routine screening by DRE until there is more definitive evidence of increased survival from early detection and of decreased adverse effects from testing and even surgery (prostatectomy carries up to a 20% risk of impotence and a 5% risk of urinary incontinence). Instead, the Task Force advises clinicians to counsel all men requesting screening about the utility of testing and "the benefits and harms of early detection and treatment."

The benefits of PSA testing are equally unclear. The PSA can be elevated in benign conditions like hyperplasia and prostatitis, and its detection rate for prostate cancer is low, about 28% to 35% in asymptomatic men. Several groups recommend annual combined screening with PSA and DRE for men over 50 and for African Americans and men over age 40 with a positive family history. Other groups, including the U.S. Preven-

---

*U.S. Preventive Health Services Task Force. Guide to Clinical Preventive Services, 2nd ed. Baltimore, Williams & Wilkins, pp. 119–134, 1996.

tive Health Services Task Force, do not recommend routine PSA screening until its benefits are more firmly established.

For men *with symptoms* of prostate disorders, the clinician's role is more straightforward. As men approach 50, risk of prostate cancer begins to increase. Review the symptoms of prostate disorders—incomplete emptying of the bladder, urinary frequency or urgency, weak or intermittent stream or straining to initiate flow, hematuria, nocturia, or even bony pains in the pelvis. Men may be reluctant to report such symptoms, but should be encouraged to seek evaluation and treatment early.

To increase detection of colorectal cancer, clinicians can make use of three screening tests that are currently available: the DRE, the fecal occult blood test (FOBT), and sigmoidoscopy. Both the DRE and the FOBT have significant limitations. The DRE permits the clinician to examine only 7 to 8 cm of the rectum (usually about 11 cm long)—only about 10% of colorectal cancers arise in this zone. The FOBT (see discussion on p. 379) detects only 2% to 11% of colorectal cancers and 20% to 30% of adenomas in individuals over age 50, and results in a high rate of false positives. Among advocates, the DRE and FOBT are usually performed annually after age 40 to 50. Flexible sigmoidoscopy (also discussed on p. 379) permits good surveillance of the distal third of the colon. It is generally recommended every 3 to 5 years for patients over 50. Patients over 40 with familial polyposis, inflammatory bowel disease, or history of colon cancer in a first-degree relative should be advised to obtain a colonoscopy or air contrast barium enema every 3 to 5 years.

TABLE 15-1   Abnormalities of the Anus, Surrounding Skin, and Rectum

Pilonidal Cyst and Sinus

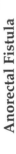

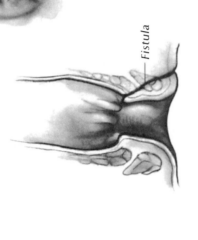

Location

A pilonidal cyst is a fairly common, probably congenital abnormality located in the midline superficial to the coccyx or the lower sacrum. It is clinically identified by the opening of a sinus tract. This opening may exhibit a small tuft of hair and be surrounded by a halo of erythema. Although pilonidal cysts are generally asymptomatic except perhaps for slight drainage, abscess formation and secondary sinus tracts may complicate the picture.

Anorectal Fistula

Opening

An anorectal fistula is an inflammatory tract or tube that opens at one end into the anus or rectum and at the other end onto the skin surface (as shown here) or into another viscus. An abscess usually antedates such a fistula. Look for the fistulous opening or openings anywhere in the skin around the anus.

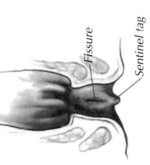

Fistula

Anal Fissure

An anal fissure is a very painful oval ulceration of the anal canal, found most commonly in the midline posteriorly, less commonly in the midline anteriorly. Its long axis lies longitudinally. Inspection may show a swollen "sentinel" skin tag just below it, and gentle separation of the anal margins may reveal the lower edge of the fissure. The sphincter is spastic; the examination painful. Local anesthesia may be required.

Fissure

Sentinel tag

(Table continues on next page)

Table 15-1   Abnormalities of the Anus, Surrounding Skin, and Rectum

TABLE 15-1 *(continued)*

Polyps of the Rectum

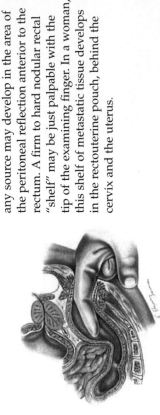

Polyps of the rectum are fairly common. Variable in size and number, they can develop on a stalk (*pedunculated*) or lie on the mucosal surface (*sessile*). They are soft and may be difficult or impossible to feel even when in reach of the examining finger. Proctoscopy is usually required for diagnosis, as is biopsy for the differentiation of benign from malignant lesions.

Cancer of the Rectum

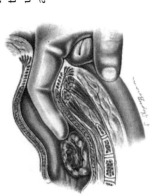

Asymptomatic carcinoma of the rectum makes routine rectal examination important for adults. Illustrated here is the firm, nodular, rolled edge of an ulcerated cancer. Polyps, as noted above, may also be malignant.

Rectal Shelf

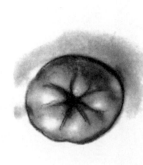

Widespread peritoneal metastases from any source may develop in the area of the peritoneal reflection anterior to the rectum. A firm to hard nodular rectal "shelf" may be just palpable with the tip of the examining finger. In a woman, this shelf of metastatic tissue develops in the rectouterine pouch, behind the cervix and the uterus.

External Hemorrhoids
(Thrombosed)

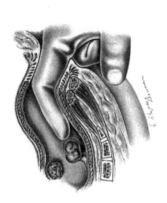

External hemorrhoids are dilated hemorrhoidal veins that originate below the pectinate line and are covered with skin. They seldom produce symptoms unless thrombosis occurs. This causes acute local pain that is increased by defecation and by sitting. A tender, swollen, bluish, ovoid mass is visible at the anal margin.

Internal Hemorrhoids
(Prolapsed)

ANTERIOR

POSTERIOR

Internal hemorrhoids are an enlargement of the normal vascular cushions that are located above the pectinate line. Here they are not usually palpable. Sometimes, especially during defecation, internal hemorrhoids may cause bright red bleeding. They may also prolapse through the anal canal and appear as reddish, moist, protruding masses, typically located in one or more of the positions illustrated.

Prolapse of the Rectum

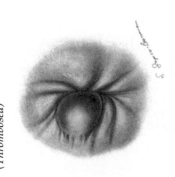

On straining for a bowel movement the rectal mucosa, with or without its muscular wall, may prolapse through the anus, appearing as a doughnut or rosette of red tissue. A prolapse involving only mucosa is relatively small and shows radiating folds, as illustrated. When the entire bowel wall is involved, the prolapse is larger and covered by concentrically circular folds.

Table 15-2 Abnormalities of the Prostate

TABLE 15-2 *Abnormalities of the Prostate*

Normal Prostate Gland

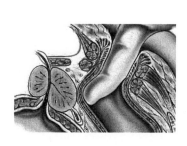

As palpated through the anterior rectal wall, the normal prostate is a rounded, heart-shaped structure about 2.5 cm in length. The median sulcus can be felt between the two lateral lobes. Only the posterior surface of the prostate is palpable. Anterior lesions, including those that may obstruct the urethra, are not detectable by physical examination.

Cancer of the Prostate

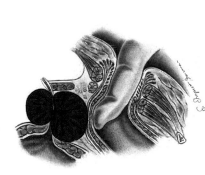

Cancer of the prostate is suggested by an area of hardness in the gland. A distinct hard nodule that alters the contour of the gland may or may not be palpable. As the cancer enlarges, it feels irregular and may extend beyond the confines of the gland. The median sulcus may be obscured. Hard areas in the prostate are not always malignant. They may also result from prostatic stones, chronic inflammation, and other conditions.

Benign Prostatic Hyperplasia

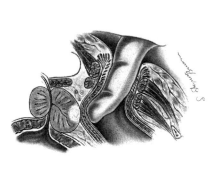

Starting in the fifth decade of life, benign prostatic hyperplasia becomes increasingly prevalent. The affected gland usually feels symmetrically enlarged, smooth, and firm though slightly elastic. It seems to protrude more into the rectal lumen. The median sulcus may be obliterated. Finding a normal-sized gland by palpation, however, does not rule out this diagnosis. Prostatic hyperplasia may obstruct urinary flow, causing symptoms, yet not be palpable.

Prostatitis

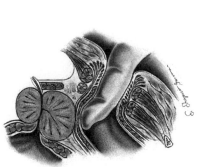

Acute prostatitis (illustrated here) is an acute, febrile condition caused by bacterial infection. The gland is very tender, swollen, firm, and warm. Examine it gently.

Chronic prostatitis does not produce consistent physical findings and must be evaluated by other methods.

The Peripheral Vascular System

CHAPTER 16

Anatomy and Physiology

This chapter focuses on the circulatory supply to the arms and legs. It includes the arteries, the veins, the capillary bed that connects them, and the lymphatic system with its lymph nodes.

Arteries

Arterial pulses are palpable when an artery lies close to the body surface. In the arms, there are two or sometimes three such locations. Pulsations of the *brachial artery* can be felt in and above the bend of the elbow, just medial to the biceps tendon and muscle. The brachial artery divides into the radial and ulnar arteries. *Radial artery* pulsations can be felt on the flexor surface of the wrist laterally. Medially, pulsations of the *ulnar artery* may be palpable, but overlying tissues frequently obscure them.

The radial and ulnar arteries are interconnected by two vascular arches within the hand. Circulation to the hand and fingers is thereby doubly protected against possible arterial occlusion.

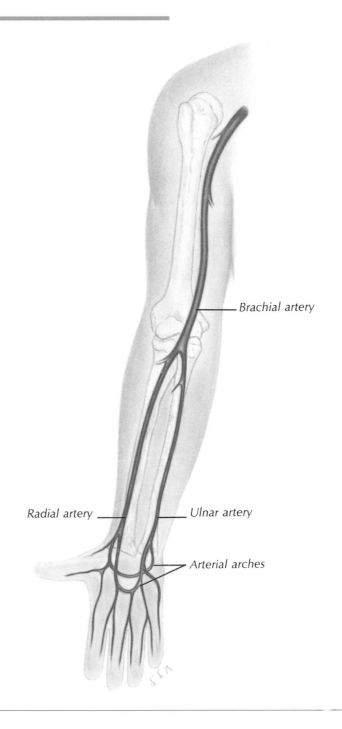

Brachial artery

Radial artery

Ulnar artery

Arterial arches

In the legs, arterial pulsations can usually be felt in four places. Those of the *femoral artery* are palpable below the inguinal ligament, midway between the anterior superior iliac spine and the symphysis pubis. The femoral artery travels downward deep within the thigh, passes medially behind the femur, and becomes the *popliteal artery.* Popliteal pulsations can be felt in the tissues behind the knee. Below the knee, the popliteal artery divides into two branches, both of which continue to the foot. There the anterior branch becomes the *dorsalis pedis artery.* Its pulsations are palpable on the dorsum of the foot just lateral to the extensor tendon of the big toe. The posterior branch, the *posterior tibial artery,* can be felt as it passes behind the medial malleolus of the ankle.

Like the hand, the foot is protected by an interconnecting arch between its two chief arterial branches.

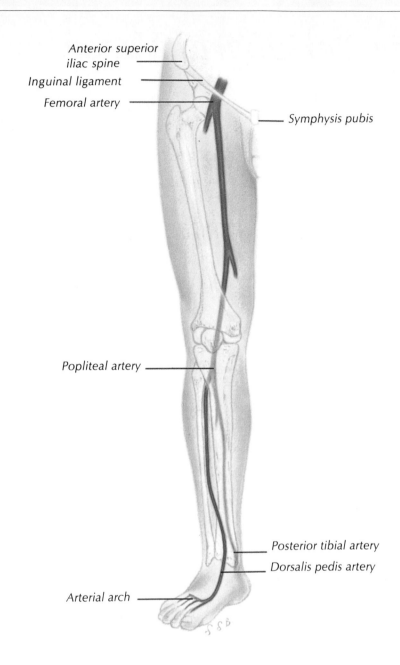

Anterior superior iliac spine

Inguinal ligament

Femoral artery

Symphysis pubis

Popliteal artery

Posterior tibial artery

Dorsalis pedis artery

Arterial arch

Veins

The veins from the arms, together with those from the upper trunk and the head and neck, drain into the superior vena cava and on into the right atrium. Veins from the legs and the lower trunk drain upward into the inferior vena cava. Because the leg veins are especially susceptible to dysfunction, they warrant special attention.

The *deep veins* of the legs carry about 90% of the venous return from the lower extremities. They are well supported by surrounding tissues.

In contrast, the *superficial veins* are located subcutaneously, and are supported relatively poorly. The superficial veins include (1) the *great saphenous vein,* which originates on the dorsum of the foot, passes just in front of the medial malleolus, and then continues up the medial aspect of the leg to join the deep venous system (the femoral vein) below the inguinal ligament; and (2) the *small saphenous vein,* which begins at the side of the foot and passes upward along the back of the leg to join the deep system in the popliteal space. Anastomotic veins connect the two saphenous veins superficially and, when dilated, are readily visible. In addition, *communicating (or perforating) veins* connect the saphenous system with the deep venous system.

Deep, superficial, and communicating veins all have one-way valves. These allow venous blood to flow from the superficial to the deep system and toward the heart, but not in the opposite directions. Muscular activity contributes importantly to venous blood flow. As calf muscles contract in walking, for example, blood is squeezed upward against gravity, and competent valves keep it from falling back again.

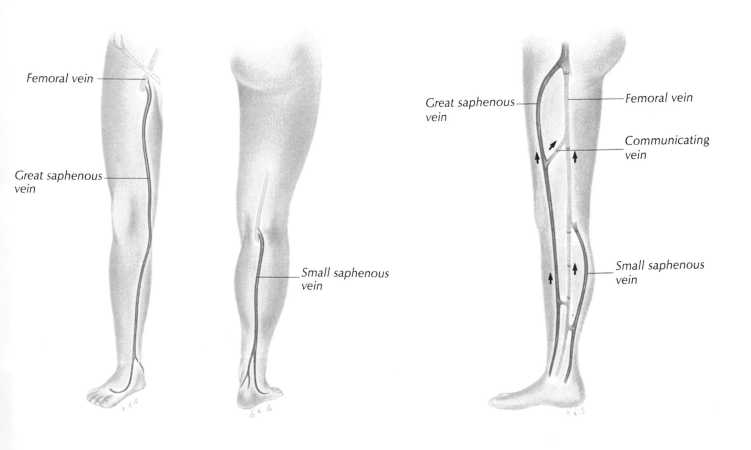

The Lymphatic System and Lymph Nodes

The lymphatic system comprises an extensive vascular network that drains fluid, called lymph, from bodily tissues and returns it to the venous circulation. The system starts peripherally as blind lymphatic capillaries, and continues centrally as thin vascular vessels and then collecting ducts that finally empty into major veins at the root of the neck. The lymph transported in these channels is filtered through lymph nodes that are interposed along the way.

Lymph nodes are round, oval, or bean-shaped structures that vary in size according to their location. Some lymph nodes, such as the preauriculars, if palpable at all, are typically very small. The inguinal nodes, in contrast, are relatively larger—often 1 cm in diameter and occasionally even 2 cm in an adult.

In addition to its vascular functions, the lymphatic system plays an important role in the body's immune system. Cells within the lymph nodes engulf cellular debris and bacteria and produce antibodies.

Only the superficial lymph nodes are accessible to physical examination. These include the cervical nodes (p. 180), the axillary nodes (p. 338), and nodes in the arms and legs.

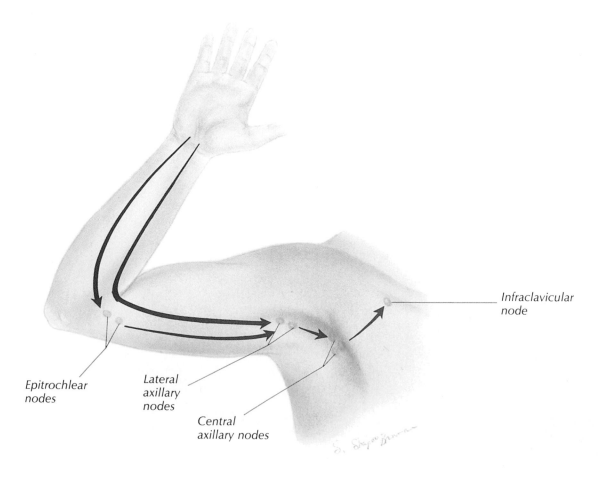

Infraclavicular node

Epitrochlear nodes

Lateral axillary nodes

Central axillary nodes

Recall that the axillary lymph nodes drain most of the arm. Lymphatics from the ulnar surface of the forearm and hand, the little and ring fingers, and the adjacent surface of the middle finger, however, drain first into the *epitrochlear nodes.* These are located on the medial surface of the arm about 3 cm above the elbow. Lymphatics from the rest of the arm drain mostly into the axillary nodes. A few may go directly to the infraclaviculars.

The lymphatics of the lower limb, following the venous supply, consist of both deep and superficial systems. Only the superficial nodes are palpable. The *superficial inguinal nodes* include two groups. The *horizontal group* lies in a chain high in the anterior thigh below the inguinal ligament. It drains the superficial portions of the lower abdomen and buttock, the external genitalia (but not the testes), the anal canal and perianal area, and the lower vagina.

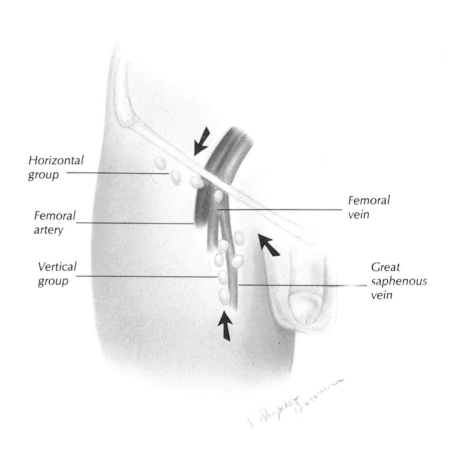

The *vertical group* clusters near the upper part of the saphenous vein and drains a corresponding region of the leg. In contrast, lymphatics from the portion of leg drained by the small saphenous vein (the heel and outer aspect of the foot) join the deep system at the level of the popliteal space. Lesions in this area, therefore, are not usually associated with palpable inguinal lymph nodes.

Fluid Exchange and the Capillary Bed

Blood circulates from arteries to veins through the capillary bed. Here fluids diffuse across the capillary membrane, maintaining a dynamic equilibrium between the vascular and interstitial spaces. Blood pressure (hydrostatic pressure) within the capillary bed, especially near the arteriolar end, forces fluid out into the tissue spaces. In effecting this movement, it is aided by the relatively weak osmotic attraction of proteins within the tissues (interstitial colloid osmotic pressure) and is opposed by the hydrostatic pressure of the tissues.

As blood continues through the capillary bed toward the venous end its hydrostatic pressure falls, and another force gains dominance. This is the colloid osmotic pressure of plasma proteins, which pulls fluid back into the vascular tree. Net flow of fluid, which was directed outward on the arteriolar side of the capillary bed, reverses itself and turns inward on the venous side. Lymphatic capillaries, which also play an important role in this equilibrium, remove excessive fluid, including protein, from the interstitial space.

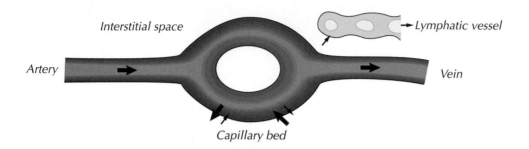

Lymphatic dysfunction or disturbances in hydrostatic or osmotic forces can all disrupt this equilibrium. The most common clinical result is the increased interstitial fluid known as edema. (See Table 16-3, Mechanisms and Patterns of Edema, pp. 480–481.)

Changes With Age

Children and young adolescents normally have larger lymph nodes relative to body size than do adults (see p. 621).

Aging itself brings relatively few clinically important changes to the peripheral vascular system. Although arterial and venous disorders, especially atherosclerosis, do afflict older people more frequently, they probably cannot be considered part of the aging process. Age lengthens the arteries, makes them tortuous, and typically stiffens their walls, but these changes develop with or without atherosclerosis and therefore lack diagnostic specificity. Loss of arterial pulsations is not a part of normal aging, however, and demands careful evaluation. Skin may get thin and dry with age, nails may grow more slowly, and hair on the legs often becomes scant. Because these changes are common, they are not specific for arterial insufficiency, although they are classically associated with it.

Techniques of Examination

Assessment of the peripheral vascular system relies primarily on inspection of the arms and legs, palpation of the pulses, and a search for edema. See Chapter 4 for a method of integrating these techniques into your examination of the limbs. Additional techniques may be useful when you suspect an abnormality.

Arms

Inspect both arms from the fingertips to the shoulders. Note:

- Their size, symmetry, and any swelling

- The venous pattern

- The color of the skin and nail beds and the texture of the skin

Palpate the *radial pulse* with the pads of your fingers on the flexor surface of the wrist laterally. Partially flexing the patient's wrist may help you feel this pulse. Compare the pulses in both arms.

Pulses here and elsewhere in the body may be described as increased, normal, diminished, or absent. If an artery is widely dilated, it is *aneurysmal.*

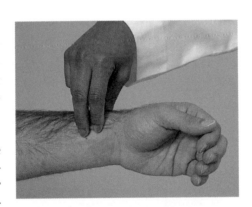

If you suspect arterial insufficiency, feel for the *brachial pulse.* Flex the patient's elbow slightly, and with the thumb of your opposite hand palpate the artery just medial to the biceps tendon at the antecubital crease. The brachial artery can also be felt higher in the arm in the groove between the biceps and triceps muscles.

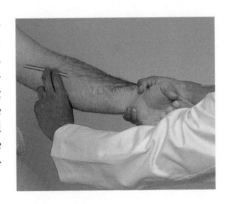

Lymphedema of arm and hand may follow axillary node dissection and radiation therapy.

Prominent veins in an edematous arm suggest venous obstruction.

In Raynaud's disease, wrist pulses are typically normal but spasm of more distal arteries causes episodes of sharply demarcated pallor of the fingers, as shown below.

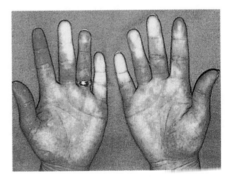

(Source of photo above: Marks R: Skin Disease in Old Age. Philadelphia, JB Lippincott, 1987)

Feel for one or more *epitrochlear nodes*. With the patient's elbow flexed to about 90° and the forearm supported by your hand, reach around behind the arm and feel in the groove between the biceps and triceps muscles, about 3 cm above the medial epicondyle. If a node is present, note its size, consistency, and tenderness.

Epitrochlear nodes are difficult or impossible to identify in most normal people.

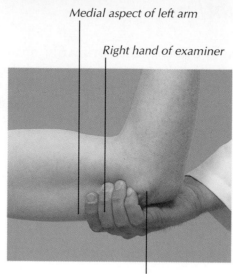

Medial aspect of left arm

Right hand of examiner

Medial epicondyle of humerus

An enlarged epitrochlear node may be secondary to a lesion in its drainage area or may be associated with generalized lymphadenopathy.

Legs

The patient should be lying down and draped so that the external genitalia are covered and the legs fully exposed. A good examination is impossible through stockings or socks!

Inspect both legs from the groin and buttocks to the feet. Note:

- Their size, symmetry, and any swelling
- The venous pattern and any venous enlargement
- Any pigmentation, rashes, scars, or ulcers
- The color and texture of the skin, the color of the nail beds, and the distribution of hair on the lower legs, feet, and toes

Palpate the *superficial inguinal nodes*, including both the horizontal and the vertical groups. Note their size, consistency, and discreteness, and note any tenderness. Nontender, discrete inguinal nodes up to 1 cm or even 2 cm in diameter are frequently palpable in normal people.

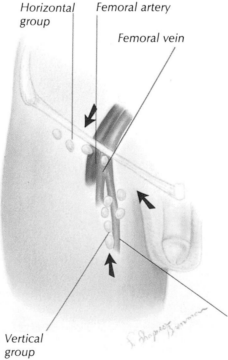

Horizontal group

Femoral artery

Femoral vein

Vertical group

Great saphenous vein

See Table 16-1, Chronic Insufficiency of Arteries and Veins (p. 478).

See Table 16-2, Common Ulcers of the Feet and Ankles (p. 479).

Lymphadenopathy refers to enlargement of the nodes, with or without tenderness. Try to distinguish between local and generalized lymphadenopathy, respectively, by finding either (1) a causative lesion in the drainage area, or (2) enlarged nodes in at least two other noncontiguous lymph node regions.

Palpate the pulses in order to assess the arterial circulation.

- *The femoral pulse.* Press deeply, below the inguinal ligament and about midway between the anterior superior iliac spine and the symphysis pubis. As in deep abdominal palpation, the use of two hands, one on top of the other, may facilitate this examination, especially in obese patients.

A diminished or absent pulse indicates partial or complete arterial occlusion proximally. A decreased or absent femoral pulse, for example, suggests disease at the aortic or iliac level. All pulses distal to the occlusion are typically affected. Chronic arterial occlusion causes intermittent claudication (pp. 96–97), postural color changes (p. 476), and trophic changes in the skin (p. 478). The most common cause is arteriosclerosis obliterans, in which fatty (atheromatous) plaques impede arterial flow.

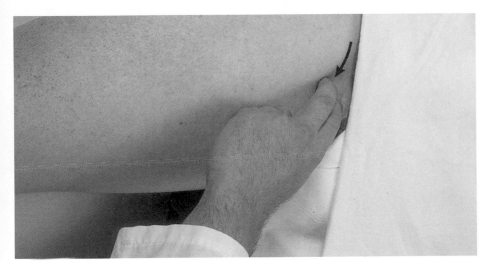

An exaggerated, widened femoral pulse suggests a femoral aneurysm, a pathologic dilatation of the artery.

- *The popliteal pulse.* The patient's knee should be somewhat flexed, the leg relaxed. Place the fingertips of both hands so that they just meet in the midline behind the knee and press them deeply into the popliteal fossa. The popliteal pulse is often more difficult to find than other pulses. It is deeper and feels more diffuse.

An exaggerated, widened popliteal pulse suggests an aneurysm of the popliteal artery. Neither popliteal nor femoral aneurysms are common. They are usually due to arteriosclerosis, and occur primarily in men over age 50.

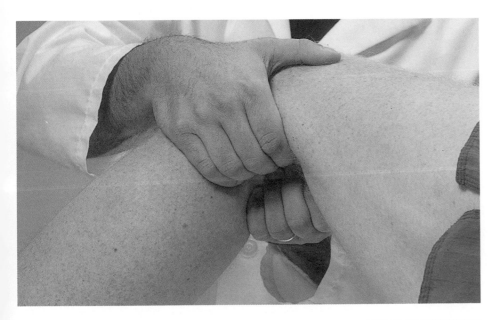

If you cannot feel the popliteal pulse with this approach, try feeling for it with the patient prone. Flex the patient's knee to about 90°, let the lower leg relax against your shoulder or upper arm, and press your two thumbs deeply into the popliteal fossa.

Arteriosclerosis obliterans most commonly obstructs arterial circulation in the thigh. The femoral pulse is then normal, the popliteal decreased or absent.

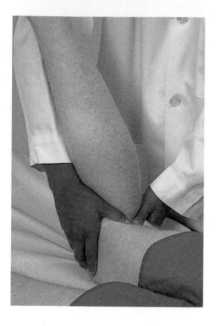
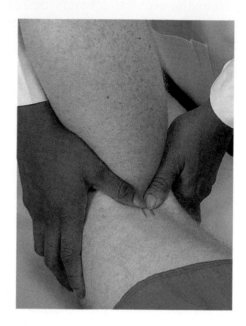

- *The dorsalis pedis pulse.* Feel the dorsum of the foot (not the ankle) just lateral to the extensor tendon of the great toe. If you cannot feel a pulse, explore the dorsum of the foot more laterally.

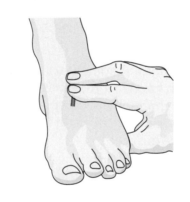

The dorsalis pedis artery may be congenitally absent or may branch higher in the ankle. Search for a pulse more laterally.

Decreased or absent foot pulses (assuming a warm environment) with normal femoral and popliteal pulses suggest occlusive disease in the lower popliteal artery or its branches—a pattern often associated with diabetes mellitus.

- *The posterior tibial pulse.* Curve your fingers behind and slightly below the medial malleolus of the ankle. (This pulse may be hard to feel in a fat or edematous ankle.)

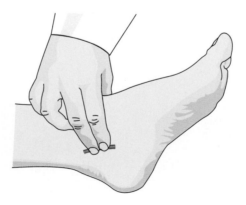

Sudden arterial occlusion, as by embolism or thrombosis, causes pain and numbness or tingling. The limb distal to the occlusion becomes cold, pale, and pulseless. Emergency treatment is required. If collateral circulation is good, only numbness and coolness may result.

Tips on feeling difficult pulses: (1) Position your own body and examining hand comfortably; awkward positions decrease your tactile sensitivity. (2) Place your hand properly and linger there, varying the pressure of your fingers to pick up a weak pulsation. If unsuccessful, then explore the area deliberately. (3) Do not confuse the patient's pulse with your own pulsating fingertips. If you are unsure, count your own heart rate and compare it with the patient's. The rates are usually different. Your carotid pulse is convenient for this comparison.

Note the temperature of the feet and legs with the backs of your fingers. Compare one side with the other. Bilateral coldness is most often due to a cold environment or anxiety.

Coldness, especially when unilateral or associated with other signs, suggests arterial insufficiency, an inadequate arterial circulation.

Look for edema. Compare one foot and leg with the other, noting their relative size and the prominence of veins, tendons, and bones.

Edema causes swelling that may obscure the veins, tendons, and bony prominences.

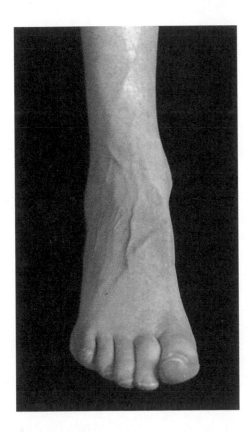

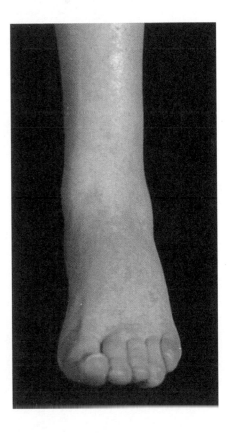

Check for pitting edema. Press firmly but gently with your thumb for at least 5 seconds (1) over the dorsum of each foot (see p. 472), (2) behind each medial malleolus, and (3) over the shins. Look for *pitting*—a depression caused by pressure from your thumb. Normally there is none. The severity of edema is graded on a four-point scale, from slight to very marked.

See Table 16-3, Mechanisms and Patterns of Edema (pp. 480–481).

See Table 16-4, Some Peripheral Causes of Edema (p. 482).

Shown below is 3+ pitting edema.

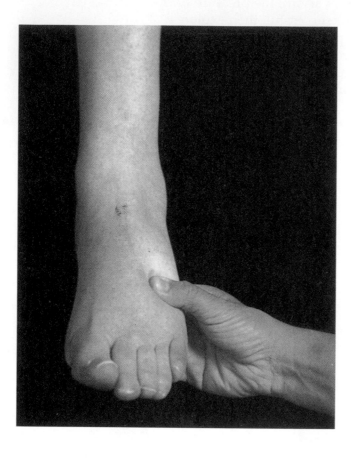

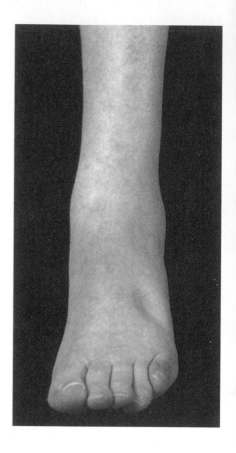

If you suspect edema, *measurement of the legs* may help you to identify it and to follow its course. With a flexible tape, measure (1) the forefoot, (2) the smallest possible circumference above the ankle, (3) the largest circumference at the calf, and (4) the midthigh a measured distance above the patella with the knee extended. Compare one side with the other. A difference of more than 1 cm just above the ankle or 2 cm at the calf is unusual in normal people and suggests edema.

Conditions such as muscular atrophy can also cause different circumferences in the legs.

If edema is present, look for possible causes in the peripheral vascular system. These include (1) recent deep venous thrombosis, (2) chronic venous insufficiency due to previous deep venous thrombosis or to incompetence of the venous valves, and (3) lymphedema. Note the extent of the swelling. How far up the leg does it go?

In deep venous thrombosis, the extent of edema suggests the location of the occlusion: the calf when the lower leg or the ankle is swollen, the iliofemoral veins when the entire leg is swollen.

Is the swelling unilateral or bilateral? Are the veins unusually prominent?

Venous distention suggests a venous cause of edema.

Try to identify any venous tenderness that may accompany deep venous thrombosis. Palpate the groin just medial to the femoral pulse for tenderness of the femoral vein. Next, with the patient's leg flexed at the

A painful, pale, swollen leg, together with tenderness of the femoral vein, suggests deep

knee and relaxed, palpate the calf. With your fingerpads, gently compress the calf muscles against the tibia, and search for any tenderness or cords. Deep venous thrombosis, however, may have no demonstrable signs, and diagnosis often depends on high clinical suspicion and other testing.

iliofemoral thrombosis. Tenderness and cords deep in the calf suggest deep thrombosis there. Calf tenderness, however, may be present without thrombosis.

Note the color of the skin.

Is there a local area of redness? If so, note its temperature, and gently try to feel the firm cord of a thrombosed vein in the area. The calf is most often involved.

Local swelling, redness, warmth, and a subcutaneous cord suggest superficial thrombophlebitis.

Are there brownish areas near the ankles?

Note any ulcers in the skin. Where are they?

A brownish color or ulcers just above the ankle suggest chronic venous insufficiency.

Feel the thickness of the skin.

Thickened (brawny) skin occurs in lymphedema and advanced venous insufficiency.

Ask the patient to stand, and *inspect the saphenous system for varicosities*. The standing posture allows any varicosities to fill with blood and makes them visible. You can easily miss them when the patient is in a supine position. Feel for any varicosities, noting any signs of thrombophlebitis.

Varicose veins are dilated and tortuous. Their walls may feel somewhat thickened. Many can be seen in the leg below.

Special Techniques

Mapping Varicose Veins. You can map out the course and connections of varicose veins by transmitting pressure waves along the blood-filled veins. With the patient standing, place your palpating fingers gently on a vein and, with your other hand below it, compress the vein sharply. Feel for a pressure wave transmitted to the fingers of your upper hand. A palpable pressure wave indicates that the two parts of the vein are connected.

A wave may also be transmitted downward, but not as easily.

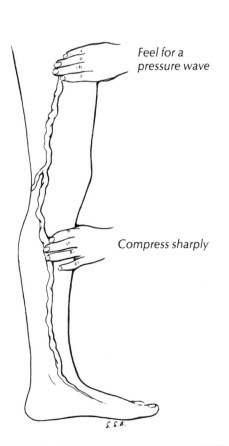

Feel for a pressure wave

Compress sharply

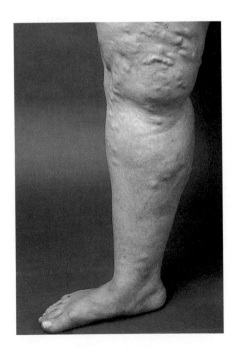

Evaluating the Competency of Venous Valves. By the *retrograde filling (Trendelenburg) test,* you can assess the valvular competency in both the communicating veins and the saphenous system. Start with the patient supine. Elevate one leg to about 90° to empty it of venous blood.

Next, occlude the great saphenous vein in the upper thigh by manual compression, using enough pressure to occlude this vein but not the deeper vessels. Ask the patient to stand. While you keep the vein occluded, watch for venous filling in the leg. Normally the saphenous vein fills from below, taking about 35 seconds as blood flows through the capillary bed into the venous system.

Rapid filling of the superficial veins while the saphenous vein is occluded indicates incompetent valves in the communicating veins. Blood flows quickly in a retrograde direction from the deep to the saphenous system.

After the patient has stood for 20 seconds, release the compression and look for any sudden additional venous filling. Normally there is none: competent valves in the saphenous vein block retrograde flow. Slow venous filling continues.

Sudden additional filling of superficial veins after release of compression indicates incompetent valves in the saphenous vein.

When both steps of this test are normal, the response is termed negative–negative. Negative–positive and positive–negative responses may also occur.

When both steps are abnormal, the test is positive–positive.

Evaluating the Bedfast Patient. People who are confined to bed, especially when they are emaciated, elderly, or neurologically impaired, are particularly susceptible to skin damage and ulceration. *Pressure sores* result when sustained compression obliterates arteriolar and capillary blood flow to the skin. Sores may also result from the shearing forces created by bodily movements. When a person slides down in bed from a partially sitting position, for example, or is dragged rather than lifted up from a supine position, the movements may distort the soft tissues of the buttocks and close off the arteries and arterioles within. Friction and moisture further increase the risk.

Assess every susceptible patient by carefully inspecting the skin that overlies the sacrum, buttocks, greater trochanters, knees, and heels. Roll the patient onto one side to see the sacrum and buttocks.

Local redness of the skin warns of impending necrosis, although some deep pressure sores develop without antecedent redness. Ulcers may be seen.

Use the side-lying position also to evaluate a patient for *sacral edema.* Press firmly for at least 5 seconds in the sacral area and look for any pitting. If you find it, check other areas higher on the back.

Dependent edema may accumulate in the back of a bed patient and not appear in the legs.

Evaluating the Arterial Supply to the Hand. If you suspect arterial insufficiency in the arm or hand, try to feel the *ulnar pulse* as well as the radial and brachial pulses. Feel for it deeply on the flexor surface of the wrist medially. Partially flexing the patient's wrist may help you. The pulse of a normal ulnar artery, however, may not be palpable.

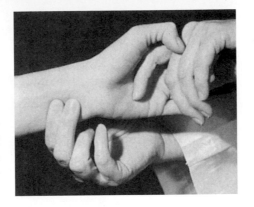

Arterial insufficiency is much less common in the arms than in the legs. Thromboangiitis obliterans (*Buerger's disease*) or acute arterial occlusion (as from an embolus) may cause it, producing diminished or absent pulses at the wrist.

The *Allen test* gives further information. This test is also useful to assure the patency of the ulnar artery before puncturing the radial artery for blood samples. The patient should rest with hands in lap, palms up.

Ask the patient to make a tight fist with one hand; then compress both radial and ulnar arteries firmly between your thumbs and fingers. Next, ask the patient to open the hand into a relaxed, slightly flexed position. The palm is pale.

Extending the hand fully may cause pallor and a falsely positive test.

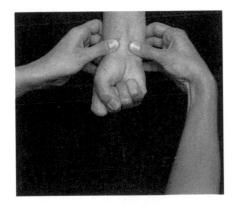
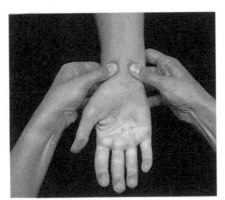

Release your pressure over the ulnar artery. If the ulnar artery is patent, the palm flushes within about 3 to 5 seconds.

Persisting pallor indicates occlusion of the ulnar artery or its distal branches.

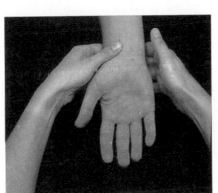
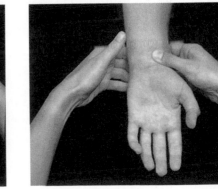

Patency of the radial artery may be tested by releasing the radial artery while still compressing the ulnar.

Postural Color Changes of Chronic Arterial Insufficiency. If pain or diminished pulses suggest arterial insufficiency (an inadequate arterial circulation), look for postural color changes. Raise both legs, as shown at the right, to about 60° until maximal pallor of the feet develops—usually within a minute. In light-skinned persons, either maintenance of normal color, as seen in this right foot, or slight pallor is normal.

Marked pallor on elevation suggests arterial insufficiency.

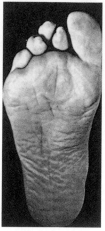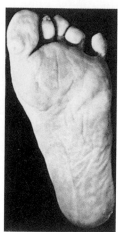

Then ask the patient to sit up with legs dangling down. Compare both feet, noting the time required for:

- Return of pinkness to the skin, normally about 10 seconds or less
- Filling of the veins of the feet and ankles, normally about 15 seconds

This right foot has normal color and the veins on the foot have filled. These normal responses, suggest an adequate circulation.

The foot below is still pale and the veins are just starting to fill—signs of arterial insufficiency.

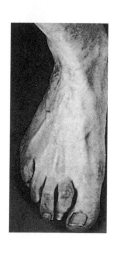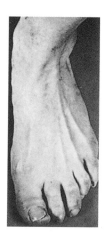

Look for any unusual *rubor* (dusky redness) to replace the pallor of the dependent foot. Rubor may take a minute or more to appear.

Normal responses accompanied by diminished arterial pulses suggest that a good collateral circulation has developed around an arterial occlusion.

Color changes may be difficult to see in darker-skinned persons. Inspect the soles of the feet for these changes, and use tangential lighting to see the veins.

(Source of foot photos: Kappert A., Winsor T: Diagnosis of Peripheral Vascular Diseases. Philadelphia, FA Davis, 1972).

Persisting rubor on dependency suggests arterial insufficiency (see p. 478). When veins are incompetent, dependent rubor and the timing of color return and venous filling are not reliable tests of arterial insufficiency.

Health Promotion and Counseling

Adoption of health-promoting behaviors such as exercise, diet, blood pressure control, and smoking cessation are the most effective ways for patients to reduce risk of peripheral vascular disease (PVD). Routine screening recommendations for the general population are limited to palpation of the peripheral pulses and inspection of the lower extremities and feet. Although PVD is relatively common in individuals over age 50, only 1% to 2% of the population develops symptoms of pain, fatigue, or weakness in the leg muscles with walking and relieved by rest. Symptoms are most likely to occur in smokers and particularly in patients with diabetes, who account for more than half of all amputations. Clinicians should establish quit dates with smokers and review strategies to aid smoking cessation (see p. 268). Patients with diabetes should pursue optimal glucose control and measures to maintain good foot care—daily inspection of feet for skin breakdown or ulcers, well fitting shoes, and regular clipping of nails by a podiatrist.

Table 16-1 Chronic Insufficiency of Arteries and Veins

TABLE 16-1 Chronic Insufficiency of Arteries and Veins

	Chronic Arterial Insufficiency (*Advanced*)	Chronic Venous Insufficiency (*Advanced*)
	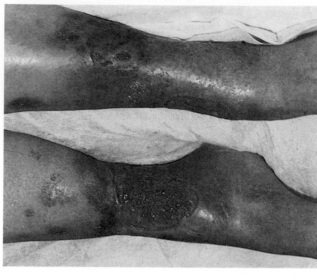 Rubor — Ischemic ulcer —	
Pain	Intermittent claudication, progressing to pain at rest	None to an aching pain on dependency
Pulses	Decreased or absent	Normal, though may be difficult to feel through edema
Color	Pale, especially on elevation; dusky red on dependency	Normal, or cyanotic on dependency. Petechiae and then brown pigmentation appear with chronicity.
Temperature	Cool	Normal
Edema	Absent or mild; may develop as the patient tries to relieve rest pain by lowering the leg	Present, often marked
Skin Changes	Trophic changes: thin, shiny, atrophic skin; loss of hair over the foot and toes; nails thickened and ridged	Often brown pigmentation around the ankle, stasis dermatitis, and possible thickening of the skin and narrowing of the leg as scarring develops
Ulceration	If present, involves toes or points of trauma on feet	If present, develops at sides of ankle, especially medially
Gangrene	May develop	Does not develop

(Sources of photos: *Arterial Insufficiency*—Kappert A., Winsor T: Diagnosis of Peripheral Vascular Disease. Philadelphia, FA Davis, 1972; *Venous Insufficiency*—Marks R: Skin Disease in Old Age. Philadelphia, JB Lippincott, 1987)

Table 16-2   Common Ulcers of the Feet and Ankles

TABLE 16-2   *Common Ulcers of the Feet and Ankles*

	Arterial Insufficiency	Chronic Venous Insufficiency	Neuropathic Ulcer
	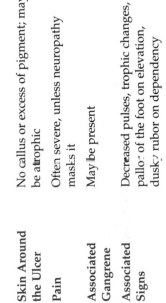	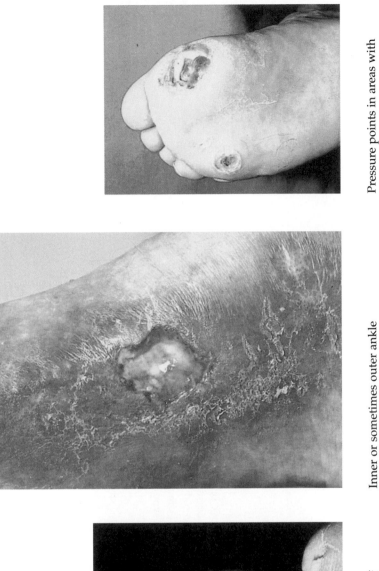	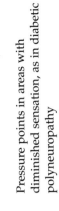
Location	Toes, feet, or possibly in areas of trauma (e.g., the shin)	Inner or sometimes outer ankle	Pressure points in areas with diminished sensation, as in diabetic polyneuropathy
Skin Around the Ulcer	No callus or excess of pigment; may be atrophic	Pigmented, sometimes fibrotic	Calloused
Pain	Often severe, unless neuropathy masks it	Not severe	Absent (and therefore the ulcer may go unnoticed)
Associated Gangrene	May be present	Absent	In uncomplicated neuropathic ulcer, absent
Associated Signs	Decreased pulses, trophic changes, pallor of the foot on elevation, dusky rubor on dependency	Edema, pigmentation, stasis dermatitis, and possibly cyanosis of the foot on dependency	Decreased sensation, absent ankle jerks

(Source of photos: Marks R: Skin Disease in Old Age. Philadelphia, JB Lippincott, 1987)

Table 16-3   Mechanisms and Patterns of Edema

TABLE 16-3   Mechanisms and Patterns of Edema

Causes of edema may be divided roughly into two groups: (1) *systemic causes*, including congestive heart failure, hypoalbuminemia, and excessive renal retention of salt and water; and (2) *local causes*, such as venous stasis, lymphatic stasis, and prolonged dependency. Increased capillary permeability may be either local or general in distribution.

	Mechanism of Edema	Distribution of Edema	Other Signs May Include—
Right-Sided Congestive Heart Failure	Decreased ability of the heart to pump venous blood forward increases the hydrostatic pressure in the veins and capillaries, producing congestion and loss of fluid into the tissues.	Edema first appears in the dependent areas of the body where hydrostatic pressure is highest (i.e., the feet and the legs). When the patient is bedridden, the low back is dependent and becomes edematous.	Increased jugular venous pressure, an enlarged and often tender liver, an enlarged heart, S_3
Hypoalbuminemia	Decreased colloid osmotic pressure in the plasma allows excessive fluid to escape into the interstitial space and remain there. Causes include cirrhosis, the nephrotic syndrome, and severe malnutrition.	Edema may appear first in the loose subcutaneous tissues of the eyelids, especially after the patient lies down at night, but may also show first in the feet and legs. In cirrhosis, ascites often appears first. When cirrhosis is more advanced, edema may become generalized.	Serum albumin is low. Signs of chronic liver disease such as ascites, spider angiomas, and jaundice. Signs of the nephrotic syndrome vary with its causes.
Excessive Renal Retention of Salt and Water	The kidneys may initiate edema by retaining excessive amounts of salt and water, some of which pass into the interstitial space. Drugs such as corticosteroids, estrogens, and some antihypertensives may be responsible.	Edema usually starts in the dependent areas and may become generalized.	Usually none

Table 16-3 Mechanisms and Patterns of Edema

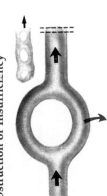

Mechanism	Description	Distribution	Appearance
Venous Stasis Secondary to Obstruction or Insufficiency	Thrombophlebitis may block venous drainage. Venous valves may be damaged by thrombophlebitis or become incompetent because of varicose veins. Less commonly, veins may be compressed from the outside, as by a tumor or fibrosis. In any case, hydrostatic pressure rises in the veins and capillaries, producing excessive loss of fluid into the tissues.	Edema is limited to the area of blockage, often one leg or, less commonly, both legs or an arm. A blocked superior vena cava may cause edema in the entire upper part of the body.	Local swelling and increased tissue turgor. When large veins such as the superior vena cava or the iliofemoral veins are involved, an increased venous pattern of dilated veins may be visible. Tenderness sometimes accompanies phlebitis. Signs of venous insufficiency, as outlined on p. 479
Lymphatic Stasis (Lymphedema)	Lymph channels may be congenitally abnormal, or may be obstructed by tumor, fibrosis, or inflammation.	Local, often involving one or both legs. Lymphedema of an arm may follow axillary node dissection and radiation therapy.	Indurated skin in the involved area. Except in the early phases, lymphedema is characteristically nonpitting.
Orthostatic Edema	Prolonged sitting or standing, without sufficient muscular activity to promote venous flow, increases the pressure in the veins and capillaries and thus increases the flow of fluid into the interstitial spaces.	The dependent areas (e.g., the legs)	None. Get a good history, including long trips. People who get up after prolonged bed rest are at first especially susceptible to orthostatic edema.
Increased Capillary Permeability	When capillary permeability increases, protein leaks into the interstitial spaces and, by increasing the interstitial colloid osmotic pressure, draws excessive fluid with it. Causes vary, including burns, snake bite, and allergy.	Usually local, depending on the cause; may be generalized	Variable

Table 16-4   Some Peripheral Causes of Edema

TABLE 16-4   Some Peripheral Causes of Edema

	Orthostatic Edema	Lymphedema	Lipedema	Chronic Venous Insufficiency*
Process	Edema from prolonged sitting or standing	Lymphatic obstruction	Fatty deposition in legs (not true edema)	Chronic obstruction or valvular incompetence of the deep veins
Nature of Edema	Soft, pits on pressure	Soft early, becomes hard and nonpitting	Minimal, if any	Soft, pits on pressure; later may become brawny (hard)
Skin Thickening	Absent	Becomes marked	Absent	May be present, especially near ankle
Ulceration	Absent	Rare	Absent	Common
Pigmentation	Absent	Absent	Absent	Common
Edema of Foot	Present	Present, including toes	Absent	Often present
Bilaterality	Always	Often	Always	Occasionally

* The advanced state described here is seen in *deep venous insufficiency*, also called postphlebitic syndrome or postthrombotic syndrome. *Superficial venous insufficiency seldom progresses to this state; mild bilateral edema that disappears overnight is its chief manifestation.*

The Musculoskeletal System

CHAPTER 17

Anatomy and Physiology

This section reviews the structure and function of the major joints and their connecting bony structures, muscles, and soft tissues, including ligaments, tendons, and bursae. Knowledge of the major bony landmarks and soft-tissue structures of each joint is essential to the systematic evaluation of musculoskeletal function. In this Anatomy and Physiology section, practice learning the important anatomic features of each joint on yourself or on a fellow student. The Overview for each joint should help orient you to its distinguishing characteristics. Then turn to Techniques of Examination to learn the fundamental steps for examining each joint—inspection; palpation to identify bony landmarks and soft-tissue structures; assessment of range of motion (the directions of joint movement); and maneuvers to test joint function.

Both sections of the chapter follow a "head-to-toe" sequence, beginning with the jaw and the joints of the upper extremities and then proceeding to the spine and hip and on to the joints of the lower extremities.

Structure and Function of Joints

To understand joint function, begin by reviewing the various types of joints and how they articulate, or interconnect, and the role of bursae in easing joint movement.

Types of Joints. There are three primary types of joint articulation—synovial, cartilaginous, and fibrous—allowing varying degrees of joint movement.

Type of Joint	Extent of Movement	Example
Synovial	Freely movable	Knee, shoulder
Cartilaginous	Slightly movable	Vertebral bodies of the spine
Fibrous	Immovable	Skull sutures

In synovial joints, the bones do not touch each other and the joint articulations are *freely movable.* The bones are covered by *articular cartilage* and separated by a *synovial cavity* that cushions joint movement, as shown below. A *synovial membrane* lines the synovial cavity and secretes a small amount of viscous lubricating fluid—the *synovial fluid.* The membrane is attached at the margins of the articular cartilage and pouched or folded to accommodate joint movement. Surrounding the synovial membrane is a fibrous *joint capsule,* which is strengthened by ligaments extending from bone to bone.

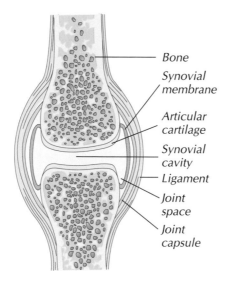

Bone
Synovial membrane
Articular cartilage
Synovial cavity
Ligament
Joint space
Joint capsule

Synovial

Cartilaginous joints, such as those between vertebrae, are *slightly movable.* The bony surfaces are separated by fibrocartilaginous discs. At the center of each disc is the *nucleus pulposus,* fibrocartilaginous material that serves as a cushion or shock absorber between bony surfaces.

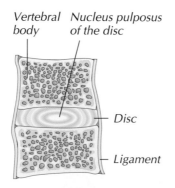

Vertebral body   Nucleus pulposus of the disc
Disc
Ligament

Cartilaginous

In fibrous joints, such as the sutures of the skull, the bones are held together by intervening layers of fibrous tissue or cartilage. The bones are almost in direct contact, which allows *no appreciable movement.*

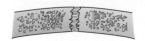

Fibrous

As you learn about the examination of the musculoskeletal system, think about how the anatomy of the joint relates to its movement. Many of the joints we examine are synovial, or movable, joints. The shape of the articulating surfaces of synovial joints determines the type of motion in the joint. *Spheroidal joints* have a ball-and-socket configuration—a rounded convex surface articulating with a cuplike cavity, allowing a wide range of rotatory movement as in the shoulder and hip. *Hinge joints* are flat, planar, or slightly curved, allowing a gliding motion in one plane only, as in flexion and extension of the digits. In *condylar joints,* such as the knee, the articulating surfaces are convex or concave, referred to as condyles.

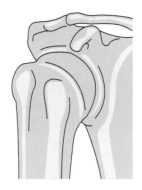

**Spheroidal joint
(Ball and socket)**

Synovial Joints

Type of Joint	Articular Shape	Movement	Example
Spheroidal (ball and socket)	Convex surface in concave cavity	Wide-ranging flexion, extension, abduction, adduction rotation, circumduction	Shoulder, hip
Hinge	Flat, planar	Motion in one plane; flexion, extension	Interphalangeal joints of hand and foot; elbow
Condylar	Convex or concave	Movement of two articulating surfaces not dissociable	Knee; temporo-mandibular joint

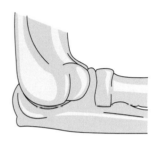

Hinge joint

Bursae. Easing joint action are *bursae,* roughly disc-shaped synovial sacs that allow adjacent muscles or muscles and tendons to glide over each other during movement. They lie between the skin and the convex surface of a bone or joint (as in the prepatellar bursa of the knee, p. 502) or in areas where tendons or muscles rub against bone, ligaments, or other tendons or muscles (as in the subacromial bursa of the shoulder, p. 490)

Knowledge of the underlying joint anatomy and movement will help you assess joints subjected to trauma. Your knowledge of the soft-tissue structures, ligaments, tendons, and bursae will help you evaluate the changes of arthritis.

Temporomandibular Joint

Overview, Bony Structures, and Joints. The temporomandibular joint is the most active joint in the body, opening and closing up to 2,000 times a day. The temporomandibular joint is formed by the fossa and articular tubercle of the temporal bone and the condyle of the mandible. It lies midway between the external acoustic meatus and the zygomatic arch.

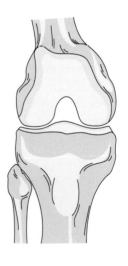

Condylar joint

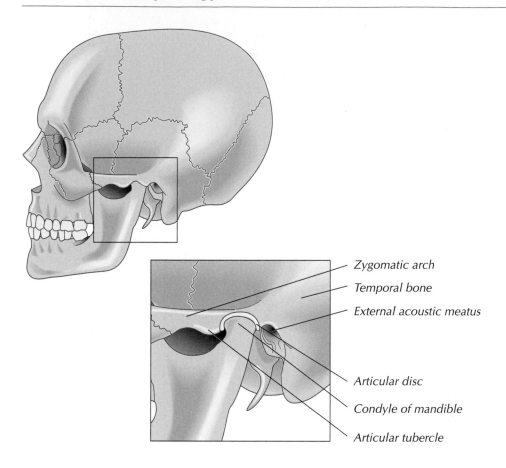

Zygomatic arch

Temporal bone

External acoustic meatus

Articular disc

Condyle of mandible

Articular tubercle

A fibrocartilaginous disc cushions the action of the condyle of the mandible against the synovial membrane and capsule of the articulating surfaces of the temporal bone. (Hence it is a condylar synovial joint.)

Muscle Groups and Additional Structures. The principal muscles opening the mouth are the *external pterygoids*. Closing the mouth are the muscles innervated by Cranial Nerve V, the trigeminal nerve (see p. 559)—the *masseter*, the *temporalis*, and the *internal pterygoids*.

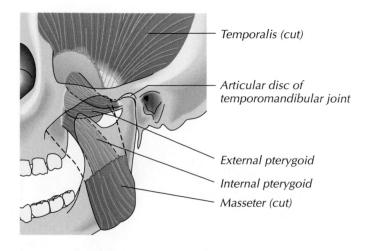

Temporalis (cut)

Articular disc of temporomandibular joint

External pterygoid

Internal pterygoid

Masseter (cut)

The Shoulder

Overview. The shoulder is distinguished by wide-ranging movement in all directions. The humerus is virtually suspended from the scapula, held against the shallow glenoid fossa by the joint capsule and a meshwork of muscles, tendons, and ligaments.

The shoulder derives its mobility from a complex interconnected structure of four joints, three large bones, and three principal muscle groups, often referred to as the *shoulder girdle.* The clavicle and acromion stabilize the shoulder girdle, allowing the humerus to swing out and away from the body, giving the shoulder its remarkable range of motion.

Bony Structures. The bony structures of the shoulder include the humerus, the clavicle, and the scapula. The scapula is anchored to the axial skeleton only by the sternoclavicular joint and inserting muscles, often called the *scapulothoracic articulation.*

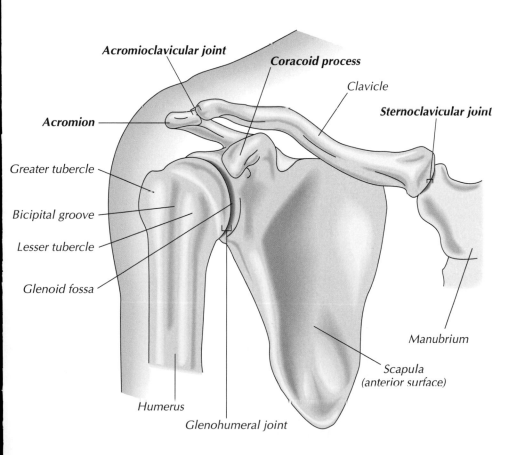

Identify the manubrium, the sternoclavicular joint, and the clavicle. With your fingers, trace the clavicle laterally. Now, from behind, follow the bony spine of the scapula laterally and upward until it becomes the *acromion,* the summit of the shoulder. Its upper surface is rough and slightly convex. Identify the anterior tip of the acromion (*A*) and mark it with ink. With your index finger on top of the acromion, just behind its tip, press medially to find the slightly elevated ridge that marks the distal end of the clavicle. This junction marks the *acromioclavicular joint* (shown by the arrow). Move your finger laterally and down a short step to the next bony prominence, the *greater tubercle of the humerus (B)*. Mark this with ink. Now sweep your finger medially a few centimeters until you feel a large bony prominence, the *coracoid process* of the scapula (*C*). Mark this also. These three points—the tip of the acromion, the greater tubercle of the humerus, and the coracoid process—orient you to the anatomy of the shoulder.

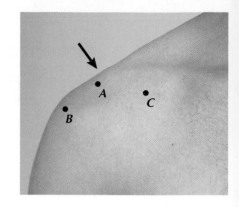

Joints. Three different joints articulate at the shoulder:

- The *glenohumeral joint.* In this joint, the head of the humerus articulates with the shallow glenoid fossa of the scapula. This joint is deeply situated and not normally palpable. It is a classic ball-and-socket joint, allowing the arm its wide arc of movement—flexion, extension, abduction (movement away from the trunk), adduction (movement toward the trunk), rotation, and circumduction.

- The *sternoclavicular joint.* The convex medial end of the clavicle articulates with the concave hollow in the upper sternum.

- The *acromioclavicular joint.* The lateral end of the clavicle articulates with the acromion process of the scapula.

Muscle Groups. Three groups of muscles attach at the shoulder:

- The *scapulohumeral group.* This group extends from the scapula to the humerus. It includes the deltoid, the teres major, and muscles inserting directly on the humerus known as the *rotator cuff* or "SITS muscles," the **S**upraspinatus, **I**nfraspinatus, **T**eres minor, and **Sub**scapularis. The fibrous capsule of the glenohumeral joint is reinforced by the tendons of the SITS muscles. The supraspinatus, which runs above the glenohumeral joint, and the infraspinatus and teres minor, which cross it posteriorly, all insert on the greater tubercle. The subscapularis (not illustrated) originates on the anterior surface of the scapula, crosses the joint anteriorly, and inserts on the lesser tubercle. The scapulohumeral group rotates the shoulder laterally (the rotator cuff), and depresses and rotates the head of the humerus.

- The *axioscapular group.* This group attaches the trunk to the scapula, and includes the trapezius, rhomboids, serratus anterior, and levator scapulae. These muscles rotate and fix the scapula and pull the shoulder backward.

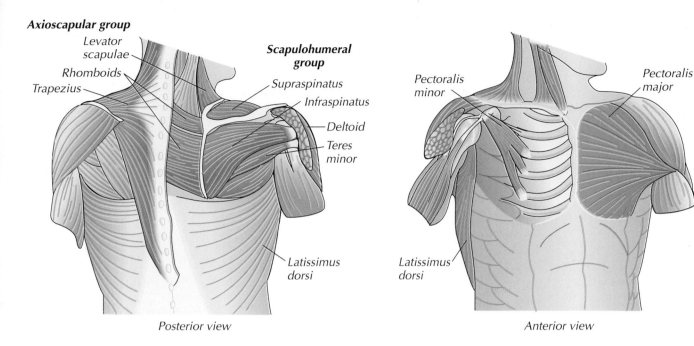

Axioscapular group
Levator scapulae
Rhomboids
Trapezius

Scapulohumeral group
Supraspinatus
Infraspinatus
Deltoid
Teres minor

Latissimus dorsi

Pectoralis minor

Pectoralis major

Latissimus dorsi

Posterior view

Anterior view

Axioscapular group *(pulls shoulder backward)*
Scapulohumeral group *(rotates shoulder laterally; includes rotator cuff)*

Axiohumeral group *(rotates shoulder internally)*

- The *axiohumeral group.* This group attaches the trunk to the humerus. In this group are the pectoralis major, the pectoralis minor, and the latissimus dorsi. These muscles produce internal rotation of the shoulder.

The biceps and triceps, which connect the scapula to the bones of the forearm, are also involved in shoulder movement, particularly abduction.

Additional Structures. Also important to shoulder movement are the *articular capsule and bursae.* Surrounding the glenohumeral joint is a fibrous articular capsule formed by the tendon insertions of the rotator cuff and other capsular muscles. The loose fit of the capsule allows the shoulder bones to separate, and contributes to the shoulder's wide range of movement. The capsule is lined by a synovial membrane with two outpouchings—the subscapular bursa and the synovial sheath of the tendon of the long head of the biceps.

To locate the biceps tendon, rotate the arm externally and find the tendinous cord that runs just medial to the greater tubercle. Roll it under your fingers. This is the tendon of the *long head of the biceps.* It runs in the bicipital groove between the greater and lesser tubercles.

The principal bursa of the shoulder is the *subacromial bursa,* positioned between the acromion and the head of the humerus and overlying the supraspinatus tendon. Abduction of the shoulder compresses this bursa. Normally, the supraspinatus tendon and the subacromial bursa are not palpable. However, if the bursal surfaces are inflamed (subacromial bursitis), there may be tenderness just below the tip of the acromion, pain with abduction and rotation, and loss of smooth movement.

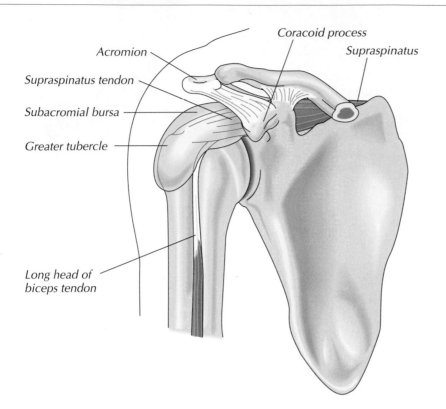

Coracoid process

Acromion

Supraspinatus

Supraspinatus tendon

Subacromial bursa

Greater tubercle

Long head of
biceps tendon

The Elbow

Overview, Bony Structures, and Joints. The elbow helps position the
hand in space and stabilizes the lever action of the forearm. The elbow
joint is formed by the humerus and the two bones of the forearm, the radius and the ulna. Identify the medial and lateral epicondyles of the
humerus and the olecranon process of the ulna.

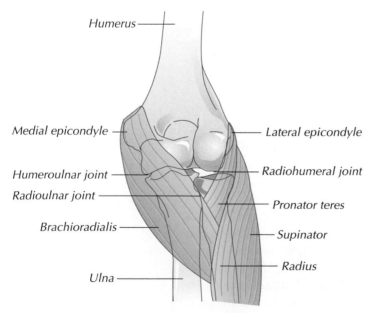

Humerus

Medial epicondyle

Lateral epicondyle

Humeroulnar joint

Radiohumeral joint

Radioulnar joint

Pronator teres

Brachioradialis

Supinator

Radius

Ulna

LEFT ELBOW – ANTERIOR VIEW

These bones have three articulations: the *humeroulnar joint*, the *radiohumeral joint*, and the *radioulnar joint*. All three share a large common articular cavity and an extensive synovial lining.

Muscle Groups and Additional Structures. Muscles traversing the elbow include the biceps and brachioradialis (flexion), the triceps (extension), the pronator teres (pronation), and the supinator (supination).

Note the location of the *olecranon bursa* between the olecranon process and the skin. The bursa is not normally palpable, but swells and becomes tender when inflamed. The *ulnar nerve* runs posteriorly between the medial epicondyle and the olecranon process. The *median nerve* is just medial to the brachial artery.

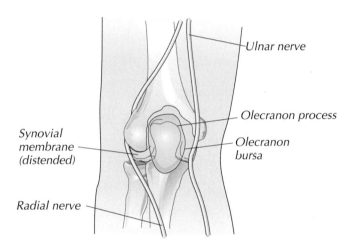

LEFT ELBOW – POSTERIOR VIEW

The Wrist and Hands

Overview. The wrist and hands form a complex unit of small, highly active joints used almost continuously during waking hours. There is little protection from overlying soft tissue, increasing vulnerability to trauma and disability.

Bony Structures. The wrist includes the distal radius and ulna and eight small carpal bones. At the wrist, identify the bony tips of the radius and the ulna.

The carpal bones lie distal to the wrist joint within each hand. Identify the carpal bones, each of the five metacarpals, and the proximal, middle, and distal phalanges. (The thumb lacks a middle phalanx.)

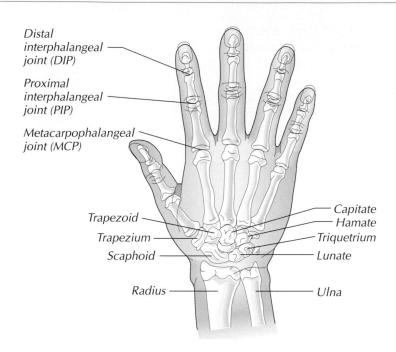

Distal interphalangeal joint (DIP)
Proximal interphalangeal joint (PIP)
Metacarpophalangeal joint (MCP)

Trapezoid
Trapezium
Scaphoid
Radius

Capitate
Hamate
Triquetrium
Lunate
Ulna

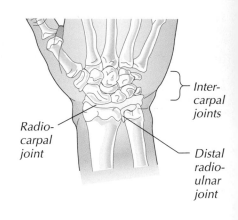

Radio-carpal joint
Inter-carpal joints
Distal radio-ulnar joint

Joints. The numerous joints of the wrist and hand lend unusual dexterity to the hands.

- *Wrist joints.* The wrist joints include the *radiocarpal (wrist) joint*, the *distal radioulnar joint*, and the *intercarpal joints*. The joint capsule, articular disc, and synovial membrane of the wrist join the radius to the ulna and to the proximal carpal bones. On the dorsum of the wrist, locate the groove of the radiocarpal joint.

- *Hand joints.* The joints of the hand include the *metacarpophalangeal joints* (MCPs), the *proximal interphalangeal joints* (PIPs), and the *distal interphalangeal joints* (DIPs). Flex the hand and find the groove marking the MCP joint of each finger. It is distal to the knuckle and is best felt on either side of the extensor tendon.

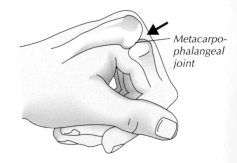

Metacarpo-phalangeal joint

Muscle Groups. Wrist flexion arises from the two carpal muscles, located on the radial and ulnar surfaces. Two radial and one ulnar muscle provide wrist extension. Supination and pronation arise from muscle contraction in the forearm.

The thumb is powered by three muscles that form the thenar eminence and provide flexion, abduction, and opposition. The muscles of extension are at the base of the thumb along the radial margin. Movement in the digits depends on action of the flexor and extensor tendons of muscles in the forearm and wrist.

The intrinsic muscles of the hand attaching to the metacarpal bones are involved in flexion (*lumbricals*), abduction (*dorsal interossei*), and adduction (*palmar interossei*) of the fingers.

Additional Structures. Soft-tissue structures, especially tendons and tendon sheaths, are especially important in the wrist and hand. Six extensor tendons and two flexor tendons pass across the wrist and hand to insert on the fingers. Through much of their course these tendons travel in tunnel-like sheaths, generally palpable only when swollen or inflamed.

Be familiar with the structures in the *carpal tunnel,* a narrow channel beneath the palmar surface of the wrist and proximal hand. The canal contains the sheath and flexor tendons of the forearm muscles and the *median nerve.*

Holding the tendons and tendon sheath in place is a transverse ligament, the *flexor retinaculum.* The median nerve lies between the tendon sheath and the flexor retinaculum. It provides sensation to the palm and the palmar surface of most of the thumb, the second and third digits, and half of the fourth digit. It also innervates the thumb muscles of flexion, abduction, and opposition.

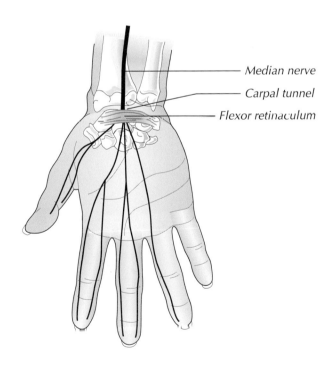

Median nerve

Carpal tunnel

Flexor retinaculum

The Spine

Overview. The vertebral column, or spine, is the central supporting structure of the trunk and back. Note the concave curves of the cervical and lumbar spine and the convex curves of the thoracic and sacrococcygeal spine. These curves help distribute upper body weight to the pelvis and lower extremities and cushion the concussive impact of walking or running.

The complex mechanics of the back arise from the coordinated action of:

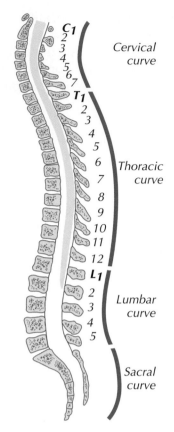

* The vertebrae and intervertebral discs

* An interconnecting system of ligaments, including longitudinal ligaments between anterior vertebrae and posterior vertebrae, ligaments between the spinous processes, and ligaments between the lamina of two adjacent vertebrae

* Large superficial muscles, deeper intrinsic muscles, and muscles of the abdominal wall.

Viewing the patient from behind, identify the following landmarks: (1) the spinous processes (unusually prominent at C7 and T1), which become more evident on forward flexion, (2) the paravertebral muscles on either side of the midline, (3) the scapulae, (4) the iliac crest, and (5) the posterior superior iliac spines, usually marked by skin dimples. A line drawn between the iliac crests crosses the spinous process of L4.

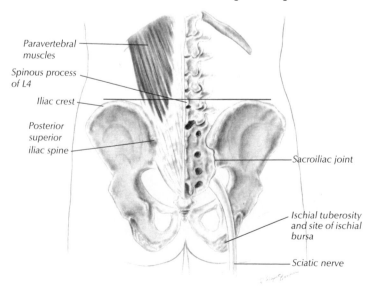

Bony Structures. The vertebral column contains 24 vertebrae stacked on the sacrum and coccyx. A typical vertebra contains sites for joint articulations, weight bearing, and muscle attachments, as well as foramina for the spinal nerve roots and peripheral nerves. Anteriorly, the *vertebral body* supports weight bearing. The posterior portion, the *vertebral arch*, encloses the spinal cord. Review the location of the vertebral processes and foramina, with particular attention to:

- The *spinous process* projecting posteriorly in the midline and the two *transverse processes* at the junction of the *pedicle* and the *lamina.* Muscle attachments occur at these processes.

- The *articular processes*—two on each side of the vertebra, one facing up and one facing down, at the junction of the pedicles and laminae (often called *articular facets*)

- The *vertebral foramen,* which encloses the spinal cord; the *intervertebral foramen* formed by the inferior and superior articulating processes of adjacent vertebrae and forming a channel for the spinal nerve roots; and, in the cervical vertebrae, the *transverse foramen* for the vertebral artery

The proximity of the spinal cord and roots to their bony vertebral casing makes them especially vulnerable to trauma and degenerative change.

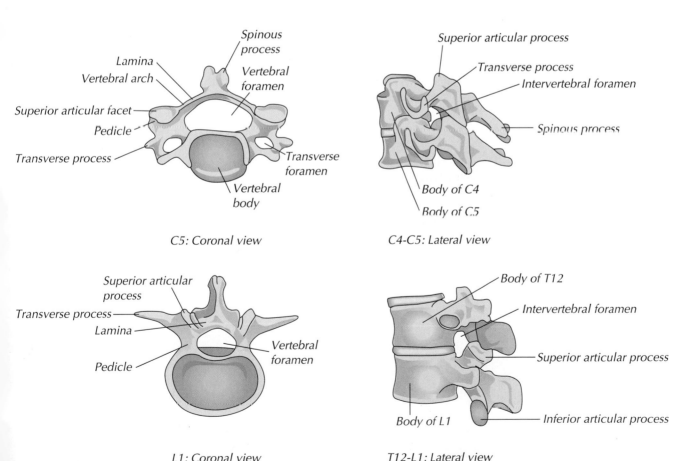

C5: Coronal view

C4-C5: Lateral view

L1: Coronal view

T12-L1: Lateral view

REPRESENTATIVE CERVICAL AND LUMBAR VERTEBRAE

Joints. The spine has cartilaginous slightly movable joints between the vertebral bodies and between the articular facets. Between the vertebral bodies are the *intervertebral discs,* each consisting of a soft mucoid central core, the *nucleus pulposus,* rimmed by the tough fibrous tissue of the *annulus fibrosis.* The intervertebral discs cushion movement between vertebrae and allow the vertebral column to curve, flex, and bend. The flexibility of the spine is largely determined by the angle of the articular facet joints relative to the plane of the vertebral body, and varies at different levels of the spine. Note that the vertebral column angles sharply posterior at the *lumbosacral junction* and becomes immovable. The mechanical stress at this angulation contributes to the risk of subluxation, or slippage, of L5 on S1.

Muscle Groups. The *trapezius* and *latissimus dorsi* form the large outer layer of muscles attaching to each side of the spine. They overlie two deeper muscle layers—a layer attaching to the head, neck, and spinous processes (splenius capitis, splenius cervicis, and sacrospinalis) and a layer of smaller intrinsic muscles between vertebrae. Muscles attaching to the anterior surface of the vertebrae, including the psoas muscle and the abdominal wall, assist with flexion. Muscles moving the neck and lower vertebral column are summarized below.

Movement	Principle Muscle Group
Cervical Spine (neck)	
Flexion	Sternocleidomastoid, scalene and prevertebral muscles
Extension	Splenius, trapezius, small intrinsic neck muscles
Rotation	Sternocleidomastoid, small intrinsic neck muscles
Lateral bending	Scalene and small intrinsic neck muscles
Lumbar Spine	
Flexion	Psoas major, psoas minor, quadratus lumborum; abdominal muscles such as the internal and external obliques and rectus abdominis, attaching to the anterior vertebrae
Extension	Intrinsic muscles of the back, sacrospinalis
Rotation	Abdominal muscles, intrinsic muscles of the back
Lateral bending	Abdominal muscles, intrinsic muscles of the back

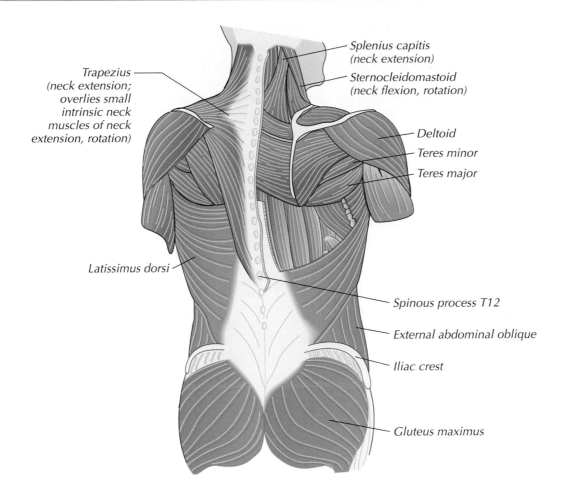

Splenius capitis
(neck extension)

Sternocleidomastoid
(neck flexion, rotation)

Trapezius
(neck extension;
overlies small
intrinsic neck
muscles of neck
extension, rotation)

Deltoid

Teres minor

Teres major

Latissimus dorsi

Spinous process T12

External abdominal oblique

Iliac crest

Gluteus maximus

The Hip

Overview. The hip joint is deeply embedded in the pelvis, and is notable for its strength, stability, and wide range of motion. The stability of the hip joint, so essential for weight bearing, arises from the deep fit of the head of the femur into the *acetabulum*, its strong fibrous articular capsule, and the powerful muscles crossing the joint and inserting below the femoral head, providing leverage for movement of the femur.

Bony Structures and Joints. The hip joint lies below the middle third of the inguinal ligament but in a deeper plane. It is a ball-and-socket joint—note how the rounded head of the femur articulates with the cuplike cavity of the acetabulum. Because of its overlying muscles and depth, it is not readily palpable. Review the bones of the pelvis— the *acetabulum*, the *ilium*, and the *ischium*—and the connection inferiorly at the symphysis pubis and posteriorly with the sacroiliac bone.

On the *anterior aspect* of the hip, identify the *iliac crest* at the upper margin of the pelvis at the level of L4. Follow the downward anterior curve and locate the *iliac tubercle*, marking the widest point of the crest, and continue tracking downward to the *anterior superior iliac spine*. Place your thumbs on the anterior superior spines and move your fingers downward from the iliac tubercles to the *greater trochanter* of the femur. Then move your thumbs medially and obliquely to the *pubic symphysis*, which lies at the same level as the greater trochanter.

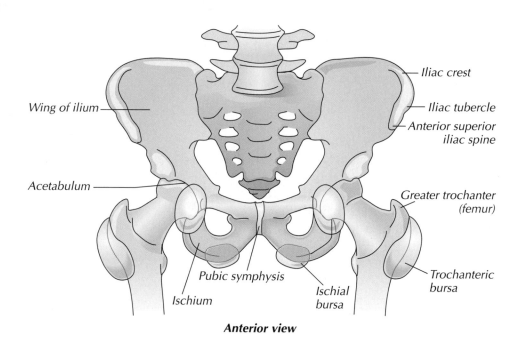

Anterior view

On the posterior aspect of the hip, locate the *posterior superior iliac spine* directly underneath the visible dimples just above the buttocks. An imaginary line along the iliac crests crosses the spinous process of L4. Placing your left thumb and index finger over the posterior superior iliac spine, next locate the *greater trochanter* laterally with your fingers at the level of the gluteal fold and place your thumb medially on the *ischial tuberosity*. The *sacroiliac joint* is not palpable. Note that an imaginary line between the posterior superior iliac spines crosses the joint at S2.

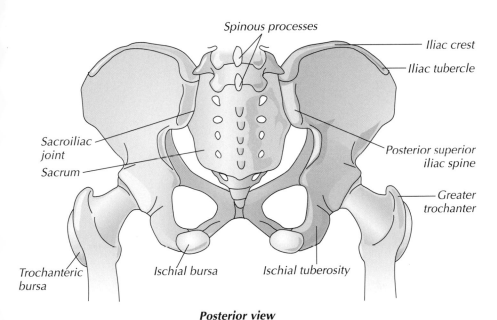

Posterior view

Muscle Groups. Four powerful muscle groups give movement to the hip. To remember these groups, try to picture where muscles need to cross joints to move limbs such as the femur in a given direction. The *flexor group* lies anteriorly and flexes the thigh. The primary hip flexor is the *iliopsoas*, extending from above the iliac crest to the lesser trochanter. The *extensor group* lies posteriorly and extends the thigh. The *gluteus maximus* is the primary extensor of the hip. It forms a band crossing from its origin along the medial pelvis to its insertion below the trochanter.

The *adductor group* is medial and swings the thigh toward the body. The muscles in this group arise from the rami of the pubis and ischium and insert on the posteromedial aspect of the femur. The *abductor group* is lateral, extending from the iliac crest to the head of the femur, and moves the thigh away from the body. This group includes the *gluteus medius* and *minimus*. These muscles help stabilize the pelvis during the stance phase of gait.

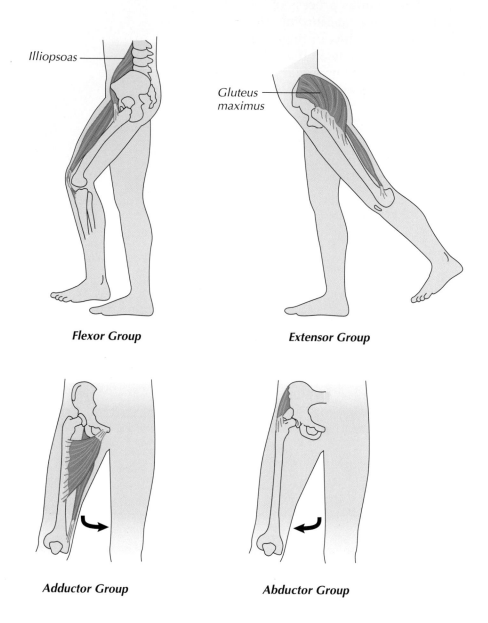

Flexor Group

Extensor Group

Adductor Group

Abductor Group

Additional Structures. A strong dense articular capsule, extending from the acetabulum to the femoral neck, encases and strengthens the hip joint, reinforced by three overlying ligaments and lined with synovial membrane. There are three bursae at the hip. Anterior to the joint is the *iliopectineal* (or *iliopsoas*) *bursa*, overlying the articular capsule and the psoas muscle. Find the bony prominence lateral to the hip joint—the *greater trochanter* of the femur. The large multilocular *trochanteric bursa* lies on its posterior surface. The *ischiogluteal bursa*—not always present—lies under the *ischeal tuberosity*, on which a person sits. Notes its proximity to the sciatic nerve, as shown on p. 494.

The Knee

Overview. The knee joint is the largest joint in the body. It involves three bones: the femur, the tibia, and the patella (or knee cap), with three articular surfaces, two between the femur and the tibia and one between the femur and the patella. Note how the two rounded condyles of the femur rest on the relatively flat tibial plateau. There is no inherent stability in the knee joint itself, making it dependent on ligaments to hold its articulating bones in place. This feature, in addition to the lever action of the femur on the tibia and lack of padding from fat or muscle, makes the knee highly vulnerable to injury.

Bony Structures. Landmarks in and around the knee will orient you to this complicated joint. Bring your fingertips firmly down the medial surface of the thigh along a line analogous to the inner seam of a pant leg. Your fingers will run up against an abrupt bony prominence, the *adductor tubercle.* Just below this is the *medial epicondyle.* The *lateral epicondyle* is comparably situated on the other side.

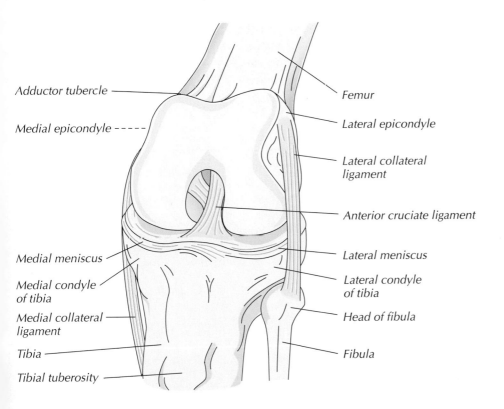

Adductor tubercle

Medial epicondyle

Medial meniscus

Medial condyle of tibia

Medial collateral ligament

Tibia

Tibial tuberosity

Femur

Lateral epicondyle

Lateral collateral ligament

Anterior cruciate ligament

Lateral meniscus

Lateral condyle of tibia

Head of fibula

Fibula

Identify the flat medial surface of the tibia—the shin. Follow its anterior border upward to the *tibial tuberosity (A)*. Mark this point with a dot of ink. Now follow the medial border of the tibia upward until it merges into a bony prominence—the *medial condyle* of the tibia *(B)*. This is somewhat higher than the tibial tuberosity. In a comparable location on the other side of the knee, find a similar prominence—the *lateral condyle (C)*. Mark both condyles with ink. These three points form an isosceles triangle. On the lateral surface of the knee, somewhat below the level of the lateral tibial condyle, find the head of the fibula.

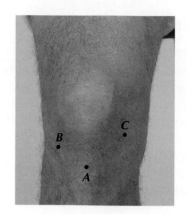

The *patella* rests on the anterior articulating surface of the femur, midway between the epicondyles, embedded in the tendon of the quadriceps muscle. This tendon continues below the knee joint as the *patellar tendon* and inserts on the tibial tuberosity.

Joints. Two of the knee joints are formed by the convex curves of the medial and lateral condyles of the femur as they articulate with the corresponding concave condyles of the tibia. The third articular surface is the patellofemoral joint. The patella slides in a groove on the anterior aspect of the distal femur, called the trochlear groove, during flexion and extension of the knee.

With the knee flexed about 90°, you can press your thumbs—one on each side of the patellar tendon—into the groove of the tibiofemoral joint. Note that the patella lies just above this joint line. As you press your thumbs downward you can feel the edge of the tibial plateau, the upper surface of the tibia. Follow it medially, then laterally until you are stopped by the converging femur and tibia. By moving your thumbs upward toward the midline to the top of the patella, you can follow the articulating surface of the femur and identify the margins of the joint.

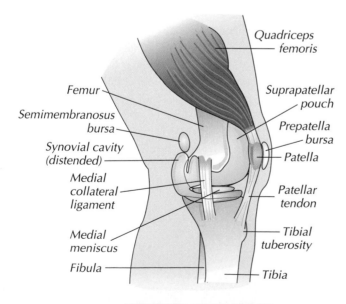

LEFT KNEE – MEDIAL VIEW

Muscle Groups. Powerful muscles move and support the knee. The *quadriceps femoris* extends the leg, covering the anterior, medial, and lateral aspects of the thigh. The *hamstring muscles* lie on the posterior aspect of the thigh and flex the knee.

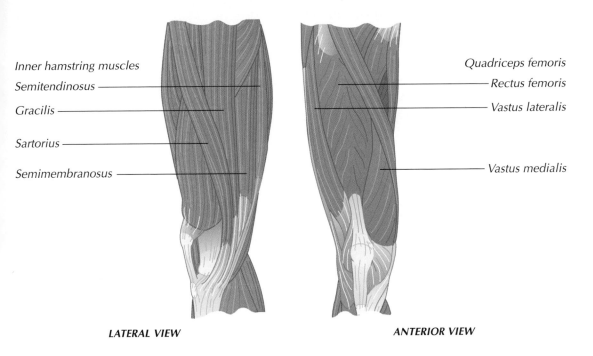

Inner hamstring muscles
Semitendinosus
Gracilis
Sartorius
Semimembranosus

Quadriceps femoris
Rectus femoris
Vastus lateralis

Vastus medialis

LATERAL VIEW   **ANTERIOR VIEW**

Additional Structures. Two important pairs of ligaments, the collateral ligaments and the cruciate ligaments, provide stability to the knee.

The *medial collateral ligament* (MCL), not easily palpable, is a broad flat ligament connecting the medial condyles of the femur and the tibia. To locate the anatomic region of the MCL, move your fingers medially and posteriorly along the joint line, then palpate along the ligament from its origin to insertion. The *lateral collateral ligament* (LCL) connects the lateral femoral condyle and the head of the fibula. To feel the LCL, cross one leg so the ankle rests on the opposite knee and find the firm cord that runs from the lateral epicondyle of the femur to the head of the fibula. The MCL and LCL provide medial and lateral stability to the knee.

The *anterior cruciate ligament* (ACL) crosses obliquely from the lateral femoral condyle to the medial tibia, preventing the tibia from sliding forward on the femur. The *posterior cruciate ligament* (PCL) crosses from the lateral tibia and lateral meniscus to the medial femoral condyle, preventing the tibia from slipping backward on the femur. Since these ligaments lie within the knee joint, they are not palpable. They are nonetheless crucial to the anteroposterior stability of the knee.

The *medial and lateral menisci* cushion the action of the femur on the tibia. These crescent-shaped fibrocartilaginous discs add a cuplike surface to the otherwise flat tibial plateau. Palpate the *medial meniscus* by pressing on the medial soft-tissue depression along the upper edge of the tibial plateau. Place the knee in slight flexion and palpate the *lateral meniscus* along the lateral joint line.

Observe the concavities that are usually evident at each side of the patella and also above it. Occupying these areas is the synovial cavity of the knee, the largest joint cavity in the body. This cavity includes an extension 6 centimeters above the upper border of the patella, lying upward and deep to the quadriceps muscle—the *suprapatellar pouch.* The joint cavity covers the anterior, medial, and lateral surfaces of the knee, as well as the condyles of the femur and tibia posteriorly. Although the synovium is not normally detectable, these areas may become swollen and tender when the joint is inflamed.

Several bursae lie near the knee. The *prepatellar bursa* lies between the patella and the overlying skin. The *anserine bursa* lies 1 to 2 inches below the knee joint on the medial surface and cannot be palpated due to overlying tendons. Now identify the large *semimembranosus bursa* that communicates with the joint cavity, also on the posterior and medial surfaces of the knee.

The Ankle and Foot

Overview. The total weight of the body is transmitted through the ankle to the foot. The ankle and foot must balance the body and absorb the impact of the heel strike and gait. Despite thick padding along the toes, sole, and heel and stabilizing ligaments at the ankles, the ankle and foot are frequent sites of sprain and bony injury.

Bony Structures and Joints. The ankle is a hinge joint formed by the *tibia,* the *fibula,* and the *talus.* The tibia and fibula act as a mortise, stabilizing the joint while bracing the talus like an inverted cup.

The principal joints of the ankle are the *tibiotalar joint,* between the tibia and the talus, and the *subtalar (talocalcaneal) joint.*

Note the principal landmarks of the ankle: the *medial malleolus,* the bony prominence at the distal end of the tibia, and the *lateral malleolus,* at the distal end of the fibula. Lodged under the talus and jutting posteriorly is the *calcaneus,* or heel.

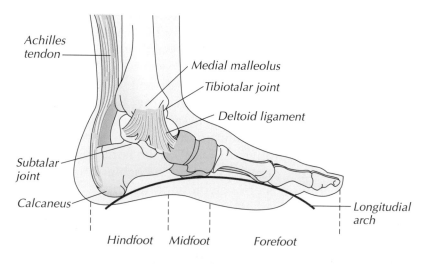

Achilles tendon

Medial malleolus

Tibiotalar joint

Deltoid ligament

Subtalar joint

Calcaneus

Hindfoot   Midfoot   Forefoot

Longitudinal arch

Medial view

An imaginary line, the *longitudinal arch*, spans the foot, extending from the calcaneus of the hind foot along the tarsal bones of the midfoot to the forefoot metatarsals and toes. The *heads of the metatarsals* are palpable in the ball of the foot. In the forefoot, identify the *metatarsophalangeal joints*, proximal to the webs of the toes, and the *proximal and distal interphalangeal joints* of the toes.

Muscle Groups and Additional Structures. Movement at the ankle joint is limited to dorsiflexion and plantar flexion. *Plantar flexion* is powered by the gastrocnemius, the posterior tibial muscle, and the toe flexors. Their tendons run behind the malleoli. The *dorsiflexors* include the anterior tibial muscle and the toe extensors. They lie prominently on the anterior surface, or dorsum, of the ankle, anterior to the malleoli.

Ligaments extend from each malleolus onto the foot. Medially, the triangle-shaped *deltoid ligament* fans out from the inferior surface of the medial malleolus to the talus and proximal tarsal bones, protecting against stress from eversion (ankle bows inward). The three ligaments on the lateral side are less substantial, with higher risk of injury: the *anterior talofibular ligament*—most at risk in injury from inversion (ankle bows outward) injuries; the *calcaneofibular ligament*; and the *posterior talofibular ligament*. The strong Achilles tendon inserts on the heel posteriorly.

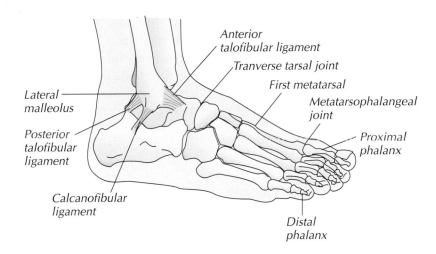

Lateral view

Changes With Age

Adolescence. The musculoskeletal system changes during adolescence in size, proportion, and strength. Between the ages of about 12.5 and 15 years, boys undergo a growth spurt, gaining an average of 8 inches in height and more than 40 pounds in weight. On the average, the growth spurt in girls occurs about 2 years earlier and is smaller in magnitude. Body proportions change in fairly regular sequence: the legs elongate, the hips and the chest widen, the shoulders broaden, and finally the trunk lengthens and the chest deepens. Shoulders broaden more in boys, while in girls an increase in the bony pelvis produces relatively greater widening of the hips. Muscles increase in size and strength, especially in boys. For illustrations of these changes, see p. 138.

As in sexual maturation, adolescents vary widely in their musculoskeletal development. Those who mature relatively late in relation to their peers face competitive disadvantages, even though they are entirely normal. Adolescent changes in height, musculoskeletal development, and sex maturity correlate well with each other and provide a better basis for counseling teenagers than chronological age alone.

Aging. Musculoskeletal changes continue through the adult years. Soon after maturity adults begin to lose height subtly, and significant shortening becomes obvious in old age. Most loss of height occurs in the trunk as intervertebral discs become thinner and the vertebral bodies shorten or even collapse because of osteoporosis. Flexion at the knees and hips may contribute to the shortened stature. The limbs of an elderly person thus tend to look long in proportion to the trunk.

The alterations in discs and vertebrae contribute too to the kyphosis of aging and increase the anteroposterior diameter of the chest, especially in women.

With aging, skeletal muscles decrease in bulk and power, and ligaments lose some of their tensile strength. Range of motion diminishes, partly because of osteoarthritis.

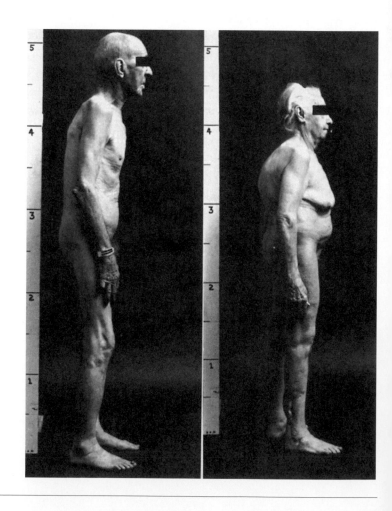

Techniques of Examination

General Approach

As you examine the musculoskeletal system, direct your attention to function as well as structure. During the interview you should have evaluated the patient's abilities to carry out normal activities of daily living. Also keep these abilities in mind during your physical examination.

In your initial survey of the patient you have assessed general appearance, body proportions, and ease of movement. Now, as you apply techniques of examination to the musculoskeletal system, visualize the underlying anatomy and recall the key elements of the history—for example, the mechanism of injury if there is trauma, or the time course of symptoms and limitations in function in arthritis.

Your examination should be systematic. It should include inspection, palpation of bony landmarks as well as related joint and soft-tissue structures, assessment of range of motion, and special maneuvers to test specific movements. These steps are described for each of the major joints. Recall that the anatomic shape of each joint determines its range of motion. This range is greatest in synovial or ball-and-socket joints.

Remember the following clues to guide your examination.

- During inspection, it is especially important to note *symmetry* of involvement. Is there a symmetric change in joints on both sides of the body, or is the change only in one or two joints?

  Involvement of only one joint increases the likelihood of bacterial arthritis. Rheumatoid athritis typically involves several joints, symmetrically distributed.

  Also note any *joint deformities* or *malalignment of bones.*

  Dupuytren's contracture (p. 549), bowlegs or knock-knees (p. 691)

- Use inspection and palpation to assess the *surrounding tissues,* noting skin changes, subcutaneous nodules, and muscle atrophy. Note any *crepitus,* an audible and/or palpable crunching during movement of tendons or ligaments over bone. This may occur in normal joints but is more significant when associated with symptoms or signs.

  Subcutaneous nodules in rheumatoid arthritis or rheumatic fever; effusions in trauma; crepitus over inflamed joints, in osteoarthritis, or inflamed tendon sheaths

- Testing range of motion and maneuvers may demonstrate *limitations in range of motion* or increased mobility and joint instability from excess mobility of joint ligaments, called *ligamentous laxity.*

  Decreased range of motion in arthritis, inflammation of tissues around a joint, fibrosis in or around a joint, or bony fixation (*ankylosis*). Ligamentous laxity of the ACL in knee trauma

507

- Finally, testing *muscle strength* may aid in the assessment of joint function (for these techniques, see Chap. 18).

Be especially alert to *signs of inflammation and arthritis.*

- *Swelling.* Palpable swelling may involve: (1) the synovial membrane, which can feel boggy or doughy; (2) effusion from excess synovial fluid within the joint space; or (3) soft-tissue structures such as bursae, tendons, and tendon sheaths.

- *Warmth.* Use the backs of your fingers to compare the involved joint with its unaffected contralateral joint, or with nearby tissues if both joints are involved.

- *Tenderness.* Try to identify the specific anatomic structure that is tender. Trauma may also cause tenderness.

- *Redness.* Redness of the overlying skin is the least common sign of inflammation near the joints.

If the person has painful joints, move the person gently. Patients may move more comfortably by themselves. Let them show you how they manage. If joint trauma is present, consider an x-ray before attempting movement.

The detail needed for examining the musculoskeletal system may vary widely. This section presents examination techniques for both comprehensive and targeted assessment of joint function. Patients with extensive or severe musculoskeletal problems will require more time. A briefer survey for those without musculoskeletal symptoms is outlined in Chapter 4.

The Temporomandibular Joint

Inspection and Palpation. Inspect the joint for swelling or redness. Swelling may appear as a rounded bulge about 1 inch anterior to the external auditory meatus.

Examples of Abnormalities (right column):

Muscle atrophy or weakness in rheumatoid arthritis

Palpable bogginess or doughiness of the synovial membrane indicates synovitis, which is often accompanied by effusion. Palpable joint fluid in effusion, tenderness over the tendon sheaths in tendinitis

Arthritis, tendinitis, bursitis, osteomyelitis

Tenderness and warmth over a thickened synovium may suggest arthritis or infection.

Redness over a tender joint suggests septic or gouty arthritis, or possibly rheumatoid arthritis.

Swelling, tenderness, and decreased range of motion suggest arthritis.

To locate and palpate the joint, place the tips of your index fingers just in front of the tragus of each ear and ask the patient to open his or her mouth. The fingertips should drop into the joint spaces as the mouth opens. Check for smooth range of motion; note any swelling or tenderness. Snapping or clicking may be felt or heard in normal people.

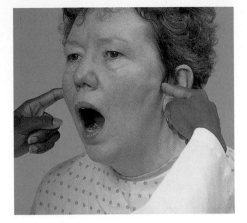

Range of Motion and Maneuvers. The temporomandibular joint has glide and hinge motions in its upper and lower portions respectively. Grinding for chewing consists primarily of gliding movements in the upper compartments.

Range of motion is three-fold: ask the patient to demonstrate opening and closing, protrusion and retraction (by jutting the jaw forward), and lateral, or side-to-side, motion. Normally as the mouth is opened wide, three fingers can be inserted between incisors. During normal protrusion of the jaw, the bottom teeth can be placed in front of the upper teeth.

Dislocation of the TMJ may be seen in trauma.

Swelling, tenderness, and decreased range of motion suggest arthritis.

Palpable crepitus or clicking may occur in poor occlusion, meniscus injury, or synovial swelling from trauma.

The Shoulder

Inspection. Observe the shoulder and shoulder girdle anteriorly, and inspect the scapulae and related muscles posteriorly. Note any swelling, deformity, or muscle atrophy or fasciculations (fine tremors of the muscles).

Inspect the contour of the shoulders and the bony landmarks of the clavicle, acromion, coracoid process, and greater tubercle of the humerus.

Absent motion may reflect paralysis (Erb's palsy).

Muscle atrophy points to lesions in the cervical nerves.

Scoliosis may cause elevation of one shoulder. With anterior dislocation of the shoulder, the rounded lateral aspect of the shoulder appears flattened.

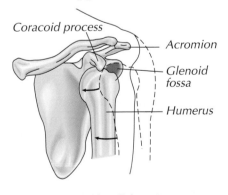

**Anterior dislocation
of humerus**

With posterior dislocation of the shoulder (relatively rare), the anterior aspect of the shoulder is flattened and the humeral head appears more prominent.

Look for swelling of the joint capsule anteriorly or a bulge in the sub-acromial bursa under the deltoid muscle. Survey the entire upper extremity for color change, skin alteration, or abnormal positioning.

A significant amount of synovial fluid is needed before the joint capsule appears distended.

Palpation. If there is a history of shoulder pain, ask the patient to point to the painful area. The location of the pain may provide clues as to its origin:

See Table 17-1, Painful Shoulders (pp. 544–545).

- Top of the shoulder, radiating toward the neck—acromioclavicular joint

- Lateral aspect of the shoulder, radiating toward the deltoid insertion—rotator cuff

- Anterior shoulder—bicipital tendon

Now identify the bony landmarks of the shoulder and then palpate the area of pain. Locate the *acromion* process and press medially to locate the distal tip of the clavicle at the *acromioclavicular joint*. Palpate laterally and down a short step to the greater tubercle of the humerus, and then press medially to locate the *coracoid process* of the scapula. Next palpate the painful area and identify the structures involved.

Range of Motion and Maneuvers. The six motions of the shoulder girdle are flexion, extension, abduction, adduction, and internal and external rotation.

Inability to perform these movements may reflect weakness or soft-tissue changes from bursitis, capsulitis, rotator cuff tears or sprains, or tendinitis.

Watch for smooth, fluid movement as you stand in front of the patient and ask the patient to (1) raise (abduct) the arms to shoulder level (90°) with palms facing down (tests pure glenohumeral motion); (2) raise the arms to a vertical position above the head with the palms facing each other (tests scapulothoracic motion for 60°, and combined glenohumeral and scapulothoracic motion during adduction for the final 30°; (3) place both hands behind the neck, with elbows out to the side (tests external rotation and abduction); and (4) place both hands behind the small of the back (tests internal rotation and adduction). (Placing your hand on the shoulder during these movements allows you to detect any crepitus.)

The examination of the shoulder often requires selective evaluation of the acromioclavicular joint, the subacromial and subdeltoid bursae, the rotator cuff, the bicipital groove and tendon, and the articular capsule and synovial membrane of the glenohumeral joint. Techniques for examining these structures are described on following pages.

Structure	Techniques of Examination
Acromioclavicular joint	Palpate and compare both joints for swelling or tenderness. Adduct the patient's arm across the chest, sometimes called the *"crossover test."*
Subacromial and subdeltoid bursae	Passively extend the shoulder by lifting the elbow posteriorly. This exposes the bursae anterior to the acromion. Palpate carefully over the subacromial and subdeltoid bursae.
Rotator cuff	With the patient's arm hanging at the side, palpate the three "SITS" muscles that insert on the greater tuberosity of the humerus. (The fourth muscle, the subscapularis, is located anteriorly and is not palpable.) • **S**upraspinatus—directly under the acromion • **I**nfraspinatus—posterior to supraspinatus • **T**eres minor—posterior and inferior to the supraspinatus

Localized tenderness or pain with adduction suggests inflammation or arthritis of the acromioclavicular joint. See Table 17-1, Painful Shoulders (pp. 544–545).

Localized tenderness arises from subacromial or subdeltoid bursitis, degenerative changes or calcific deposits in the rotator cuff.

Swelling suggests a bursal tear with communication into the articular cavity.

Tenderness over the "SITS" muscle insertions and inability to lift the arm above shoulder level are seen in sprains, tears, and tendon rupture of the rotator cuff, most commonly the *supraspinatus*. See Table 17-1, Painful Shoulders (pp. 544–545).

Structure	Techniques of Examination
	Passively extend the shoulder by lifting the elbow posteriorly. This maneuver also moves the rotator cuff out from under the acromion. Palpate the rounded SITS muscle insertions near the greater tuberosity of the humerus. 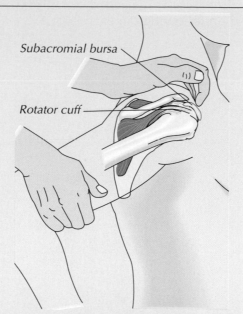

Check the *"drop-arm" sign.* Ask the patient to fully abduct the arm to shoulder level (or up to 90°) and lower it slowly. (Note that abduction above shoulder level, from 90° to 120°, reflects action of the deltoid muscle.)

If the patient is unable to hold the arm fully abducted at shoulder level, the "drop arm" test is positive, indicating a tear in the rotator cuff.

Bicipital groove and tendon

Rotate the arm and forearm externally and locate the biceps muscle distally near the elbow. Track the muscle and its tendon proximally into the bicipital groove along the anterior aspect of the humerus. As you check for tendon tenderness, rolling the tendon under the fingertips may be helpful.

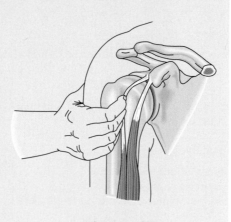

Palpation of the bicipital groove and tendon

See also Bicipital Tendinitis in Table 17-1 Painful Shoulders (pp. 544–545).

Finally, hold the patient's elbow against the body with the forearm flexed at a right angle. Ask the patient to supinate the forearm against resistance.

Tenderness or pain against resistance occurs with tenosynovitis of the bicipital tendon sheath, tendonitis, or biceps tendon rupture.

Articular capsule, synovial membrane, and glenohumeral joint

The fibrous articular capsule and the broad flat tendons of the rotator cuff are so closely associated that they must be examined simultaneously. Swelling in the capsule and synovial membrane is often best detected by looking down on the shoulder from above. Palpate the capsule and synovial membrane beneath the anterior and posterior acromion.

Tenderness and effusion suggest synovitis of the glenohumeral joint. If the margins of the capsule and synovial membrane are palpable, a moderate to large effusion is present. Minimal degrees of synovitis at the glenohumeral joint cannot be detected on palpation.

The following maneuvers test individual muscles of the shoulder girdle and help localize pain. Note that medial rotation against resistance also tests the pectoralis major, teres major, and latissimus dorsi.

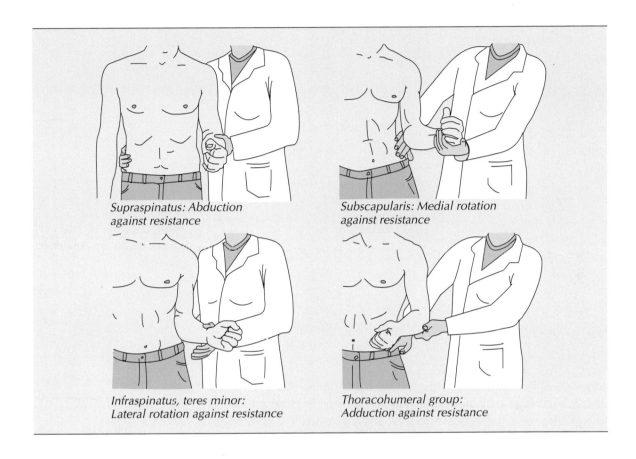

Supraspinatus: Abduction against resistance

Subscapularis: Medial rotation against resistance

Infraspinatus, teres minor: Lateral rotation against resistance

Thoracohumeral group: Adduction against resistance

The Elbow

Inspection and Palpation. Support the patient's forearm with your opposite hand so the elbow is flexed to about 70°. Identify the medial and lateral epicondyles and the olecranon process of the ulna. Inspect the contours of the elbow, including the extensor surface of the ulna and the olecranon process. Note any nodules or swelling.

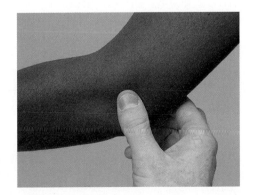

See Table 17-2, Swollen or Tender Elbows (p. 546).

Swelling over the olecranon process seen in olecranon bursitis; inflammation, or synovial fluid in arthritis.

Palpate the olecranon process and press on the epicondyles for tenderness.

Tenderness in *lateral epicondylitis* (tennis elbow) and in *medial epicondylitis* (pitcher's or golfer's elbow)

The olecranon is displaced posteriorly in *posterior dislocation of the elbow* and *supracondylar fracture.*

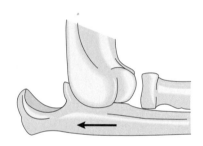

Posterior dislocation of the elbow

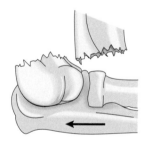

Supracondylar fracture

Palpate the grooves between the epicondyles and the olecranon, noting any tenderness, swelling, or thickening. The synovium is most accessible to examination between the olecranon and the epicondyles. (Normally neither synovium nor bursa is palpable.) The sensitive ulnar nerve can be felt posteriorly between the olecranon process and the medial epicondyle.

Range of Motion and Maneuvers. Range of motion includes flexion and extension at the elbow and pronation and supination of the forearm. To test flexion and extension, ask the patient to bend and straighten the elbow.

With the arms at the sides and elbows flexed (to minimize shoulder movement), the patient should turn the palms up (supination) and down (pronation).

The Wrist and Hand

Inspection. Observe the position of the hands in motion to see if movements are smooth and natural. At rest the fingers should be slightly flexed and aligned almost in parallel.

Guarded movement suggests injury. Poor finger alignment is seen in flexor tendon damage.

Inspect the palmar and dorsal surfaces of the wrist and hand carefully for swelling over the joints.

Diffuse swelling in arthritis or infection; localized swelling or ganglia from cystic enlargement. See Table 17-3, Swellings and Deformities of the Hands (pp. 547–549).

Note any deformities of the wrist, hand, or finger bones, as well as any angulation from radial or ulnar deviation.

In osteoarthritis, Heberden's nodes at the DIP joints, Bouchard's nodes at the PIP joints

In rheumatoid arthritis, symmetrical deformity in the PCP, MCP, and wrist joints, with ulnar deviation

Observe the contours of the palm, namely the thenar and hypothenar eminences.

Thenar atrophy is seen in median nerve compression from carpal tunnel syndrome; hypothenar atrophy in ulnar nerve compression.

Note any thickening of the flexor tendons or flexion contractures in the fingers.

Flexion contractures in the ring, 5th and 3rd fingers, or *Dupuytren's contractures*, arise from thickening of the palmar fascia (see p. 549).

Palpation. At the wrist, palpate the distal radius and ulna on the lateral and medial surfaces. Palpate the groove of each wrist joint with your thumbs on the dorsum of the wrist, your fingers beneath it. Note any swelling, bogginess, or tenderness.

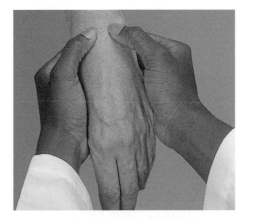

Tenderness over the ulnar styloid in *Colles' fracture*, any tenderness or bony step-offs are suspicious for fracture.

Swelling and/or tenderness suggests rheumatoid arthritis if it is bilateral and of several weeks' duration.

Gonococcal infection may involve the wrist joint (arthritis) or the tendon sheaths at the wrist (gonococcal tenosynovitis).

Palpate the *anatomic snuffbox*, a hollowed depression just distal to the radial styloid process formed by the abductor and extensor muscles of the thumb. The "snuffbox" becomes more visible with lateral extension of the thumb away from the hand.

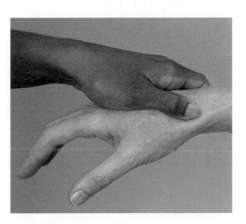

Tenderness over the "snuffbox" suggests a scaphoid fracture.

Palpate the eight carpal bones lying distal to the wrist joint, and then each of the five metacarpals and the proximal, middle, and distal phalanges.

Palpate any other area where you suspect an abnormality.

Compress the MCP joints by squeezing the hand from each side between the thumb and fingers. Alternatively, use your thumb to palpate each MCP joint just distal to and on each side of the knuckle as your index finger feels the head of the metacarpal in the palm. Note any swelling, bogginess, or tenderness.

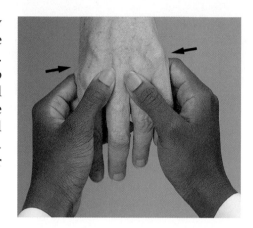

Synovitis in the MCPs is painful with this pressure—a point to remember when shaking hands.

The MCPs are often boggy or tender in rheumatoid arthritis (but rarely involved in osteoarthritis).

Now examine the fingers. Palpate the medial and lateral aspects of each PIP joint between your thumb and index finger, again checking for swelling, bogginess, bony enlargement, or tenderness.

PIP changes seen in rheumatoid arthritis; Bouchard's nodes in osteoarthritis

Using the same techniques, examine the DIP joints.

Hard dorsolateral nodules on the DIP joints, or *Heberden's nodes*, in osteoarthritis

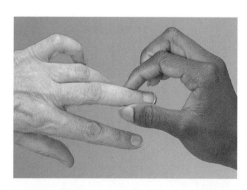

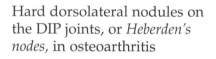

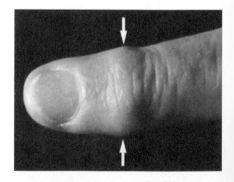

In any area of swelling or inflammation, palpate along the tendons inserting on the thumb and fingers.

Tenderness and swelling in *tenosynovitis*, or inflammation of the tendon sheaths. *DeQuervain's tenosynovitis* over the extensor and abductor tendons of the thumb as they cross the radial styloid

Range of Motion and Maneuvers.
Now assess range of motion for the wrists, fingers, and thumb. At the wrist, test flexion, extension, and ulnar and radial deviation.

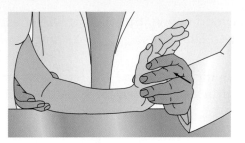

Flexion

- *Flexion.* With the patient's forearm stabilized, place his wrist in extension and place your fingertips in the patient's palm. Ask the patient to flex the wrist against gravity, then against graded resistance.

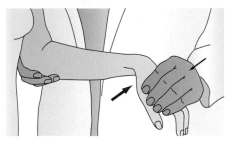

Extension

- *Extension.* With the patient's forearm stabilized, place his wrist in flexion and put your hand on the patient's dorsal metacarpals. Ask the patient to extend the wrist against gravity, then against graded resistance.

- *Ulnar and radial deviation.* With palms down, ask the patient to move the wrists laterally and medially.

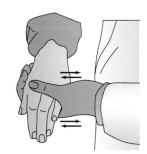

*Ulnar and radial
deviation*

Test flexion, extension, abduction, and adduction of the fingers:

- *Flexion and extension.* Ask the patient to make a tight fist with each hand, thumb across the knuckles, and then extend and spread the fingers. The fingers should close and open smoothly and easily. At the

Conditions that impair range of motion include arthritis, tenosynovitis, Dupuytren's contracture. See Table 17-3, Swelling and Deformities of the Hands (pp. 547–549).

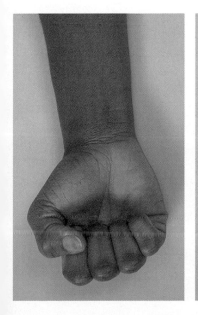

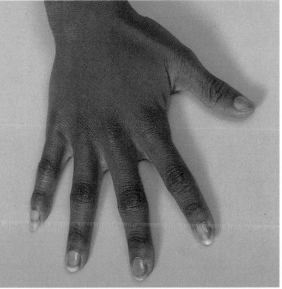

MCPs, the fingers may extend beyond the neutral position. Also test flexion and extension at the PIP and DIP joints.

- *Abduction and adduction.* Ask the patient to spread the fingers apart (abduction) and back together (adduction). Check for smooth, coordinated movement.

For the thumb, assess flexion, extension, abduction, adduction, and opposition. Ask the patient to move the thumb across the palm and touch the base of the 5th finger (*flexion*), and then to move the thumb back across the palm and away from the fingers (*extension*).

Next ask the patient to place the fingers and thumb in the neutral position with the palm up, and then to move the thumb anteriorly away from the palm (*abduction*) and back down (*adduction*). To test *opposition*, or movements of the thumb across the palm, ask the patient to touch the thumb to each of the other fingertips.

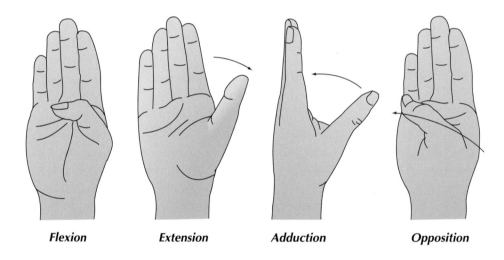

Flexion   **Extension**   **Adduction**   **Opposition**

Test sensation in the fingers only along the lateral and medial surfaces to isolate any alterations in the digital nerves. Test median, ulnar, and radial nerve function by checking sensation as follows:

- Pulp of the index finger—median nerve

- Pulp of the 5th finger—ulnar nerve

- Dorsal web space of the thumb and index finger—radial nerve

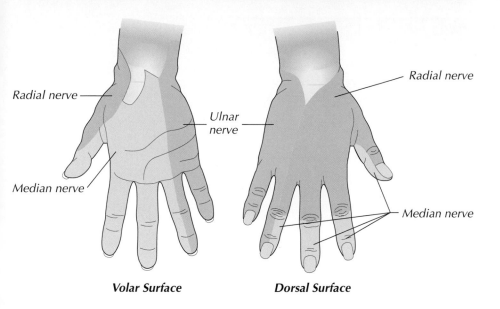

Volar Surface   **Dorsal Surface**

Radial nerve —
Ulnar nerve
Median nerve
Radial nerve
Median nerve

The Spine

Inspection. Begin by observing the patient's posture, including the position of both neck and trunk, when entering the room.

Assess the patient for erect position of the head, smooth, coordinated neck movement, and ease of gait.

Drape or gown the patient to expose the entire back for complete inspection. If possible, the patient should be upright in the patient's natural standing position—with feet together and arms hanging at the sides. The head should be midline in the same plane as the sacrum, and the shoulders and pelvis should be level.

Inspect the patient from the side. Note any spinal curvatures.

Neck stiffness signals arthritis, muscle strain, or other underlying pathology that should be pursued.

Lateral deviation of the head suggests *torticollis*, from contraction of the sternocleidomastoid muscle.

See Table 17-4, Spinal Curvatures (pp. 550–551).

Inspection of the Spine

View of Patient	Focus of Inspection	
From the side	Cervical, thoracic, and lumbar curves.	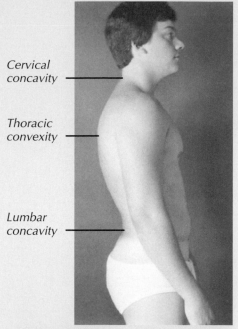 Cervical concavity — Thoracic convexity — Lumbar concavity —
From behind	Upright spinal column (an imaginary line should fall from C7 through the gluteal cleft) Alignment of the shoulders, the iliac crests, and the skin creases below the buttocks (gluteal folds)	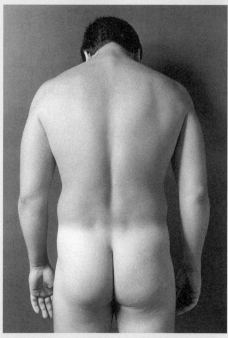
	Skin markings, tags, or masses	

Increased thoracic kyphosis occurs with aging. In children a correctible structural deformity should be pursued. See Table 17-4, Spinal Curvatures (pp. 550–551).

In scoliosis, there is lateral and rotatory curvature of the spine to bring the head back to midline. Scoliosis often becomes evident during adolescence, before symptoms appear.

Unequal shoulder heights seen in Sprengel's deformity of the scapula (from the attachment of an extra bone or band between the upper scapula and C7); in "winging" of the scapula (from loss of innervation of the serratus anterior muscle by the long thoracic nerve), and in contra-lateral weakness of the trapezius.

Unequal heights of the iliac crests (a *pelvic tilt*) suggest unequal lengths of the legs and disappear when a block is placed under the short leg and foot. Scoliosis and hip abduction or adduction may also cause a pelvic tilt. "Listing" of the trunk to one side is seen with a herniated lumbar disc.

Birthmarks, port-wine stains, hairy patches, and lipomas often overlie bony defects such as *spina bifida*.

Café-au-lait spots (discolored patches of skin), skin tags, and fibrous tumors in *neurofibromatosis*

Palpation. From a sitting or standing position, palpate the spinous processes of each vertebra with your thumb.

Tenderness suggests fracture or dislocation if preceded by trauma, underlying infection, or arthritis.

In the neck, also palpate the facet joints that lie between the cervical vertebrae about 1 inch lateral to the spinous processes of C2–C7. These joints lie deep to the trapezius muscle and may not be palpable unless the neck muscles are relaxed.

Tenderness occurs with arthritis, especially at the facet joints between C5 and C6.

In the lower lumbar area, check carefully for any vertebral "step-offs" to determine if one spinous process seems unusually prominent (or recessed) in relation to the one above it. Identify any tenderness.

Step-offs in *spondylolisthesis,* or forward slippage of one vertebra, which may compress the spinal cord. Vertebral tenderness is suspicious for fracture or infection.

Palpate over the sacroiliac joint, often identified by the dimple overlying the posterior superior iliac spine.

Tenderness over the sacroiliac joint pinpoints a common cause of low back pain. Ankylosing spondylitis may produce sacroiliac tenderness.

You may wish to percuss the spine for tenderness by thumping (not too roughly) with the ulnar surface of your fist.

Pain in percussion may arise from osteoporosis, infection, or malignancy.

Inspect and palpate the paravertebral muscles for tenderness and spasm. Muscles in spasm feel firm and knotted and may be visible.

Spasm occurs in degenerative and inflammatory processes of muscles, prolonged contraction from abnormal posture, or anxiety.

With the hip flexed and the patient lying on the opposite side, palpate the sciatic nerve, the largest nerve in the body, consisting of nerve roots from L4, L5, S1, S2, and S3. The nerve lies midway between the greater trochanter and the ischial tuberosity as it leaves the pelvis through the sciatic notch.

Sciatic nerve tenderness suggests a herniated disc or mass lesion impinging on the contributing roots.

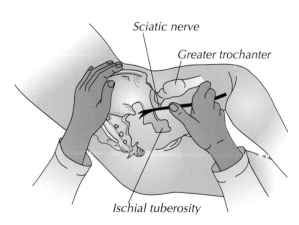

Sciatic nerve

Greater trochanter

Ischial tuberosity

Palpate for tenderness in any other areas that are suggested by the patient's symptoms. Recall that low back pain warrants careful assessment for cord compression, the most serious cause of pain due to risk of paralysis of the affected limb.

Herniated invertebral discs, most common between L5 and S1 or between L4 and L5, may produce tenderness of the spinous processes, the intervertebral joints, the paravertebral muscles, the sacrosciatic notch, and the sciatic nerve.

Rheumatoid arthritis may also cause tenderness of the intervertebral joints.

Remember that tenderness in the costovertebral angles may signify kidney infection rather than a musculoskeletal problem.

See Table 2-15, Low Back Pain (p. 100).

Range of Motion and Maneuvers. The neck is the most mobile portion of the spine, remarkable for its seven fragile vertebrae supporting the 10- to 15-pound ball of the head. Flexion and extension occur primarily between the skull and C1 (the atlas), rotation at C1–C2 (the axis), and lateral bending at C2–C7.

Limitations in range of motion may reflect stiffness from arthritis, pain from trauma, or muscle spasm such as *torticollis.*

Ask the patient to perform the following maneuvers, and check for smooth, coordinated motion:

- *Flexion.* Touch the chin to the chest.

- *Extension.* Look up at the ceiling.

- *Rotation.* Turn the head to each side, looking directly over the shoulder.

- *Lateral bending.* Tilt the head, touching each ear to the corresponding shoulder.

Tenderness, loss of sensation, or impaired movement warrants careful neurologic testing of the neck and upper extremities.

It is important to assess any complaints of neck, shoulder, or arm pain or numbness for possible cervical cord or nerve root compression. See Table 2-16, Pains in the Neck (p. 101).

Now assess range of motion in the spinal column.

• *Flexion.* Ask the patient to bend forward to touch the toes (flexion). Note the smoothness and symmetry of movement, the range of motion, and the curve in the lumbar area. As flexion proceeds, the lumbar concavity should flatten out.

Deformity of the thorax on forward bending in scoliosis. See Table 17-4, Spinal Curvatures (pp. 550–551).

Persistence of lumbar lordosis suggests muscle spasm or ankylosing spondylitis.

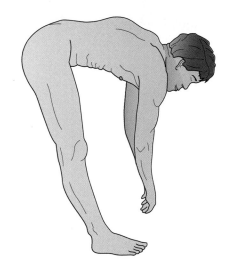

You may wish to measure the degree of flexion of the spine with the patient standing and bending forward. Mark the spine at the lumbosacral junction, then 10 cm above and 5 cm below this point. A 4-cm increase between the two upper marks is normally seen. (The distance between the lower two marks should be unchanged).

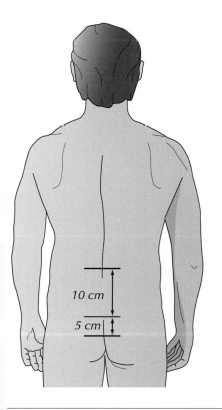

10 cm

5 cm

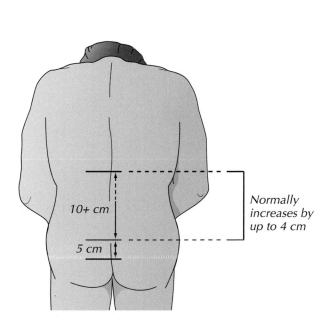

10+ cm

5 cm

Normally increases by up to 4 cm

- *Extension.* Place your hand on the posterior superior iliac spine, with your fingers pointing toward the midline, and ask the patient to bend backward as far as possible.

Decreased spinal mobility in osteoarthritis and ankylosing spondylitis, among other conditions

- *Rotation.* Stabilize the pelvis by placing one hand on the patient's hip and the other on the opposite shoulder. Then rotate the trunk by pulling both the shoulder and the hip posteriorly. Repeat the maneuver for the opposite side.

- *Lateral bending.* Again stabilize the pelvis by placing your hand on the patient's hip. Ask the patient to lean to both sides as far as possible.

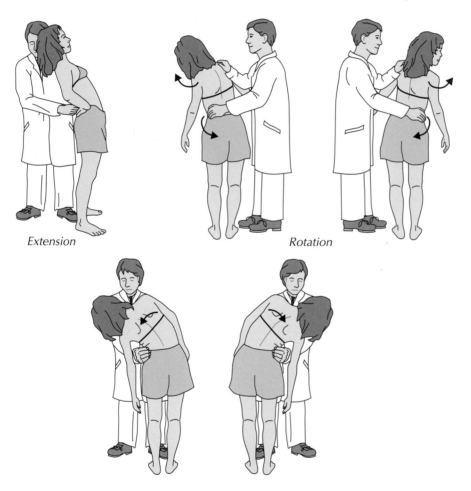

Extension

Rotation

Lateral bending

As with the neck, pain or tenderness with these maneuvers, particularly with radiation into the leg, warrants careful neurologic testing of the lower extremities.

Underlying cord or nerve root compression should be considered. Note that arthritis or infection in the hip, rectum, or pelvis may cause symptoms in the lumbar spine. See Table 2-15, Low Back Pain, (p. 100).

The Hip

Inspection. Inspection of the hip begins with careful observation of the patient's gait on entering the room. Observe the two phases of gait:

- *Stance*—when the foot is on the ground and bears weight (60% of the walking cycle)

Most problems appear during the weight-bearing stance phase.

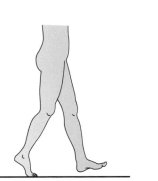

| Heelstrike | Foot flat | Midstance | Push-off |

The Stance Phase of Gait

- *Swing*—when the foot moves forward and does not bear weight (40% of the cycle)

Observe the gait for the width of the base, the shift of the pelvis, and flexion of the knee. The width of the base should be 2 to 4 inches from heel to heel. Normal gait has a smooth, continuous rhythm, achieved in part by contraction of the abductors of the weight-bearing limb. Abductor contraction stabilizes the pelvis and helps maintain balance, raising the opposite hip. The knee should be flexed throughout the stance phase, except when the heel strikes the ground to counteract motion at the ankle.

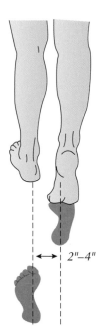

2"–4"

A wide base suggests cerebellar disease or foot problems.

Hip dislocation, arthritis, or abductor weakness can cause the pelvis to drop on the opposite side, producing a waddling gait.

Lack of knee flexion interrupts the smooth pattern of gait.

Observe the lumbar portion of the spine for slight lordosis and, with the patient supine, assess the length of the legs for symmetry. (To measure leg length, see Special Techniques, p. 540).

Loss of lordosis may reflect paravertebral spasm; excess lordosis suggests a flexion deformity of the hip.

Changes in leg length are seen in abduction or adduction deformities and scoliosis. Leg shortening and external rotation suggest hip fracture.

Inspect the anterior and posterior surfaces of the hip for any areas of muscle atrophy or bruising.

Palpation. Review the surface landmarks of the hip. On the anterior surface locate the iliac crest, the iliac tubercle, and the anterior superior iliac spine. On the posterior surface identify the posterior superior iliac spine, the greater trochanter, the ischial tuberosity, and the sciatic nerve.

With the patient supine, ask the patient to place the heel of the leg being examined on the opposite knee. Then palpate along the *inguinal ligament,* extending from the anterior superior iliac spine to the pubic tubercle. The femoral nerve, artery, and vein bisect the overlying inguinal ligament; lymph nodes lie medially. (The mnemonic NAVEL may be helpful for remembering the lateral to medial sequence of *n*erve–*a*rtery–*v*ein–*e*mpty space–*l*ymph node.) If the hip is painful, palpate the *iliopectineal (iliopsoas) bursa,* below the inguinal ligament but on a deeper plane.

Bulges along the ligament may suggest an inguinal hernia or, on occasion, an *aneurysm.*

Enlarged lymph nodes suggest infections in the lower extremity or pelvis.

Tenderness may be due to synovitis of the hip joint, bursitis, or possibly psoas abscess.

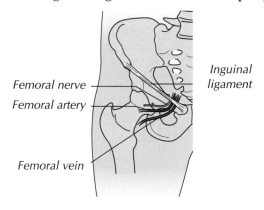

Femoral nerve

Femoral artery

Inguinal ligament

Femoral vein

With the patient resting on one side and the hip flexed and internally rotated, palpate the *trochanteric bursa* lying over the greater trochanter. Normally the *ischiogluteal bursa,* over the ischial tuberosity, is not palpable unless inflamed.

Swelling with tenderness suggests *trochanteric bursitis.* Tenderness without swelling on the posterolateral surface of the greater trochanter suggests localized tendinitis or muscle spasm from referred hip pain. Tenderness and swelling in ischiogluteal bursitis ("weaver's bottom"). Because of the adjacent sciatic nerve, pain from this bursitis may mimic sciatica.

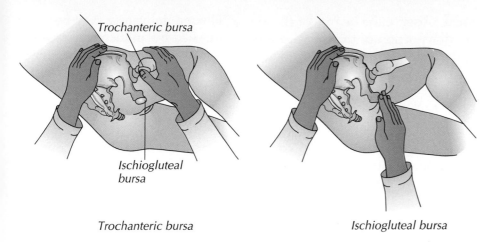

Trochanteric bursa

Ischiogluteal bursa

Range of Motion and Maneuvers. Range of motion at the hip includes flexion, extension, abduction, adduction, and rotation. Note that the hip can flex farther when the knee is also flexed. Rotation at the hip while the knee is flexed may be confusing at first. When the foot swings laterally, the femur rotates externally. It is the motion of the femur at the hip joint that identifies these movements.

Flexion. With the patient supine, place your hand under the patient's lumbar spine. Ask the patient to bend each knee in turn up to the chest and pull it firmly against the abdomen. Note when the back touches your hand, indicating normal flattening of the lumbar lordosis—further flexion must arise from the hip joint itself.

In flexion deformity of the hip, as the opposite hip is flexed (with the thigh against the chest), the affected hip does not allow full leg extension and the affected thigh appears flexed.

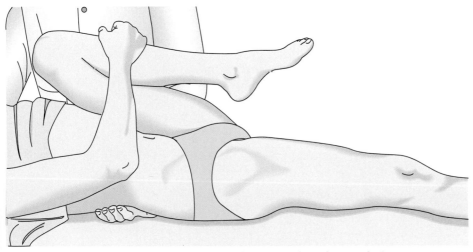

Hip Flexion and Flattening of Lumbar Lordosis

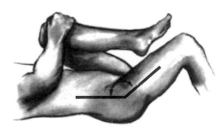

As the thigh is held against the abdomen, observe the degree of flexion at the hip and knee. Normally the anterior portion of the thigh can almost touch the chest wall. Note whether the opposite thigh remains fully extended, resting on the table.

Extension. With the patient lying face down, extend the thigh backward (or upward).

Abduction. Stabilize the pelvis by pressing down on the opposite anterior superior iliac spine with one hand. With the other hand, grasp the ankle and abduct the extended leg until you feel the iliac spine move. This movement marks the limit of hip abduction.

Flexion deformity may be masked by an increase, rather than flattening, in lumbar lordosis and an anterior pelvic tilt.

Restricted abduction is common in hip disease from osteoarthritis.

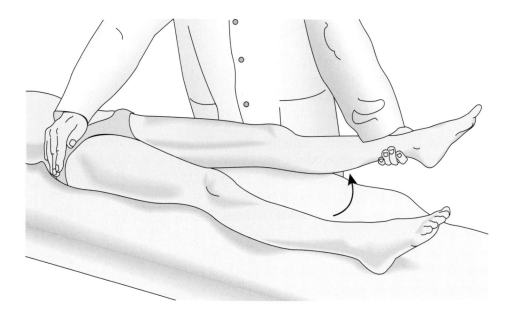

Alternatively, stand at the foot of the table, grasp both ankles, and spread them maximally, abducting both extended legs at the hips. This method provides easy comparison of two sides when movements are restricted, but it is impractical when range of motion is full.

Adduction. With the patient supine, stabilize the pelvis, hold one ankle, and move the leg medially across the body and over the opposite extremity.

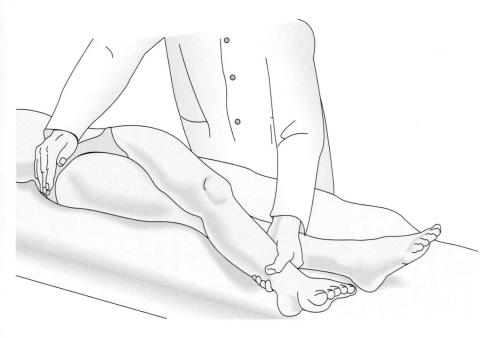

Rotation. Flex the leg to 90° at hip and knee, stabilize the thigh with one hand, grasp the ankle with the other, and swing the lower leg—medially for external rotation at the hip and laterally for internal rotation.

Restriction of internal rotation is an especially sensitive indicator of hip disease such as arthritis. External rotation is also often restricted.

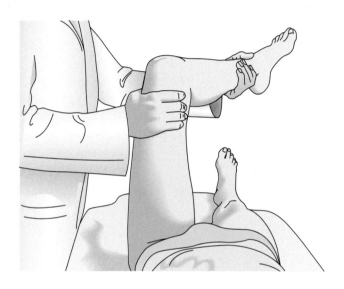

The Knee

Inspection. Observe the gait for a smooth, rhythmic flow as the patient enters the room. The knee should be extended at heel strike and flexed at all other phases of swing and stance.

Stumbling or pushing the knee into extension with the hand during heel strike suggests quadriceps weakness.

Check the alignment and contours of the knees. Observe any atrophy of the quadriceps muscles.

Bowlegs (genu varum), knock-knees (genu valgum), or flexion contracture (inability to extend fully)

Look for loss of the normal hollows around the patella (a sign of swelling in the knee joint and suprapatellar pouch), and note any other swelling in or around the knee.

Swelling over the patella suggests *prepatellar bursitis.* Swelling over the tibial tubercle suggests *infrapatellar* or, if more medial, *pes anserine bursitis.*

Palpation. Ask the patient to sit on the edge of the examining table with the knees in flexion. In this position, bony landmarks are more visible and the muscles, tendons, and ligaments are more relaxed, making them easier to palpate.

First review the important bony landmarks of the knee. Facing the knee, place your thumbs in the soft-tissue depressions on either side of the *patellar tendon.* On the medial aspect, move your thumb upward and then downward and identify the *medial femoral condyle* and the upper margin of the *medial tibial plateau.* Trace the patellar tendon distally to the *tibial tubercle.* The *adductor tubercle* is posterior to the *medial femoral condyle.*

Lateral to the patellar tendon, identify the *lateral femoral condyle* and the *lateral tibial plateau.* The medial and lateral femoral *epicondyles* are lateral to the condyles with the knee in flexion. Locate the *patella.*

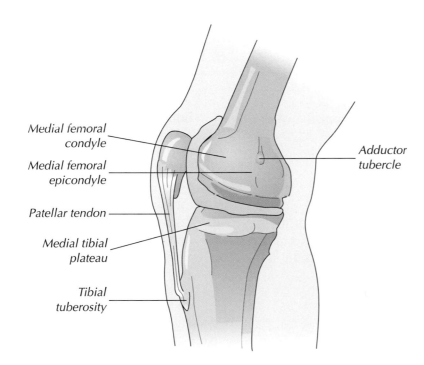

Medial femoral
condyle

Medial femoral
epicondyle

Patellar tendon

Medial tibial
plateau

Tibial
tuberosity

Adductor
tubercle

Palpate the ligaments, the menisci, and the bursae of the knee, paying special attention to any areas of tenderness. Pain is a common complaint in knee problems, and localizing the structure causing pain is important for accurate evaluation.

In the *patellofemoral compartment,* palpate the patellar tendon and ask the patient to extend the leg to make sure the tendon is intact.

Tenderness over the tendon or inability to extend the leg suggests a partial or complete tear of the patellar tendon.

With the patient supine and the knee extended, push the patella against the underlying femur. Ask the patient to tighten the quadriceps as the patella moves distally in the trochlear groove. Check for a smooth sliding motion (the patellofemoral grinding test).

Pain and crepitus suggest roughening of the patellar undersurface that articulates with the femur. Similar pain may occur with climbing stairs or getting up from a chair.

Pain with patellar movement during quadriceps contraction suggests *chondromalacia,* or degenerative patella.

Now assess the *medial and lateral compartments* of the *tibiofemoral joint.* Flex the patient's knee to about 90°. The patient's foot should rest on the examining table. Palpate the *medial collateral ligament* (MCL) between the medial femoral epicondyle and the femur; then palpate the cordlike *lateral collateral ligament* (LCL) between the lateral femoral epicondyle and the fibular head.

MCL tenderness after injury is suspicious for an MCL tear. (The LCL is less subject to injury.)

Palpate the *medial and lateral menisci* along the medial and lateral joint lines. It is easier to palpate the medial meniscus if the tibia is internally rotated. Note any swelling or tenderness.

Tenderness from tears following injury more common in the medial than in the lateral meniscus.

Note any irregular bony ridges along the joint margins.

Bony ridges along the joint margins may be felt in osteoarthritis.

Try to feel any thickening or swelling in the suprapatellar pouch and along the sides of the patella. Start 10 centimeters above the superior border of the patella (well above the pouch) and feel the soft tissues between your thumb and fingers. Move your hand distally in progressive steps, trying to identify the pouch. Continue your palpation along the

Swelling above and adjacent to the patella suggests synovial thickening or effusion in the knee joint.

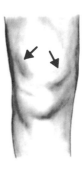

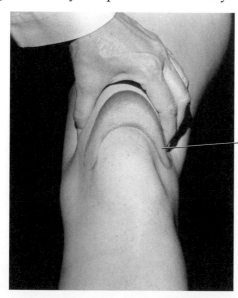

Suprapatellar pouch

sides of the patella. Note any tenderness or warmth greater than in the surrounding tissues.

Check three other bursae for bogginess or swelling. Palpate the prepatellar bursa, and over the anserine bursa on the posteromedial side of the knee between the medial collateral ligament and the tendons inserting on the medial tibial and plateau. On the posterior surface, with the leg extended, check the medial aspect of the popliteal fossa.

Three further tests will help you detect fluid in the knee joint.

- The *Bulge Sign* (*for minor effusions*). With the knee extended, place the left hand above the knee and apply pressure on the suprapatellar pouch, displacing or "milking" fluid downward. Stroke downward on the medial aspect of the knee and apply pressure to force fluid into the lateral area. Tap the knee just behind the lateral margin of the patella with the right hand.

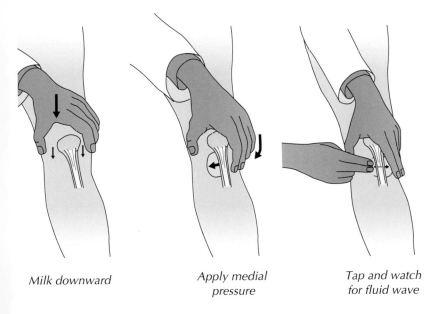

Milk downward *Apply medial pressure* *Tap and watch for fluid wave*

- The *Balloon Sign (for major effusions).* Place the thumb and index finger of your right hand on each side of the patella; with the left hand, compress the suprapatellar pouch against the femur. Feel for fluid entering (or ballooning into) the spaces next to the patella under your right thumb and index finger.

Thickening, bogginess, or warmth in these areas indicates synovitis or nontender effusions in osteoarthritis.

Prepatellar bursitis ("housemaid's knee") from excessive kneeling. Anserine bursitis from running, valgus knee deformity, fibromyalgias, osteoarthritis. A popliteal or "baker's" cyst from distention of the gastrocnemius semimembranosus bursa.

A fluid wave or bulge on the medial side between patella and femur confirms an effusion.

When the knee joint contains a large effusion, suprapatellar compression ejects fluid into the spaces adjacent to the patella. A palpable fluid wave signifies a positive "balloon sign." A returning fluid wave into the suprapatellar pouch confirms an effusion.

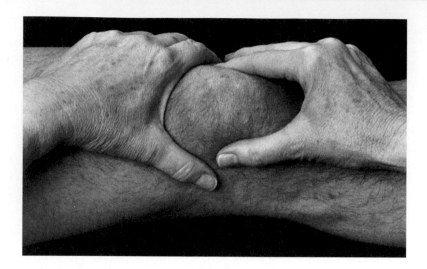

- *Ballotting the patella.* To further detect large effusions, compress the suprapatellar pouch and "ballotte" or push the patella sharply against the femur. Watch for fluid returning to the suprapatellar pouch.

Palpable fluid returning into the pouch further confirms presence of a large effusion.

A palpable patellar click with compression may also occur, but yields more false positives.

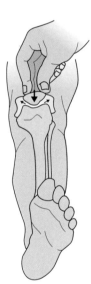

Range of Motion and Maneuvers. The principal movements of the knee are flexion, extension, and internal and external rotation. Ask the patient to flex and extend the knee while sitting. To check internal and external rotation, instruct the patient to rotate the foot medially and laterally. Knee flexion and extension can also be assessed by asking the patient to squat and stand up.

You will often need to test ligamentous stability and integrity of the menisci, particularly when there is a history of trauma or palpable tenderness. Always examine both knees and compare findings.

Structure	Maneuver	
Medial collateral ligament (MCL)	*Abduction Stress Test.* With the patient supine, move the thigh about 30° laterally to the side of the table. Place one hand against the lateral knee to stabilize the femur and the other hand around the medial ankle. Push medially against the knee and pull laterally at the ankle to open the knee joint on the medial side (*valgus stress*).	Pain or a gap in the medial joint line points to ligamentous laxity and a partial tear of the medial collateral ligament. Most injuries are on the medial side.
Lateral collateral ligament (LCL)	*Adduction Stress Test.* Now, with the thigh in the same position, change your position so you can place one hand against the medial surface of the knee and the other around the lateral ankle. Push medially against the knee and pull laterally at the ankle to open the knee joint on the lateral side (*varus stress*).	Pain or a gap in the lateral joint line points to ligamentous laxity and a partial tear of the lateral collateral ligament.
Anterior cruciate ligament (ACL)	*Anterior Drawer Sign.* With the patient supine, hips and knees flexed and feet flat on the table, cup your hands around the knee with the thumbs on the medial and lateral joint line and the fingers on the medial and lateral insertions of the hamstrings. Draw the tibia forward and observe if it slides forward (like a drawer) from under the femur. Compare the degree of forward movement with that of the opposite knee.	A few degrees of forward movement are normal if equally present on the opposite side. A forward jerk showing the contours of the upper tibia is a *positive anterior drawer sign* and suggests a tear of the ACL.
	Lachman Test. Place the knee in 15° of flexion and external rotation. Grasp the distal femur with one hand and the upper tibia with the other. With the thumb of the tibial hand on the joint line, simultaneously move the tibia forward and the femur back. Estimate the degree of forward excursion.	Significant forward excursion suggests an ACL tear.

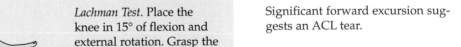

Structure	Maneuver
Posterior cruciate ligament (PCL)	*Posterior Drawer Sign.* Position the patient and place your hands in the positions described for the anterior drawer test. Push the tibia posteriorly and observe the degree of backward movement in the femur.
Medial meniscus and lateral meniscus	*McMurray Test.* If a click is felt or heard at the joint line during flexion and extension of the knee, or if tenderness is noted along the joint line, further assess the meniscus for a posterior tear. With the patient supine, grasp the heel and flex the knee. Cup your other hand over the knee joint with fingers and thumb along the medial and lateral joint line. From the heel, rotate the lower leg internally and externally. Then push on the lateral side to apply a valgus stress on the medial side of the joint. At the same time, rotate the leg externally and slowly extend it.

Isolated PCL tears are rare.

A click or pop along the medial joint with valgus stress, external rotation, and leg extension suggests a probable tear of the posterior portion of the medial meniscus.

The Ankle and Foot

Inspection. Observe all surfaces of the ankles and feet, noting any deformities, nodules, or swellings, and any calluses or corns.

See Table 17-5, Abnormalities of the Feet and Toes (pp. 552–553).

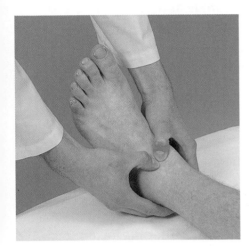

Palpation. With your thumbs, palpate the anterior aspect of each *ankle joint,* noting any bogginess, swelling, or tenderness.

Localized tenderness in arthritis, ligamentous injury, or infection of the ankle

Feel along the *Achilles tendon* for nodules and tenderness.

Rheumatoid nodules; tenderness in Achilles tendinitis, bursitis, or partial tear from trauma

Palpate the heel, especially the posterior and inferior calcaneus, and the plantar fascia for tenderness.

Bone spurs may be present on the calcaneus; pain over the plantar fascia suggests *plantar fasciitis.*

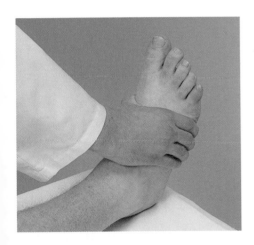

Palpate the *metatarsophalangeal joints* for tenderness. Compress the forefoot between the thumb and fingers. Exert pressure just proximal to the heads of the 1st and 5th metatarsals.

Tenderness on compression is an early sign of rheumatoid arthritis. Acute inflammation of the first metatarsophalangeal joint in gout

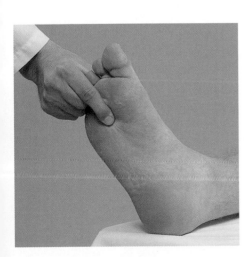

Palpate the heads of the five metatarsals and the grooves between them with your thumb and index finger. Place your thumb on the dorsum of the foot and your index finger on the plantar surface.

Pain and tenderness, called *metatarsalgia,* seen in trauma, arthritis, vascular compromise

Range of Motion and Maneuvers. Range of motion at the ankle includes flexion and extension at the ankle (tibiotalar) joint and, in the foot inversion and eversion at the subtalar and transverse tarsal joints.

- *The Ankle (Tibiotalar) Joint.* Dorsiflex and plantar flex the foot at the ankle.

Pain during movements of the ankle and the foot helps to localize possible arthritis.

- *The Subtalar (Talocalcaneal) Joint.* Stabilize the ankle with one hand, grasp the heel with the other, and invert and evert the foot.

An arthritic joint is frequently painful when moved in any direction, while a ligamentous sprain produces maximal pain when the ligament is stretched. For example, in a common form of sprained ankle, inversion and plantar flexion of the foot cause pain, while eversion and plantar flexion are relatively pain free.

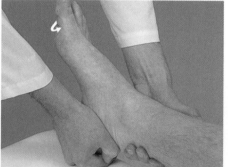 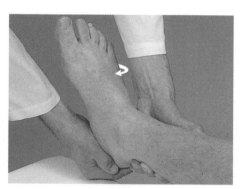

INVERSION   **EVERSION**

- *The Transverse Tarsal Joint.* Stabilize the heel and invert and evert the forefoot.

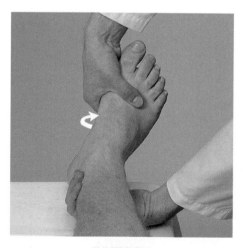 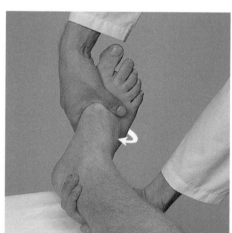

INVERSION   **EVERSION**

- *The Metatarsophalangeal Joints.* Flex the toes in relation to the feet.

Special Techniques

For the Carpal Tunnel Syndrome. Pain and numbness in the hand, especially at night, suggest compression of the median nerve in the carpal tunnel, lying between the carpal bones dorsally and a band of more superficial fascia ventrally. Two clinical tests are used:

Phalen's Test. Hold the patient's wrists in acute flexion for 60 seconds. Alternatively, ask the patient to press the backs of both hands together to form right angles. These maneuvers compress the median nerve.

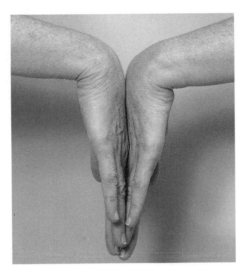

If numbness and tingling develop over the distribution of the median nerve (e.g., the palmar surface of the thumb, and the index, middle, and part of the ring fingers), the sign is positive, suggesting the carpal tunnel syndrome.

Tinel's Sign. With your finger, percuss lightly over the course of the median nerve in the carpal tunnel at the spot indicated by the arrow.

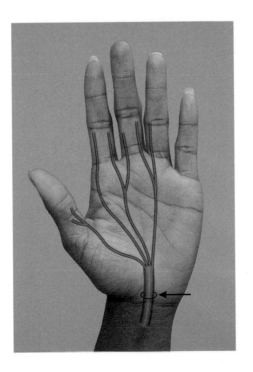

Tingling or electric sensations in the distribution of the median nerve constitute a positive test, suggesting the carpal tunnel syndrome.

For Low Back Pain with Radiation into the Leg. If the patient has noted low back pain that radiates down the leg, check straight leg raising on each side in turn. The patient should be lying supine. Raise the patient's relaxed and straightened leg until pain occurs. Then dorsiflex the foot.

Record the degree of elevation at which pain occurs, the quality and distribution of the pain, and the effects of dorsiflexion. Tightness and mild discomfort in the hamstrings with these maneuvers are common and do not indicate radicular pain.

Sharp pain radiating from the back down the leg in an L5 or S1 distribution (*radicular pain*) suggests tension on or compression of the nerve root(s), often caused by a herniated lumbar disc. Dorsiflexion of the foot increases the pain. Increased pain in the affected leg when the opposite leg is raised strongly confirms radicular pain and constitutes a positive *crossed straight leg-raising sign.*

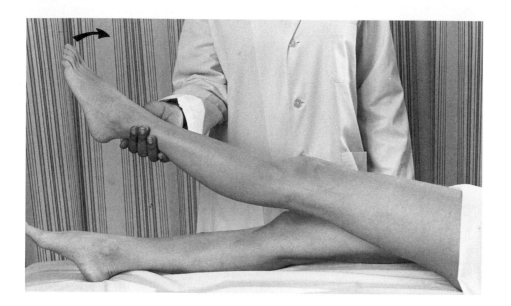

Examine the patient neurologically, focusing on the motor and sensory functions and the reflexes at the lumbosacral levels. These are outlined in the next chapter.

See Table 2-15 Low Back Pain (p. 100).

Measuring the Length of Legs. If you suspect that the patient's legs are unequal in length, measure them. Get the patient relaxed in the supine position and symmetrically aligned with legs extended. With a tape, measure the distance between the anterior superior iliac spine and the medial malleolus. The tape should cross the knee on its medial side.

Unequal leg length may explain a scoliosis.

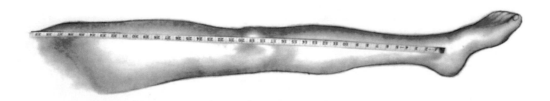

Decribing Limited Motion of a Joint. Although measurement of motion is seldom necessary, limitations can be described in degrees. Pocket goniometers are available for this purpose. In the two examples shown below, the red lines indicate the range of the patient's movement and the black lines suggest the normal range.

Observations may be described in several ways. The numbers in parentheses are suitably abbreviated recordings.

A.

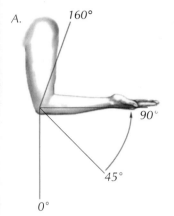

B.

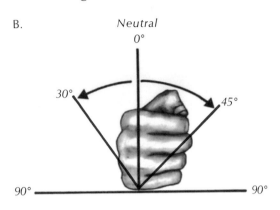

A. The elbow flexes from 45° to 90° (45° → 90°),

-or-

The elbow has a flexion deformity of 45° and can be flexed farther to 90° (45° → 90°).

B. Supination at elbow = 30° (0° → 30°)
Pronation at elbow = 45° (0° → 45°)

Health Promotion and Counseling

Maintaining the integrity of the musculoskeletal system brings many features of daily life into play—balanced nutrition, regular exercise, appropriate weight. As shown in this chapter, each joint has its specific vulnerabilities to trauma and wear. Care with lifting, avoidance of falls, household safety measures, and, for selected older women, hormone replacement therapy help to protect and preserve well-functioning muscles and joints.

The habits of a healthy lifestyle convey direct benefit to the skeleton. Good nutrition supplies calcium needed for bone mineralization and bone density. Exercise appears to maintain and possibly increase bone mass, in addition to improving outlook and management of stress. Weight appropriate to height and body frame reduces excess mechanical wear on weight-bearing joints such as hips and knees. (For further discussion of these topics, see pp. 318–319.)

One of the most vulnerable parts of the skeleton is the low back, especially L5–S1, where the sacral vertebrae angle sharply posterior. More than 80% of the population experiences low back pain at least once in a lifetime. Usually symptoms are short lived, but there is a pattern of recurrence in 30% to 60% of individuals when onset is work related. Exercises to strengthen the low back, especially in flexion and extension, are often recommended (although studies have not consistently demonstrated a reduction in sick days from work). Alternatively, general fitness exercises appear equally effective. Education on lifting strategies, posture, and the biomechanics of injury is prudent for patients doing repetitive lifting such as nurses, heavy-machinery operators, and construction workers.

Among U.S. elderly persons falls exact a heavy toil in morbidity and mortality. They are the leading cause of nonfatal injuries and account for a dramatic rise in death rates after age 65, increasing from ~5/100,000 in the general population to ~10/100,000 between the ages of 65 and 74 to ~147/100,000 after age 85.* Approximately 5% of falls result in fractures, usually of the wrist, hip, pelvis, or femur. Risk factors are both cognitive and physiological, including unstable gait, imbalanced posture, reduced strength, cognitive loss as in dementia, deficits in vision and proprioception, and osteoporosis. Poor lighting, stairs, chairs at awkward heights, slippery or irregular surfaces, and ill-fitting shoes are environmental dangers that can often be corrected. Clinicians should work with patients and families to help modify such risks whenever possible. Medications affecting balance, especially benzodiazepines, vasodilators, and diuretics, should be scrutinized. Home

---

* U.S. Preventive Services Task Force: In *Guide to Clinical Preventive Services*. Baltimore: Williams & Wilkins, 1996, pp. 659–685.

health assessments have proven useful in reducing environmental hazards, as have exercise programs to improve patient balance and strength.

Finally, it is important to counsel postmenopausal women about hormone replacement therapy and osteoporosis, defined as bone density >2.5 standard deviations below normal bone mass in young women.[†] Bone density reflects the interaction between bone mass (highest in the second decade), new bone formation, and bone resorption. A 10% drop in bone mineral density, equivalent to one standard deviation, is associated with a 20% increase in risk of fracture. Most fractures in patients over age 45 are attributable to postmenopausal osteoporosis. The decline in bone mass begins in the third decade and then accelerates in early menopause, especially in the trabecular bone of the vertebrae. At highest risk are women of Caucasian origin, slender build, or prior history of bilateral oophorectomy before menopause. A number of agents inhibit bone resorption—calcium, vitamin D, calcitonin, bisphosphonates, and estrogen—but consensus on several clinical management decisions has yet to emerge. Criteria are unclear for identifying those women at menopause at greatest risk of bone loss and fractures one to two decades later. In addition, guidelines for tailoring dosage of medication to level of bone density have yet to be determined. Estrogen therapy appears to prevent vertebral trabecular bone resorption, and is most beneficial when started near menopause. Lifetime use is recommended because bone loss resumes once therapy is discontinued. Although hormone replacement is protective against osteoporosis and cardiovascular disease, use of estrogen must be weighed carefully in each patient against risk of breast cancer, endometrial cancer (risk is decreased by progesterone), and thrombosis. Cognitive, environmental, and other physiological risk factors for falls and fractures should also be addressed.

† U.S. Preventive Services Task Force: In *Guide to Clinical Preventive Services.* Baltimore: Williams & Wilkins, 1996, pp. 509–516.

Table 17-1   Painful Shoulders

TABLE 17-1   *Painful Shoulders*

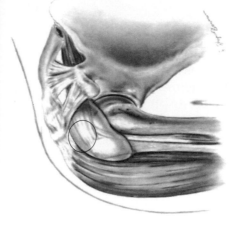

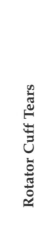

Shoulder-shrugging effort

Normal abduction

Limited abduction

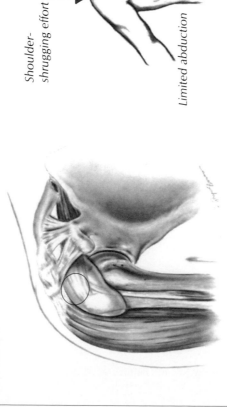

Rotator Cuff Tendinitis
(Impingement Syndrome)

When the arm is raised, the rotator cuff may impinge against the undersurface of the acromion and the coracoacromial ligament. Repeated impingement of this kind, as in throwing or swimming, can cause edema and hemorrhage followed by inflammation and fibrosis, most often involving the supraspinatus tendon. Acute, recurrent, or chronic pain may result, often aggravated by activity. Sharp catches of pain may occur as the arm is elevated into an overhead position. When the supraspinatus tendon is involved, tenderness is maximal just below the tip of the acromion. The patients tend to be young (teens to 40 years) and are often, though not necessarily, athletically active.

Rotator Cuff Tears

Repeated impingement (or other conditions) may weaken the rotator cuff and eventually cause partial or complete tears in it, usually after the age of 40 years. Injury, such as falling, may precipitate a tear. Manifestations include weakness, atrophy of the supraspinatus and infraspinatus muscles, pain, and tenderness. In a complete tear of the supraspinatus tendon (illustrated), active abduction at the glenohumeral joint is severely impaired. Efforts to abduct the arm produce a characteristic shoulder shrugging instead.

Calcific Tendinitis

Calcific tendinitis refers to a degenerative process in the tendon that is associated with the deposition of calcium salts. Like rotator cuff tendinitis, it usually involves the supraspinatus tendon. Acute, disabling attacks of shoulder pain may occur, usually in patients over 30 years of age and more often in women. The arm is held close to the side, and all motions are severely limited by pain. Tenderness is maximal below the tip of the acromion. The subacromial bursa, which overlies the supraspinatus tendon, may become involved in the inflammation. Chronic, less severe pain may also occur.

Table 17-1 Painful Shoulders

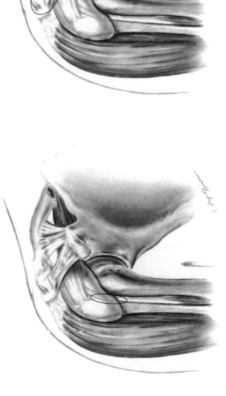

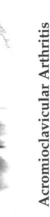

Bicipital Tendinitis

Inflammation of the long head of the biceps tendon and its sheath causes anterior shoulder pain that may resemble rotator cuff tendinitis and may coexist with it. This tendon, like the cuff, may suffer impingement injury. Tenderness is maximal in the bicipital groove. By externally rotating and abducting the arm, you can more easily separate this area from the subacromial tenderness of supraspinatus tendinitis. With the patient's arm at the side, elbow flexed to 90°, ask the patient to supinate the forearm against your resistance. Increased pain in the bicipital groove confirms this condition.

Acromioclavicular Arthritis

Acromioclavicular arthritis is not a common cause of shoulder pain. When present, it usually is the result of direct injury to the shoulder girdle with resulting degenerative changes. Tenderness is localized over the acromioclavicular joint. Although motion in the glenohumeral joint is not painful in acromioclavicular arthritis, as it is in many other painful conditions of the shoulder, movements of the scapula, such as shoulder shrugging, are.

Adhesive Capsulitis (Frozen Shoulder)

Adhesive capsulitis refers to a mysterious fibrosis of the glenohumeral joint capsule, manifested by diffuse, dull, aching pain in the shoulder and progressive restriction of motion, but usually no localized tenderness. The condition is usually unilateral and occurs in persons aged 50 to 70. There is often an antecedent painful disorder of the shoulder or possibly another condition (such as myocardial infarction) that has decreased shoulder movements. The course is chronic, lasting months to years, but the disorder often resolves spontaneously, at least partially.

Table 17-2 Swollen or Tender Elbows

TABLE 17-2 *Swollen or Tender Elbows*

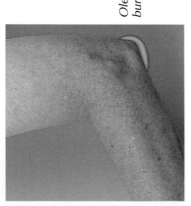

Olecranon bursitis

Olecranon Bursitis

Swelling and inflammation of the olecranon bursa may result from trauma or may be associated with rheumatoid or gouty arthritis. The swelling is superficial to the olecranon process.

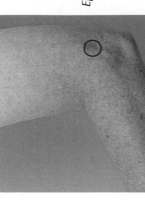

Arthritis

Arthritis of the Elbow

Synovial inflammation or fluid is felt best in the grooves between the olecranon process and the epicondyles on either side. Palpate for a boggy, soft, or fluctuant swelling and for tenderness.

Rheumatoid nodules

Rheumatoid Nodules

Subcutaneous nodules may develop at pressure points along the extensor surface of the ulna in patients with rheumatoid arthritis or acute rheumatic fever. They are firm and nontender, and are not attached to the overlying skin. They may or may not be attached to the underlying periosteum. Although they may develop in the area of the olecranon bursa, they often occur more distally.

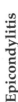

Epicondylitis

Epicondylitis

Lateral epicondylitis (tennis elbow) follows repetitive extension of the wrist or pronation–supination of the forearm. Pain and tenderness develop at the lateral epicondyle and possibly in the extensor muscles close to it. When the patient tries to extend the wrist against resistance, pain increases.
Medial epicondylitis (pitcher's, golfer's, or Little League elbow) follows repetitive wrist flexion, as in throwing. Tenderness is maximal at the medial epicondyle. Wrist flexion against resistance increases the pain.

Table 17-3   Swellings and Deformities of the Hands

TABLE 17 - 3   Swellings and Deformities of the Hands

Osteoarthritis (Degenerative Joint Disease)

Nodules on the dorsolateral aspects of the distal interphalangeal joints (*Heberden's nodes*) are due to the bony overgrowth of osteoarthritis. Usually hard and painless, they affect the middle-aged or elderly and often, although not always, are associated with arthritic changes in other joints. Flexion and deviation deformities may develop. Similar nodules on the proximal interphalangeal joints (*Bouchard's nodes*) are less common. The metacarpophalangeal joints are spared.

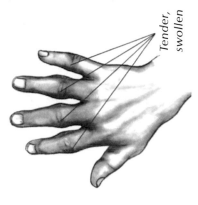

Radial deviation of distal phalanx

Heberden's node

Bouchard's node

Metacarpophalangeal joints uninvolved

Acute Rheumatoid Arthritis

Tender, painful, stiff joints characterize rheumatoid arthritis. Symmetrical involvement on both sides of the body is typical. The proximal interphalangeal, metacarpophalangeal, and wrist joints are frequently affected; the distal interphalangeal joints are rarely so. Patients with acute disease often have fusiform or spindle-shaped swelling of the proximal interphalangeal joints.

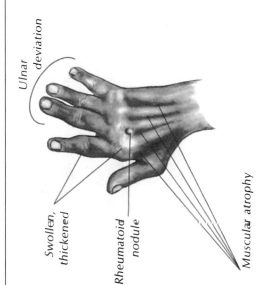

Tender, swollen

Boutonniere deformity

Swan neck deformity

Chronic Rheumatoid Arthritis

As the arthritic process continues and worsens, chronic swelling and thickening of the metacarpophalangeal and proximal interphalangeal joints appear. Range of motion becomes limited and the fingers may deviate toward the ulnar side. The interosseous muscles atrophy. The fingers may show *"swan neck" deformities* (i.e., hyperextension of the proximal interphalangeal joints with fixed flexion of the distal interphalangeal joints). Less common is a *boutonniere deformity* (i.e., persistent flexion of the proximal interphalangeal joint with hyperextension of the distal interphalangeal joint). Rheumatoid nodules may accompany either the acute or the chronic stage.

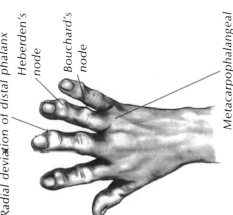

Ulnar deviation

Swollen, thickened

Rheumatoid nodule

Muscular atrophy

Continued

Table 17-3 Swellings and Deformities of the Hands

TABLE 17-3 *(continued)*

Chronic Tophaceous Gout

The deformities that develop in longstanding chronic tophaceous gout can sometimes mimic those of rheumatoid and osteoarthritis. Joint involvement is usually not so symmetrical as in rheumatoid arthritis. Acute inflammation may be present. Knobby swellings around the joints sometimes ulcerate and discharge white chalklike urates.

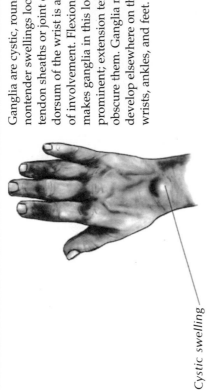

Swollen

Knobby swelling

Draining tophus

Ganglion

Ganglia are cystic, round, usually nontender swellings located along tendon sheaths or joint capsules. The dorsum of the wrist is a frequent site of involvement. Flexion of the wrist makes ganglia in this location more prominent; extension tends to obscure them. Ganglia may also develop elsewhere on the hands, wrists, ankles, and feet.

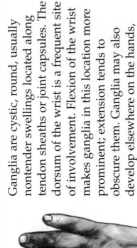

Cystic swelling

Tendon Sheath and Palmar Space Infections

Acute Tenosynovitis

Infection of the flexor tendon sheaths (acute tenosynovitis) may follow local injury, even of apparently trivial nature. Unlike in arthritis, tenderness and swelling develop not in the joint but along the course of the tendon sheath, from the distal phalanx to the level of the metacarpophalangeal joint. The finger is held in slight flexion; attempts to extend it are very painful.

Pain on extension

Swelling and tenderness along tendon sheath

Finger held in slight flexion

Acute Tenosynovitis and Thenar Space Involvement

If the infection progresses, it may escape the bounds of the tendon sheath to involve one of the adjacent fascial spaces within the palm. Infections of the index finger and thenar space are illustrated. Early diagnosis and treatment are important.

Puncture wound

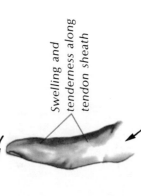

Tender, swollen

Table 17-3   Swellings and Deformities of the Hands

Felon

Injury to the fingertip may result in infection in the enclosed fascial spaces of the finger pad. Severe pain, localized tenderness, swelling, and dusky redness are characteristic. Early diagnosis and treatment are important.

Puncture wound

Swollen, tender, dusky red

Dupuytren's Contracture

The first sign of a Dupuytren's contracture is a thickened plaque overlying the flexor tendon of the ring finger and possibly the little finger at the level of the distal palmar crease. Subsequently the skin in this area puckers, and a thickened fibrotic cord develops between palm and finger. Flexion contracture of the fingers may gradually ensue.

Flexion contraction

Cord

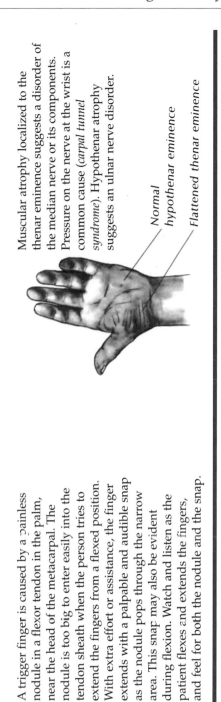

Thenar Atrophy

Muscular atrophy localized to the thenar eminence suggests a disorder of the median nerve or its components. Pressure on the nerve at the wrist is a common cause (*carpal tunnel syndrome*). Hypothenar atrophy suggests an ulnar nerve disorder.

Normal hypothenar eminence

Flattened thenar eminence

Trigger Finger

A trigger finger is caused by a painless nodule in a flexor tendon in the palm, near the head of the metacarpal. The nodule is too big to enter easily into the tendon sheath when the person tries to extend the fingers from a flexed position. With extra effort or assistance, the finger extends with a palpable and audible snap as the nodule pops through the narrow area. This snap may also be evident during flexion. Watch and listen as the patient flexes and extends the fingers, and feel for both the nodule and the snap.

Table 17-4   Spinal Curvatures

T A B L E   1 7 - 4   *Spinal Curvatures*

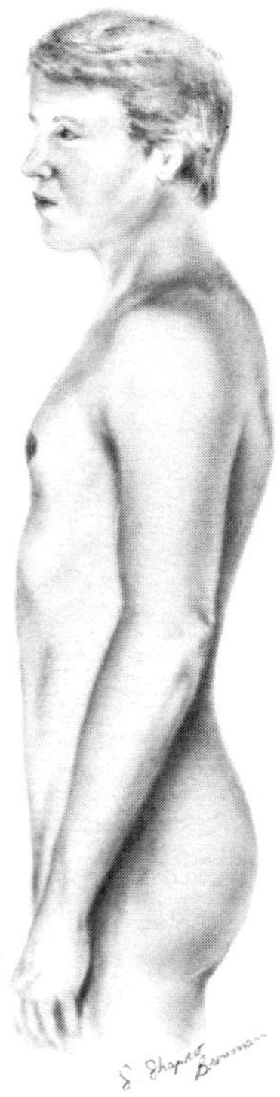

Normal Spinal Curvatures

Note the gentle curves of the normal spine—concavities in the cervical and lumbar regions and a convexity in the thorax.

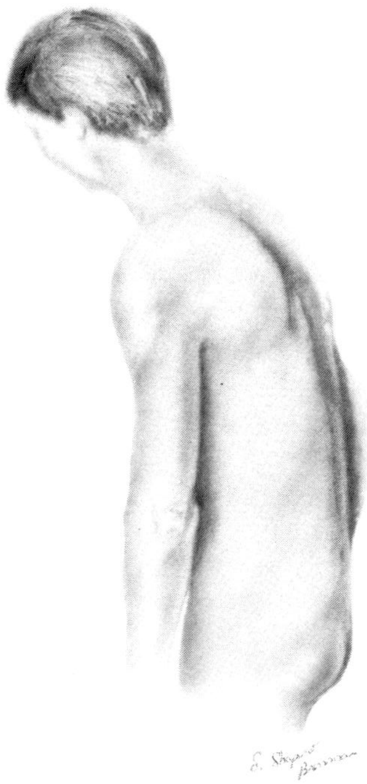

Flattening of the Lumbar Curve

When you see flattening of the lumbar curve, look for muscle spasm in the lumbar area and for decreased spinal mobility. This combination of signs suggests the possibility of a herniated lumbar disc or, especially in men, ankylosing spondylitis.

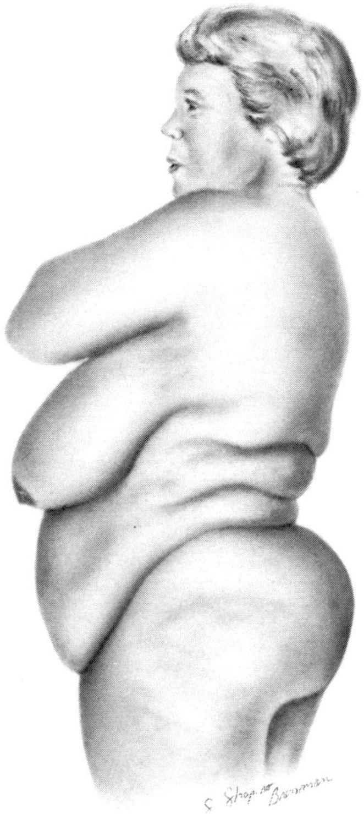

Lumbar Lordosis

Lordosis—an accentuation of the normal lumbar curve—develops to compensate for the protuberant abdomen of pregnancy or marked obesity (as illustrated here). It may also compensate for kyphosis and flexion deformities of the hips. A deep midline furrow may be seen between the lumbar paravertebral muscles.

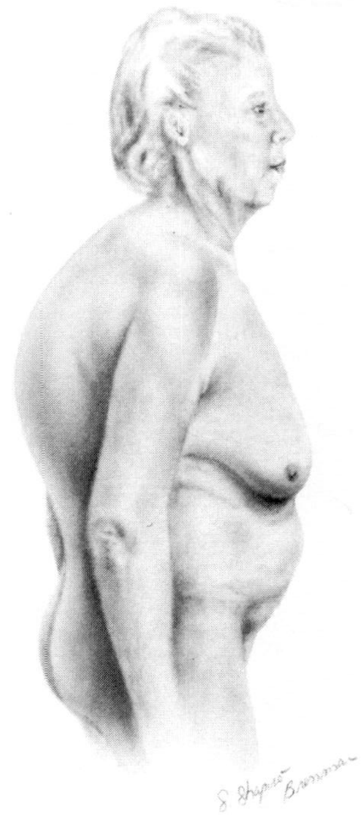

Kyphosis

Kyphosis—a rounded thoracic convexity—is common in aging, especially in women. In adolescent patients, consider Scheuermann's disease.

Table 17-4 *Spinal Curvatures*

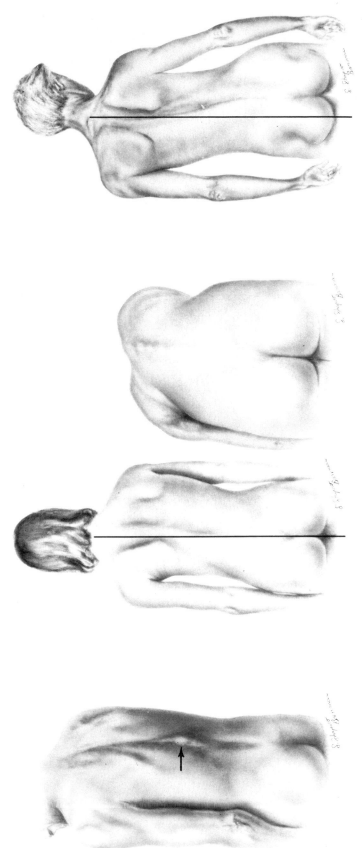

Gibbus

Gibbus is an angular deformity of a collapsed vertebra. Causes include metastatic cancer and tuberculosis of the spine.

Scoliosis

Scoliosis—a lateral curvature of the spine—is shown here with a thoracic convexity to the right. The body has compensated for the curve and a plumb line from T1 drops through the gluteal cleft. Scoliosis may be structural, as illustrated, or functional.

Structural scoliosis is typically associated with rotation of the vertebrae upon each other, and the rib cage is accordingly deformed. This deformity is seen best when the patient flexes forward. On the side of the thoracic convexity, the ribs bulge posteriorly and are widely separated. On the opposite side, they are displaced anteriorly and are close together.

Functional scoliosis compensates for other abnormalities such as unequal leg lengths. It involves neither vertebral rotation nor thoracic deformity. The scoliosis disappears with forward flexion.

List

List is a lateral tilt of the spine. When a plumb line dropped from the spinous process of T1 falls to one side of the gluteal cleft, a list is present. Causes include a herniated disc and painful spasms of the paravertebral muscles. Scoliosis is inherent in list but has not been fully compensated for by a spinal deviation in the opposite direction.

Table 17-5   Abnormalities of the Feet and Toes

TABLE 17-5   Abnormalities of the Feet and Toes

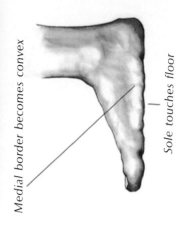

Medial border becomes convex

Sole touches floor

Flat Feet

Signs of flat feet may be apparent only when the patient stands, or they may become permanent. The longitudinal arch flattens so that the sole approaches or touches the floor. The normal concavity on the medial side of the foot becomes convex. Tenderness may be present from the medial malleolus down along the medial-plantar surface of the foot. Swelling may develop anterior to the malleoli. Inspect the shoes for excess wear on the inner side of the soles and heels.

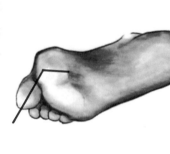

Hallux Valgus

In hallux valgus, the great toe is abnormally abducted in relationship to the first metatarsal, which itself is deviated medially. The head of the first metatarsal may enlarge on its medial side and a bursa may form at the pressure point. This bursa may become inflamed.

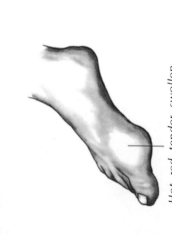

Hot, red, tender, swollen

Acute Gouty Arthritis

The metatarsophalangeal joint of the great toe may be the first joint involved in acute gouty arthritis. It is characterized by a very painful and tender, hot, dusky red swelling that extends beyond the margin of the joint. It is easily mistaken for a cellulitis. Acute gout may also involve the dorsum of the foot.

Table 17-5   Abnormalities of the Feet and Toes

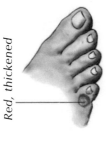

Red, tender

Granulation tissue

Ingrown Toenail

The sharp edge of a toenail may dig into and injure the lateral nail fold, resulting in inflammation and infection. A tender, reddened, overhanging nail fold, sometimes with granulation tissue and purulent discharge, results. The great toe is most often affected.

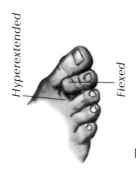

Hyperextended

Flexed

Hammer Toe

Most commonly involving the second toe, a hammer toe is characterized by hyperextension at the metatarsophalangeal joint with flexion at the proximal interphalangeal joint. A corn frequently develops at the pressure point over the proximal interphalangeal joint.

Red, thickened

Corn

A corn is a painful conical thickening of skin that results from recurrent pressure on normally thin skin. The apex of the cone points inward and causes pain. Corns characteristically occur over bony prominences (e.g., the 5th toe). When located in moist areas (e.g., at pressure points between the 4th and 5th toes), they are called soft corns.

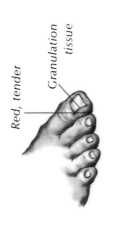

Callus

Like a corn, a callus is an area of greatly thickened skin that develops in a region of recurrent pressure. Unlike a corn, however, a callus involves skin that is normally thick, such as the sole, and is usually painless. If a callus is painful, suspect an underlying plantar wart.

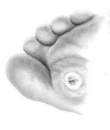

Plantar Wart

A plantar wart is a common wart (verruca vulgaris) located in the thickened skin of the sole. It may look somewhat like a callus or even be covered by one. Look for the characteristic small dark spots that give a stippled appearance to a wart. Normal skin lines stop at the wart's edge.

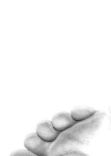

Neuropathic Ulcer

When pain sensation is diminished or absent (as in diabetic neuropathy, for example), neuropathic ulcers may develop at pressure points on the feet. Although often deep, infected, and indolent, they are painless. Callus formation about the ulcer is diagnostically helpful. Like the ulcer itself, it results from chronic pressure.

The Nervous System

CHAPTER 18

Anatomy and Physiology

This section deals briefly with structures, functions, and concepts that relate directly to the neurologic examination. After a short description of the brain, spinal cord, cranial and peripheral nerves, and reflexes, it summarizes important motor and sensory pathways.

As you review this material, note that the *central nervous system* consists of the brain and the spinal cord. The *peripheral nervous system* consists of the 12 pairs of cranial nerves and the spinal and peripheral nerves. Most of the peripheral nerves contain both motor and sensory fibers.

Central Nervous System

The Brain

The brain has four regions: the cerebrum, the diencephalon, the brainstem, and the cerebellum. The cerebral hemispheres contain the greatest mass of brain tissue. Each hemisphere is subdivided into frontal, parietal, temporal, and occipital lobes.

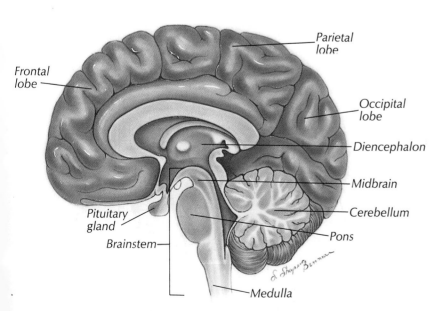

RIGHT HALF OF THE BRAIN, MEDIAL VIEW

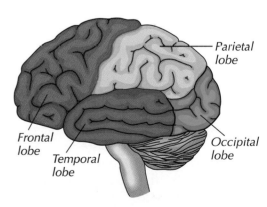

LEFT LATERAL VIEW OF THE BRAIN

The brain is a vast network of interconnecting *neurons* (nerve cells). These consist of cell bodies and their *axons*—single long fibers that conduct impulses to other parts of the nervous system.

Brain tissue may be gray or white. *Gray matter* consists of aggregations of neuronal cell bodies. It rims the surfaces of the cerebral hemispheres, forming the cerebral cortex. *White matter* consists of neuronal axons that are coated with myelin. The myelin sheaths, which create the white color, allow nerve impulses to travel more rapidly.

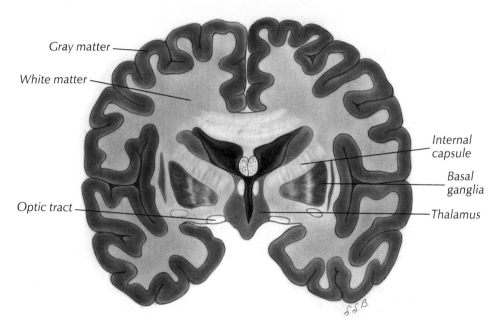

CORONAL SECTION, BRAIN

Deep in the brain lie additional clusters of gray matter. These include the *basal ganglia,* which affect movement, and the thalamus and the hypothalamus (structures in the deincephalon). The *thalamus* processes sensory impulses and relays them to the cerebral cortex. The *hypothalamus* maintains homeostasis and regulates temperature, heart rate, and blood pressure. The hypothalamus affects the endocrine system and governs emotional behaviors such as anger and sexual drive. Hormones secreted in the hypothalamus act directly on the pituitary gland.

In contrast, note the *internal capsule,* a white matter structure where myelinated fibers converge from all parts of the cerebral cortex and descend into the brainstem. The *brainstem,* which connects the upper part of the brain with the spinal cord, has three sections: the midbrain, the pons, and the medulla.

Consciousness depends on the interaction between intact cerebral hemispheres and an important structure in the diencephalon and upper brainstem, the *reticular activating (arousal) system.*

The *cerebellum,* which lies at the base of the brain, coordinates all movement and helps maintain the body upright in space.

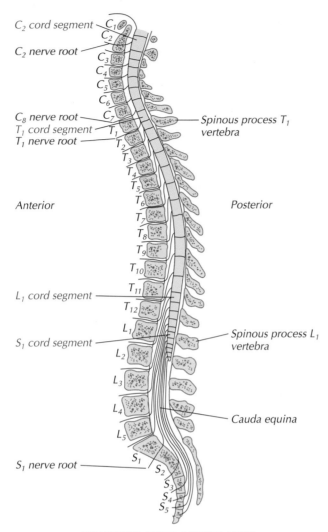

C_2 cord segment — C_1
C_2
C_2 nerve root — C_3
C_4
C_5
C_6
C_8 nerve root — C_7
T_1 cord segment — T_1
T_1 nerve root — T_2
T_3
T_4
T_5
T_6
T_7
T_8
T_9
T_{10}
L_1 cord segment — T_{11}
T_{12}
L_1
S_1 cord segment — L_2
L_3
L_4
L_5
S_1 nerve root — S_1
S_2
S_3
S_4
S_5

Spinous process T_1 vertebra

Anterior

Posterior

Spinous process L_1 vertebra

Cauda equina

THE SPINAL CORD, LATERAL VIEW

The Spinal Cord

The *spinal cord* is a cylindrical mass of nerve tissue encased within the bony vertebral column, extending from the medulla to the first or second lumbar vertebra. It contains important motor and sensory nerve pathways that exit and enter the cord via anterior and posterior nerve roots and spinal and peripheral nerves. The spinal cord also mediates reflex activity of the deep tendon (or spinal nerve) reflexes. (Motor and sensory tracts and the deep tendon reflexes are further discussed on pp. 560–565).

The spinal cord is divided into five segments: cervical (C1–8), thoracic (T1–12), lumbar (L1–5), sacral (S1–5), and coccygeal.

Note that the spinal cord is not as long as the vertebral canal. The level of the nerve roots exiting the cord differs from the adjacent vertebral level. The lumbar and sacral roots travel the longest intraspinal distance. These roots fan out like a horse's tail at L1–2, giving rise to the term *cauda equina.* (To avoid injury to the cord, most lumbar punctures are performed at the L3–4 vertebral interspace.)

Peripheral Nervous System

The Cranial Nerves

Twelve pairs of special nerves called cranial nerves emerge from within the skull (cranium). Cranial Nerves II through XII arise from the diencephalon and the brainstem, as illustrated below. (Cranial Nerves I and II are actually fiber tracts emerging from the brain.) Some cranial nerves are limited to general motor or sensory functions, whereas others are specialized, producing smell, vision, or hearing (I, II, VIII).

Functions of the cranial nerves (CN) most relevant to physical examination are summarized on the next page.

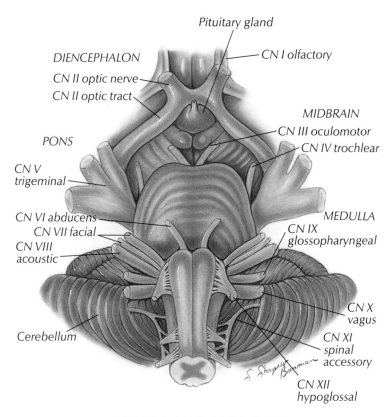

INFERIOR SURFACE OF THE BRAIN

No.	Cranial Nerve	Function
I	Olfactory	Sense of smell
II	Optic	Vision
III	Oculomotor	Pupillary constriction, opening the eye, and most extraocular movements
IV	Trochlear	Downward, inward movement of the eye
VI	Abducens	Lateral deviation of the eye
V	Trigeminal	*Motor*—temporal and masseter muscles (jaw clenching), also lateral movement of the jaw *Sensory*—facial. The nerve has three divisions: (1) ophthalmic, (2) maxillary, and (3) mandibular.

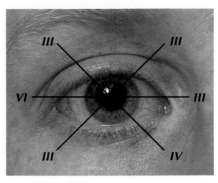

RIGHT EYE (CN III, IV, VI)

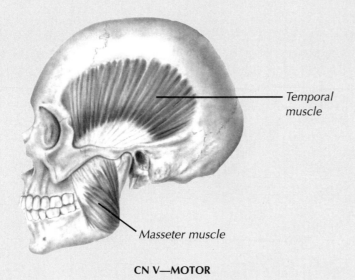

CN V—MOTOR

Temporal muscle

Masseter muscle

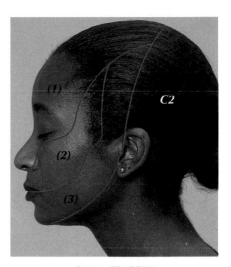

CN V—SENSORY

No.	Cranial Nerve	Function
VII	Facial	*Motor*—facial movements, including those of facial expression, closing the eye, and closing the mouth *Sensory*—taste for salty, sweet, sour, and bitter substances on the anterior two thirds of the tongue
VIII	Acoustic	Hearing (cochlear division) and balance (vestibular division)
IX	Glossopharyngeal	*Motor*—pharynx *Sensory*—posterior portions of the eardrum and ear canal, the pharynx, and the posterior tongue, including taste (salty, sweet, sour, bitter)
X	Vagus	*Motor*—palate, pharynx, and larynx *Sensory*—pharynx and larynx
XI	Spinal accessory	*Motor*—the sternomastoid and upper portion of the trapezius
XII	Hypoglossal	*Motor*—tongue

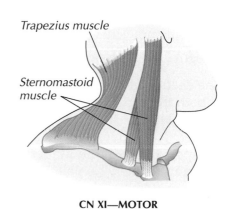

Trapezius muscle

Sternomastoid muscle

CN XI—MOTOR

The Peripheral Nerves

In addition to cranial nerves, the peripheral nervous system also includes spinal and peripheral nerves that carry impulses to and from the cord. Thirty-one pairs of nerves attach to the spinal cord: 8 cervical, 12 thoracic, 5 lumbar, 5 sacral, and 1 coccygeal. Each nerve has an anterior (ventral) root containing motor fibers, and a posterior (dorsal) root containing sensory fibers. The anterior and posterior roots merge to form a short (<5 mm) *spinal nerve.* Spinal nerve fibers commingle with similar fibers from other levels to form *peripheral nerves.* Most peripheral nerves contain both *sensory* (afferent) and *motor* (efferent) fibers.

Like the brain, the spinal cord contains both gray matter and white matter. Nuclei of gray matter (aggregations of nerve cell bodies) are surrounded by white tracts of nerve fibers connecting the brain to the peripheral nervous system. Note the butterfly appearance of the gray matter nuclei, with anterior and posterior horns.

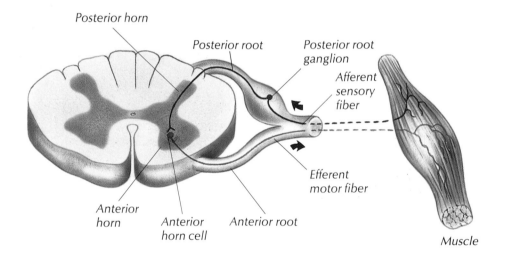

THE SPINAL CORD, CROSS SECTION

Spinal Reflexes: The Deep Tendon Response

The deep tendon (or muscle stretch) reflexes are relayed over structures of both the central and peripheral nervous systems. Recall that a *reflex* is an involuntary stereotypical response that may involve as few as two neurons, one afferent (sensory) and one efferent (motor), across a single synapse. The deep tendon reflexes in the arms and legs are such monosynaptic reflexes. They illustrate the simplest unit of sensory and motor function. (Other reflexes are polysynaptic, involving interneurons interposed between sensory and motor neurons.)

To elicit a deep tendon reflex, briskly tap the tendon of a partially stretched muscle. For the reflex to fire, all components of the reflex arc must be intact: sensory nerve fibers, spinal cord synapse, motor nerve fibers, neuromuscular junction, and muscle fibers. Tapping the tendon activates special sensory fibers in the partially stretched muscle, triggering a sensory impulse that travels to the spinal cord via a peripheral nerve. The stimulated sensory fiber synapses directly with the anterior horn cell innervating the same muscle. When the impulse crosses the neuromuscular junction, the muscle suddenly contracts, completing the reflex arc.

Because each deep tendon reflex involves specific spinal segments, together with their sensory and motor fibers, an abnormal reflex can help you to locate a pathologic lesion. You should know the segmental levels of the deep tendon reflexes. You can remember them easily by their numerical sequence in ascending order from ankle to triceps: S1—L2, 3, 4,—C5, 6, 7.

Ankle reflex	Sacral 1 primarily
Knee reflex	Lumbar 2, 3, 4
Supinator (brachioradialis) reflex	Cervical 5, 6
Biceps reflex	Cervical 5, 6
Triceps reflex	Cervical 6, 7

Reflexes may be initiated by stimulating skin as well as muscle. Stroking the skin of the abdomen, for example, produces a localized muscular twitch. These superficial (cutaneous) reflexes and their corresponding spinal segments include:

Abdominal reflexes—upper	Thoracic 8, 9, 10
—lower	Thoracic 10, 11, 12
Plantar responses	Lumbar 5, Sacral 1

Motor Pathways

Motor pathways contain upper motor neurons, synapses in the brainstem or spinal cord, and lower motor neurons. Nerve cell bodies or *upper motor neurons* lie in the motor strip of the cerebral cortex and in several brainstem nuclei; their axons synapse with motor nuclei in the brainstem (for cranial nerves) and in the spinal cord (for peripheral nerves). *Lower motor neurons* have cell bodies in the spinal cord, termed anterior horn cells; their axons transmit impulses through the anterior roots and spinal nerves into peripheral nerves, terminating at the neuromuscular junction.

Three kinds of motor pathways impinge on the anterior horn cells: the corticospinal tract, the basal ganglia system, and the cerebellar system. There are additional pathways originating in the brainstem that mediate flexor and extensor tone in limb movement and posture (most notable in coma; see Table 18-9 p. 620).

- The *corticospinal (pyramidal) tract.* The corticospinal tracts mediate voluntary movement and integrate skilled, complicated, or delicate movements by stimulating selected muscular actions and inhibiting others. They also carry impulses that inhibit muscle tone, the slight tension maintained by normal muscle even when it is relaxed. The corticospinal tracts originate in the motor cortex of the brain. Motor fibers travel down into the lower medulla, where they form an anatomical structure resembling a pyramid. There most of these fibers cross to the opposite (contralateral) side of the medulla, continue downward, and synapse with anterior horn cells or with intermediate neurons. (Tracts synapsing in the brainstem with motor nuclei of the cranial nerves are termed *corticobulbar.*)

- The *basal ganglia system.* This exceedingly complex system includes motor pathways between the cerebral cortex, basal ganglia, brainstem, and spinal cord. It helps to maintain muscle tone and to control body movements, especially gross automatic movements such as walking.

- The *cerebellar system.* The cerebellum receives both sensory and motor input and coordinates motor activity, maintains equilibrium, and helps to control posture.

All of these higher motor pathways affect movement only through the lower motor neurons—sometimes called the "final common pathway." Any movement, whether initiated voluntarily in the cortex, "automatically" in the basal ganglia, or reflexly in the sensory receptors, must ultimately be translated into action via the anterior horn cells. A lesion in any of these areas will affect movement or reflex activity.

When the corticospinal tract is damaged or destroyed, its functions are reduced or lost below the level of injury. When upper motor neurons are damaged above the crossover of its tracts in the medulla, motor impairment develops on the opposite (contralateral) side. In damage below the crossover, motor impairment occurs on the same (ipsilateral) side of the body. The affected limb becomes weak or paralyzed, and skilled, complicated, or delicate movements are performed especially poorly when compared to gross movements. Muscle tone is increased and deep tendon reflexes are exaggerated.

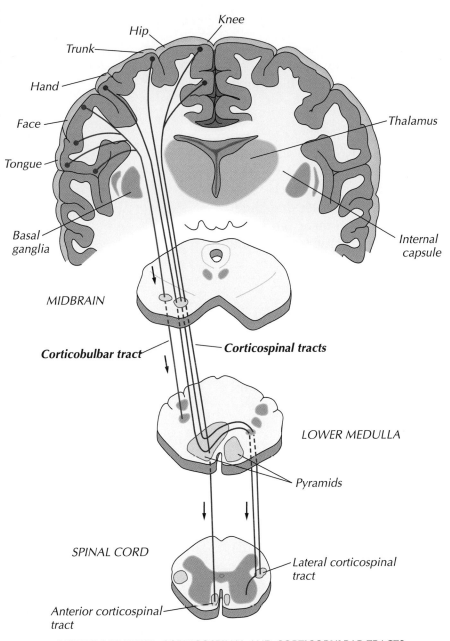

Hip

Knee

Trunk

Hand

Face

Tongue

Thalamus

Basal
ganglia

Internal
capsule

MIDBRAIN

Corticobulbar tract

Corticospinal tracts

LOWER MEDULLA

Pyramids

SPINAL CORD

Lateral corticospinal
tract

Anterior corticospinal
tract

MOTOR PATHWAYS: CORTICOSPINAL AND CORTICOBULBAR TRACTS

Damage to the lower motor neurons causes ipsilateral weakness and paralysis, but in this case muscle tone and reflexes are decreased or absent.

Disease of the basal ganglia system or cerebellar system does not cause paralysis, but can be disabling. Damage to the basal ganglia system produces changes in muscle tone (most often an increase), disturbances in posture and gait, a slowness or lack of spontaneous and automatic movements (*bradykinesia*), and a variety of involuntary movements. Cerebellar damage impairs coordination, gait, and equilibrium, and decreases muscle tone.

Sensory Pathways

Sensory impulses not only participate in reflex activity, as previously described, but also give rise to conscious sensation, calibrate body position in space, and help regulate internal autonomic functions like blood pressure, heart rate, and respiration.

A complex system of sensory receptors relays impulses from skin, mucous membranes, muscles, tendons, and viscera. Sensory fibers registering sensations such as pain, temperature, position, and touch, pass through the peripheral nerves and posterior roots and enter the spinal cord. Once inside the cord, sensory impulses reach the sensory cortex of the brain via one of the two pathways: the spinothalamic tracts or the posterior columns.

Within one or two spinal segments from their entry into the cord, fibers conducting the sensations of *pain* and *temperature* pass into the posterior horn of the spinal cord and synapse with secondary sensory neurons. Fibers conducting *crude touch*—a sensation perceived as light touch but without accurate localization—also pass into the posterior horn and synapse with secondary neurons. The secondary neurons then cross to the opposite side and pass upward in the *spinothalamic tract* into the thalamus.

Fibers conducting the sensations of *position* and *vibration* pass directly into the *posterior columns* of the cord and travel upward to the medulla, together with fibers transmitting *fine touch*—touch that is accurately localized and finely discriminating. These fibers synapse in the medulla with secondary sensory neurons. Fibers projecting from secondary neurons cross to the opposite side at the medullary level and continue on to the thalamus.

At the *thalamic level,* the general quality of sensation is perceived (e.g., pain, cold, pleasant and unpleasant), but fine distinctions are not made. For full perception, a third group of sensory neurons sends impulses from the thalamus to the *sensory cortex* of the brain. Here stimuli are localized and discriminations made among them.

Lesions at different points in the sensory pathways produce different kinds of sensory loss. Patterns of sensory loss, together with their associated motor findings, help you to identify where the causative lesions might be. A lesion in the sensory cortex may not impair the perception of pain, touch, and position, for example, but does impair finer discrimination. A person so affected cannot appreciate the size, shape, or tex-

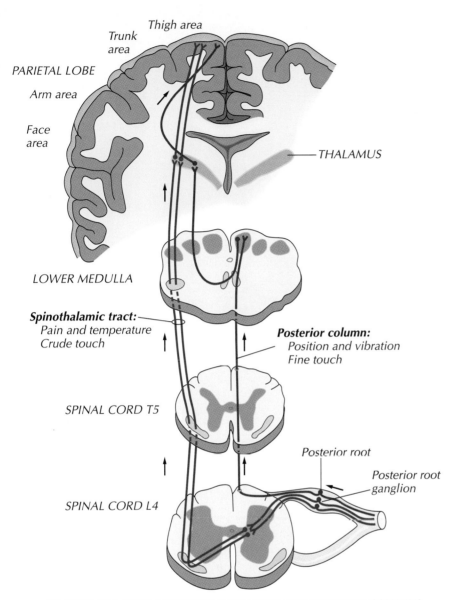

SENSORY PATHWAYS: SPINOTHALAMIC TRACT AND POSTERIOR COLUMNS

ture of an object by feeling it and therefore cannot identify it. Loss of position and vibration sense with preservation of other sensations points to disease of the posterior columns, while loss of all sensations from the waist down, together with paralysis and hyperactive reflexes in the legs, indicates transection of the spinal cord (see Table 18-5, pp. 613–615). Crude and light touch are often preserved despite partial damage to the cord because impulses originating on one side of the body travel up both sides of the cord.

A knowledge of *dermatomes* also aids in localizing neurologic lesions. A dermatome is the band of skin innervated by the sensory root of a single spinal nerve. Dermatome patterns are mapped in the next two figures. Their levels are considerably more variable than the diagrams suggest, and dermatomes overlap each other. The sensory nerves from each side of the body overlap slightly across the midline. The distribution of a few key peripheral nerves is shown in the inserts on the left.

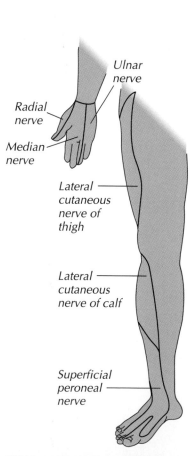

Ulnar nerve

Radial nerve

Median nerve

Lateral cutaneous nerve of thigh

Lateral cutaneous nerve of calf

Superficial peroneal nerve

AREAS INNERVATED BY PERIPHERAL NERVES

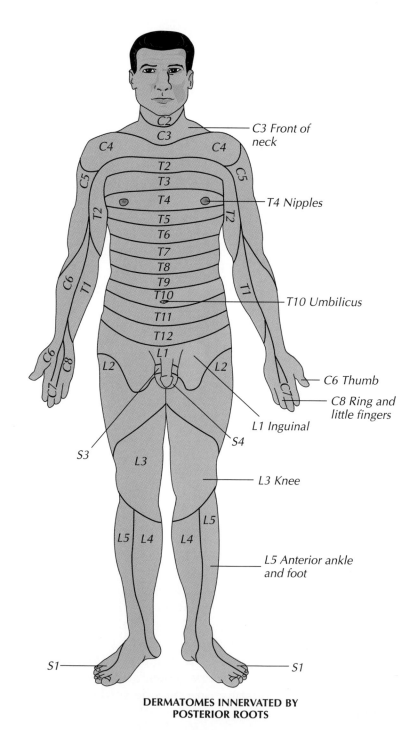

C2
C3
C4
C4
C5
C5
T2
T3
T4
T5
T6
T7
T8
T9
T10
T11
T12
T2
T2
C6
T1
T1
L1
L2
L2
C6
C8
C7
C7
S3
S4
L3
L5
L5
L4
L4
S1
S1

C3 Front of neck

T4 Nipples

T10 Umbilicus

C6 Thumb

C8 Ring and little fingers

L1 Inguinal

L3 Knee

L5 Anterior ankle and foot

DERMATOMES INNERVATED BY POSTERIOR ROOTS

Do not try to memorize all the dermatomes. It is useful, however, to remember the locations of some, such as those shaded in green on the right side of the diagrams.

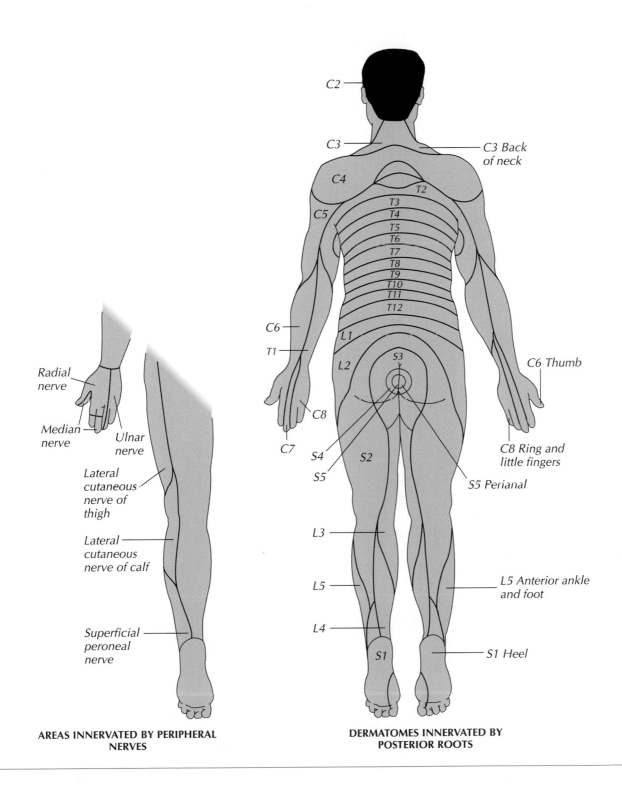

AREAS INNERVATED BY PERIPHERAL NERVES

DERMATOMES INNERVATED BY POSTERIOR ROOTS

Changes With Age

Aging. In assessing the nervous system of an elderly person, it is some-times difficult to distinguish the changes of normal aging from those of age-related or other diseases. Some findings that you would consider abnormal in younger people, however, occur often enough in the el-derly that you may attribute them to aging alone. Alterations in hearing, vision, extraocular movements, and pupillary size, shape, and reactivity have been described in Chapter 7 (see pp. 181–183).

Changes in the motor system are common. Elderly persons move and react with less speed and agility than younger ones, and skeletal mus-cles decrease in bulk. The hands of an aged person often look thin and bony because their small muscles have atrophied. Look for such mus-cular wasting in the backs of the hands, where atrophy of the dorsal in-terosseous muscles may leave concavities or grooves. As illustrated on page 575, this change is often most evident between the thumb and the hand (1st and 2nd metacarpals) but may also be seen between the other metacarpals. Atrophy of small muscles may also flatten the thenar and hypothenar eminences of the palms. Muscle strength, though dimin-ished, is relatively well maintained. Arm and leg muscles may also show atrophy. This sometimes exaggerates the apparent size of adjacent joints.

Occasionally, an aged person develops a benign essential tremor (p. 610). Head, jaw, lips, or hands may tremble at a rate and amplitude suggest-ing parkinsonism (p. 610). The tremor is usually slightly faster, however, and there is no muscular rigidity.

Old age may also alter some of the reflexes. The gag reflex may be di-minished or absent. Ankle reflexes may be symmetrically decreased or absent, even when reinforced. Less commonly, knee reflexes are simi-larly affected. Abdominal reflexes may diminish or disappear and, partly because of musculoskeletal changes in the feet, the plantar re-sponses become less obvious and more difficult to interpret.

Vibration sense is frequently decreased or lost in the feet and ankles (but not in the fingers or over the shins). Less commonly, position sense may diminish or disappear.

If changes such as those described are accompanied by other neurologic abnormalities, or if atrophy and reflex changes are asymmetrical, you should search for an explanation other than age alone.

Techniques of Examination

General Approach

Two important questions govern the neurologic examination: Are right- and left-sided findings symmetrical? And, if the findings are asymmetrical or otherwise abnormal, does the causative lesion lie in the central nervous system or in the peripheral nervous system?

The detail of an appropriate neurologic examination varies widely. It is important to master the techniques for a thorough examination, and to feel comfortable evaluating neurologic symptoms and disease. As you gain experience, you will find that in healthy persons your examination will be relatively brief. In this section you will learn the techniques for a practicable and reasonably comprehensive examination of neurologic function. Be aware that neurologists may use many other techniques in specific situations.

For efficiency, you should integrate certain portions of the neurologic assessment with other parts of your examination. Survey the patient's mental status and speech during the interview, for example, even though you may wish to do further testing during your neurologic evaluation. Assess some of the cranial nerves as you examine the head and neck, and inspect the arms and legs for neurologic abnormalities while you also observe the peripheral vascular and musculoskeletal systems. Chapter 4 provides an outline for this kind of integrated approach. Think about and describe your findings, however, in terms of the nervous system as a unit.

Organize your thinking into five categories: (1) mental status and speech (see Chap. 3), (2) cranial nerves, (3) the motor system, (4) the sensory system, and (5) reflexes. If your findings are abnormal, begin to group them into patterns of central or peripheral disorders.

The Cranial Nerves

Overview. The examination of the cranial nerves (often abbreviated as CN) can be summarized as follows:

I	Smell
II	Visual acuity, visual fields, and ocular fundi
II, III	Pupillary reactions
III, IV, VI	Extraocular movements
V	Corneal reflexes, facial sensation, and jaw movements
VII	Facial movements
VIII	Hearing
IX, X	Swallowing and rise of the palate, gag reflex
V, VII, X, XII	Voice and speech
XI	Shoulder and neck movements
XII	Tongue symmetry and position

Cranial Nerve I—Olfactory. Test the *sense of smell* by presenting the patient with familiar and nonirritating odors. First be sure that each nasal passage is open by compressing one side of the nose and asking the patient to sniff through the other. The patient should then close both eyes. Occlude one nostril and test smell in the other with such substances as cloves, coffee, soap, or vanilla. Ask if the patient smells anything and, if so, what. Test the other side. A person should normally perceive odor on each side, and can often identify it.

Loss of smell has many causes, including nasal disease, head trauma, smoking, and the use of cocaine. It may be congenital.

Cranial Nerve II—Optic. Test *visual acuity.* (See pp. 184–185.)

Inspect the *optic fundi* with your ophthalmoscope, paying special attention to the optic discs. (See pp. 191–195.)

Optic atrophy, papilledema

Screen the visual fields by confrontation. (See pp. 185–186.) Occasionally—in a stroke patient, for example—screening indicates a visual field defect, such as a homonymous hemianopsia, that you cannot confirm by testing one eye at a time. This screening observation, nevertheless, is significant.

These findings suggest visual *extinction*, a subtle impairment detectable only when testing both eyes simultaneously. It suggests a lesion in the parietal cortex.

Cranial Nerves II and III—Optic and Oculomotor. Inspect the size and shape of the pupils, and compare one side with the other. Test the *pupillary reactions to light*; if these are abnormal, examine the *near response* also. (See pp. 188–189.)

See Table 7-7, Pupillary Abnormalities (p. 217).

Cranial Nerves III, IV, and VI—Oculomotor, Trochlear, and Abducens. Test the *extraocular movements* in the six cardinal directions of gaze, and look for loss of conjugate movements in any of the six directions. Check convergence of the eyes. Identify any nystagmus, noting the direction of gaze in which it appears, the plane in which movements occur (horizontal, vertical, rotary, or mixed), and the direction of the quick and slow components. (See pp. 189–191.)

See Table 7-8, Deviations of the Eyes (p. 218).

See Table 18-1, Nystagmus (pp. 606–607).

Look for *ptosis* (drooping of the upper eyelids). A slight difference in the width of the palpebral fissures may be noted in about one third of all normal people.

Ptosis in 3rd nerve palsy, Horner's syndrome, myasthenia gravis

Cranial Nerve V—Trigeminal

Motor. While palpating the temporal and masseter muscles in turn, ask the patient to clench his or her teeth. Note the strength of muscle contraction.

Weak or absent contraction of the temporal and masseter muscles on one side suggests a lesion of CN V. Bilateral weakness may result from peripheral or central involvement. When the patient has no teeth, this test may be difficult to interpret.

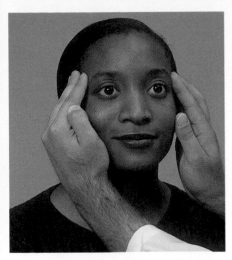

PALPATING TEMPORAL MUSCLES

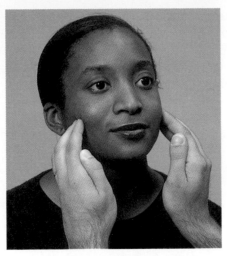

PALPATING MASSETER MUSCLES

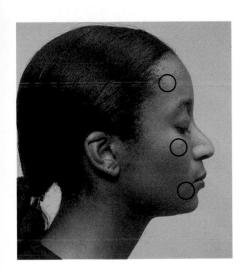

Sensory. After explaining what you plan to do, test the forehead, cheeks, and jaw on each side for *pain sensation.* Suggested areas are indicated by the circles. The patient's eyes should be closed. Use a safety pin or other suitable sharp object,* occasionally substituting the blunt end for the point as a stimulus. Ask the patient to report whether it is "sharp" or "dull" and to compare sides.

Unilateral decrease in or loss of facial sensation suggests a lesion of CN V or of interconnecting higher sensory pathways. Such a sensory loss may also be associated with a conversion reaction.

If you find an abnormality, confirm it by testing *temperature sensation.* Two test tubes, filled with hot and ice-cold water, are the traditional stimuli. A tuning fork may also be used. It usually feels cool. If you are near running water, the fork is easily made colder or warm. Dry it before use. Touch the skin and ask the patient to identify "hot" or "cold."

Then test for *light touch,* using a fine wisp of cotton. Ask the patient to respond whenever you touch the skin.

*To avoid transmitting infection, use a new object with each patient. You can create a sharp wood splinter by breaking or twisting a cotton swab. The cotton end of the swab can also be used as a dull stimulus.

Test *the corneal reflex.* Ask the patient to look up and away from you. Approaching from the other side, out of the patient's line of vision, and avoiding the eyelashes, touch the cornea (not just the conjunctiva) lightly with a fine wisp of cotton. If the patient is apprehensive, however, first touching the conjunctiva may allay fear.

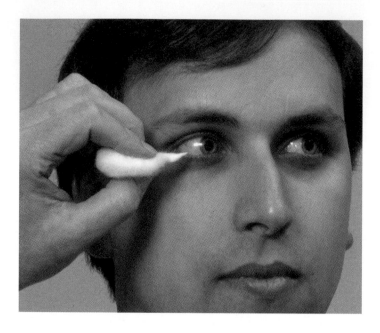

Look for blinking of the eyes, the normal reaction to this stimulus. (The sensory limb of this reflex is carried in CN V, the motor response in CN VII.) Use of contact lenses frequently diminishes or abolishes this reflex.

Absence of blinking suggests a lesion of CN V. A lesion of CN VII (the nerve to the muscles that close the eyes) may also impair this reflex.

Cranial Nerve VII—Facial. Inspect the face, both at rest and during conversation with the patient. Note any asymmetry (e.g., of the nasolabial folds), and observe any tics or other abnormal movements.

Flattening of the nasolabial fold and drooping of the lower eyelid suggest facial weakness.

Ask the patient to:

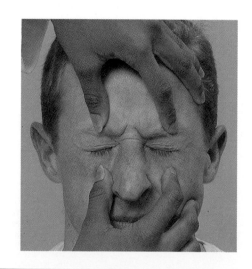

1. Raise both eyebrows.
2. Frown.
3. Close both eyes tightly so that you cannot open them. Test muscular strength by trying to open them, as illustrated.
4. Show both upper and lower teeth.
5. Smile.
6. Puff out both cheeks.

Note any weakness or asymmetry.

A peripheral injury to the CN VII, such as Bell's palsy, affects both the upper and the lower face; a central lesion affects mainly the lower face. See Table 18-2, Types of Facial Paralysis (pp. 608–609).

In unilateral facial paralysis, the mouth droops on the paralyzed side when the patient smiles or grimaces.

Cranial Nerve VIII—Acoustic. Assess _hearing._ If hearing loss is present, (1) test for _lateralization,_ and (2) compare _air and bone conduction._ (See pp. 197–198.)

Specific tests of _vestibular function_ are seldom included in the usual neurologic examination. Consult textbooks of neurology or otolaryngology as the need arises.

Cranial Nerves IX and X—Glossopharyngeal and Vagus. Listen to the patient's _voice._ Is it hoarse or does it have a nasal quality?

Is there difficulty in swallowing?

Ask the patient to say "ah" or to yawn as you watch the _movements of the soft palate and the pharynx._ The soft palate normally rises symmetrically, the uvula remains in the midline, and each side of the posterior pharynx moves medially, like a curtain. The slightly curved uvula seen occasionally in a normal person should not be mistaken for a uvula deviated by a 10th nerve lesion.

Warn the patient that you are going to test the _gag reflex._ Stimulate the back of the throat lightly on each side in turn and note the gag reflex. It may be symmetrically diminished or absent in some normal people.

Cranial Nerve XI—Spinal Accessory. From behind, look for atrophy or fasciculations in the trapezius muscles, and compare one side with the other. Ask the patient to shrug both shoulders upward against your hands. Note the strength and contraction of the trapezii.

See Table 7-17, Patterns of Hearing Loss (p. 232).

Nystagmus may indicate vestibular dysfunction. See Table 18-1, Nystagmus (pp. 606–607).

Hoarseness in vocal cord paralysis; a nasal voice in paralysis of the palate

Pharyngeal or palatal weakness

The palate fails to rise with a bilateral lesion of the vagus nerve. In unilateral paralysis, one side of the palate fails to rise and, together with the uvula, is pulled toward the normal side (see p. 202).

Unilateral absence of this reflex suggests a lesion of CN IX, perhaps CN X.

Weakness with atrophy and fasciculations indicates a peripheral nerve disorder. When the trapezius is paralyzed, the shoulder droops and the scapula is displaced downward and laterally.

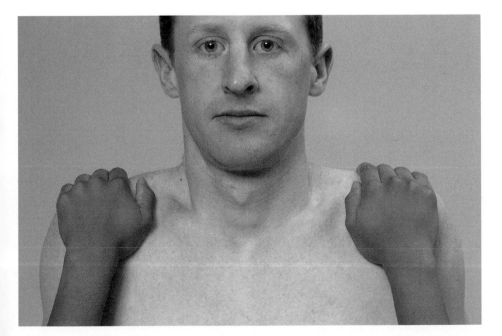

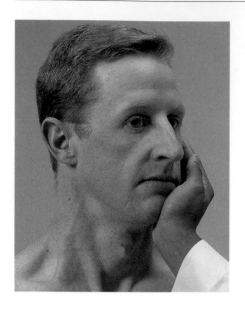

Ask the patient to turn his or her head to each side against your hand. Observe the contraction of the opposite sternomastoid and note the force of the movement against your hand.

A supine patient with bilateral weakness of the sternomastoids has difficulty raising the head off the pillow.

Cranial Nerve XII—Hypoglossal. Listen to the articulation of the patient's words. This depends on Cranial Nerves V, VII, and X as well as XII. Inspect the patient's tongue as it lies on the floor of the mouth. Look for any atrophy or *fasciculations* (fine, flickering, irregular movements in small groups of muscle fibers). Some coarser restless movements are often seen seen in a normal tongue. Then, with the patient's tongue protruded, look for asymmetry, atrophy, or deviation from the midline. Ask the patient to move the tongue from side to side, and note the symmetry of the movement. In ambiguous cases, ask the patient to push the tongue against the inside of each cheek in turn as you palpate externally for strength.

For poor articulation (*dysarthria*), see Table 3-1, Disorders of Speech (p. 123). Atrophy and fasciculations in amyotrophic lateral sclerosis, polio

With unilateral cortical lesions, the protruded tongue deviates toward the *affected* (weaker) side (see p. 201). When pushing, the tongue muscles of the unaffected side are stronger and thrust more firmly against the cheek of the affected side.

The Motor System

As you assess the motor system, focus on body position, involuntary movements, characteristics of the muscles (bulk, tone, and strength), and coordination. These components are described below in sequence. You may either use this sequence or check each component in the arms, legs, and trunk in turn. If you see an abnormality, identify the muscle(s) involved. Think about whether the abnormality is central or peripheral in origin, and begin to learn which nerves innervate the affected muscles.

Body Position. Observe the patient's body position during movement and at rest.

Abnormal positions alert you to neurologic deficits such as paralysis.

Involuntary Movements. Watch for involuntary movements such as tremors, tics, or fasciculations. Note their location, quality, rate, rhythm, and amplitude, and their relation to posture, activity, fatigue, emotion, and other factors.

See Table 18-3, Involuntary Movements (pp. 610–611).

Muscle Bulk. Compare the size and contours of muscles. Do the muscles look flat or concave, suggesting atrophy? If so, is the process unilateral or bilateral? Is it proximal or distal?

When looking for atrophy, pay particular attention to the hands, shoulders, and thighs. The thenar and hypothenar eminences should be full and convex, and the spaces between the metacarpals, where the dorsal interosseous muscles lie, should be full or only slightly depressed. Atrophy of hand muscles may occur with normal aging, however, as shown on the right below.

Muscular *atrophy* refers to a loss of muscle bulk (wasting). It results from diseases of the peripheral nervous system such as diabetic neuropathy, as well as diseases of the muscles themselves. *Hypertrophy* refers to an increase in bulk with proportionate strength, while increased bulk with diminished strength is called *pseudohypertrophy* (seen in the Duchenne form of muscular dystrophy).

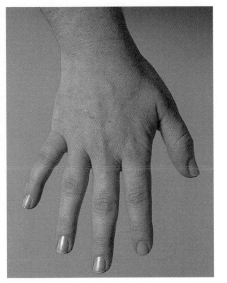

Hand of a 44-year-old woman

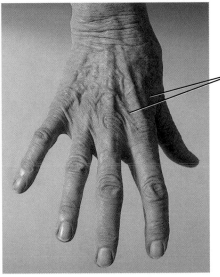

Hand of an 84-year-old woman

Atrophy

Flattening of the thenar and hypothenar eminences and furrowing between the metacarpals suggest atrophy. Localized atrophy of the thenar and hypothenar eminences suggests damage to the median and ulnar nerves, respectively.

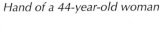

Hand of a 44-year-old woman

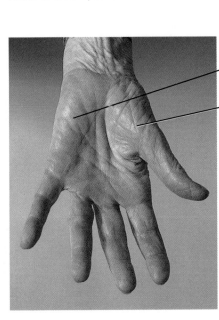

Hand of an 84-year-old woman

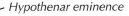

Hypothenar eminence

Flattening of the thenar eminence due to mild atrophy

Other causes of muscular atrophy include motor neuron diseases, disuse of the muscles, rheumatoid arthritis, and protein-calorie malnutrition.

Be alert for fasciculations in atrophic muscles. If you see none, a tap on the muscle with a reflex hammer may stimulate them.

Muscle Tone. When a normal muscle with an intact nerve supply is re-laxed voluntarily, it maintains a slight residual tension known as mus-cle tone. This can be assessed best by feeling the muscle's resistance to passive stretch. Persuade the patient to relax. Take one hand with yours and, while supporting the elbow, flex and extend the patient's fingers, wrist, and elbow, and put the shoulder through a moderate range of mo-tion. With practice, these actions can be combined into a single smooth movement. On each side, note muscle tone—the resistance offered to your movements. Tense patients may show increased resistance. You will learn the feel of normal resistance only with repeated practice.

If you suspect decreased resistance, hold the forearm and shake the hand loosely back and forth. Normally the hand moves back and forth freely but is not completely floppy.

If resistance is increased, determine whether it varies as you move the limb or whether it persists throughout the range of movement and in both directions, e.g., during both flexion and extension. Feel for any jerkiness in the resistance.

To assess muscle tone in the legs, support the patient's thigh with one hand, grasp the foot with the other, and flex and extend the patient's knee and ankle on each side. Note the resistance to your movements.

Muscle Strength. Normal individuals vary widely in their strength, and your standard of normal, while admittedly rough, should allow for such variables as age, sex, and muscular training. A person's dominant side is usually slightly stronger than the other side. Keep this difference in mind when you compare sides.

Test muscle strength by asking the patient to move actively against your resistance or to resist your movement. Remember that a muscle is strongest when shortest, and weakest when longest.

If the muscles are too weak to overcome resistance, test them against gravity alone or with gravity eliminated. When the forearm rests in a pronated position, for example, dorsiflexion at the wrist can be tested against gravity alone. When the forearm is midway between pronation and supination, extension at the wrist can be tested with gravity elimi-nated. Finally, if the patient fails to move the body part, watch or feel for weak muscular contraction.

Fasciculations suggest lower motor neuron disease as a cause of atrophy.

Decreased resistance suggests disease of the peripheral ner-vous system, cerebellar disease, or the acute stages of spinal cord injury. See Table 18-4, Dis-orders of Muscle Tone (p. 612).

Marked floppiness indicates hypotonic (flaccid) muscles.

Increased resistance that varies, commonly worse at the extremes of the range, is called *spasticity*. Resistance that persists through-out the range and in both direc-tions is called *lead-pipe rigidity*.

Impaired strength is called weakness (*paresis*). Absence of strength is called paralysis (*plegia*). *Hemiparesis* refers to weakness of one half of the body; *hemiplegia* to paralysis of one half of the body. *Paraplegia* means paralysis of the legs; *quadriplegia*, paralysis of all four limbs.

See Table 18-5, Disorders of the Central and Peripheral Nervous Systems (pp. 613–615).

Muscle strength is graded on a 0 to 5 scale:

0—No muscular contraction detected
1—A barely detectable flicker or trace of contraction
2—Active movement of the body part with gravity eliminated
3—Active movement against gravity
4—Active movement against gravity and some resistance
5—Active movement against full resistance without evident fatigue.
This is normal muscle strength.

Many clinicians make further distinctions by using plus or minus signs toward the stronger end of this scale. Thus 4+ indicates good but not full strength, while 5− means a trace of weakness.

Methods for testing the major muscle groups are described below. The spinal root innervations and the muscles affected are shown in parentheses. To localize lesions in the spinal cord or the peripheral nervous system more precisely, additional testing may be necessary. For these specialized methods, refer to detailed texts of neurology.

Test flexion (C5, C6—biceps) *and extension* (C6, C7, C8—triceps) *at the elbow* by having the patient pull and push against your hand.

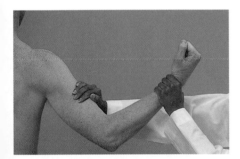
FLEXION

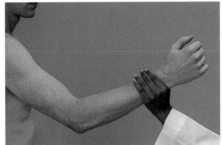
EXTENSION

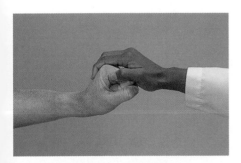
EXTENSION AT WRIST

Test extension at the wrist (C6, C7, C8, radial nerve) by asking the patient to make a fist and resist your pulling it down.

Weakness of extension is seen in peripheral nerve disease (e.g., radial nerve damage) and in central nervous system disease producing hemiplegia (e.g., stroke or multiple sclerosis).

Test the grip (C7, C8, T1). Ask the patient to squeeze two of your fingers as hard as possible and not let them go. (To avoid getting hurt by hard squeezes, place your own middle finger on top of your index finger.) You should normally have difficulty removing your fingers from the patient's grip. (Testing both grips simultaneously with arms extended or in lap facilitates comparison.)

A weak grip may be due to either central or peripheral nervous system disease. It may also result from painful disorders of the hands.

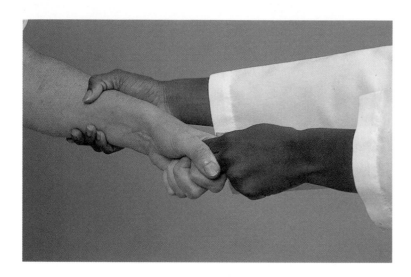

Test finger abduction (C8, T1, ulnar nerve). Position the patient's hand with palm down and fingers spread. Instructing the patient not to let you move the fingers, try to force them together.

Weak finger abduction in ulnar nerve disorders

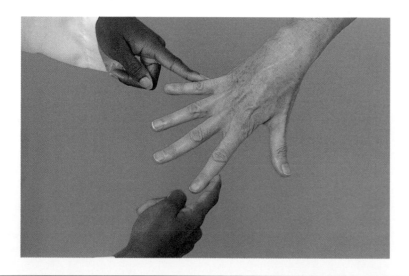

Test opposition of the thumb (C8, T1, median nerve). The patient should try to touch the tip of the little finger with the thumb, against your resistance.

Weak opposition of the thumb in median nerve disorders such as the carpal tunnel syndrome

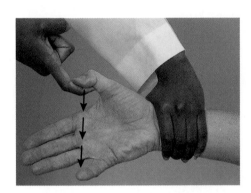

Assessment of *muscle strength of the trunk* may already have been made in other segments of the examination. It includes:

• Flexion, extension, and lateral bending of the spine, and
• Thoracic expansion and diaphragmatic excursion during respiration

Test flexion at the hip (L2, L3, L4—iliopsoas) by placing your hand on the patient's thigh and asking the patient to raise the leg against your hand.

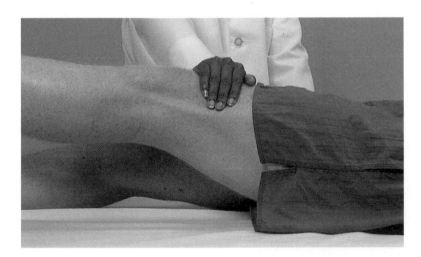

Test adduction at the hips (L2, L3, L4—adductors). Place your hands firmly on the bed between the patient's knees. Ask the patient to bring both legs together.

Symmetrical weakness of the proximal muscles suggests a *myopathy* (a disorder of mus-

Test abduction at the hips (L4, L5, S1—gluteus medius and minimus). Place your hands firmly on the bed outside the patient's knees. Ask the patient to spread both legs against your hands.

Test extension at the hips (S1—gluteus maximus). Have the patient push the posterior thigh down against your hand.

Test extension at the knee (L2, L3, L4—quadriceps). Support the knee in flexion and ask the patient to straighten the leg against your hand. The quadriceps is the strongest muscle in the body, so expect a forceful response.

cles); symmetrical weakness of distal muscles suggests a *polyneuropathy* (a disorder of peripheral nerves).

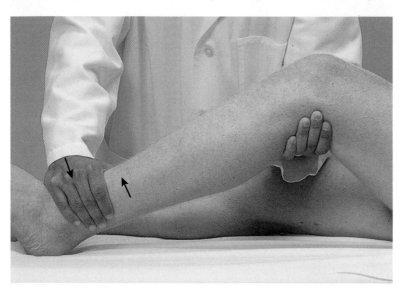

EXTENSION AT THE KNEE

Test flexion at the knee (L4, L5, S1, S2—hamstrings) as shown below. Place the patient's leg so that the knee is flexed with the foot resting on the bed. Tell the patient to keep the foot down as you try to straighten the leg.

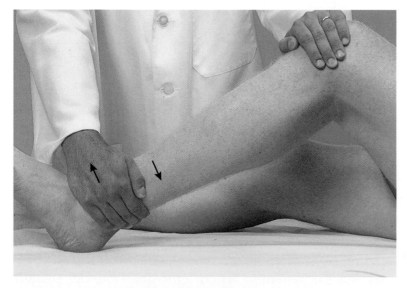

FLEXION AT THE KNEE

Test dorsiflexion (mainly L4, L5) *and plantar flexion* (mainly S1) *at the ankle* by asking the patient to pull up and push down against your hand.

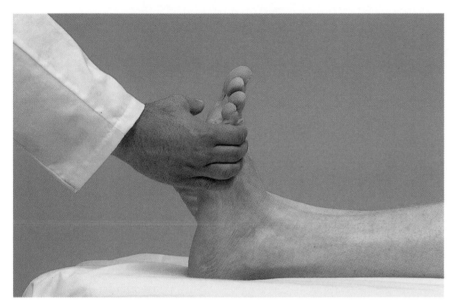

DORSIFLEXION

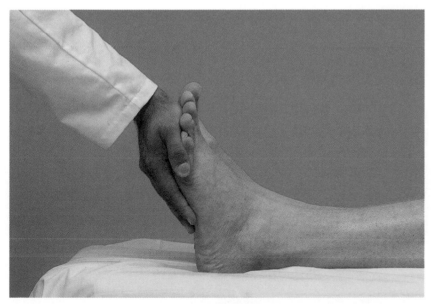

PLANTAR FLEXION

Coordination. Coordination of muscle movement requires that four areas of the nervous system function in an integrated way:

- The motor system, for muscle strength
- The cerebellar system (also part of the motor system), for rhythmic movement and steady posture
- The vestibular system, for balance and for coordinating eye, head, and body movements
- The sensory system, for position sense

To assess coordination, observe the patient's performance in:

- Rapid alternating movements
- Point-to-point movements
- Gait and other related body movements
- Standing in specified ways

Rapid Alternating Movements

Arms. Show the patient how to strike one hand on the thigh, raise the hand, turn it over, and then strike the back of the hand down on the same place. Urge the patient to repeat these alternating movements as rapidly as possible.

Observe the speed, rhythm, and smoothness of the movements. Repeat with the other hand. The nondominant hand often performs somewhat less well.

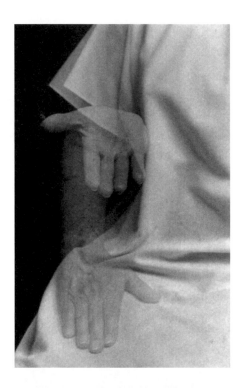

In cerebellar disease, one movement cannot be followed quickly by its opposite and movements are slow, irregular, and clumsy. This abnormality is called *dysdiadochokinesis.* Upper motor neuron weakness and basal ganglia disease may also impair rapid alternating movements, but not in the same manner.

Show the patient how to tap the distal joint of the thumb with the tip of the index finger, again as rapidly as possible. Again, observe the speed, rhythm, and smoothness of the movements. The nondominant side often performs less well.

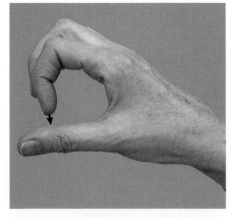

Legs. Ask the patient to tap your hand as quickly as possible with the ball of each foot in turn. Note any slowness or awkwardness. The feet normally perform less well than the hands.

Dysdiadochokinesis in cerebellar disease

Point-To-Point Movements

Arms. Ask the patient to touch your index finger and then his or her nose alternately several times. Move your finger about so that the patient has to alter directions and extend the arm fully to reach it. Observe the accuracy and smoothness of movements and watch for any tremor. Normally the patient's movements are smooth and accurate.

In cerebellar disease, movements are clumsy, unsteady, and inappropriately varying in their speed, force, and direction. The finger may initially overshoot its mark, but finally reaches it fairly well. Such movements are termed *dysmetria.* An intention tremor may appear toward the end of the movement (see p. 610).

Now hold your finger in one place so that the patient can touch it with one arm and finger outstretched. Ask the patient to raise the arm overhead and lower it again to touch your finger. After several repeats, ask the patient to close both eyes and try several more times. Repeat on the other side. Normally a person can touch the examiner's finger successfully with eyes open or closed. These maneuvers test position sense and the functions of both the labyrinth and the cerebellum.

Cerebellar disease causes incoordination that may get worse with eyes closed. Inaccuracy that appears with eyes closed suggests loss of position sense. Repetitive and consistent deviation to one side (referred to as *past pointing*), worse with the eyes closed, suggests cerebellar or vestibular disease.

Legs. Ask the patient to place one heel on the opposite knee, and then run it down the shin to the big toe. Note the smoothness and accuracy of the movements. Repetition with the patient's eyes closed tests for position sense. Repeat on the other side.

In cerebellar disease, the heel may overshoot the knee and then oscillate from side to side down the shin. When position sense is lost, the heel is lifted too high and the patient tries to look. With eyes closed, performance is poor.

Gait. Ask the patient to:

- *Walk across the room* or down the hall, then turn, and come back. Observe posture, balance, swinging of the arms, and movements of the legs. Normally balance is easy, the arms swing at the sides, and turns are accomplished smoothly.

A gait that lacks coordination, with reeling and instability, is called *ataxic.* Ataxia may be due to cerebellar disease, loss of position sense, or intoxication. See Table 18-6, Abnormalities of Gait and Posture (pp. 616–617).

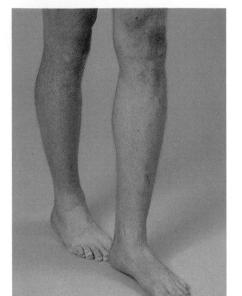

- *Walk heel-to-toe* in a straight line—a pattern called *tandem walking.*

Tandem walking may reveal an ataxia not previously obvious.

- *Walk on the toes,* then *on the heels*—sensitive tests respectively for plantar flexion and dorsiflexion of the ankles, as well as for balance.

Walking on toes and heels may reveal distal muscular weakness in the legs. Inability to heel-walk is a sensitive test for corticospinal tract weakness.

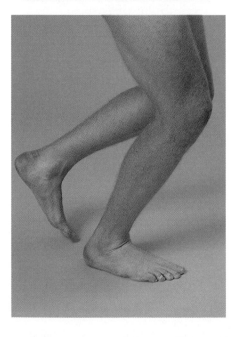

- *Hop in place* on each foot in turn (if the patient is not too old or ill). Hopping involves the proximal muscles of the legs as well as the distal ones and requires both good position sense and normal cerebellar function.

Difficulty with hopping may be due to weakness, lack of position sense, or cerebellar dysfunction.

- *Do a shallow knee bend,* first on one leg, then on the other. Support the patient's elbow if you think the patient is in danger of falling.

Difficulty here suggests proximal weakness (extensors of the hip), weakness of the quadriceps (the extensor of the knee), or both.

- *Rising from a sitting position* without arm support and *stepping up* on a sturdy stool are more suitable tests than hopping or knee bends when patients are old or less robust.

People with proximal muscle weakness involving the pelvic girdle and legs have difficulty with both these activities.

Stance. The following two tests can often be performed concurrently. They differ only in the patient's arm position and in what you are looking for. In each case, stand close enough to the patient to prevent a fall.

The Romberg Test. This is mainly a test of position sense. The patient should first stand with feet together and eyes open and then close both eyes for 20 to 30 seconds without support. Note the patient's ability to maintain an upright posture. Normally only minimal swaying occurs.

In ataxia due to loss of position sense, vision compensates for the sensory loss. The patient stands fairly well with eyes open but loses balance when they are closed, a *positive Romberg sign.* In cerebellar ataxia, the patient has difficulty standing with feet together whether the eyes are open or closed.

Test for Pronator Drift. The patient should stand for 20 to 30 seconds with both arms straight forward, palms up, and with eyes closed. A person who cannot stand may be tested for a pronator drift in the sitting position. In either case, a normal person can hold this arm position well.

The pronation of one forearm suggests a contralateral lesion in the corticospinal tract; downward drift of the arm with flexion of fingers and elbow may also occur. These movements are called a *pronator drift,* shown below.

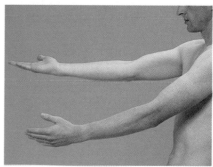

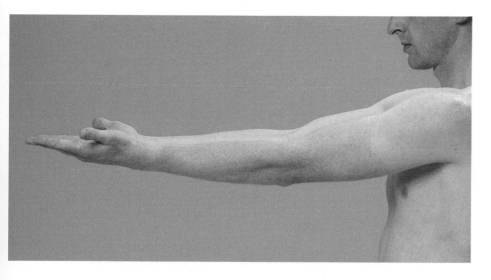

A sideward or upward drift, sometimes with searching, writhing movements of the hands, suggests loss of position sense.

Now, instructing the patient to keep the arms up and eyes shut, as shown above, *tap the arms briskly downward.* The arms normally return smoothly to the horizontal position. This response requires muscular strength, coordination, and a good sense of position.

A weak arm is easily displaced and often remains so. A patient lacking position sense may not recognize the displacement and, if told to correct it, does so poorly. In cerebellar incoordination, the arm returns to its original position but overshoots and bounces.

The Sensory System

To evaluate the sensory system, you will test several kinds of sensation:

• Pain and temperature (spinothalamic tracts)

• Position and vibration (posterior columns)

• Light touch (both of these pathways)

• Discriminative sensations, which depend on some of the above sensations but also involve the cortex

Familiarize yourself with each kind of test so that you can use it as indicated. When you detect abnormal findings, correlate them with motor and reflex activity. Is the underlying lesion central or peripheral?

See Table 18-5, Disorders of the Central and Peripheral Nervous Systems (pp. 613–615).

Patterns of Testing. Because sensory testing quickly fatigues many patients and then produces unreliable results, conduct the examination as efficiently as possible. Pay special attention to those areas (1) where there are symptoms such as numbness or pain, (2) where there are motor or reflex abnormalities that suggest a lesion of the spinal cord or peripheral nervous system, and (3) where there are trophic changes (e.g., absent or excessive sweating, atrophic skin, or cutaneous ulceration). Repeated testing at another time is often required to confirm abnormalities.

Meticulous sensory mapping helps to establish the level of a spinal cord lesion and to determine if a more peripheral lesion is in a nerve root, a major peripheral nerve, or one of its branches.

The following patterns of testing help you to identify sensory deficits accurately and efficiently.

1. Compare symmetrical areas on the two sides of the body, including the arms, legs, and trunk.

Hemisensory loss due to a lesion in the spinal cord or higher pathways

2. When testing pain, temperature, and touch sensation, also compare the distal with the proximal areas of the extremities. Further, scatter the stimuli so as to sample most of the dermatomes and major peripheral nerves (see pp. 566–567). One suggested pattern includes both shoulders (C4), the inner and outer aspects of the forearms (C6 and T1), the thumbs and little fingers (C6 and C8), the fronts of both thighs (L2), the medial and lateral aspects of both calves (L4 and L5), the little toes (S1), and the medial aspect of each buttock (S3).

Symmetrical distal sensory loss suggests a polyneuropathy, as described in the example on the next page. You may miss this finding unless you compare distal and proximal areas.

3. When testing vibration and position sensation, first test the fingers and toes. If these are normal, you may safely assume that more proximal areas will also be normal.

4. Vary the pace of your testing so that the patient does not merely respond to your repetitive rhythm.

5. When you detect an area of sensory loss or hypersensitivity, map out its boundaries in detail. Stimulate first at a point of reduced sensation, and move by progressive steps until the patient detects the change. An example is shown at right.

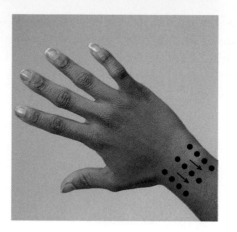

Here all sensation in the hand is lost. Repetitive testing in a proximal direction reveals a gradual change to normal sensation at the wrist. This pattern fits neither a peripheral nerve nor a dermatome (see p. 567). If bilateral, it suggests the "glove and stocking" sensory loss of a polyneuropathy, often seen in alcoholism and diabetes.

By identifying the distribution of sensory abnormalities and the kinds of sensations affected, you can infer where the causative lesion might be. Any motor deficit or reflex abnormality also helps in this localizing process.

Before each test below, show the patient what you plan to do and what responses you want. Unless otherwise specified, the patient's eyes should be closed during actual testing.

Pain. Use a sharp safety pin or other suitable tool, as described on p. 571. Occasionally, substitute the blunt end for the point. Ask the patient, "Is this sharp or dull?" or, when making comparisons, "Does this feel the same as this?" Apply the lightest pressure needed for the stimulus to feel sharp, and try not to draw blood.

Analgesia refers to absence of pain sensation, *hypalgesia* to decreased sensitivity to pain, and *hyperalgesia* to increased sensitivity.

To prevent transmitting a blood-borne infection, discard the pin or other device safely. Do not reuse it on another person.

Temperature. (This is often omitted if pain sensation is normal, but include it if there is any question.) Use two test tubes, filled with hot and cold water, or a tuning fork heated or cooled by water. Touch the skin and ask the patient to identify "hot" or "cold."

Light Touch. With a fine wisp of cotton, touch the skin lightly, avoiding pressure. Ask the patient to respond whenever a touch is felt, and to compare one area with another. Calloused skin is normally relatively insensitive and should be avoided.

Anesthesia is absence of touch sensation, *hypesthesia* is decreased sensitivity, and *hyperesthesia* is increased sensitivity.

Vibration. Use a relatively low-pitched tuning fork of 128 Hz or 256 Hz. Tap it on the heel of your hand and place it firmly over a distal interphalangeal joint of the patient's finger, then over the interphalangeal joint of the big toe. Ask what the patient feels. If you are uncertain whether it is pressure or vibration, ask the patient to tell you when the vibration stops, and then touch the fork to stop it. If vibration sense is

Vibration sense is often the first sensation to be lost in a peripheral neuropathy. Common causes include diabetes and alcoholism. Vibration sense is also lost in posterior column

impaired, proceed to more proximal bony prominences (e.g., wrist, elbow, medial malleolus, patella, anterior superior iliac spine, spinous processes, and clavicles).

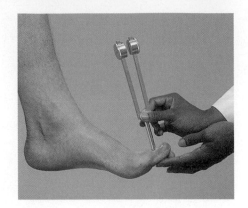

disease, as in tertiary syphilis or vitamin B_{12} deficiency.

Testing vibration sense in the trunk may be useful in estimating the level of a cord lesion.

Position. Grasp the patient's big toe, holding it by its sides between your thumb and index finger, and then pull it away from the other toes

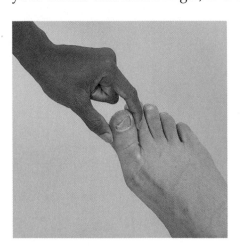

so as to avoid friction. (These precautions prevent extraneous tactile stimuli from revealing position changes that might not otherwise be detected.) Demonstrate "up" and "down" as you move the patient's toe clearly upward and downward. Then, with the patient's eyes closed, ask for a response of "up" or "down" when moving the toe in a small arc.

Loss of position sense, like loss of vibration sense, suggests either posterior column disease or a lesion of the peripheral nerve or root.

Repeat several times on each side, avoiding simple alternation of the stimuli. If position sense is impaired, move proximally to test it at the ankle joint. In a similar fashion, test position in the fingers, moving proximally if indicated to the metacarpophalangeal joints, wrist, and elbow.

Discriminative Sensations. Several additional techniques test the ability of the sensory cortex to correlate, analyze, and interpret sensations. Because discriminative sensations are dependent on touch and position sense, they are useful only when these sensations are either intact or only slightly impaired.

Screen a patient with stereognosis, and proceed to other methods if indicated. The patient's eyes should be closed during all these tests.

When touch and position sense are normal or only slightly impaired, a disproportionate decrease in or loss of discriminative sensations suggests disease of the sensory cortex. Stereognosis, number identification, and two-point discrimination are also impaired by posterior column disease.

1. *Stereognosis.* Stereognosis refers to the ability to identify an object by feeling it. Place in the patient's hand a familiar object such as a coin, paper clip, key, pencil, or cotton ball, and ask the patient to tell you what it is. Normally a patient will manipulate it skillfully and identify it correctly. Asking the patient to distinguish "heads" from "tails" on a coin is a sensitive test of stereognosis.

Astereognosis refers to the inability to recognize objects placed in the hand.

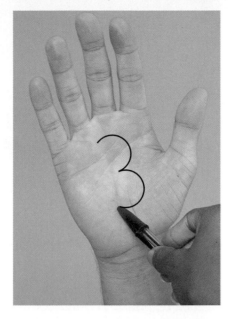

2. *Number identification (graphesthesia).* When motor impairment, arthritis, or other conditions prevent the patient from manipulating an object well enough to identify it, test the ability to identify numbers. With the blunt end of a pen or pencil, draw a large number in the patient's palm. A normal person can identify most such numbers.

The inability to recognize numbers, like astereognosis, suggests a lesion in the sensory cortex.

3. *Two-point discrimination.* Using the two ends of an opened paper clip, or the sides of two pins, touch a finger pad in two places simultaneously. Alternate the double stimulus irregularly with a one-point touch. Be careful not to cause pain.

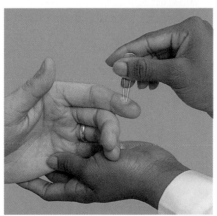

Find the minimal distance at which the patient can discriminate one from two points (normally less than 5 mm on the finger pads). This test may be used on other parts of the body, but normal distances vary widely from one body region to another.

Lesions of the sensory cortex increase the distance between two recognizable points.

4. *Point localization.* Briefly touch a point on the patient's skin. Then ask the patient to open both eyes and point to the place touched. Normally a person can do so accurately. This test, together with the test for extinction, is especially useful on the trunk and the legs.

Lesions of the sensory cortex impair the ability to localize points accurately.

5. *Extinction.* Simultaneously stimulate corresponding areas on both sides of the body. Ask where the patient feels your touch. Normally both stimuli are felt.

With lesions of the sensory cortex, only one stimulus may be recognized. The stimulus on the side opposite the damaged cortex is extinguished.

Deep Tendon Reflexes

To elicit a *deep tendon reflex*, persuade the patient to relax, position the limbs properly and symmetrically, and strike the tendon briskly, using a rapid wrist movement. Your strike should be quick and direct, not glancing. You may use either the pointed or the flat end of the hammer. The pointed end is useful in striking small areas, such as your finger as it overlies the biceps tendon, while the flat end gives the patient less discomfort over the brachioradialis. Hold the reflex hammer between your thumb and index finger so that it

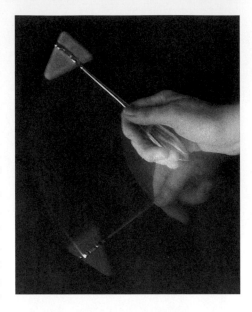

swings freely within the limits set by your palm and other fingers. Note the speed, force, and amplitude of the reflex response. Always compare one side with the other.

Reflexes are usually graded on a 0 to 4+ scale:

4+ Very brisk, hyperactive, with *clonus* (rhythmic oscillations between flexion and extension)
3+ Brisker than average; possibly but not necessarily indicative of disease
2+ Average; normal
1+ Somewhat diminished; low normal
0   No response

Hyperactive reflexes suggest central nervous system disease. Sustained clonus confirms it. Reflexes may be diminished or absent when sensation is lost, when the relevant spinal segments are damaged, or when the peripheral nerves are damaged. Diseases of muscles and neuromuscular junctions may also decrease reflexes.

Reflex response depends partly on the force of your stimulus. Use no more force than you need to provoke a definite response. Differences between sides are usually easier to assess than symmetrical changes. Symmetrically diminished or even absent reflexes may be found in normal people.

If the patient's reflexes are symmetrically diminished or absent, use *reinforcement*, a technique involving isometric contraction of other muscles that may increase reflex activity. In testing arm reflexes, for example, ask the patient to clench his or her teeth or to squeeze one thigh with the opposite hand. If leg reflexes are diminished or absent, reinforce them by asking the patient to lock fingers and pull one hand against the other. Tell the patient to pull just before you strike the tendon.

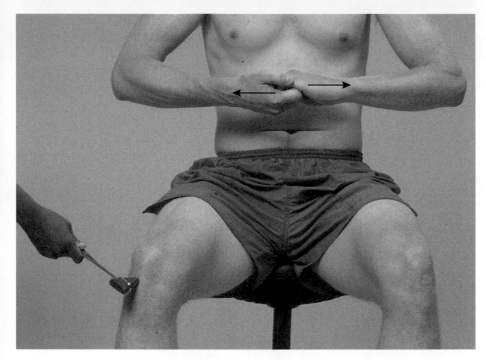

REINFORCEMENT OF KNEE REFLEX

The Biceps Reflex (C5, C6). The patient's arm should be partially flexed at the elbow with palm down. Place your thumb or finger firmly on the biceps tendon. Strike with the reflex hammer so that the blow is aimed directly through your digit toward the biceps tendon.

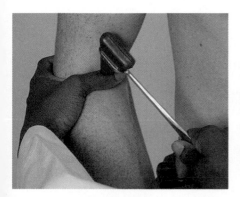

PATIENT SITTING

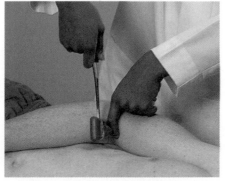

PATIENT LYING DOWN

Observe flexion at the elbow, and watch for and feel the contraction of the biceps muscle.

The Triceps Reflex (C6, C7). Flex the patient's arm at the elbow, with palm toward the body, and pull it slightly across the chest. Strike the triceps tendon above the elbow. Use a direct blow from directly behind it. Watch for contraction of the triceps muscle and extension at the elbow.

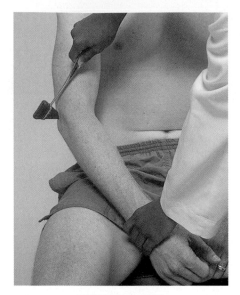

PATIENT SITTING

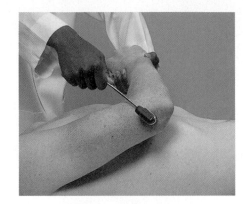

PATIENT LYING DOWN

If you have difficulty getting the patient to relax, try supporting the upper arm as illustrated on the right. Ask the patient to let the arm go limp, as if it were "hung up to dry." Then strike the triceps tendon.

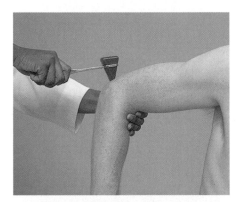

The Supinator or Brachioradialis Reflex (C5, C6). The patient's hand should rest on the abdomen or the lap, with the forearm partly pronated. Strike the radius about 1 to 2 inches above the wrist. Watch for flexion and supination of the forearm.

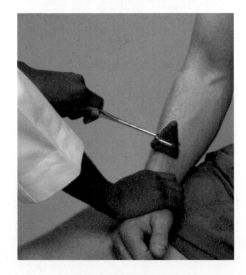

The Abdominal Reflexes. Test the abdominal reflexes by lightly but briskly stroking each side of the abdomen, above (T8, T9, T10) and below (T10, T11, T12) the umbilicus, in the directions illustrated. Use a key, the wooden end of a cotton-tipped applicator, or a tongue blade twisted and split longitudinally. Note the contraction of the abdominal muscles and deviation of the umbilicus toward the stimulus. Obesity may mask an abdominal reflex. In this situation, use your finger to retract the patient's umbilicus away from the side to be stimulated. Feel with your retracting finger for the muscular contraction.

Abdominal reflexes may be absent in both central and peripheral nervous system disorders.

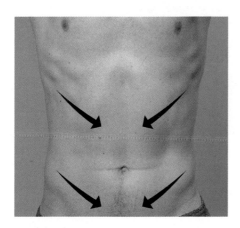

The Knee Reflex (L2, L3, L4). The patient may be either sitting or lying down as long as the knee is flexed. Briskly tap the patellar tendon just below the patella. Note contraction of the quadriceps with extension at the knee. A hand on the patient's anterior thigh lets you feel this reflex.

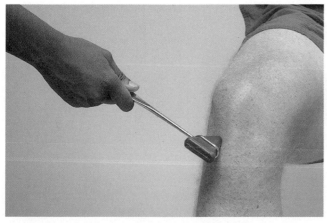

PATIENT SITTING

Two methods are useful in examining the supine patient. Supporting both knees at once, as shown below on the left, allows you to assess small differences between knee reflexes by repeatedly testing one reflex and then the other. Sometimes, however, supporting both legs is uncomfortable for both the examiner and the patient. You may wish to rest your supporting arm under the patient's opposite leg, as shown below on the right. Some patients find it easier to relax with this method.

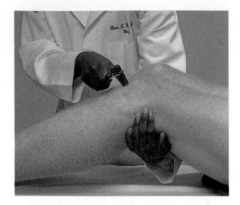
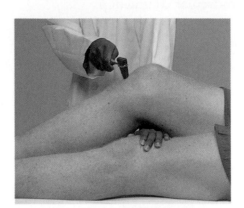

The Ankle Reflex (primarily S1). If the patient is sitting, dorsiflex the foot at the ankle. Persuade the patient to relax. Strike the Achilles tendon. Watch and feel for plantar flexion at the ankle. Note also the speed of relaxation after muscular contraction.

The slowed relaxation phase of reflexes in hypothyroidism is often easily seen and felt in the ankle reflex.

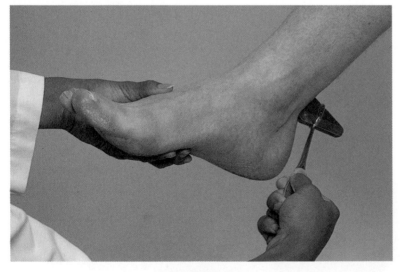

PATIENT SITTING

When the patient is lying down, flex one leg at both hip and knee and rotate it externally so that the lower leg rests across the opposite shin. Then dorsiflex the foot at the ankle and strike the Achilles tendon.

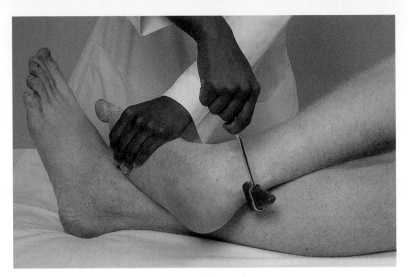

PATIENT LYING DOWN

The Plantar Response (L5, S1). With an object such as a key or the wooden end of an applicator stick, stroke the lateral aspect of the sole from the heel to the ball of the foot, curving medially across the ball. Use the lightest stimulus that will provoke a response, but be increasingly firm if necessary. Note movement of the toes, normally flexion.

Dorsiflexion of the big toe, often accompanied by fanning of the other toes, constitutes a Babinski response. It often indicates a central nervous system lesion in the corticospinal tract.

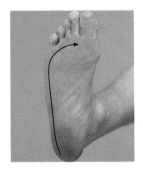

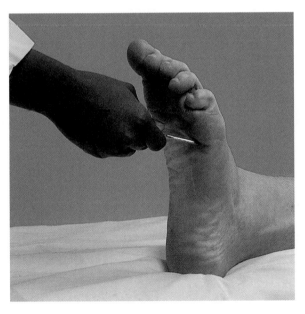

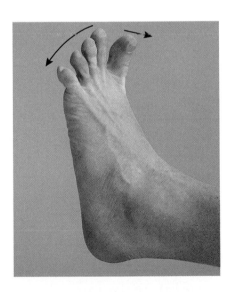

A Babinski response may also be seen in unconscious states due to drug or alcohol intoxication or in the postictal period following a seizure.

Some patients withdraw from this stimulus by flexing the hip and the knee. Hold the ankle, if necessary, to complete your observation. It is sometimes difficult to distinguish withdrawal from a Babinski response.

Clonus. If the reflexes seem hyperactive, test for *ankle clonus.* Support the knee in a partly flexed position. With your other hand, dorsiflex and plantar flex the foot a few times while encouraging the patient to relax, and then sharply dorsiflex the foot and maintain it in dorsiflexion. Look and feel for rhythmic oscillations between dorsiflexion and plantar flexion. In most normal people, the ankle does not react to this stimulus. A few clonic beats may be seen and felt, especially when the patient is tense or has exercised.

A marked Babinski response is occasionally accompanied by reflex flexion at hip and knee.

Sustained clonus indicates central nervous system disease. The ankle plantar flexes and dorsiflexes repetitively and rhythmically.

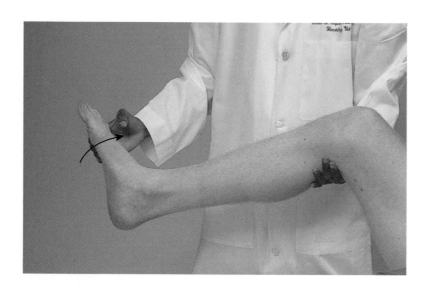

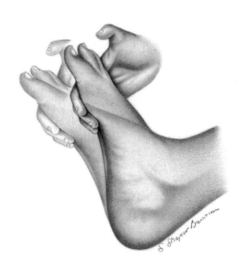

Clonus may also be elicited at other joints. A sharp downward displacement of the patella, for example, may elicit patellar clonus in the extended knee.

Special Techniques

Aphasia. If the patient's speech lacks meaning or has a disturbance in fluency, test the patient more carefully for aphasia, a disorder of the comprehension or use of words or symbolic language arising from anatomical lesions in the dominant hemisphere of the brain. A method for testing aphasia is outlined on p. 113.

See also Table 3-1, Disorders of Speech (p. 123).

Asterixis. Asterixis is useful in identifying a metabolic encephalopathy in patients whose mental functions are impaired. Ask the patient to "stop traffic" by extending both arms, with hands cocked up and fingers spread. Watch for 1 to 2 minutes, coaxing the patient as necessary to maintain this position.

Sudden, brief, nonrhythmic flexion of the hands and fingers indicates asterixis.

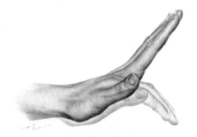

Winging of the Scapula. When the shoulder muscles seem weak or atrophic, look for winging. Ask the patient to extend both arms and push against your hand or against a wall. Observe the scapulae. Normally they lie close to the thorax.

In winging, shown below, the medial border of the scapula juts backward. It suggests weakness of the serratus anterior muscle, as in muscular dystrophy or injury to the long thoracic nerve.

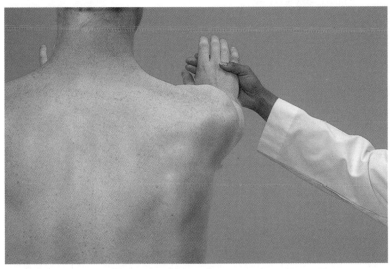

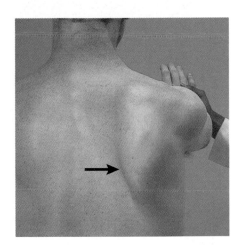

In very thin but normal people, the scapulae may appear "winged" even when the musculature is intact.

Meningeal Signs. Testing for these signs is important if you suspect meningeal inflammation from infection or subarachnoid hemorrhage.

Neck Mobility. First make sure there is no injury to the cervical vertebrae or cervical cord. (In settings of trauma, this may require evaluation by x-ray.) Then, with the patient supine, place your hands behind the patient's head and flex the neck forward, until the chin touches the chest if possible. Normally the neck is supple and the patient can easily bend the head and neck forward.

Pain in the neck and resistance to flexion can arise from meningeal inflammation, arthritis, or neck injury.

Brudzinski's Sign. As you flex the neck, watch the hips and knees in reaction to your maneuver. Normally they should remain relaxed and motionless.

Flexion of the hips and knees is a *positive Brudzinski's sign* and suggests meningeal inflammation.

Kernig's Sign. Flex the patient's leg at both the hip and the knee, and then straighten the knee. Discomfort behind the knee during full extension occurs in many normal people, but this maneuver should not produce pain.

Pain and increased resistance to extending the knee are a *positive Kernig's sign.* When bilateral, it suggests meningeal irritation.

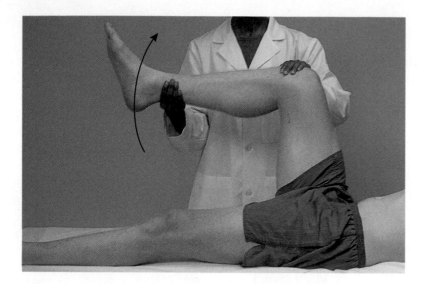

Compression of a lumbosacral nerve root may also cause resistance, together with pain in the low back and the posterior thigh. Only one leg is usually involved.

Anal Reflex. Using a dull object, such as a cotton swab, stroke outward in the four quadrants from the anus. Watch for reflex contraction of the anal musculature.

Loss of the anal reflex suggests a lesion in the S2–3–4 reflex arc, as in a cauda equina lesion.

The Stuporous or Comatose Patient. Coma signals a potentially life-threatening event affecting the two hemispheres, the brainstem, or both. The usual sequence of history, physical examination, and laboratory evaluation does not apply. Instead, you must:

* First assess the ABCs (airway, breathing, and circulation)

* Establish the patient's level of consciousness, and

* Examine the patient neurologically. Look for focal or asymmetrical findings, and determine whether impaired consciousness arises from a metabolic or a structural cause.

See Table 18-7, Metabolic and Structural Coma (p. 618).

Interview relatives, friends, or witnesses to establish the speed of onset and duration of unconsciousness, any warning symptoms, precipitating factors, or previous episodes, and the prior appearance and behavior of the patient. Any history of past medical and psychiatric illnesses is also useful.

As you proceed to the examination, remember two cardinal DON'Ts:

1. *Don't* dilate the pupils, the single most important clue to the underlying cause of coma (structural vs. metabolic), and
2. *Don't* flex the neck if there is any question of trauma to the head or neck. Immobilize the cervical spine and get an x-ray first to rule out fractures of the cervical vertebrae that could compress and damage the spinal cord.

Airway, Breathing, and Circulation. Quickly check the patient's color and pattern of breathing. Inspect the posterior pharynx and listen over the trachea for stridor to make sure the airway is clear. If respirations are slowed or shallow, or if the airway is obstructed by secretions, consider intubating the patient as soon as possible while stabilizing the cervical spine.

Assess the remaining vital signs: pulse, blood pressure, and *rectal* temperature. If hypotension or hemorrhage is present, establish intravenous access and begin intravenous fluids. (Further emergency management and laboratory studies are beyond the scope of this text.)

Level of Consciousness. Level of consciousness primarily reflects the patient's capacity for arousal, or wakefulness. It is determined by the level of activity that the patient can be aroused to perform in response to escalating stimuli from the examiner.

Five clinical levels of consciousness are described in the table on p. 600, together with the techniques that may be used to elicit their characteristics. Increase your stimuli in a stepwise manner, depending on the patient's response.

When you examine patients with an altered level of consciousness, describe and record exactly what you see and hear. Summary terms such as lethargy, obtundation, stupor, or coma may have different meanings for other examiners.

Level of Consciousness (Arousal): Techniques and Patient Response

Level	Technique	Abnormal Response
Alertness	Speak to the patient in a normal tone of voice. An alert patient opens the eyes, looks at you, and responds fully and appropriately to stimuli (arousal intact).	
Lethargy	Speak to the patient in a loud voice. For example, call the patient's name or ask "How are you?"	A lethargic patient appears drowsy but opens the eyes and looks at you, responds to questions, and then falls asleep.
Obtundation	Shake the patient gently as if awakening a sleeper.	An obtunded patient opens the eyes and looks at you, but responds slowly and is somewhat confused. Alertness and interest in the environment are decreased.
Stupor	Apply a painful stimulus. For example, pinch a tendon, rub the sternum, or roll a pencil across a nail bed. (No stronger stimuli needed!)	A stuporous patient arouses from sleep only after painful stimuli. Verbal responses are slow or even absent. The patient lapses into an unresponsive state when the stimulus ceases. There is minimal awareness of self or the environment.
Coma	Apply repeated painful stimuli.	A comatose patient remains unarousable with eyes closed. There is no evident response to inner need or external stimuli.

Neurologic Evaluation

Respirations. Observe the rate, rhythm, and pattern of respirations. Because neural structures that govern breathing in the cortex and brainstem overlap those that govern consciousness, abnormalities of respiration often occur in coma.

See Table 18-7, Metabolic and Structural Coma (p. 618), and Table 8-1, Abnormalities in Rate and Rhythm of Breathing (p. 269).

Pupils. Observe the size and equality of the pupils and test their reaction to light. The presence or absence of the light reaction is one of the most important signs distinguishing structural from metabolic causes of coma. The light reaction often remains intact in metabolic coma.

See Table 18-8, Pupils in Comatose Patients (p. 619).

Structural lesions such as stroke may lead to asymmetrical pupils and loss of light reaction.

Ocular Movement. Observe the position of the eyes and eyelids at rest. Check for horizontal deviation of the eyes to one side (*gaze preference*). When the oculomotor pathways are intact, the eyes look straight ahead.

In structural hemispheric lesions, the eyes "look at the lesion" in the affected hemisphere.

In irritative lesions due to epilepsy or early cerebral hemorrhage, the eyes "look away" from the affected hemisphere.

Oculocephalic Reflex (Doll's-Eye Movements). This reflex helps to assess brainstem function in a comatose patient. Holding open the upper eyelids so that you can see the eyes, turn the head quickly, first to one side and then to the other. (Make sure the patient has no neck injury before performing this test.)

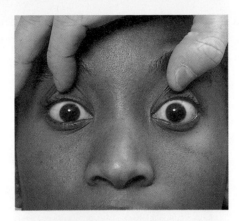

In a comatose patient with an intact brainstem, as the head is turned the eyes move toward the opposite side (the doll's eye movements). In the adjacent photo, for example, the patient's head has been turned to the right; her eyes have moved to the left. Her eyes still seem to gaze at the camera. The doll's eye movements are intact.

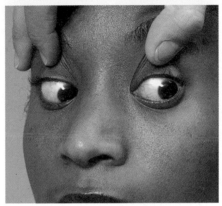

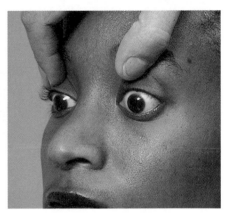

In a comatose patient with absence of doll's eye movements, shown above, the ability to move both eyes to one side is lost, suggesting a lesion of midbrain or pons.

Oculovestibular Reflex (With Caloric Stimulation). If the oculocephalic reflex is absent and you seek further assessment of brainstem function, test the oculovestibular reflex. Note that this test is almost never performed in an awake patient.

Make sure the eardrums are intact and the canals clear. You must elevate the patient's head to 30° to perform the test accurately. Place a kidney basin under the ear to catch any overflowing water. With a large syringe, inject ice water through a small catheter that is lying in (but not plugging) the ear canal. Watch for deviation of the eyes in the horizontal plane. You may need to use up to 120 ml of ice water to elicit a response. In the comatose patient with an intact brainstem, the eyes drift *toward* the irrigated ear. Repeat on the opposite side, waiting 3 to 5 minutes if necessary for the first response to disappear.

No response to stimulation suggests brainstem injury.

Posture and Muscle Tone. Observe the patient's posture. If there is no spontaneous movement, you may need to apply a painful stimulus (see p. 600). Classify the resulting pattern of movement as:

See Table 18-9, Abnormal Postures in the Comatose Patient (p. 620).

- *Normal–avoidant*—the patient pushes the stimulus away or withdraws.

- *Stereotypic*—the stimulus evokes abnormal postural responses of the trunk and extremities.

Two stereotypic responses predominate: *decorticate rigidity* and *decerebrate rigidity*.

- *Flaccid paralysis or no response*

No response on one side suggests a corticospinal tract lesion.

Test muscle tone by grasping each forearm near the wrist and raising it to a vertical position. Note the position of the hand, usually only slightly flexed at the wrist.

The hemiplegia of sudden cerebral accidents is usually flaccid at first. The limp hand drops to form a right angle with the wrist.

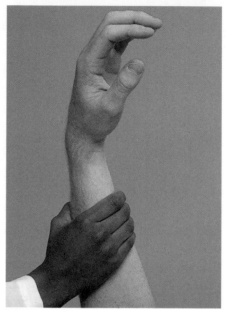
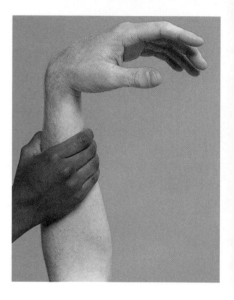

Then lower the arm to about 12 or 18 inches off the bed and drop it. Watch how it falls. A normal arm drops somewhat slowly.

A flaccid arm drops rapidly, like a flail.

Support the patient's flexed knees. Then extend one leg at a time at the knee and let it fall. Compare the speed with which each leg falls.

In acute hemiplegia, the flaccid leg falls more rapidly.

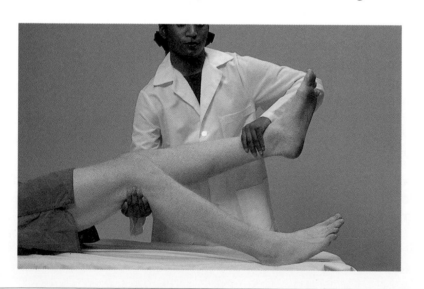

Flex both legs so that the heels rest on the bed and then release them. The normal leg returns slowly to its original extended position.

In acute hemiplegia, the flaccid leg falls rapidly into extension, with external rotation at the hip.

Further Examination

As you complete the neurologic examination, check for facial asymmetry and asymmetries in motor, sensory, and reflex function. Test for meningeal signs if indicated.

Meningitis, subarachnoid hemorrhage.

As you proceed to the general physical examination, check for unusual odors.

Alcohol, liver failure, uremia

Look for abnormalities of the skin, including color, moisture, evidence of bleeding disorders, needle marks, and other lesions.

Jaundice, cyanosis, cherry red color of carbon monoxide poisoning

Examine the scalp and skull for signs of trauma.

Bruises, lacerations, swelling

Examine the fundi carefully.

Papilledema, hypertensive retinopathy

Check to make sure the corneal reflexes are intact. (Remember that use of contact lenses may abolish these reflexes.)

Reflex loss in coma and lesions affecting CN V or CN VII

Inspect the ears and nose, and examine the mouth and throat.

Blood or cerebrospinal fluid in the nose or the ears suggests a skull fracture; otitis media suggests a possible brain abscess.

Tongue injury suggests a seizure.

Be sure to evaluate the heart, lungs, and abdomen.

Health Promotion and Counseling

For counseling and health promotion related to the nervous system, direct clinical attention to averting cerebrovascular accidents (CVAs) and screening for dementia. Risks to mental health—abuse of alcohol and drugs, depression, and suicide—should also be addressed. (see Chap. 3, pp. 121–122.)

Strokes, or CVAs, are the third leading cause of death in the United States and contribute to extensive disability in the workforce and general population. The incidence of stroke increases with age and is 60% higher in African Americans compared to Caucasians. The clinician's first task in stroke prevention is to control hypertension. Hypertension accelerates atherosclerotic changes in the carotid, vertebral, and cerebral arteries and disturbs autoregulation of cerebral blood pressure. It is the leading risk factor for both ischemic and hemorrhagic stroke, which account for approximately 85% and approximately 10% of all CVAs, respectively. In addition, clinicians should counsel patients to modify conditions contributing to atherosclerosis: smoking, hyperlipidemia, and diabetes. Drug users should be warned of the link between stroke and cocaine.

Clinicians should be alert to symptoms of transient ischemic attacks (TIAs), generally defined as neurologic events that resolve within 24 hours. TIAs can be viewed as CVA warning signals, the anginal equivalent of the brain. In the first year after a TIA, risk of CVA is 6%–7%, usually occurring in the same vascular distribution as the TIA. Common symptoms of TIAs include visual loss (especially transient monocular blindness from emboli), aphasia, dysarthria, and changes in facial movement or sensation. For TIAs affecting motor or sensory pathways, watch for clumsiness, weakness, paralysis, or tingling or paresthesias of the arm, leg, or hemibody.

As the population ages, clinicians need to sharpen skills for detection of dementia, particularly in its early stages. Couple cognitive and behavioral assessment, as discussed in Chap. 3, Mental Status, with a careful neurologic examination during your evaluation of the patient. Review the patient's medications and be sure to look for other medical and psychiatric conditions that could be contributing to changes in behavior or level of daily activity. If dementia is identified, provide guidance for community services and specialty referrals that may be needed. Support both patient and family as they make what are often difficult decisions about patient care.

Table 18-1 Nystagmus

T A B L E   1 8 - 1   Nystagmus

Nystagmus is a rhythmic oscillation of the eyes, analogous to a tremor in other parts of the body. Its causes are multiple, including impairment of vision in early life, disorders of the labyrinth and the cerebellar system, and drug toxicity. Nystagmus occurs normally when a person watches a rapidly moving object (e.g., a passing train). Observe the three characteristics of nystagmus listed below and on the following page. Then refer to textbooks of neurology for differential diagnosis.

Direction of the Quick and Slow Components

Example: Nystagmus to the Left—A Slow Drift to the Right, Then a Quick Jerk to the Left in Each Eye

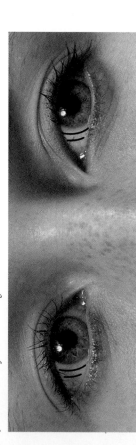

Nystagmus usually has both fast and slow movements, but is defined by its fast phase. For example, if the eyes jerk quickly to the patient's left and drift back slowly to the right, the patient is said to have nystagmus to the left.

Occasionally, nystagmus consists only of coarse oscillations without quick and slow components. It is then said to be *pendular*.

The movements of nystagmus may occur in one or more planes (i.e., horizontal, vertical, or rotary). It is the plane of the movements, not the direction of the gaze, that defines this variable.

Plane of the Movements

Horizontal Nystagmus

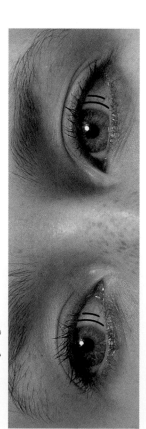

Vertical Nystagmus

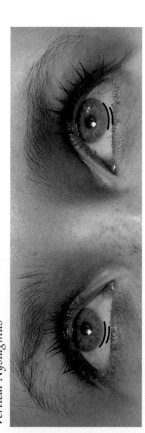

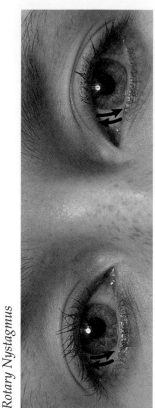
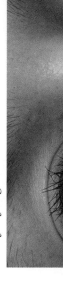

Rotary Nystagmus

Table 18-1   Nystagmus

Direction of Gaze in Which Nystagmus Appears

Example: Nystagmus on Right Lateral Gaze

Nystagmus may be present in all directions of gaze, it may appear or become accentuated only on deviation of the eyes (e.g., to the side or upward). On extreme lateral gaze, the normal person may show a few beats resembling nystagmus. Avoid making assessments in such extreme positions, and observe for nystagmus only within the field of full binocular vision.

Nystagmus Present (Right Lateral Gaze)

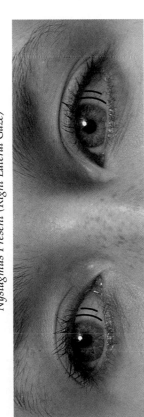

Nystagmus Not Present (Left Lateral Gaze)

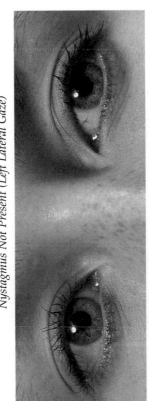

Table 18-2   Types of Facial Paralysis

TABLE 18-2   *Types of Facial Paralysis*

Facial weakness or paralysis may result either (1) from a peripheral lesion of the facial nerve, anywhere from its origin in the pons to its periphery in the face, or (2) from a central lesion involving the upper motor neurons anywhere between the cortex and the pons. A peripheral lesion of the facial nerve, exemplified here by a Bell's palsy, is compared with a central lesion, exemplified by a left hemispheric cerebrovascular accident. Note their different effects on the upper part of the face, by which they can be distinguished.

Peripheral Nervous System Lesion

Damage to the right facial nerve paralyzes the entire right side of the face, including the forehead.

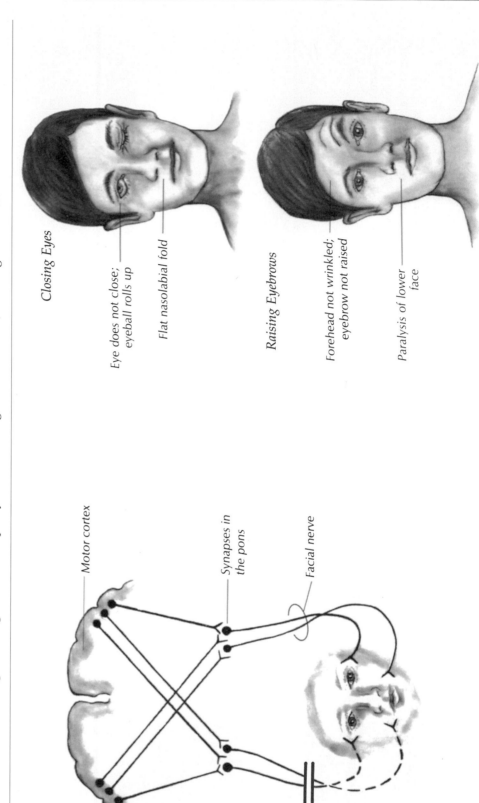

Closing Eyes

Eye does not close;
eyeball rolls up

Flat nasolabial fold

Raising Eyebrows

Forehead not wrinkled;
eyebrow not raised

Paralysis of lower
face

Motor cortex

Synapses in
the pons

Facial nerve

CN VII
Peripheral
lesion

Table 18-2   Types of Facial Paralysis

Central Nervous System Lesion

The lower part of the face normally is controlled by upper motor neurons located on only one side of the cortex—the opposite side. Left-sided damage to these pathways, as in a stroke, paralyzes the right lower face. The upper face, however, is controlled by pathways from both sides of the cortex. Even though the upper motor neurons on the left are destroyed, others on the right remain and the right upper face continues to function fairly well.

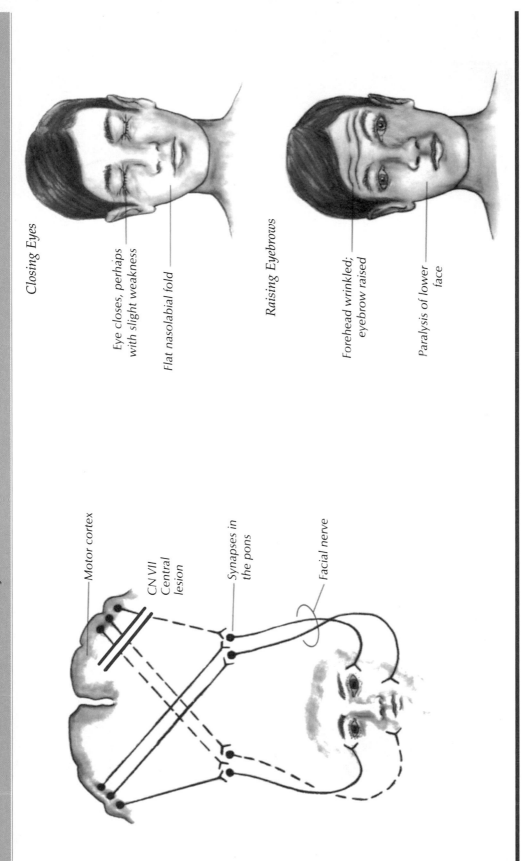

Closing Eyes

Eye closes, perhaps with slight weakness

Flat nasolabial fold

Raising Eyebrows

Forehead wrinkled; eyebrow raised

Paralysis of lower face

Motor cortex

CN VII
Central lesion

Synapses in the pons

Facial nerve

Table 18-3   Involuntary Movements

TABLE 18-3   Involuntary Movements

Tremors

Tremors are relatively rhythmic oscillatory movements which may be roughly subdivided into three groups: resting (or static) tremors, intention tremors, and postural tremors.

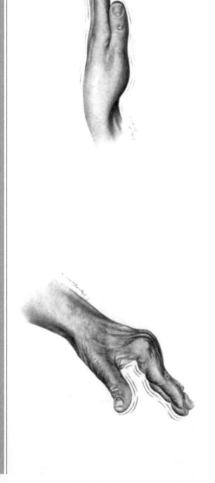

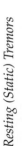

Resting (Static) Tremors

These tremors are most prominent at rest, and may decrease or disappear with voluntary movement. Illustrated is the common, relatively slow, fine, pill-rolling tremor of parkinsonism, about 5 per second.

Postural Tremors

These tremors appear when the affected part is actively maintaining a posture. Examples include the fine, rapid tremor of hyperthyroidism, the tremors of anxiety and fatigue, and benign essential (and sometimes familial) tremor. Tremor may worsen somewhat with intention.

Intention Tremors

Intention tremors, absent at rest, appear with activity and often get worse as the target is neared. Causes include disorders of cerebellar pathways, as in multiple sclerosis.

Oral–Facial Dyskinesias

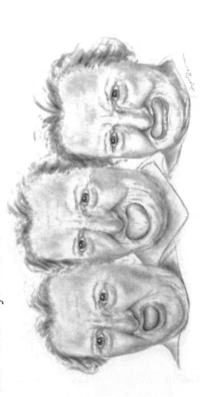

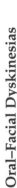

Oral–facial dyskinesias are rhythmic, repetitive, bizarre movements that chiefly involve the face, mouth, jaw, and tongue: grimacing, pursing of the lips, protrusions of the tongue, opening and closing of the mouth, and deviations of the jaw. The limbs and trunk are involved less often. These movements may be a late complication of psychotropic drugs such as phenothiazines, and have then been termed *tardive* (late) dyskinesias. They also occur in longstanding psychoses, in some elderly individuals, and in some edentulous persons.

Table 18-3   Involuntary Movements

Tics

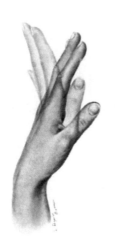

Tics are brief, repetitive, stereotyped, coordinated movements occurring at irregular intervals. Examples include repetitive winking, grimacing, and shoulder shrugging. Causes include Tourette's syndrome and drugs such as phenothiazines and amphetamines.

Chorea

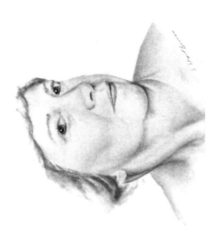

Choreiform movements are brief, rapid, jerky, irregular, and unpredictable. They occur at rest or interrupt normal coordinated movements. Unlike tics, they seldom repeat themselves. The face, head, lower arms, and hands are often involved. Causes include Sydenham's chorea (with rheumatic fever) and Huntington's disease.

Athetosis

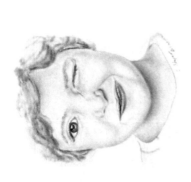

Athetoid movements are slower and more twisting and writhing than choreiform movements, and have a larger amplitude. They most commonly involve the face and the distal extremities. Athetosis is often associated with spasticity. Causes include cerebral palsy.

Dystonia

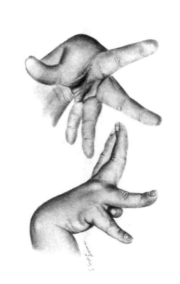

Dystonic movements are somewhat similar to athetoid movements, but often involve larger portions of the body, including the trunk. Grotesque, twisted postures may result. Causes include drugs such as phenothiazines, primary torsion dystonia and, as illustrated, spasmodic torticollis.

Table 18-4   Disorders of Muscle Tone

TABLE 18-4   *Disorders of Muscle Tone*

	Spasticity	Rigidity	Flaccidity	Paratonia
Location of Lesion	Upper motor neuron of the corticospinal tract at any point from the cortex to the spinal cord	Basal ganglia system	Lower motor neuron at any point from the anterior horn cell to the peripheral nerves	Both hemispheres, usually in the frontal lobes
Description	Increased muscle tone (*hypertonia*) that is rate-dependent. Tone is greater when passive movement is rapid, and less when passive movement is slow. Tone is also greater at the extremes of the movement arc. During rapid passive movement, initial hypertonia may give way suddenly as the limb relaxes. This spastic "catch" and relaxation is known as "clasp-knife" resistance.	Increased resistance that persists throughout the movement arc, independent of rate of movement, is called *lead-pipe rigidity*. With flexion and extension of the wrist or forearm, a superimposed rachetlike jerkiness is called *cogwheel rigidity*.	Loss of muscle tone (*hypotonia*), causing the limb to be loose or floppy. The affected limbs may be hyperextensible or even flail-like.	Sudden changes in tone with passive range of motion. Sudden loss of tone that increases the ease of motion is called *mitgehen* (moving with). Sudden increase in tone making motion more difficult is called *gegenhalten* (holding against).
Common Cause	Stroke, especially late or chronic stage	Parkinsonism	Guillain–Barré syndrome; also initial phase of spinal cord injury (spinal shock) or stroke	Dementia

Table 18-5   Disorders of the Central and Peripheral Nervous Systems

T A B L E   1 8 - 5 *Disorders of the Central and Peripheral Nervous System*

Central Nervous System Disorders

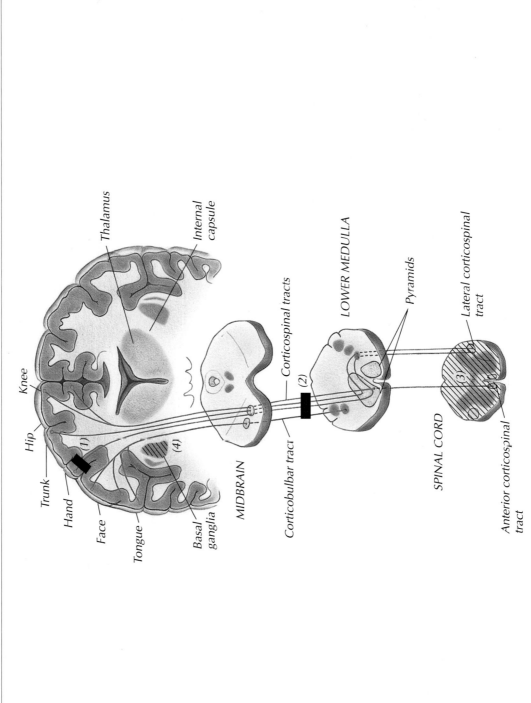

Table 18-5　Disorders of the Central and Peripheral Nervous Systems

T A B L E 1 8 - 5 *(continued)*

Central Nervous System Disorders

Location of Lesion	Typical Findings			Examples of Cause
	Motor	*Sensory*	*Deep Tendon Reflexes*	
Cerebral Cortex (1)	Chronic contralateral upper motor neuron weakness and spasticity. Flexion is stronger than extension in the arm, plantar flexion is stronger than dorsiflexion in the foot, and the leg is externally rotated at the hip.	Contralateral sensory loss on the limbs and trunk on the same side as the motor deficits	↑	Cortical stroke
Brainstem (2)	Weakness and spasticity as above, plus cranial nerve deficits such as diplopia (from weakness of the extraocular muscles) and dysarthria	Variable. No typical sensory findings	↑	Brainstem stroke, acoustic neuroma
Spinal Cord (3)	Weakness and spasticity, as above, but often affecting both sides (when cord damage is bilateral), causing paraplegia or quadriplegia depending on the level of injury	Dermatomal sensory deficit on the trunk bilaterally at the level of the lesion, and sensory loss from tract damage below the level of the lesion	↑	Trauma, causing cord compression
Subcortical Gray Matter: Basal Ganglia (4)	Slowness of movement (bradykinesia), rigidity, and tremor	Sensation not affected	Normal or ↓	Parkinsonism
Cerebellar (not illustrated)	Hypotonia, ataxia, and other abnormal movements, including nystagmus, dysdiadochokinesis, and dysmetria	Sensation not affected	Normal or ↓	Cerebellar stroke, brain tumor

Table 18-5   Disorders of the Central and Peripheral Nervous Systems

Peripheral Nervous System Disorders

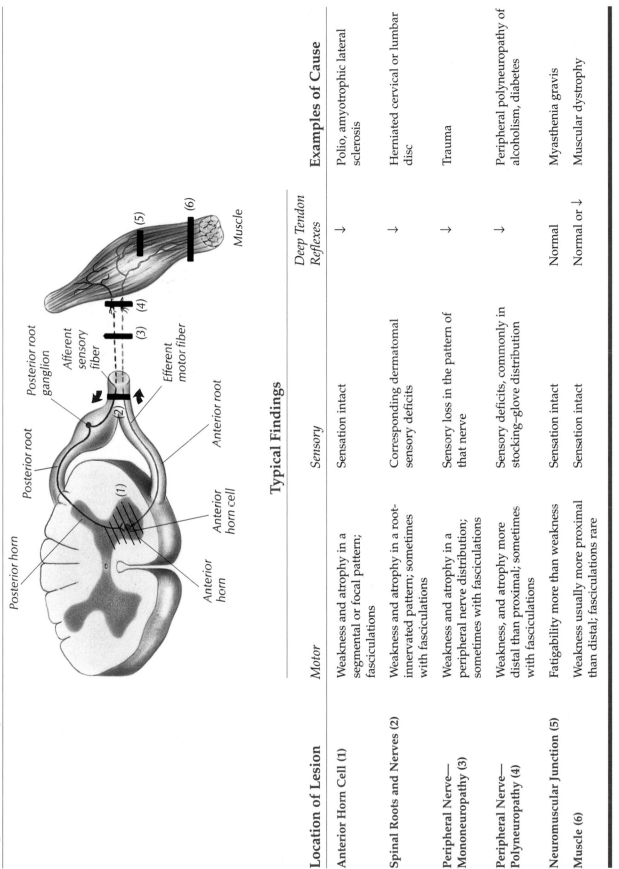

Typical Findings

Location of Lesion	Motor	Sensory	Deep Tendon Reflexes	Examples of Cause
Anterior Horn Cell (1)	Weakness and atrophy in a segmental or focal pattern; fasciculations	Sensation intact	↓	Polio, amyotrophic lateral sclerosis
Spinal Roots and Nerves (2)	Weakness and atrophy in a root-innervated pattern; sometimes with fasciculations	Corresponding dermatomal sensory deficits	↓	Herniated cervical or lumbar disc
Peripheral Nerve—Mononeuropathy (3)	Weakness and atrophy in a peripheral nerve distribution; sometimes with fasciculations	Sensory loss in the pattern of that nerve	↓	Trauma
Peripheral Nerve—Polyneuropathy (4)	Weakness, and atrophy more distal than proximal; sometimes with fasciculations	Sensory deficits, commonly in stocking–glove distribution	↓	Peripheral polyneuropathy of alcoholism, diabetes
Neuromuscular Junction (5)	Fatigability more than weakness	Sensation intact	Normal	Myasthenia gravis
Muscle (6)	Weakness usually more proximal than distal; fasciculations rare	Sensation intact	Normal or ↓	Muscular dystrophy

Table 18-6   Abnormalities of Gait and Posture

TABLE 18-6   Abnormalities of Gait and Posture

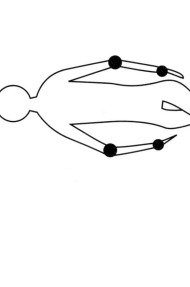
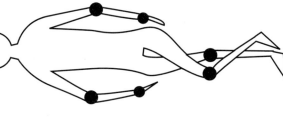
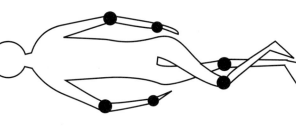
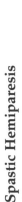

	Spastic Hemiparesis	**Scissors Gait**	**Steppage Gait**
Underlying Defect	Associated with corticospinal tract disease, as with stroke	Associated with bilateral spastic paresis of the legs	Associated with foot drop, usually secondary to lower motor neuron disease
Description	One arm is held immobile and close to the side, with elbow, wrist, and interphalangeal joints flexed. The leg is extended, with plantar flexion of the foot. On walking, the patient either drags the foot, often scraping the toe, or circles it stiffly outward and forward (*circumduction*).	The gait is stiff. Each leg is advanced slowly, and the thighs tend to cross forward on each other at each step. The steps are short. The patient appears to be walking through water.	These patients either drag their feet or lift them high, with knees flexed, and bring them down with a slap onto the floor, thus appearing to be walking up stairs. They are unable to walk on their heels. The steppage gait may involve one or both sides.

Table 18-6   Abnormalities of Gait and Posture

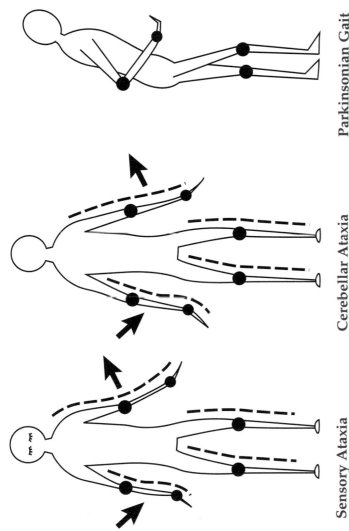

	Sensory Ataxia	**Cerebellar Ataxia**	**Parkinsonian Gait**	**Gait of Old Age**
Underlying Defect	Associated with loss of position sense in the legs, as from polyneuropathy or posterior column damage	Associated with disease of the cerebellum or associated tracts	Associated with the basal ganglia defects of Parkinson's disease	The aging process
Description	The gait is unsteady and wide based (with feet wide apart). These patients throw their feet forward and outward and bring them down, first on the heels and then on the toes, with a double tapping sound. They watch the ground for guidance while walking. With eyes closed, they cannot stand steadily with feet together (a positive Romberg sign) and the staggering gait worsens.	The gait is staggering, unsteady, and wide based, with exaggerated difficulty on the turns. These patients cannot stand steadily with feet together, whether their eyes are open or closed.	The posture is stooped, with head and neck forward and hips and knees slightly flexed. Arms are flexed at elbows and wrists. The patient is slow in getting started. Steps are short and often shuffling. Arm swings are decreased and the patient turns around stiffly—"all in one piece."	Speed, balance, and grace decrease with aging. Steps become short, uncertain, and even shuffling. The legs may be flexed at hips and knees. A cane may bolster lost confidence.

Table 18-7   Metabolic and Structural Coma

TABLE 18-7   *Metabolic and Structural Coma*

Although there are many causes of coma, most can be classified as either structural or metabolic. Findings vary widely in individual patients; the features listed are general guidelines rather than strict diagnostic criteria. Remember that psychiatric disorders may mimic coma.

	Toxic–Metabolic	Structural
Pathophysiology	Arousal centers poisoned or critical substrates depleted	Lesion destroys or compresses brainstem arousal areas, either directly or secondary to more distant expanding mass lesions.
Clinical Features		
• Respiratory pattern	If regular, may be normal or hyperventilation. If irregular, usually Cheyne–Stokes	Irregular, especially Cheyne–Stokes or ataxic breathing
• Pupillary size and reaction	Equal, reactive to light. If *pinpoint* from opiates or cholinergics, you may need a magnifying glass to see the reaction.	Unequal or unreactive to light (fixed)
	May be unreactive if *fixed and dilated* from anticholinergics or hypothermia	*Midposition, fixed*—suggests midbrain compression
		Dilated, fixed—suggests compression of CN III from herniation
• Level of consciousness	Changes after pupils change	Changes before pupils change
Examples of Cause	Uremia, hyperglycemia	Epidural, subdural, or intracerebral hemorrhage
	Alcohol, drugs, liver failure	Cerebral infarct or embolus
	Hypothyroidism, hypoglycemia	Tumor, abscess
	Anoxia, ischemia	Brainstem infarct, tumor, or hemorrhage
	Meningitis, encephalitis	Cerebellar infarct, hemorrhage, tumor, or abscess
	Hyperthermia, hypothermia	

Table 18-8   Pupils in Comatose Patients

TABLE 18-8   Pupils in Comatose Patients

Pupillary size, equality, and light reactions help in assessing the cause of coma and in determining the region of the brain that is impaired. Remember that unrelated pupillary abnormalities, including miotic drops for glaucoma or mydriatic drops for a better view of the ocular fundi, may have preceded the coma.

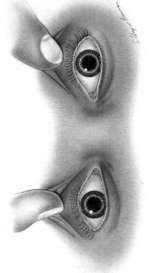

Small or Pinpoint Pupils

Bilaterally small pupils (1–2.5 mm) suggest (1) damage to the sympathetic pathways in the hypothalamus, or (2) metabolic encephalopathy (a diffuse failure of cerebral function that has many causes, including drugs). Light reactions are usually normal.

Pinpoint pupils (<1 mm) suggest (1) a hemorrhage in the pons, or (2) the effects of morphine, heroin, or other narcotics. The light reactions may be seen with a magnifying glass.

Midposition Fixed Pupils

Pupils that are in the *midposition or slightly dilated* (4–6 mm) and are *fixed to light* suggest structural damage in the midbrain.

Large Pupils

Bilaterally fixed and dilated pupils may be due to severe anoxia and its sympathomimetic effects, as seen after cardiac arrest. They may also result from atropinelike agents, phenothiazines, or tricyclic antidepressants.

Bilaterally large reactive pupils may be due to cocaine, amphetamine, LSD, or other sympathetic nervous system agonists.

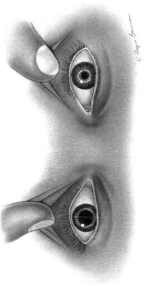

One Large Pupil

A *pupil that is fixed and dilated* warns of herniation of the temporal lobe, causing compression of the oculomotor nerve and midbrain.

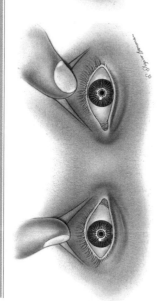

Table 18-9   Abnormal Postures in the Comatose Patient

TABLE 18-9   *Abnormal Postures in the Comatose Patient*

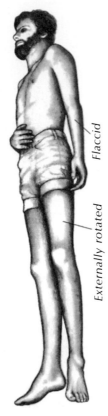

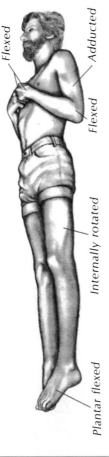

Flexed

Flexed   *Adducted*

Internally rotated

Plantar flexed

Decorticate Rigidity (Abnormal Flexor Response)

In decorticate rigidity, the upper arms are held tight to the sides with elbows, wrists, and fingers flexed. The legs are extended and internally rotated. The feet are plantar flexed. This posture implies a destructive lesion of the corticospinal tracts within or very near the cerebral hemispheres. When unilateral, this is the posture of chronic spastic hemiplegia.

Flaccid

Externally rotated

Hemiplegia (Early)

Sudden unilateral brain damage involving the corticospinal tract may produce a hemiplegia (one-sided paralysis), which early in its course is flaccid. Spasticity will develop later. The paralyzed arm and leg are slack. They fall loosely and without tone when raised and dropped to the bed. Spontaneous movements or responses to noxious stimuli are limited to the opposite side. The leg may lie externally rotated. One side of the lower face may be paralyzed, and that cheek puffs out on expiration. Both eyes may be turned away from the paralyzed side.

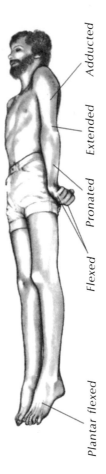

Adducted

Flexed   *Pronated*   *Extended*

Plantar flexed

Decerebrate Rigidity (Abnormal Extensor Response)

In decerebrate rigidity, the jaws are clenched and the neck is extended. The arms are adducted and stiffly extended at the elbows, with forearms pronated, wrists and fingers flexed. The legs are stiffly extended at the knees, with the feet plantar flexed. This posture may occur spontaneously or only in response to external stimuli such as light, noise, or pain. It is caused by a lesion in the diencephalon, midbrain, or pons, although severe metabolic disorders such as hypoxia or hypoglycemia may also produce it.

The Physical Examination of Infants and Children

CHAPTER 19

Robert A. Hoekelman

The anatomy and physiology, the techniques of examination, and the normal and abnormal findings presented in the foregoing chapters of this book primarily focus on the adult patient. Developmentally, however, children are anatomically and physiologically unique. Consequently, many of the techniques, the physical findings, and the significance of the findings differ in younger patients.

This chapter describes the approaches and techniques of the physical examination of infants and children that differ from those used for adults. Emphasis is placed on findings that are normal and variations of normal, and on findings that accompany common pathologic conditions of infancy and childhood. A few examination techniques that are specific to uncommon pathologic conditions are also presented. Readers are encouraged to consult the texts listed in the Bibliography for complete differential diagnoses of abnormal physical findings.

Assessing Child Development

When assessing an infant or a child, consider where the individual fits on the continuum of growth and development, compared to the age range for normal growth and development.

You must be well acquainted, therefore, with the normal and abnormal patterns of growth and development. You should be aware, for example, that a physical finding such as a Babinski response is abnormal beyond the age of 2 years, but may be found in as many as 10% of normal subjects before that age.

Also take into account the different rates of growth of the various systems of the body. For example, growth and development of the central nervous system, the lymphatic system, and the reproductive system parallel neither general somatic growth nor each other. The figure at the right illustrates these differences.

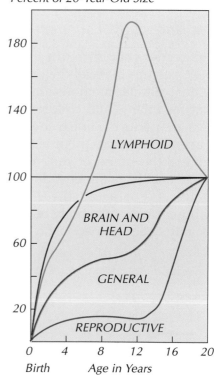

Growth Patterns of Various Systems

Percent of 20-Year-Old Size

The developmental milestones measured by the Denver Developmental Screening Test are discussed on p. 631 and illustrated on pp. 632 and 633. For more comprehensive developmental information, refer to texts listed in the Bibliography.

Measurement of length, weight, and head circumference allows clinicians to compare physical growth at different ages with norms for infants, children, and adolescents. The growth charts for length and weight for females and males are on pp. 647 and 648. Grids for head circumference are on p. 649. Measurements should be entered on these grids at each well child visit. Record measurements more often when a patient lags behind or exceeds expected patterns of growth, and at any initial examination, whatever the child's age. Recommendations for Preventive Pediatric Health care are on p. 623.

Organization of the Chapter

The examination described in this chapter is divided into regions or systems similar to those in the rest of the book. Within each section, discussion is tailored to the three somewhat different approaches needed for different *developmental levels: infancy* (the first year), *early childhood* (years 1 through 4), and *late childhood* (years 5 through 12). The physical examination of adolescents (years 13 through 20) is similar to that of adults.

Because discussion of individual systems here is brief, sections on *techniques of examination* are set off in boldface rather than presented separately, as in the earlier chapters.

Sequence of the Examination

The reader should return to Chapter 4, *Physical Examination: Approach and Overview,* to recall the methods and sequence of examining an adult patient. Similar methods are used to examine infants and children. Note that for infants and children potentially painful or distressing maneuvers are performed near the end of the examination and nondisturbing maneuvers early on. For example, palpating the head and neck, determining the range of motion of the extremities, and auscultating the heart and lungs are best done early, whereas looking into the ears and mouth and palpating the abdomen are done near the end of the examination. Areas of the body in which the patient, by history, is having pain usually are examined last.

Recommendations for Preventive Pediatric Health Care

Each child and family is unique; therefore, these Recommendations are designed for the care of children who are receiving competent parenting; have no manifestations of any important health problems, and are growing and developing in satisfactory fashion. Additional visits may become necessary if circumstances suggest variations from normal.

	INFANCY								EARLY CHILDHOOD					MIDDLE CHILDHOOD				ADOLESCENCE									
AGE	2-4 days¹	By 1 mo	2 mo	4 mo	6 mo	8 mo	10 mo	12 mo	15 mo	18 mo	24 mo	3 y	4 y	5 y	6 y	8 y	10 y	11 y	12 y	13 y	14 y	15 y	16 y	17 y	18 y	19 y	20 y+
HISTORY Initial / Interval	•	•	•	•	•	•	•	•	•	•	•	•	•	•	•	•	•	•	•	•	•	•	•	•	•	•	•
MEASUREMENTS Height and weight	•	•	•	•	•	•	•	•	•	•	•	•	•	•	•	•	•	•	•	•	•	•	•	•	•	•	•
Head Circumference	•	•	•	•	•	•	•	•	•	•	•																
Blood Pressure												•	•	•	•	•	•	•	•	•	•	•	•	•	•	•	•
SENSORY SCREENING Vision	S	S	S	S	S	S	S	S	S	S	S	O	O	O	S	S	O	S	O	S	S	O	S	S	O	S	S
Hearing	S	S	S	S	S	S	S	S	S	S	S	O	O	O	S	S	O	S	O	S	S	O	S	S	O	S	S
DEVELOPMENTAL / BEHAVIORAL ASSESSMENT²	•	•	•	•	•	•	•	•	•	•	•	•	•	•	•	•	•	•	•	•	•	•	•	•	•	•	•
PHYSICAL EXAMINATION³	•	•	•	•	•	•	•	•	•	•	•	•	•	•	•	•	•	•	•	•	•	•	•	•	•	•	•

1. For newborns discharged in less than 48 hours after delivery
2. By history and appropriate physical examination: if suspicious, by specific objective development testing
3. At each visit, a complete physical examination is essential, with infant totally unclothed, older child undressed and suitably draped

Key: • = to be performed   S = subjective, by history
      O = objective, by a standard testing method

Adapted from Recommendations For Preventive Pediatric Health Care promulgated by the American Academy of Pediatrics Committee on Practice and Ambulatory Medicine. Pediatrics 96:373, 1995. Additional recommendations made by the Committee regarding screening for metabolic disorders, tuberculosis, anemia and urinary tract diseases, administration of immunizations, provision of anticipatory guidance, and initial dental referral are not included in the above summation.

Techniques of Examination

APPROACH TO THE NEWBORN, CHILD, AND ADOLESCENT

Often, neophyte (and some veteran) examiners are intimidated by approaching a tiny baby or a screaming child, especially if the physical examination is performed under the critical eyes of anxious parents. Although it takes a bit of courage to overcome this feeling, one soon comes to accept this challenge easily and to enjoy almost all such encounters. This section provides guidelines for a reassuring yet thorough approach to children in three age groups: infancy (both newborn and older infants), early and late childhood, and adolescence. Note that the approach to the newborn includes important information on techniques of physical assessment. For older children, techniques of examination are detailed in the Physical Examination sections beginning on p. 638.

Approach to the Newborn

General Approach

The first year of life, infancy, is divided into the neonatal period (the first 28 days) and the postneonatal period (29 days to 1 year). This distinction is important for reporting mortality rates for those age groups.

The next few pages deal with (1) the immediate adaptation of newborn infants to extrauterine life, using basic clinical signs to predict immediate survival and long-term morbidity, (2) classification of infants according to birth weight and gestational age, and (3) special techniques used in general assessment. The examination of newborns is for the most part identical to that of infants.

Immediate Assessment at Birth: Adaptation to Extrauterine Life

The newborn should be examined briefly immediately after birth to determine the general condition of the cardiorespiratory, neurologic, and gastrointestinal systems and to detect any gross congenital abnormalities.

Determine the Apgar Score and classify the infant according to birth weight and gestational age.

The Apgar Scoring System. **Assess the infant's immediate adaptation to extrauterine life by making the five observations shown in Table 19-1, p. 625. Score each infant at 1 minute and 5 minutes after birth.** Each observation is scored on a three-point scale (0,1, or 2). The total Apgar score may range from 0 to 10.

If at 5 minutes the Apgar score is 8 or more, proceed to a more complete examination.

One-minute Apgar scores of 7 or less usually indicate nervous system depression. Scores of 4 or less indicate severe depression requiring immediate resuscitation. Five-minute Apgar scores of less than 7 place the infant at high risk for subsequent central nervous system and other organ system dysfunction.

TABLE 19-1	*The Apgar Scoring System*		
	Assigned Score		
Clinical Sign	*0*	*1*	*2*
Heart Rate	Absent	<100	>100
Respiratory Effort	Absent	Slow and irregular	Good; crying
Muscle Tone	Flaccid	Some flexion of the arms and legs	Active movement
Reflex Irritability*	No responses	Crying	Crying vigorously, sneeze, or cough
Color	Blue, pale	Pink body, blue extremities	Pink all over

* Reaction to suction of nares with bulb syringe

Classification of Newborn Infants by Birth Weight and Gestational Age
Newborn infants may be classified according to their birth weight, their gestational age (maturity), or a combination of these two dimensions.

• Classification by Birth Weight

   Extremely low birth weight = <1000 grams
   Very low birth weight = 1000–1499 grams
   Low birth weight = 1500–2499 grams
   Normal birth weight = ≥2500 grams

• Classification by Gestational Age

   The clinical assessment of gestational age is used to determine whether an infant should be categorized as pre-term, term, or post-term.

      Pre-term = gestational age <37 weeks
      Term = gestational age 37 to 42 weeks
      Post-term = gestational age ≥ 42 weeks

   Gestational age is based on specific neuromuscular signs and physical characteristics that change with gestational maturity. Several scores have been developed to estimate an infant's gestational age using these neuromuscular and physical characteristics. The Ballard scoring system enables estimates of gestational age to within 1 week, even in extremely premature infants.

Ballard scoring system for determining gestational age in weeks.

Neuromuscular Maturity

	-1	0	1	2	3	4	5
Posture							
Square Window (wrist)	>90°	90°	60°	45°	30°	0°	
Arm Recoil		180°	140°-180°	110°-140°	90°-110°	<90°	
Popliteal Angle	180°	160°	140°	120°	100°	90°	<90°
Scarf Sign							
Heel to Ear							

Physical Maturity

Skin	sticky friable transparent	gelatinous red, translucent	smooth pink, visible veins	superficial peeling &/or rash. few veins	cracking pale areas rare veins	parchment deep cracking no vessels	leathery cracked wrinkled
Lanugo	none	sparse	abundant	thinning	bald areas	mostly bald	
Plantar Surface	heel-toe 40-50mm:-1 <40 mm:-2	>50mm no crease	faint red marks	anterior transverse crease only	creases ant. 2/3	creases over entire sole	
Breast	imperceptible	barely perceptible	flat areola no bud	stippled areola 1-2mm bud	raised areola 3-4mm bud	full areola 5-10mm bud	
Eye/Ear	lids fused loosely:-1 tightly:-2	lids open pinna flat stays folded	sl. curved pinna; soft; slow recoil	well-curved pinna; soft but ready recoil	formed &firm instant recoil	thick cartilage ear stiff	
Genitals male	scrotum flat, smooth	scrotum empty faint rugae	testes in upper canal rare rugae	testes descending few rugae	testes down good rugae	testes pendulous deep rugae	
Genitals female	clitoris prominent labia flat	prominent clitoris small labia minora	prominent clitoris enlarging minora	majora & minora equally prominent	majora large minora small	majora cover clitoris & minora	

Maturity Rating

score	weeks
-10	20
-5	22
0	24
5	26
10	28
15	30
20	32
25	34
30	36
35	38
40	40
45	42
50	44

The Neuromuscular Maturity Criteria *are depicted in the top half of the figure. The techniques for assessing each of the neuromuscular maturity criteria are described in Table 19-2, page 627. The scores for each criterion are indicated at the top of the vertical columns. Asphyxiated neonates or neonates obtunded by anesthetic agents or drugs will score lower on neuromuscular maturity criteria. In such instances, scoring should be repeated at 24 to 48 hours of age. The Physical Maturity Criteria are shown in the bottom half of the figure and are self explanatory. The scores for each criterion are again the numbers at the top of the columns. The sum of the scores for all of the neuromuscular and physical maturity items provides an estimate of gestational age in weeks, using the maturity rating scale at the lower right portion of the figure. (Figure from Ballard JL, et. al. J Pediatr 119:417, 1991.)*

TABLE 19-2   *Techniques for Assessment of Neuromuscular Maturity*

Posture

With the infant supine and quiet, score as follows:
  Arms and legs extended = 0
  Slight or moderate flexion of hips and knees = 1
  Moderate to strong flexion of hips and knees = 2
  Legs flexed and abducted, arms slightly flexed = 3
  Full flexion of arms and legs = 4

Square Window

Flex the hand at the wrist (exert pressure sufficient to get as much flexion as possible); do not rotate the wrist. Measure and score the angle between the hypothenar eminence and the anterior aspect of the forearm according to chart.

Arm Recoil

With the infant supine, fully flex the forearm for 5 seconds, then fully extend by pulling the hands and releasing. Score the reaction according to the following:
  Remains extended or random movements = 0
  Up to 40° flexion = 1
  Between 40° and 70° flexion = 2
  From 70° through 90° flexion = 3
  Brisk return to 90° flexion = 2

Popliteal Angle

With the infant supine and the pelvis flat on the examining surface, use one hand to flex the leg on the thigh and then fully flex the thigh; use the other hand to extend the leg. Score the angle attained as in the chart.

Scarf Sign

With the infant supine, take the infant's hand and draw it across the neck and as far across the opposite shoulder as possible (assistance to the elbow is permissible by lifting it across the body). Score according to the location of the elbow:
  Elbow reaches beyond the opposite anterior axillary line = 0
  Elbow reaches to the opposite anterior axillary line = 1
  Elbow is between opposite anterior axillary line and midline of thorax = 2
  Elbow is at midline of thorax = 3
  Elbow does not reach midline of thorax = 4

Heel-to-Ear Maneuver

With the infant supine, hold the infant's foot with one hand and move it as near to the head as possible without forcing it. Keep the pelvis flat on the examining surface. Score as in the chart.

Adapted from Amiel-Tison C: *Arch Dis Child* 43:89, 1968; Dubowitz LMS, Dubowitz V, Goldberg C: *J Pediatr* 77: 1, 1970; and Ballard, JL, et al, *J Pediatr* 119; 417, 1991.

- Classification by Birth Weight and Gestational Age

    Weight Small for Gestational Age (SGA) = birth weight <10th percentile on the intrauterine growth curve

    Weight Appropriate for Gestational Age (AGA) = birth weight within the 10th and 90th percentiles on the intrauterine growth curve

    Weight Large for Gestational Age (LGA) = birth weight > 90th percentile on the intrauterine growth curve

The three babies shown below are all at 32 weeks' gestational age. They weighed 600 g (SGA), 1400 g (AGA), and 2,750 g (LGA), respectively.

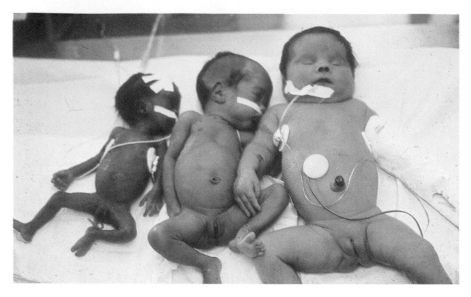

(Reprinted with permission from Korones SB: High-Risk Newborn Infants: The Basis for Intensive Nursing Care, 4th ed. St. Louis, CV Mosby, 1986.)

The figure on p. 629 shows the intrauterine growth curves for the 10th and 90th percentiles, and depicts nine possible categories of maturity for newborn infants based on birth weight and gestational age: pre-term (<37 weeks) SGA, AGA, and LGA; term (37 to 42 weeks) SGA, AGA, and LGA; and post-term (≥42 weeks) SGA, AGA, and LGA.

Each of these categories has a different mortality rate, highest for pre-term SGA and AGA infants and lowest for term AGA infants. Furthermore, pre-term AGA infants are more prone to respiratory distress syndrome, apnea, patent ductus arteriosus with left-to-right shunt, and infection, while pre-term SGA infants are more likely to experience asphyxia, hypoglycemia, and hypocalcemia.

Further Techniques Used in Newborn Assessment

Listen to the anterior thorax with your stethoscope, palpate the abdomen, and inspect the head, face, oral cavity, extremities, genitalia, and perineum.

Pass a small tube through the nose, nasopharynx, and esophagus into the stomach to establish their patency. To be sure that the tube is in the stomach, palpate the epigastrium for the tip itself; if the tip cannot be felt, feel or listen there for the emergence of an air bubble injected with a 5 cc–10 cc syringe through the tube into the stomach.

Failure to pass the tube through the nasopharynx suggests *posterior nasal*(choanal) *atresia.*

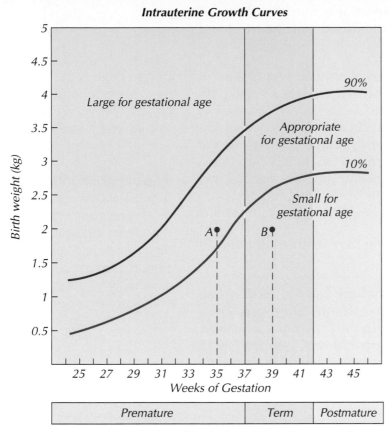

Intrauterine Growth Curves

Level of intrauterine growth based on birth weight and gestational age of liveborn, single, white infants. Point A represents a premature infant, while point B indicates an infant of similar birth weight who is mature but small for gestational age; the growth curves are representative of the 10th and 90th percentiles for all of the newborns in the sampling (Adapted from Sweet YA: Classification of the low-birth-weight infant. In Klaus MH, Fanaroff AA: Care of the High-Risk Neonate, 3rd ed. Philadelphia, WB Saunders, 1986. Reproduced with permission.)

Aspirate the gastric contents in premature babies, in babies born with meconium-stained amniotic fluid, and in babies born by cesarean section, in order to prevent regurgitation and aspiration.

A more extensive examination of the newborn should be conducted within 12 hours of birth, and again at approximately 72 hours of age when the effects of anesthesia and shock of birth have subsided.

Examination at 2 to 3 Hours After Birth
Best results, in terms of responsiveness, are obtained 2 or 3 hours after a feeding when the baby is neither too satiated (and therefore less responsive) nor too hungry (and therefore more agitated).

Inspection. **Observe the baby, first as it is lying undisturbed in the bassinet and then completely undressed on an examining table.**

Failure to pass the tube into the stomach suggests *esophageal atresia*, usually with an associated *tracheoesophageal fistula*.

Observe the baby's color, size, body proportions, nutritional status, and posture, as well as respirations and movements of the head and extremities.

Normal full-term newborns lie in a symmetrical position with the limbs semiflexed and the legs partially abducted at the hip. The head is slightly flexed and positioned in the midline or turned to one side. Normal newborns have spontaneous motor activity of flexion and extension, alternating between the arms and the legs. The forearms supinate with flexion at the elbow and pronate with extension. The fingers are usually flexed in a tight fist, but may extend in slow athetoid posturing movements. Low-amplitude and high-frequency tremors of the arms, legs, and body are seen with vigorous crying and even at rest during the first 48 hours of life.

In *breech babies* the legs and head are extended, and the legs of a *frank breech baby* are abducted and externally rotated.

Most newborn infants are cooperative during the examination unless it is close to feeding time.

Auscultation and Palpation. **Make sure that the baby is quiet when you auscultate the heart and lungs and palpate the abdomen, since these maneuvers are more difficult to perform if the baby is crying. Place a pacifier, a bottle of formula, or the tip of one of your fingers in a crying baby's mouth to silence the baby long enough to complete these portions of the examination.**

By 4 days after birth, however, tremors occurring at rest signal central nervous system disease. Asymmetrical movements of the arms or legs at any time should alert the clinician to the possibility of central or peripheral neurologic deficits, birth injuries, or congenital anomalies.

Hereafter, the order of examination is relatively unimportant, except that painful components, such as hip abduction (pp. 692–693), should be performed at the end because they usually cause the baby to cry.

Approach to Older Infants

General Approach

After the newborn period and throughout the rest of infancy, you should encounter little difficulty when performing the complete physical examination. The key to success is distraction. Since infants usually attend to only one thing at a time, it is relatively easy to bring the baby's attention to something other than the examination being performed.

Use a moving object, a flashing light, a game of peek-a-boo, tickling, or any sort of noise to distract the baby.

Infants usually do not object to removal of their clothing. Indeed, most seem to prefer being nude, perhaps because it allows for greater tactile stimulation. It is wise, however, in the interest of keeping yourself and your surroundings dry, to leave the diaper in place throughout the examination, removing it only to examine the genitalia, rectum, lower spine, and hips.

You can perform much of the examination with the infant lying or sitting in the parent's lap or held in an upright position against the parent's chest, although this usually is not necessary except with tired, hungry, or acutely ill babies. Occasionally, most of the physical examination can be completed without waking a sleeping infant.

Observe the parent–infant interactions.

Note the parent's affect in talking about the infant, manner of holding, moving, and dressing the baby, and response to situations that may produce discomfort for the infant. A breast or a bottle feeding should be observed.

Such observations may identify maladaptive nurturing patterns on the parent's part and are important in assessing *"failure to thrive,"* malnutrition, colic, chronic regurgitation, and suspected parental neglect.

Testing for Developmental Milestones

Before performing the general physical examination of older infants, test for attainment of developmental milestones, such as the ability to reach for a toy, transfer a cube from one hand to the other, and use the thumb and forefinger pincer grasp in picking up a small object.

The standard for measuring the attainment of developmental milestones throughout infancy and childhood is the Denver Developmental Screening Test (DDST). The DDST is designed to reveal developmental delays in personal–social, fine motor-adaptive, language, and gross motor dimensions from birth through 6 years of age. It is easy and rapid to administer.

The form used for recording specific observations is shown on p. 632, and directions for its use are on p. 633. Each test item is represented on the form under the appropriate age by a bar, which indicates when 25%, 50%, 75%, and 90% of children attain the milestone depicted. It must be emphasized that the DDST is only a measure of developmental attainment in the categories indicated, and not a measure of intelligence. It is a highly specific test (i.e., most normal children score as normal), but it is not very sensitive (i.e., many children with mild developmental delay also score as normal). While the DDST is a useful screening test, other more sophisticated tests are available to assess motor, language, and social development when, despite normal DDST results, it is suspected that these are delayed.

Approach in Early Childhood

General Approach
One of the most difficult challenges facing the professional who cares for children in this age group is completing the examination without producing a physical struggle, a crying child, or a distraught parent. When this is accomplished successfully, it provides a great measure of satisfaction to all involved and comes close to "art" in the practice of pediatrics.

Gaining the confidence and dispersing the fears of the child begin at the moment of encounter and continue throughout the visit. The approach may vary with the place and circumstances of the visit; however, a health-supervision visit for a well child probably allows greater development of rapport than a visit at the office, in the home, or in the hospital emergency room when the child is acutely ill.

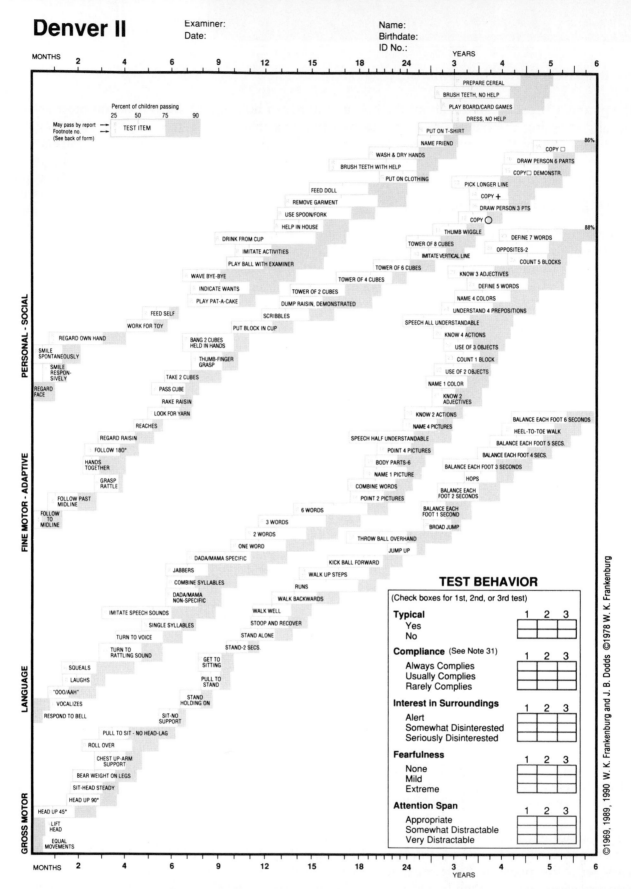

Denver II

Examiner:
Date:

Name:
Birthdate:
ID No.:

Testing kits, test forms, and reference manuals (which must be used to ensure accuracy in administration of the test) for the DDST may be ordered from Denver Developmental Materials Incorporated, P.O. Box 6919, Denver, CO 80206-0919 (Reprinted with permission from William K. Frankenburg, M.D.)

DIRECTIONS FOR ADMINISTRATION

1. Try to get child to smile by smiling, talking or waving. Do not touch him/her.
2. Child must stare at hand several seconds.
3. Parent may help guide toothbrush and put toothpaste on brush.
4. Child does not have to be able to tie shoes or button/zip in the back.
5. Move yarn slowly in an arc from one side to the other, about 8″ above child's face.
6. Pass if child grasps rattle when it is touched to the backs or tips of fingers.
7. Pass if child tries to see where yarn went. Yarn should be dropped quickly from sight from tester's hand without arm movement.
8. Child must transfer cube from hand to hand without help of body, mouth, or table.
9. Pass if child picks up raisin with any part of thumb and finger.
10. Line can vary only 30 degrees or less from tester's line. ⋁
11. Make a fist with thumb pointing upward and wiggle only the thumb. Pass if child imitates and does not move any fingers other than the thumb.

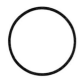   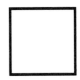

12. Pass any enclosed form. Fail continuous round motions.

13. Which line is longer? (Not bigger.) Turn paper upside down and repeat. (pass 3 of 3 or 5 of 6)

14. Pass any lines crossing near midpoint.

15. Have child copy first. If failed, demonstrate.

When giving items 12, 14, and 15, do not name the forms. Do not demonstrate 12 and 14.

16. When scoring, each pair (2 arms, 2 legs, etc.) counts as one part.
17. Place one cube in cup and shake gently near child's ear, but out of sight. Repeat for other ear.
18. Point to picture and have child name it. (No credit is given for sounds only.)
    If less than 4 pictures are named correctly, have child point to picture as each is named by tester.

  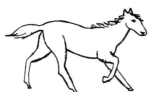 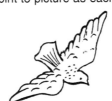 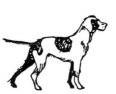 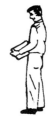

19. Using doll, tell child: Show me the nose, eyes, ears, mouth, hands, feet, tummy, hair. Pass 6 of 8.
20. Using pictures, ask child: Which one flies?... says meow?... talks?... barks?... gallops? Pass 2 of 5, 4 of 5.
21. Ask child: What do you do when you are cold?... tired?... hungry? Pass 2 of 3, 3 of 3.
22. Ask child: What do you do with a cup? What is a chair used for? What is a pencil used for?
    Action words must be included in answers.
23. Pass if child correctly places <u>and</u> says how many blocks are on paper. (1, 5)
24. Tell child: Put block **on** table; **under** table; **in front of** me, **behind** me. Pass 4 of 4.
    (Do not help child by pointing, moving head or eyes.)
25. Ask child: What is a ball?... lake?... desk?... house?... banana?... curtain?... fence?... ceiling? Pass if defined in terms of use, shape, what it is made of, or general category (such as banana is fruit, not just yellow). Pass 5 of 8, 7 of 8.
26. Ask child: If a horse is big, a mouse is __? If fire is hot, ice is __? If the sun shines during the day, the moon shines during the __? Pass 2 of 3.
27. Child may use wall or rail only, not person. May not crawl.
28. Child must throw ball overhand 3 feet to within arm's reach of tester.
29. Child must perform standing broad jump over width of test sheet (8½ inches).
30. Tell child to walk forward, ⚬⟞⚬⟞⚬⟞ ➤ heel within 1 inch of toe. Tester may demonstrate.
    Child must walk 4 consecutive steps.
31. In the second year, half of normal children are noncompliant.

OBSERVATIONS:

Instructions printed on the back of the DDST form (p. 632) for administering some of the items contained in the Denver Developmental Screening Test. (Reprinted with permission from William K. Frankenburg, M.D.)

During the interview, children usually should remain dressed. This may prolong the visit, but avoids apprehension on their part and affords the opportunity later to observe their response to being undressed or their ability to undress and dress themselves. Children also are more apt to play quietly and interact more appropriately with the parent and examiner if fully clothed.

Engage children in conversation appropriate to their ages and ask simple questions about their health or illness. Compliment them about their appearance, dress, or performance, tell a story, or play a simple trick to help "break the ice."

This dialogue will indicate the child's level of receptive and expressive function and will direct the approach by the examiner.

If children respond to conversation and questions directed to them by silence, shielding of the eyes, or apprehension, it is wise to ignore them temporarily.

Careful observation of the parent's response to the child's verbal and nonverbal signals may reveal problems such as overly anxious parents, disengaged parents who provide insufficient stimulation, stressed families, enmeshed families, and even possibly abusive parents.

Include in your observations during the interview a general assessment of the degree of sickness or wellness, mood, state of nutrition, speech, cry, respiratory pattern, facial expression, apparent chronologic and emotional age, posture (particularly as it may reflect discomfort), and developmental skills. In addition, closely observe the parent–child interaction, including the amount of separation tolerated, displays of affection, and response to discipline.

Abusing parents often pay little or no attention to their abused child, treating him or her more like a piece of property than a person. By the same token, an abused child usually demonstrates no separation anxiety when removed physically and environmentally from the parents. On the other hand, both child and parents may appear overaffectionate to one another in an attempt to hide the abuse.

Specific developmental testing (such as building towers with blocks, playing ball with the examiner, and performing hop, skip, and jump maneuvers) is best accomplished at the end of the interview, just before the formal physical examination. This "fun and games" interlude is likely to improve the child's view of the examiner and enhance cooperation during the examination.

Preparing the Child for the Examination

The actual performance of the physical examination, with certain exceptions, need not take place on the examining table. In fact, some parts of the examination can best be accomplished with the child standing, sitting on the parent's lap, or even sitting on the examiner's lap. It is not essential that the child be completely undressed throughout the examination; often, exposing only the part of the body being examined will suffice and may avert objection by the child. Occasionally, a child is reluctant to undress because the examining room is cool and the examining table and instruments (including the examiner's hands) are cold, rather than because of apprehension or modesty.

Actually, only a few children resist undressing. Most will allow themselves to be stripped to their underpants and placed, sitting, on the examining table without objection.

When two or more siblings are to be examined, it is wise to begin with the oldest, who is most likely to cooperate and set a good example for the younger children.

During the examination, ask the parent to stand at the head of the examining table, to the right of the child and to your left as you face the examining table. As with infants, distraction is the key to gaining the patient's cooperation. The child in this age group, however, is not as easily distracted as the infant; therefore, approach the patient pleasantly and, whenever possible, explain each step of the examination before performing it. Demonstrate the procedure on yourself or on a doll or toy animal. This also helps the child understand what is to be done. For example, you can place the otoscope in your ear, flash the light into your open mouth, or place the stethoscope on your chest. Allow the child to play with the examining instruments to create an atmosphere of trust. Play at blowing out the examining light or use the stethoscope bell as a telephone to create attractive diversions.

Tips to the Examiner. The initial "laying on of the hands" is the most crucial point of the examination; if resistance is encountered, it will most likely be at this point. Therefore, the first contact should be in non-vulnerable areas.

Hold the patient's hand, count the fingers, and palpate the wrist and elbow while talking gently to place the patient at ease.

Having both of the examiner's hands in contact with the patient's body whenever possible has a comforting effect on the patient and is less apt to produce involuntary withdrawal than is the use of one hand or a few probing fingers.

For example, when examining the heart, place your left hand on the patient's right shoulder while your right hand, holding the stethoscope, makes contact with the chest wall.

In a sense, the left hand acts as both a distracting and a comforting force. The examiner who moves unhesitatingly, firmly, and gracefully, and who talks pleasantly and reassuringly throughout the examination is not apt to provoke apprehension. Most children increase their resistance when spoken to sharply.

Use a firm voice and unequivocal instructions when asking a child to perform an act pertaining to the examination. Tell the child what to do rather than asking the child to do it. For example, say "Roll over on your belly" rather than "Will you roll over on your belly for me?"

Often children will sit or lie passively on the examining table covering both eyes with their hands, because they think the examiner cannot see them if they cannot see the examiner. This posture can be tolerated, because it does not interfere with the examination. The eyes can easily be examined after the child has dressed.

During this initial part of the examination, careful observation can reveal a variety of abnormalities, including tachypnea, tachycardia, skin rashes, birthmarks, bruises, asymmetrical eye movements, decreased or increased muscle tone, speech impediments, and diminished fine motor skills.

Base the order of your examination on performing the least distressing procedures first and the most distressing last. Thus, perform those parts of the examination that can be accomplished while the child is sitting—for example, palpation, percussion, and auscultation of the heart and lungs—before the child lies down. Since lying down may make the child feel more vulnerable and resist further examination, accomplish this with great care. Often you can avert apprehension by supporting the head and back with your arm while the child lies down. Once the child is supine, examine the abdomen first, the throat and ears next to last, and the genitalia and rectum last. Examination of the genitalia and perineum, when a rectal examination is not performed, is usually less disturbing to the child than is the examination of the throat. However, in light of the fastidious and perhaps modest nature of some parents, leave these portions of the examination to last.

The child's comfort should be paramount in conducting the examination. Immediately before an examination maneuver the child should be told kindly, but matter-of-factly, of the likelihood of pain or other unpleasant sensations that might result. In instances when the child is extremely apprehensive about one portion of the examination (e.g., the examination of the throat), it is helpful to do this first. Indeed, to ensure a reasonable interview, it may be necessary to complete the entire physical examination before obtaining the entire history. Distasteful portions of the examination should be accomplished quickly to minimize the child's discomfort. The examiner should remember, however, that the physical examination is designed to gather essential information and that the child's comfort may need to be sacrificed at times to achieve this end. A completed examination is a comfort and reassurance to the parent and examiner; an incomplete examination is a frustration and a source of dissatisfaction to both.

Resistance to the Examination. Obviously there sometimes will be resistance to the examination. Some children will scream throughout the examination but offer no physical resistance. Most toddlers will fight the examination and strive to gain an upright position and the comfort and security of a parent's arms. Parents can be helpful here in orally reassuring children and in actually restraining their movements for certain parts of the examination, such as the ears and throat.

Rarely, for the child's sake or the parent's, it is necessary to discontinue the examination before it is completed and return to it another time.

Using another person, in addition to the parent, to restrain the child is often helpful under ordinary circumstances; however, using other kinds of restraints or mummying methods has no place in the physical examination procedure.

The examiner should not convey feelings of frustration or anger, but should reassure the parent that the child's resistance is developmentally normal. Embarrassment may cause the parent to compound the problem by scolding the child. Some parents feel that the examiner is at fault when their child is uncooperative while being examined. Others feel that such resistance is a reflection of the child's level of independence.

If this resistance is inappropriate for the child's age, the examiner should consider the possibility of underlying developmental, emotional, or parent–child interactional difficulties.

Neophyte examiners are apt to be less successful in examining very young children than in examining older ones. However, with practice, perseverance, and patience they should succeed. While it is difficult to teach "how to approach a reluctant child," flexibility, enthusiasm, and an informal caring but firm approach are key factors. Examiners must learn which techniques work best for them as individuals and which approach they find most comfortable.

Approach in Late Childhood

General Approach

There usually is little difficulty in examining most children after they reach school age. Some, however, may have unpleasant memories of previous encounters with examiners and offer resistance.

Question children to determine their orientation to time and place, their knowledge, and their language and number skills. Use intelligence screening tests, such as the Goodenough draw-a-man, the Durrell, and the Bender, when there is some element of doubt concerning the child's intellectual capacity. Keep these tests to a minimum, however, to avoid errors due to familiarity with their content, should formal psychological testing be necessary later on. Observe motor skills involved in writing, tying shoelaces, buttoning shirt fronts, and using scissors, and determine right–left discrimination for self (attained at age 6 or 7 years) and for others (attained at age 8 or 9 years).

The Physical Examination

A child's modesty may be the greatest deterrent to a successful examination. Therefore girls, as early as age 6 or 7, should be gowned. For both boys and girls, leave underpants on until their removal is required, even if the lower half of the body is draped. It is usually wise for examiners who are of the opposite sex from their preadolescent and adolescent patients to leave the room while the patient disrobes. Younger children often request that siblings of the opposite sex depart; older boys often prefer that their mothers leave during the examination, and older girls that their fathers leave.

The order of examination in late childhood can follow that used with adults. At any age, it is important to examine painful areas last.

Approach in Adolescence

General Approach

The key to a successful physical examination of adolescents is a comfortable environment in which they feel safe. It is important to establish a trusting relationship. This will allow for a more relaxed and informative physical examination. The clinician must consider the cognitive development of adolescents when examining them. Most are developing a sense of identity and autonomy, and the examiner must consider these points when deciding on issues of privacy, parental involvement, and confidentiality during the examination.

As for the older child, modesty is often an issue for the adolescent. The patient should remain dressed until the time of the physical examination, and the examiner should leave the room while the patient undresses and gowns. Most older adolescents prefer to be examined alone without a parent or guardian in the examination room, but younger adolescents may prefer to have a familiar person with them, particularly if that person is of the same sex and the examiner is of the opposite sex.

The Physical Examination

The physical examination of the adolescent is very similar to that of the adult, and should progress in much the same manner; however, particular attention should be given to issues unique to the adolescent population. It is important to understand normal pubertal maturation, and to assess it in all adolescents to ensure that normal growth and development are occurring. For the same reason, height and weight should be plotted at all visits. The spine should be examined, particularly in younger adolescents in whom scoliosis tends to be progressive.

Regardless of age, any sexually active female adolescent should have periodic pelvic examinations and Pap smears.

New clinicians often find the examination of adolescents anxiety provoking because of the possible perceived invasion of privacy on the part of the patient; however, with practice, straightforwardness, and understanding, these interactions can be very rewarding for both the adolescent and the clinician.

TECHNIQUES OF PHYSICAL EXAMINATION
The General Survey

Observing infants and children carefully over time is extremely rewarding, as is noting general physical and behavioral changes. This section covers the measurement of vital signs and body size, which is particularly important in infants and children because deviations from the normal may be the first and only indicators of disease.

For example, *parental neglect, chronic renal disease, and juvenile hypothyroidism* may present as growth failure.

Temperature

Take the patient's body temperature whenever an infectious, collagen vascular, or malignant disease is suspected. Where no disease is suspected (e.g., during well-child visits), the temperature need not be taken.

The techniques for obtaining auditory canal, oral, and electronic oral and rectal temperatures in adults are described on pp. 143 and 144. Axillary and thermal-tape skin temperature recordings are not accurate enough to be clinically useful. Electronic dermal thermometers for continuous temperature recordings are used in neonatal intensive care units.

For children and adolescents, auditory canal temperature recordings are preferable because they can be obtained quickly with essentially no discomfort. However, for infants and children under 3 years of age, rectal temperature recordings are preferred. This is because clinical guidelines for evaluation for the presence of serious bacterial infections (SBI), based upon dozens of studies, have used the rectal temperature level as a major criterion. Until studies that establish the level of auditory canal temperature as a criterion for SBI have been conducted, rectal temperatures should be taken in this age group.

The Rectal Temperature. The technique of obtaining the rectal temperature is relatively simple. **Place the infant or child prone on the examining table, on the parent's lap, or on your own lap. While you separate the buttocks with the thumb and forefinger of one hand, with the other hand gently insert a well lubricated rectal thermometer (inclined approximately 20° from the table or lap) through the anal sphincter to a depth of approximately 1 inch. Keep the thermometer in place for at least 2 minutes. One method for holding a child while obtaining the rectal temperature is illustrated on the right.**

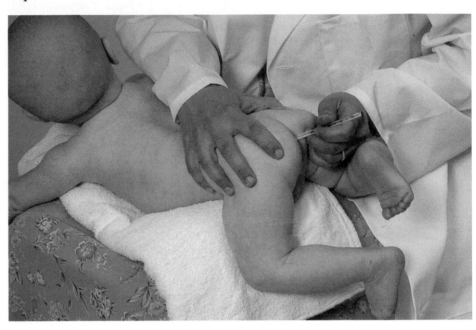

Body temperature in infants and children is less constant than that in adults. The average rectal temperature is higher in infancy and early childhood, usually not falling below 99.0° F (37.2° C) until after the third year. Ranges in body temperature of children may be as much as 3 or more degrees Fahrenheit during the course of a single day. Rectal temperature recordings may approach 101° F (38.3° C) in normal children, particularly in late afternoon after a full day of activity.

Anxiety may elevate the body temperature, as demonstrated by the frequency with which elevated temperatures are found in children on elective hospital admission. Bundling of infants may elevate their skin temperature, but not their core body temperature.

While fever is usually present with an overwhelming infection, an infant with such an infection may have a normal or subnormal temperature. On the other hand, during early childhood extremely high temperature recordings (103° to 105° F, 39.5° to 40.5° C) are common, even with minor infections.

Pulse

The heart rate in infants and children is quite labile, and more sensitive to the effects of illness, exercise, and emotion than that in adults. Average heart rates according to age are shown in Table 19-3.

Obtain the heart rate in infants by observing the pulsations of the anterior fontanelle, by palpating the femoral arteries in the inguinal area and the brachial arteries in the mid-upper arm, or by directly auscultating the heart if the rate is very rapid. Palpate the radial artery at the wrist in older children and in young children who are cooperative.

Beyond the first month, a pulse greater than 180 usually indicates *paroxysmal atrial tachycardia*

Age	Average Rate	Range (Two Standard Deviations)
Birth	140	90–190
1st 6 months	130	80–180
6–12 months	115	75–155
1–2 years	110	70–150
2–6 years	103	68–138
6–10 years	95	65–125
10–14 years	85	55–115

TABLE 19-3 *Average Heart Rate of Infants and Children at Rest*

Respiratory Rate

As with the heart rate, the respiratory rate in infants and children has a greater range and is more responsive to illness, exercise, and emotion than that in adults. The rate of respirations per minute ranges between 30 and 60 in the newborn, 20 and 40 during early childhood, and 15 and 25 during late childhood, reaching adult levels at age 15 years.

Respiratory rates that exceed 100 per minute are seen in diseases associated with lower respiratory tract obstruction (e.g., *bronchiolitis, pneumonia,* and *bronchial asthma*).

The respiratory rate may vary appreciably from moment to moment in premature and full-term newborn infants, with alternating periods of rapid and slow breathing. The respiratory pattern should be observed for more than the usual 30 to 60 seconds to determine the true rate; the sleeping respiratory rate is most reliable. In infancy and early childhood, diaphragmatic breathing is predominant and thoracic excursion is minimal.

Ascertain the respiratory rate by observing abdominal rather than chest excursions. Auscultation of the chest and placement of the stethoscope in front of the mouth and external nares are also useful for counting respirations in this age group. In older children, observe the thoracic movement directly or place your hand on the thorax to determine the respiratory rate.

Blood Pressure

Measuring the blood pressure in infants and children often is omitted because it has erroneously been judged to be too difficult to do with an active child. When the procedure is explained and demonstrated beforehand, however, most children 3 years of age and older are fascinated by the sphygmomanometer and are very cooperative. Obtaining the blood pressure measurement should be part of the physical examination of every child over 2 years of age, and of any younger child whose history or physical examination suggests that the blood pressure may be high or low (rare).

Elevations of blood pressure levels in normal individuals occur due to exercise, crying, and emotional upset. Because children may be anxious about the entire physical examination as well as the blood pressure procedure *per se,* some clinicians prefer to obtain the blood pressure near the end of the examination. Others repeat the determination at the end of the formal examination if the initial pressure was high.

Anxiety may produce elevated systolic blood pressure readings.

Use the sphygmomanometer to determine blood pressures in children as you would in adults. The inflatable rubber bag cuff should be long enough to encircle 80% to 100% of the upper arm or the thigh. Its width should be approximately 90% of the circumference of the arm at a point midway between the acromion and olecranon processes. A narrower cuff elevates the pressure reading, while a wider cuff lowers it and may interfere with proper placement of the stethoscope's bell over the artery as it traverses the antecubital fossa or the popliteal fossa.

With children, as with adults, the point at which the Korotkoff sounds disappear is recorded as the diastolic pressure. At times, especially in early childhood, the Korotkoff sounds are not audible due to a narrow or deeply placed brachial artery.

In infants, blood pressure readings from the thigh are approximately 10 mm Hg higher than those from the upper arm. If they are the same or lower, *coarctation of the aorta* should be suspected.

In such instances, determine the systolic blood pressure by palpation (see page 295). This is approximately 10 mm Hg lower than the systolic pressure determined by auscultation.

The Flush Technique. In infants and very young children, small extremities and lack of cooperation preclude the use of these techniques to determine the blood pressure. However, a value lying somewhere between the systolic and the diastolic pressures can be obtained by using the *flush technique.*

With the cuff in place, wrap an elastic bandage snugly around the elevated arm, proceeding from the fingers to the antecubital space. This essentially empties the capillary and venous network. Inflate the cuff to a pressure above the expected systolic reading, remove the bandage, and place the pallid arm at the patient's side. Allow the cuff pressure to fall slowly until the sudden flush of color returns to the forearm, hand, and fingers. The endpoint is strikingly clear. This method may also be used in the leg.

A more accurate measure of the systolic blood pressure of infants and very young children is obtained with an electronic sphygmomanometer (Doppler), which senses arterial blood flow vibrations, converts them to systolic blood pressure levels, and transmits them to a digital read-out device. Purchase and maintenance costs essentially limit use of these instruments to hospitals and cardiac diagnostic centers.

The level of systolic blood pressure gradually increases throughout infancy and childhood. Measured in mm Hg, normal systolic pressure in males is in the vicinity of 70 mm Hg at birth, 85 at 1 month, and 90 at 6 months.

The 1995 National Heart, Lung, and Blood Institute's National High Blood Pressure Working Group on Hypertension Control in Children and Adolescents defined *Normal Blood Pressure* as systolic and diastolic BPs <90th percentile for age, sex, and height; *High Normal Blood Pressure* as average systolic and/or average diastolic BPs between the 90th and 95th percentiles for age, sex, and height; and *High Blood Pressure* (hypertension) as average systolic and/or diastolic BPs ≥95th percentile for age, sex, and height with measurements obtained on at least three occasions. Table 19-4 and Table 19-5 on pp. 643 and 644 provide the age and height-specific percentiles needed to make those assessments for boys and girls, respectively.

Children who have hypertension should be evaluated extensively to determine its cause. For infants and young children, a specific cause usually can be found. In older children and adolescents, however, the etiology may be obscure, and in many instances observed elevated blood pressure may be a developmental phenomenon that disappears over time.

Renal disease (78%), renal arterial disease (12%), coarctation of the aorta (2%), and pheochromocytoma are the most common causes of *hypertension* during infancy and early childhood. Primary hypertension becomes increasingly prevalent beyond age 6 years. In adolescents, hypertension frequently accompanies obesity.

Somatic Growth

Growth, reflected in increases in body weight and length and head circumference along expected pathways and within certain limits, is probably the best indicator of health. The significance of any measure is determined by relating it to prior measurements of the same dimension, to mean values and standard deviations for that dimension as they occur in other individuals, and to measures of other dimensions in the same patient. Measures of somatic growth in infants and children, therefore, should be plotted on standard growth charts so that those comparisons can be made. (See pp. 647–649.)

Measurements of height and weight above the 97th percentile or below the 3rd percentile on standard growth charts may indicate a growth disturbance and require investigation.

Height. **Measure the body length of infants by placing them supine on a measuring board or in a measuring tray, as illustrated on p. 645. If**

TABLE 19-4 *Blood Pressure Levels for the 90th and 95th Percentiles of Blood Pressure for Boys Aged 1 to 17 Years by Percentiles of Height*

Age, y	Blood Pressure Percentile*	Systolic Blood Pressure by Percentile of Height, mm Hg†							Diastolic Blood Pressure by Percentile of Height, mm Hg†						
		5%	10%	25%	50%	75%	90%	95%	5%	10%	25%	50%	75%	90%	95%
1	90th	94	95	97	98	100	102	102	50	51	52	53	54	54	55
	95th	98	99	101	102	104	106	106	55	55	56	57	58	59	59
2	90th	98	99	100	102	104	105	106	55	55	56	57	58	59	59
	95th	101	102	104	106	108	109	110	59	59	60	61	62	63	63
3	90th	100	101	103	105	107	108	109	59	59	60	61	62	63	63
	95th	104	105	107	109	111	112	113	63	63	64	65	66	67	67
4	90th	102	103	105	107	109	110	111	62	62	63	64	65	66	66
	95th	106	107	109	111	113	114	115	66	67	67	68	69	70	71
5	90th	104	105	106	108	110	112	112	65	65	66	67	68	69	69
	95th	108	109	110	112	114	115	116	69	70	70	71	72	73	74
6	90th	105	106	108	110	111	113	114	67	68	69	70	70	71	72
	95th	109	110	112	114	115	117	117	72	72	73	74	75	76	76
7	90th	106	107	109	111	113	114	115	69	70	71	72	72	73	74
	95th	110	111	113	115	116	118	119	74	74	75	76	77	78	78
8	90th	107	108	110	112	114	115	116	71	71	72	73	74	75	75
	95th	111	112	114	116	118	119	120	75	76	76	77	78	79	80
9	90th	109	110	112	113	115	117	117	72	73	73	74	75	76	77
	95th	113	114	116	117	119	121	121	76	77	78	79	80	80	81
10	90th	110	112	113	115	117	118	119	73	74	74	75	76	77	78
	95th	114	115	117	119	121	122	123	77	78	79	80	80	81	82
11	90th	112	113	115	117	119	120	121	74	74	75	76	77	78	78
	95th	116	117	119	121	123	124	125	78	79	79	80	81	82	83
12	90th	115	116	117	119	121	123	123	75	75	76	77	78	78	79
	95th	119	120	121	123	125	126	127	79	79	80	81	82	83	83
13	90th	117	118	120	122	124	125	126	75	76	76	77	78	79	80
	95th	121	122	124	126	128	129	130	79	80	81	82	83	83	84
14	90th	120	121	123	125	126	128	128	76	76	77	78	79	80	80
	95th	124	125	127	128	130	132	132	80	81	81	82	83	84	85
15	90th	123	124	125	127	129	131	131	77	77	78	79	80	81	81
	95th	127	128	129	131	133	134	135	81	82	83	83	84	85	86
16	90th	125	126	128	130	132	133	134	79	79	80	81	82	82	83
	95th	129	130	132	134	136	137	138	83	83	84	85	86	87	87
17	90th	128	129	131	133	134	136	136	81	81	82	83	84	85	85
	95th	132	133	135	136	138	140	140	85	85	86	87	88	89	89

* Blood pressure percentile was determined by a single measurement.

† Height percentile was determined by standard growth curves.

Reproduced with permission from Update on the 1987 Task Force Report on High Blood Pressure in Children and Adolescents: A Working Group Report from the National High Blood Pressure Education Program. *Pediatrics* 98:649, 1996.

TABLE 19-5 Blood Pressure Levels for the 90th and 95th Percentiles of Blood Pressure for Girls Aged 1 to 17 Years by Percentiles of Height

Age, y	Blood Pressure Percentile*	Systolic Blood Pressure by Percentile of Height, mm Hg[†]							Diastolic Blood Pressure by Percentile of Height, mm Hg[†]						
		5%	10%	25%	50%	75%	90%	95%	5%	10%	25%	50%	75%	90%	95%
1	90th	97	98	99	100	102	103	104	53	53	53	54	55	56	56
	95th	101	102	103	104	105	107	107	57	57	57	58	59	60	60
2	90th	99	99	100	102	103	104	105	57	57	58	58	59	60	61
	95th	102	103	104	105	107	108	109	61	61	62	62	63	64	65
3	90th	100	100	102	103	104	105	106	61	61	61	62	63	63	64
	95th	104	104	105	107	108	109	110	65	65	65	66	67	67	68
4	90th	101	102	103	104	106	107	108	63	63	64	65	65	66	67
	95th	105	106	107	108	109	111	111	67	67	68	69	69	70	71
5	90th	103	103	104	106	107	108	109	65	66	66	67	68	68	69
	95th	107	107	108	110	111	112	113	69	70	70	71	72	72	73
6	90th	104	105	106	107	109	110	111	67	67	68	69	69	70	71
	95th	108	109	110	111	112	114	114	71	71	72	73	73	74	75
7	90th	106	107	108	109	110	112	112	69	69	69	70	71	72	72
	95th	110	110	112	113	114	115	116	73	73	73	74	75	76	76
8	90th	108	109	110	111	112	113	114	70	70	71	71	72	73	74
	95th	112	112	113	115	116	117	118	74	74	75	75	76	77	78
9	90th	110	110	112	113	114	115	116	71	72	72	73	74	74	75
	95th	114	114	115	117	118	119	120	75	76	76	77	78	78	79
10	90th	112	112	114	115	116	117	118	73	73	73	74	75	76	76
	95th	116	116	117	119	120	121	122	77	77	77	78	79	80	80
11	90th	114	114	116	117	118	119	120	74	74	75	75	76	77	77
	95th	118	118	119	121	122	123	124	78	78	79	79	80	81	81
12	90th	116	116	118	119	120	121	122	75	75	76	76	77	78	78
	95th	120	120	121	123	124	125	126	79	79	80	80	81	82	82
13	90th	118	118	119	121	122	123	124	76	76	77	78	78	79	80
	95th	121	122	123	125	126	127	128	80	80	81	82	82	83	84
14	90th	119	120	121	122	124	125	126	77	77	78	79	79	80	81
	95th	123	124	125	126	128	129	130	81	81	82	83	83	84	85
15	90th	121	121	122	124	125	126	127	78	78	79	79	80	81	82
	95th	124	125	126	128	129	130	131	82	82	83	83	84	85	86
16	90th	122	122	123	125	126	127	128	79	79	79	80	81	82	82
	95th	125	126	127	128	130	131	132	83	83	83	84	85	86	86
17	90th	122	123	124	125	126	128	128	79	79	79	80	81	82	82
	95th	126	126	127	129	130	131	132	83	83	83	84	85	86	86

* Blood pressure percentile was determined by a single reading.

† Height percentile was determined by standard growth curves.

Reproduced with permission from Update on the 1987 Task Force Report on High Blood Pressure in Children and Adolescents: A Working Group Report from the National High Blood Pressure Education Program. *Pediatrics* 98:649, 1996.

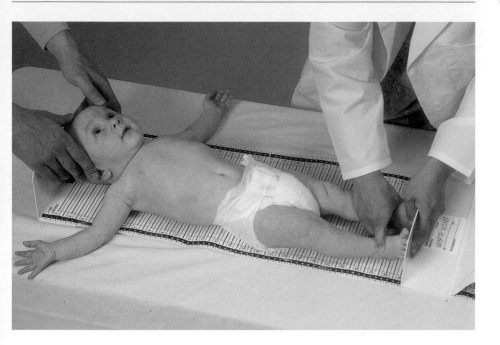

these are not available, measure the distance between marks made on the examining table paper indicating the crown and the heel of the infant. Direct measurement of the infant in this way with a tape is inaccurate, unless an assistant holds the baby still with its legs extended. Measure the height in older children by standing the child with heels, back, and head against a wall marked with a centimeter or inch rule. Hold a small board flat against the top of the child's head and at right angles to the rule to complete the measure.

Weighing scales equipped with a height measure are not as satisfactory because children are less likely to stand erect when not against a wall; many younger children also fear standing on a scale's slightly raised, unsteady base.

Weight. Weigh infants directly with an infant scale, rather than indirectly by holding them while you stand on the scale and subtracting your weight from the total weight registered. Remove all clothing, except for underpants in children beyond infancy and dressing gowns provided for girls in late childhood. Use balance rather than spring scales, and whenever possible weigh the child on the same scale at each visit.

Head Circumference. The head circumference should be measured at every physical examination during the first 2 years of life, and at any *initial* examination at whatever age, to determine the rate of growth and the size of the head.

A cloth or soft plastic tape is preferred for this procedure, but disposable paper tapes are satisfactory.

Place the tape over the occipital, parietal, and frontal prominences to obtain the greatest circumference. During infancy and early childhood this is done best with the patient supine.

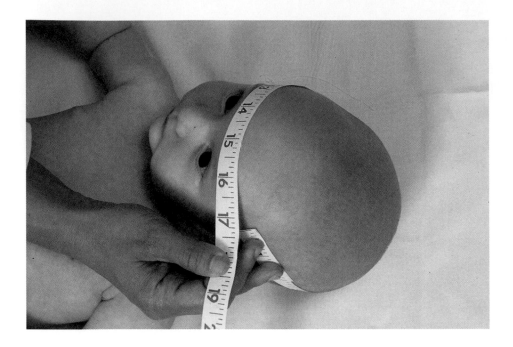

The head circumference reflects the rate of growth of the cranium and its contents.

Measurements of chest circumference and the abdominal circumference are, in general, inaccurate and have no clinical use.

If growth is delayed, consider *premature closure of the sutures* or *microcephaly.* Microcephaly may be familial or due to a variety of chromosomal abnormalities, congenital infections, maternal metabolic disorders, and neurologic insults. When growth is too rapid, suspect *hydrocephalus, subdural hematoma,* or *brain tumor.*

GIRLS: 2 TO 18 YEARS
PHYSICAL GROWTH
NCHS PERCENTILES

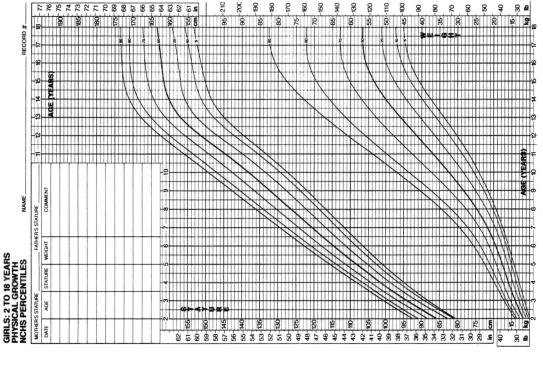

GIRLS: BIRTH TO 36 MONTHS
PHYSICAL GROWTH
NCHS PERCENTILES

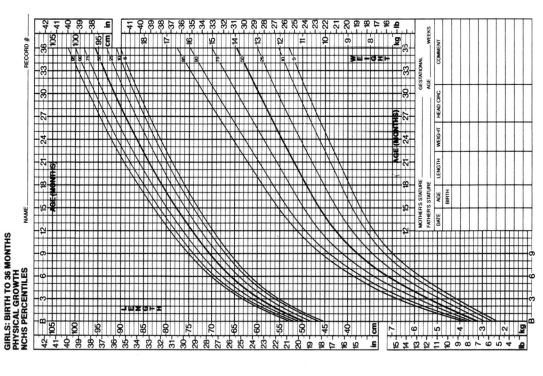

(Adapted from Hamill PVV, Drizd TA, Johnson CL, Reed RB, Roche AF, Moore AM: Physical growth: National Center for Health Statistics percentiles. Am J Clin Nutr 32:607–629, 1979. Data from the National Center for Health Statistics [NCHS], Hyattsville, MD. Figures provided through the courtesy of Ross Laboratories, Columbus, OH).

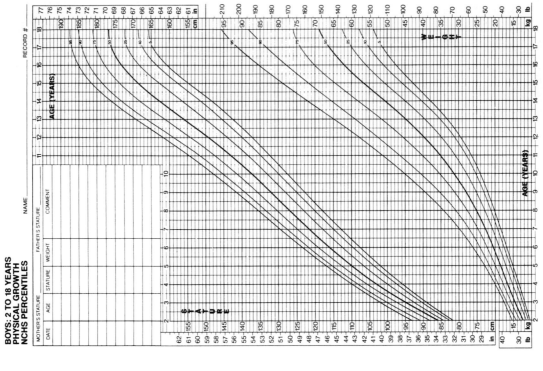

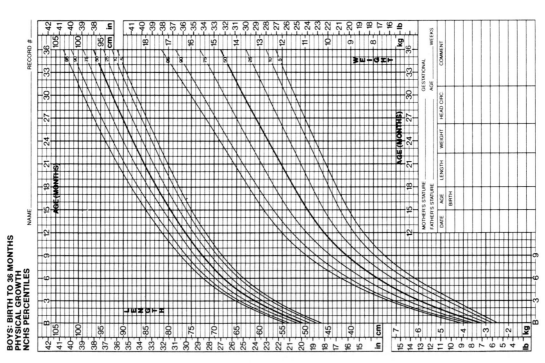

(Adapted from Hamill PVV, Drizd TA, Johnson CL, Reed RB, Roche AF, Moore AM: Physical growth: National Center for Health Statistics percentiles. Am J Clin Nutr 32:607–629, 1979. Data from the National Center for Health Statistics [NCHS], Hyattsville, MD. Figures provided through the courtesy of Ross Laboratories, Columbus, OH).

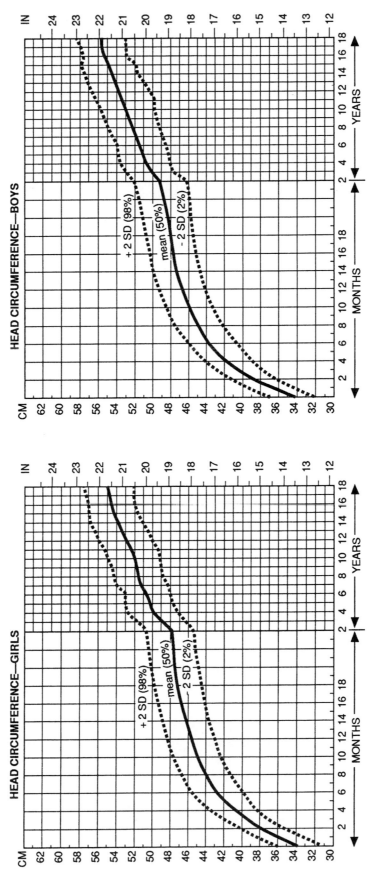

Girls: Birth to 18 Years
Head Circumference Growth

Boys: Birth to 18 Years
Head Circumference Growth

(Adapted with permission from Wellhaus G: Head circumference from birth to eighteen years. Pediatrics 41:106–114, 1968)

The Skin

Infancy

Texture and Appearance. The newborn infant's skin has many unique characteristics. The texture is soft and smooth because it is thinner than the skin of older children. In white infants an erythematous flush, giving the entire surface of the skin the appearance of a "boiled lobster," is present during the first 8 to 24 hours, after which the normal pale pink coloring predominates. Vasomotor changes in the dermis and subcutaneous tissue—a response to cooling or chronic exposure to radiant heat—produce a mottled appearance (*cutis marmorata*), particularly on the trunk, arms, and legs. In normal newborns a striking color change is often seen: one side of the body is red, the other pale, and an abrupt border separates the two sides at the midline. This phenomenon (*harlequin dyschromia*) is transient and its etiology is unknown. The hands and feet may be "blue" (*acrocyanosis*) at birth and may remain so for several days. This may recur throughout early infancy when the baby is cold. After 4 or 5 hours, the cyanosis becomes less marked in the hands than in the feet.

Pigmentation. Melanotic pigmentation of the skin is not as great as it will become in most African American newborns, except in the nail beds and the skin of the scrotum or labia majora. Ill-defined blackish blue areas located over the buttocks and lower lumbar regions are often seen, especially in African American, Native American, and Asian babies. These areas, called *Mongolian spots*, are due to the presence of pigmented cells in the deeper layers of the skin. The spots become less noticeable as the pigment in the overlying cells becomes more prominent, and they eventually disappear in early childhood.

Lanugo and Hair. There is a fine, downy growth of hair called *lanugo* over the entire body, but mostly on the shoulders and back. The amount and length vary from baby to baby, and are unusually prominent in premature infants. Most of this hair is shed within 2 weeks. The amount of hair on the head of a newborn varies considerably, being absent entirely in some and abundant in others. All the original hair is shed within a few months and replaced with a new crop, sometimes of a different color.

Features at Birth. Superficial desquamation of the skin is often noticeable 24 to 36 hours after birth. Also, a cheesy white material, composed of sebum and desquamated epithelial cells and called *vernix caseosa*, covers the body in varying degrees at birth. It is almost always present in the vaginal labial folds and under the fingernails. A certain amount of puffiness and edema, even to the point of pitting over the hands, feet, lower legs, pubis, and sacrum, may be present but usually disappears by the second or third day.

Generalized pallor may indicate either *anoxia,* in which the pulse will be slowed, or *severe anemia,* in which the pulse will be very rapid.

This marbled, or dappled, reticular pattern is especially prominent in premature infants and in infants with *congenital hypothyroidism* and *Down's syndrome.*

If acrocyanosis does not disappear within 8 hours or with warming, cyanotic congenital heart disease should be considered.

Skin desquamation at birth occurs in babies born after 40 weeks of gestation, in those with placental circulatory insufficiency, and in various forms of *congenital ichthyosis.*

Three dermatologic conditions are seen in newborns often enough to deserve description. None is of clinical significance. *Milia,* pinhead-sized, smooth, white, raised areas without surrounding erythema, on the nose, chin, and forehead, are caused by retention of sebum in the openings of the sebaceous glands. Milia may be present at birth but more often appear within the first few weeks of life and disappear spontaneously over several weeks. *Miliaria rubra* consists of scattered vesicles on an erythematous base, usually on the face and the trunk, caused by sweat gland duct obstruction. This rash also disappears spontaneously within 1 to 2 weeks. *Erythema toxicum,* which usually appears on the second or third day of life, consists of erythematous macules with central urticarial wheals or vesicles scattered diffusely over the entire body, appearing much like flea bites. The cause is unknown and the lesions disappear spontaneously within a week.

Physiologic Jaundice. Normal "physiologic" jaundice, which occurs in approximately 50% of all babies, appears on the second or third day, peaks during the fourth and fifth days, and usually disappears within a week but may persist for as long as a month.

In general, jaundice that appears within 24 hours of birth should alert one to the possible presence of hemolytic disease (*erythroblastosis fetalis*) and its accompanying hyperbilirubinemia; jaundice that persists beyond 2 weeks of age should raise suspicions of biliary obstruction. Jaundice may indicate severe infection at any time in infancy, particularly in the newborn.

Use natural daylight rather than artificial light when evaluating for the presence of jaundice at any age. In borderline cases, press a glass slide against the infant's cheek to help you detect the presence of jaundice by producing a blanched background for contrast.

Older infants who are fed yellow vegetables (carrots, sweet potatoes, and squash) may develop a pale, yellow to orange color that is sometimes mistaken for jaundice. However, the pigmentation in this condition, called *carotenemia,* is most prominent on the palms, soles, nose, and nasolabial folds. The scleras are not involved.

Vascular Markings. Irregular pink areas frequently are found over the nape of the neck ("stork's beak" mark) and on the upper eyelids, the forehead, and the upper lip ("angel kisses"). This redness is due to proliferation of the skin's capillary bed, and is variously called *capillary hemangioma, nevus flammeus, nevus vasculosus,* and *telangiectatic nevus.* The lesions invariably disappear at about a year of age, although they may occasionally reappear, even in adulthood, when the skin is flushed from anger or embarrassment. Such lesions appearing on other areas of the skin are larger, darker (purplish), and more sharply demarcated, and may involve the mucosa of the mouth or the vagina. These "port wine stains" are not likely to fade.

When a port wine stain affects the skin innervated by the ophthalmic portion of the trigeminal nerve, the vascular network of the meninges and ocular orbit may also be affected. This can result in seizures, hemiparesis, mental retardation, and glaucoma—the *Sturge–Weber syndrome.*

Turgor. The examination of the skin should go beyond observation and include palpation.

651

Roll a fold of loosely adherent skin on the abdominal wall between your thumb and forefinger to determine its consistency, the amount of subcutaneous tissue, and the degree of hydration (turgor).

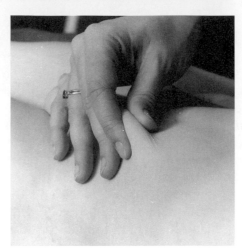

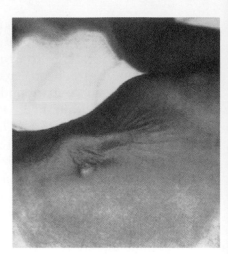

From Zitelli BJ and Davis HW: Atlas of Pediatric Diagnosis, ed. 3, St. Louis, 1997, Mosby-Year Book.

The skin in well-hydrated infants and children returns to its normal position immediately upon release.

Delay in return, a phenomenon called *tenting*, as shown above, usually occurs in dehydrated patients.

Early and Late Childhood

The normal child's skin beyond the first year does not vary significantly. The techniques of examination and the general classification of pathologic lesions for this age are the same as the adult.

The Head and Neck

Examining the head and neck in infants and children requires a wide array of skills, often tailored to the child's specific stage of growth and development. The examining instruments, the ophthalmoscope, otoscope, and tongue blade, may evoke fear. The active child may be unwilling to settle into one position, so a calm and reassuring manner is important.

To guide the examiner, the important features of the examination are described in this section.

Infancy

Sutures and Fontanelles. The *head* accounts for one fourth of the body length and one third of the body weight at birth, whereas at full maturity it only accounts for one eighth of the body length and, for most, one tenth of the body weight. The bones of the skull are separated from one another by membranous tissue spaces called *sutures.* The areas where the major sutures intersect in the anterior and posterior portions of the skull are known as *fontanelles*. The sutures and fontanelles, shown in this figure, form the basis for much of the physical assessment of the infant's head.

The sutures feel like slightly depressed ridges and the fontanelles like soft concavities. The anterior fontanelle at birth measures 4 cm to 6 cm in its largest diameter and normally closes between 4 and 26 months of age; 90% close between 7 and 19 months. The posterior fontanelle measures 1 cm to 2 cm at birth and usually closes by 2 months of age. The intracranial pressure is reflected in the amount of tenseness and fullness seen and felt in the anterior fontanelle. Increased intracranial pressure produces a bulging, full anterior fontanelle. This is normally seen when a baby cries, coughs, or vomits. Pulsations of the fontanelle reflect the peripheral pulse.

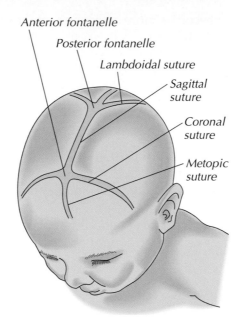

Anterior fontanelle
Posterior fontanelle
Lambdoidal suture
Sagittal suture
Coronal suture
Metopic suture

Increased intracranial pressure is found in infectious and neoplastic diseases of the central nervous system and with obstruction to the circulation of cerebrospinal fluid within the ventricles of the brain. Decreased intracranial pressure, reflected in a depressed fontanelle, is a sign of dehydration in infants. A large posterior fontanelle may be present in *congenital hypothyroidism*.

Palpate the anterior fontanelle for tenseness and fullness while the baby is sitting quietly or being held upright.

Inspect the scalp for dilated veins.

Dilated scalp veins are indicative of longstanding increased intracranial pressure.

The anterior fontanelle is such an important indicator of high or low intracranial pressure and of serious disease of the central nervous system that seasoned clinicians palpate it before doing any other part of the physical examination on an acutely ill baby.

The newborn infant's cranial bones may overlap at the sutures to a certain degree. This phenomenon, called *molding*, results from passage of the head through the birth canal and disappears within 2 days. It is not seen in babies born by cesarean section.

Symmetry of the Skull and Face. A newborn baby's scalp often is swollen from edema and bruising over the occipitoparietal region. This is the *caput succedaneum*, caused by the drawing of that portion of the scalp into the cervical os when the amniotic sac ruptures. The negative pressure or vacuum effect caused by the loss of amniotic fluid produces distended capillaries with local extravasation of blood and fluid. These findings subside within the first 24 hours of life.

A second type of localized swelling involving the scalp, the *cephalhematoma*, often is seen in newborns (see Table 19-6, Abnormal Enlargement of the Head in Infancy, p. 656).

Ascertain the shape and symmetry of the skull and the face.

Asymmetry of the cranial vault (*plagiocephaly*) occurs when an infant lies constantly on one side. Such positioning results in a flattening of the occiput on the dependent side and a prominence of the frontal region on the

Plagiocephaly is apt to be more prominent in infants with *torticollis* secondary to injury to the

opposite side. It disappears as the baby becomes more active and spends less time in one position. In almost all instances, symmetry is restored when the position of the head becomes less constant. In utero positioning may result in transient facial asymmetries. If the head is flexed on the sternum, a shortened chin (*micrognathia*) may result; pressure of the shoulder on the jaw may create a temporary lateral displacement of the mandible.

The premature infant's head at birth is relatively long in the occipitofrontal diameter and narrow in the bitemporal diameter (*dolichocephaly*). This relationship continues for most of the first year; in some it lasts indefinitely. An abnormally large head (*hydrocephaly*, see Table 19-6, Abnormal Enlargement of the Head in Infancy, p. 656, or *megacephaly*) and an abnormally small head (*microcephaly*) should be recognized easily, but either condition initially requires frequent observation, including measurements, for early diagnosis and treatment.

If, in palpating the newborn's skull, you press your thumb or forefinger too firmly over the temporoparietal or parietooccipital areas, you may feel the underlying bone give momentarily, much as a ping-pong ball responds to similar pressure. This condition, known as *craniotabes*, is due to osteoporosis of the outer table of the involved membranous bone. It may be found in some normal infants. Purposeful elicitation of this finding is not recommended.

Percuss the parietal bone on each side by tapping your index or middle finger directly against its surface.

This will produce a "cracked pot" sound (*Macewen's sign*) in normal infants prior to closure of their cranial sutures.

Check for Chvostek's sign. Percuss at the top of the cheek just below the zygomatic bone in front of the ear, using the tip of your index or middle finger.

sternomastoid muscle at birth, in the mentally and physically handicapped, and in understimulated infants.

The shape of the head may be altered by premature closure of one or more of the cranial sutures (*craniosynostosis*). The nature of the resultant skull deformity depends on the sutures involved. For example, sagittal suture synostosis is associated with a long, narrow head, because the parietal bones do not grow laterally to their full extent. Although palpation of affected sutures may reveal a raised bony ridge in the final stages, early diagnosis is made by roentgenogram.

Craniotabes may result from increased intracranial pressure, as in *hydrocephaly*, from metabolic disturbances such as *rickets*, and from infection such as *congenital syphilis*.

Macewen's sign can be elicited in older infants and children who have increased intracranial pressure that causes closed cranial sutures to separate, e.g., in *lead encephalopathy* and *brain tumor*.

Chvostek's sign is quite striking; its elicitation produces repeated contractions of the facial muscle in most cases of *hypocalcemic tetany* and *tetanus*

One or two contractions of the facial muscles in response to percussion (*Chvostek's sign*) are present in many newborn infants and can persist normally throughout infancy and early childhood.

and *tetany due to hyperventilation.*

Transillumination of the Skull. **Transilluminate the skull during the initial examination of every infant suspected of having central nervous system disease.**

In a completely darkened room, place a standard 3-battery flashlight, with a soft rubber collar attached to the lighted end, flush against the skull at various points. (See Table 19-6, Abnormal Enlargement of the Head in Infancy, p. 656.)

Uniform transillumination of the entire head occurs when the cerebral cortex is partially absent or thinned. Localized bright spots may be seen with *subdural effusion* and *porencephalic cysts.*

In normal infants a 2-cm halo of light is present around the circumference of the flashlight when it is placed over the frontoparietal area, and a 1-cm halo is present when the flashlight is placed over the occipital area.

Routine auscultation of the skull over its front, back, and sides to detect the presence of a *bruit* is of little use until late childhood because a systolic or continuous bruit may be heard over the temporal areas in normal children until the age of 5. Similar findings may be found in older children who are significantly anemic.

Bruits heard in nonanemic older children suggest increased intracranial pressure, an intracranial *arteriovenous shunt,* or an *aneurysm.*

The Neck and Clavicles. The *neck* of the newborn is relatively short.

While the infant is supine, palpate the neck with your thumb and forefinger, feeling for lymph nodes, masses, cysts, and the position of the thyroid cartilage and the trachea.

A *thyroglossal duct fistula or cyst* may be seen or felt in the midline just above the thyroid cartilage. Cysts, rarely found at birth, may appear in early infancy, are usually small, rounded, and firm, and move with swallowing.

Remnants of the three lower branchial clefts may be seen as skin tags, cysts, or fistulas along the anterior border of the sternomastoid muscle.

Cervical lymphadenopathy is not seen often during infancy.

When present, the cause is usually a viral or a bacterial infection. Human immunodeficiency virus infection is the most common cause and is associated with generalized lymphadenopathy.

Palpate the clavicles for evidence of a fracture (shortening, break in contour, and crepitus at the fracture site).

Fracture of the clavicle may occur in vertex and breech deliveries, during difficult shoulder or arm extractions.

Table 19-6   Abnormal Enlargement of the Head in Infancy

TABLE 19-6 *Abnormal Enlargement of the Head in Infancy*

Cephalhematoma

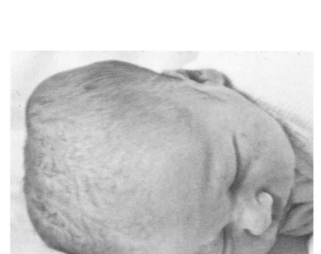

Although not present at birth, cephalhematomas appear within the first 24 hours and are due to subperiosteal hemorrhage involving the outer table of one of the cranial bones. The swelling (see illustration above, which shows a cephalhematoma overlying the left parietal bone), unlike the caput succedaneum and hematomas associated with skull fractures, does not extend across a suture. It may be small and well localized or may involve the entire bone. Occasionally, bilateral symmetrical swellings occur after difficult deliveries. Although initially soft, the swellings develop a raised bony margin within 2 to 3 days, due to the rapid deposition of calcium at the edges of the elevated periosteum. The entire process usually disappears within a few weeks, but may remain as a residual osteoma that is not resorbed for a year or two.

Hydrocephaly

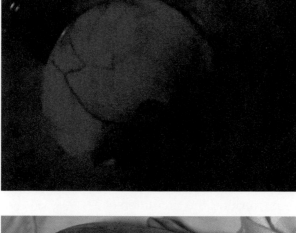

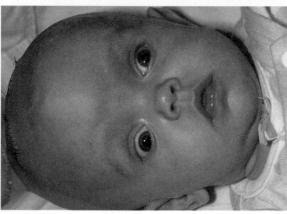

In hydrocephaly the anterior fontanelle is bulging and the eyes may be deviated downward, revealing the upper scleras and creating the *"setting sun"* sign, as shown in the figure above. The setting sun sign is also seen briefly in some normal newborns. (From Zitelli, BJ & Davis, HW. [1997]. Atlas of Pediatric Physical Diagnosis, 3rd ed. St. Louis: Mosby–Year Book. Courtesy of Dr. Albert Briglan, Children's Hospital of Pittsburgh.)

Transillumination of the skull in advanced cases of hydrocephaly produces a glow of light over the entire cranium, as illustrated above. (From Gellis, SS & Feingold, M. [1968]. Atlas of Mental Retardation Syndromes. U.S. Dept. of Health, Education, and Welfare. Washington: U.S. Government Printing Office.)

Move the head through its full range of motion at the neck (extension, flexion, lateral bending, and rotation 90° to the left and right).

The neck is supple and easily mobile in all directions throughout infancy. Its musculature is not developed sufficiently to enable the infant to turn its head from side to side until 2 weeks of age, to lift its head 90° when lying prone until 2 months of age, or to hold its head upright when sitting until 3 months of age.

Injury with bleeding into the sternomastoid muscle as it is stretched during the birth process results in wry neck (*torticollis*). The head is tilted toward and twisted away from the injured side; in 2 or 3 weeks a firm fibrous mass is felt within the muscle. This ordinarily disappears in 3 to 4 months.

Early and Late Childhood

Beyond infancy the head and neck, except as previously mentioned, should be examined with the procedures used in examining the adult. There are diagnostic facies in childhood that reflect chromosomal abnormalities, endocrine defects, social disease, chronic illness, and other categories of disease. (See Table 19-7, Diagnostic Facies in Infancy and Childhood, pp. 658–659, for examples).

The Parotid Gland

A swollen parotid gland may be difficult to detect during the early stages of mumps.

Parotid swelling and tenderness suggest *mumps,* a bacterial infection, or a stone in the parotid duct.

With your index finger, palpate along a line extending from the outer canthus of the eye to the lower tip of the pinna.

Parotid tenderness is elicited when mumps is present.

Inspect the orifice of the parotid (Stensen's) duct, which emerges from the midportion of the buccal mucosa.

Redness and swelling are usually present in the conditions noted above.

Parotid gland swelling, from any cause, extends above and below the mandible at the angle of the jaw; swelling due to *cervical adenitis* occurs only below these landmarks.

The Lymphatics

The adult lymphatic system, including the lymph nodes, is described on pp. 180–181 (head and neck), 338–339 (axillae and breasts), 388 (male genitalia), 407 (female genitalia), and 464–465 (arms and legs).

As shown in the figure on p. 621, the child's lymphatic system reaches its zenith of growth at 12 years of age; the size of its various components (lymph nodes and the tonsils and adenoids, in particular) is greater between the ages of 6 and 20 years than at other ages. Parents and clinicians who are unaware of this may become unduly concerned that large and even not so large visible nodes, especially in the neck, may be malignant.

Lymphadenopathy involving the head and neck may occur in a variety of circumstances, as shown in Table 19-8, Lymphadenopathy of the Head and Neck, p. 660.

Table 19-7 Diagnostic Facies in Infancy and Childhood

TABLE 19-7 Diagnostic Facies in Infancy and Childhood

Fetal Alcohol Syndrome	Congenital Syphilis	Congenital Hypothyroidism	Facial Nerve Palsy
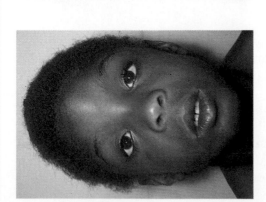	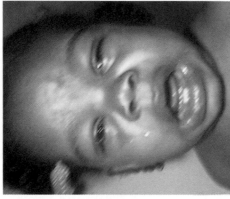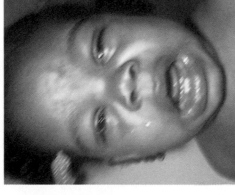	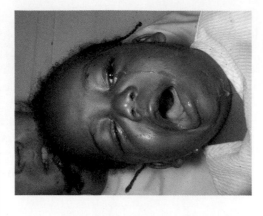	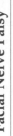

Fetal Alcohol Syndrome

Babies born to women who are chronic alcoholics are at increased risk for growth deficiency, microcephaly, and mental retardation. Facial characteristics shown here include short palpebral fissures, a wide and flattened philtrum (the vertical groove in the midline of the upper lip), and thin lips.

Congenital Syphilis

In utero infection by *Treponema pallidum* usually occurs after the 16th week of gestation and affects virtually all fetal organs. If it is not treated, 25% of infected babies will die before birth and another 30% shortly thereafter. Signs of illness appear in survivors within the first month of life. Facial stigmata shown here include bulging of the frontal bones and nasal bridge depression (*saddle nose*), both due to periostitis; rhinitis from weeping nasal mucosal lesions (*snuffles*); and a circumoral rash. Mucocutaneous inflammation and fissuring of the mouth and lips (*rhagades*), not shown here, may also occur as stigmata of congenital syphilis, as may craniotabes tibial periostitis (*saber shins*) and dental dysplasia (*Hutchinson's teeth*—see p. 241).

Congenital Hypothyroidism

The child with congenital hypothyroidism (cretinism) has coarse facial features, a low-set hair line, sparse eyebrows, and an enlarged tongue. Associated features include a hoarse cry, umbilical hernia, dry and cold extremities, myxedema, mottled skin, and mental retardation. It is important to note that the majority of infants with congenital hypothyroidism have no physical stigmata; this has led to screening of all newborns in the United States and in most other developed countries, for depressed thyroxin or elevated thyroid-stimulating hormone levels.

Facial Nerve Palsy

Peripheral (lower motor neuron) paralysis of the facial nerve may be due to (1) an injury to the nerve from pressure during labor and delivery, (2) inflammation of the middle ear branch of the nerve during episodes of acute or chronic otitis media, or (3) unknown causes (Bell's palsy). See p. 572 and pp. 608–609. The nasolabial fold on the affected left side is flattened and the eye does not close. This is accentuated during crying, as shown here. Full recovery occurs in ≥90% of those affected, usually within a few weeks.

Table 19-7   Diagnostic Facies in Infancy and Childhood

Down's Syndrome

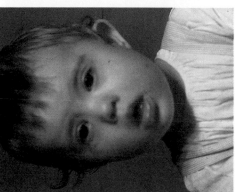
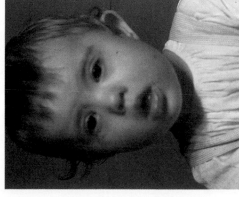

The child with Down's syndrome (Trisomy 21) usually has a small, rounded head, a flattened nasal bridge, oblique palpebral fissures, prominent epicanthal folds, small, low-set, shell-like ears, and a relatively large tongue. Associated features include generalized hypotonia, transverse palmar creases (*simian lines*), shortening and incurving of the 5th fingers (*clinodactyly*), Brushfield's spots (see p. 663), and mental retardation.

Battered-Child Syndrome

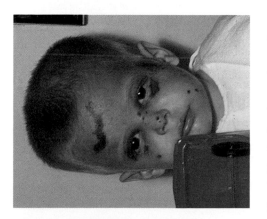

The child who has been physically abused (battered) may have old *and* fresh bruises about the head and face and may either look sad and forlorn or be actively seeking to please, sometimes even particularly involved with and attentive to the abusing parent. Other stigmata include: bruises in areas (axilla and groin) not usually subject to injury rather than the bony prominences, x-ray evidence of fractures of the skull, ribs, and long bones in various stages of healing, and skin lesions that are morphologically similar to implements used to inflict trauma (hand, belt buckle, strap, rope, coat hanger, or lighted cigarette).

Perennial Allergic Rhinitis

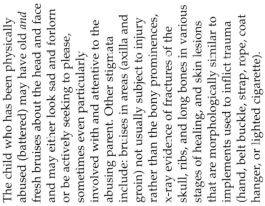

The child suffering from perennial allergic rhinitis has an open mouth (cannot breathe through the nose) and edema and discoloration of the lower orbitopalpebral grooves ("allergic shiners"). Such a child is often seen to push the nose upward and backward with a hand ("allergic salute") and to grimace (wrinkle the nose and mouth) to relieve nasal itching and obstruction. (Illustration reproduced with permission from Marks MB: Allergic shiners: Dark circles under the eyes in children. *Clin Pediatr* 5:656, 1966)

Hyperthyroidism

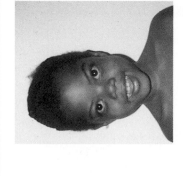
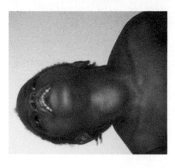

Thyrotoxicosis (*Graves' disease*) occurs in approximately 2 per 1,000 children under the age of 10 years. Affected children exhibit hypermetabolism and accelerated linear growth. Facial characteristics shown in this 6-year-old girl are "staring" eyes (not true exophthalmos, which is rare in children) and an enlarged thyroid gland (*goiter*). See pp. 204, 244.

Table 19-8 Lymphadenopathy of the Head and Neck

TABLE 19-8 *Lymphadenopathy of the Head and Neck*

Cervical

Viral Upper Respiratory Tract Infections	Enlarged anterior and posterior cervical lymph nodes are usually not tender.
Infectious Mononucleosis	Caused by Epstein–Barr virus; generalized lymphadenopathy may occur, but cervical lymph nodes are most prominently involved and may be quite tender.
Malignant Disease	These include *leukemia, Hodgkin's disease, non-Hodgkin's lymphoma,* and *metastatic cancer,* with or without enlarged lymph nodes in other regions.
Acute Bacterial Tonsillitis or Pharyngitis	Usually involves tonsillar lymph nodes, notable for swelling and tenderness. Figure below shows bilateral tonsillar lymph node enlargement due to acute tonsillitis.

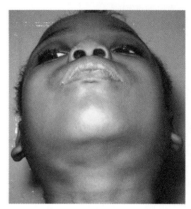

Acute Posterior Cervical Lymphadenitis	Secondary to *acute otitis externa, acute* or *chronic mastoiditis* (rare), and various scalp lesions (*pediculosis capitis, tinea capitis*)
Kawasaki's Disease (Mucocutaneous Lymph Node Syndrome)	Of unknown cause, this disease is potentially life threatening, characterized by fever, conjunctivitis, oral mucosal lesions, rash, cervical lymphadenitis, carditis, and coronary artery vasculitis.
Tuberculosis, Atypical Mycobacterium Infection, and Cat-Scratch Disease	May cause anterior or posterior cervical lymphadenitis, depending on the site of the initial lesion

Occipital

Scalp Infections from Various Causes and *Rubella* and *Roseola Infantum*	It is usually present in *rubella* and helps to establish the diagnosis

Preauricular

Chronic Conjunctivitis and Blepharitis	When preauricular lymph nodes are enlarged and tender, look for an eye infection first.
Bacterial Infections of the Ipsilateral Cheek and the Temporal Scalp	These are usually quite obvious.
Cat-Scratch Fever	The scratch on the face, usually around the ipsilateral eye, may be completely healed. The lymph node is usually markedly enlarged and tender, and can become fluctuant.

Submaxillary

Infections of the Tongue, Teeth, Gums, Lips, and Cheek	These infections are easily detected, but submaxillary lymphadenopathy is not usually very prominent.

Submental

Infections of the Tip of the Tongue and of the Lower Lip	Submental lymphadenopathy is not usually very prominent.

Most enlarged lymph nodes in children, cervical or otherwise, are either "normally so" or due to local infections (mostly viral) and not to malignant disease. Malignancy is less likely if the node is less than 2 cm in diameter, if it is not hard or fixed to the skin or underlying tissues, and, in the case of cervical lymph nodes, if the chest x-ray findings are normal. Suspicion of malignancy increases when a supraclavicular lymph node is enlarged, when fever lasting more than a week without apparent cause accompanies the lymphadenopathy, and when there has been a weight loss of 5 pounds or more within the previous 6 months.

Neck Mobility

Neck mobility is important when central nervous system diseases, especially meningitis, are suspected, because the neck may be less supple than normal when such diseases are present.

With the child supine, cradle the head in your hands so that you provide complete support as shown below. Move the head gently in all directions to determine any resistance to motion, especially to flexion.

In infancy and early childhood, this is a more reliable test for nuchal rigidity and meningeal irritation than *Brudzinski's sign* or *Kernig's sign* (see pp. 597–598). However, the infant's neck may retain its mobility, even when meningeal irritation, as with meningitis, is present.

Nuchal rigidity, or marked resistance to movement of the head in any direction, suggests meningeal irritation, as from central nervous system infections, bleeding, and tumors.

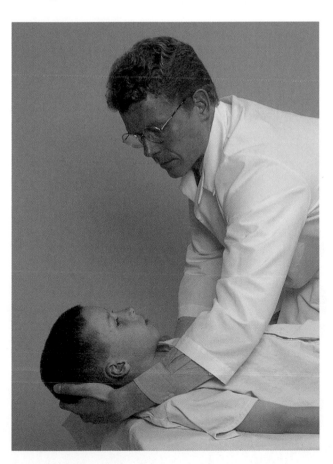

To detect nuchal rigidity in early and late childhood, ask the child to sit with legs extended on the examining table. Normally children should be able to sit upright and touch their chins to their chests. Younger children may be persuaded to flex their necks forward by getting them to look at a small toy or a light beam placed on their upper sternum.

When meningeal irritation is present, the child assumes the *tripod position* and is unable to assume a full upright position to perform the chin-to-chest manuever.

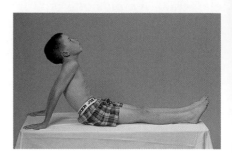

The Eye

Infancy

Inspection

Inspecting the newborn's eyes is somewhat difficult because the lids are ordinarily held tightly closed. Attempts at separating the lids usually increase the contraction of the orbicularis oculi muscles. Because bright light causes infants to blink their eyes, the newborn's eyes should be examined in subdued lighting.

Eye Movements. **Hold the baby upright in your extended arms, fixing the head in the midline with your thumbs as illustrated below. Rotate yourself with the baby slowly in one direction. This usually causes the baby's eyes to open, providing a clear view of the scleras, pupils, irises, and extraocular movements. The eyes look in the direction you**

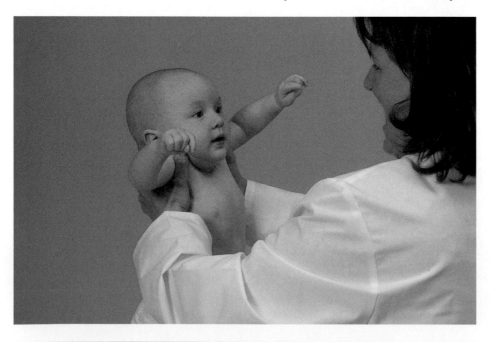

are turning. **When the rotation stops, the eyes look in the opposite direction, following a few unsustained nystagmoid movements.**

Conjugate eye movements develop rapidly after birth, and most newborns will regard a face. While some will follow a face or a bright light, definitive following movements are not seen for a few weeks in most newborns. *Nystagmus* in one or many directions is common immediately after birth. During the first 10 days of life the eyes remain fixed, staring in one direction as the head is moved slowly through the full range of motion (*doll's eye test*). *Intermittent alternating convergent strabismus* (crossed eyes) is frequently seen or reported by parents during the first 6 months of life.

Nystagmus present after a few days may indicate blindness.

Alternating convergent strabismus persisting beyond 6 months or becoming unilateral sooner, or divergent strabismus (laterally deviated eyes) occurring at any time, may indicate ocular muscle weakness or diminished visual acuity.

Scleras and Pupils. **Look at the scleras carefully.** Small subconjunctival and scleral hemorrhages are common in newborns.

Observe the pupillary reactions by covering each eye with your hand, and then uncovering it. Pupillary reactivity to light is poor during the first 4 to 5 months. Inequality of pupil size in both bright and subdued light is common, but should be considered significant if constant over time and associated with other ocular or central nervous system findings. The corneal reflex is normally present at birth, but is not tested for unless a neurologic deficit is suspected.

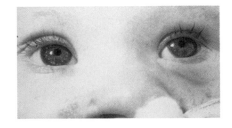

Inspect each iris for the presence of Brushfield's spots. These appear as white specks, usually scattered around a good portion of the circumference of the iris, and may be present in some normal infants.

Brushfield's spots, illustrated above, strongly suggest *Down's syndrome.* Epicanthal folds in non-Asian people also suggest this malady. (See Table 19-6, Diagnostic Facies in Infancy and Childhood, p. 656).

The Conjunctivas. *Chemical conjunctivitis* may occur following placement of silver nitrate in the eyes at birth as a prophylaxis against gonorrheal conjunctivitis (*ophthalmia neonatorum*). The latter is characterized by edema of the lids and inflammation of the conjunctivas with a purulent discharge. Many newborn nurseries now use erythromycin instead of silver nitrate because it produces much less irritation.

Dacryocystitis and *nasolacrimal duct obstruction* with ocular discharge and tearing may follow chemical conjunctivitis due to silver nitrate instillation.

Visual Acuity. The development of central vision progresses from birth, when only light perception is thought to be present, to adult visual levels, which are attained at approximately 6 years of age.

Vision assessment in the newborn is based on the presence of visual reflexes—direct and consensual pupillary constriction in response to light, blinking and extending the head in response to bright light (*optical blink reflex*), and blinking in response to quick movement of an object toward the eyes.

Those visual reflexes imply that both light perception and some degree of visual acuity are present shortly after birth. That this acuity improves is evident even without specific refractive measurement. At 2 to 4 weeks of age, fixation on objects occurs; at 5 to 6 weeks, coordinated eye movements in following an object are seen; at 3 months, the eyes converge and the baby begins to reach for various-sized objects at various distances as eye–hand coordination and the ability to focus are accomplished. At the age of 1 year, normal visual acuity is in the range of 20/200.

Failure to progress along these lines may indicate developmental delay, as well as diminished or absent vision.

The Ophthalmoscopic Examination

The Red Reflex. Demonstrate the red retinal (or fundus) reflex by setting the ophthalmoscope at 0 diopters and viewing the pupil at a distance of approximately 10 inches. Normally a red or orange color is reflected from the fundus through the pupil.

***Examining the Fundus.* Perform an ophthalmoscopic examination on all infants.** Usually this examination can be postponed until between 2 and 6 months of age, when the infant is most cooperative, unless the ocular or neurologic examination indicates that it should be done immediately. Such examinations are not difficult to perform if one exercises patience and persistence. Occasionally, a mydriatic solution may be required to examine the fundus successfully.

Both retinal anomalies and opacities of the cornea, anterior chamber, or lens interrupt the light pathway and give a partial red or a completely dark reflex. In infants, *cataracts,* a *persistent posterior lenticular fibrovascular sheath,* and *retinopathy of prematurity* may cause a dark light reflex. During and beyond infancy, *retinal detachment, chorioretinitis,* and *retinoblastoma* should be suspected when a white retinal reflex (*leukokoria*) is encountered.

To dilate the pupils, instill a sterile mydriatic (2.5% phenylephrine with 0.5% cyclopentolate—one drop in each eye). This can be repeated after 45 minutes if pupillary dilatation has not occurred. Place the baby supine on the examining table or on the parent's lap, or have the parent hold the baby upright over his or her shoulder. If the baby needs calming, use a pacifier. If necessary, retract the lids with your thumb and first finger. Funduscopic examination is otherwise the same as in adults. The cornea can ordinarily be seen at +20 diopters, the lens at +15 diopters, and the fundus at 0 diopters.

Be aware that babies with acute central nervous system disease should not have their pupils dilated, except as directed by a child neurologist or an ophthalmologist.

Look for retinal hemorrhages.

The optic disc is pale in infants, the peripheral vessels are not well developed, and the foveal light reflection is absent. *Papilledema* is rarely seen, even with markedly increased intracranial pressure, because the

Small retinal hemorrhages are often present. If they are extensive, severe *anoxia, subdural hematoma,* or *subarachnoid hemorrhage* should be suspected.

fontanelles and open sutures absorb the increased pressure, sparing the optic discs. Until age 3 years, the sutures will separate sufficiently to prevent papilledema. If vascular or optic disc anomalies are found, the parents' fundi should be examined to determine a possible genetic origin and a prognosis.

Retinal hemorrhages associated with intracranial bleeding are accompanied by dilated, congested, tortuous retinal veins. Pigmentary changes occur in the retina in newborns with congenital *toxoplasmosis*, *cytomegalovirus*, and *rubella* infections.

Early Childhood

Amblyopia and Conjugate Gaze. In this age group, the most important condition to detect is *amblyopia ex anopsia. Amblyopia* means reduced vision in an otherwise normal eye, and is caused by disuse. Because of disconjugate fixation, one of the two images received by the optic cortex is suppressed to avoid *diplopia,* or images of unequal clarity. One eye then becomes "lazy" and stops functioning to its full capacity; visual acuity in that eye is reduced markedly by suppression of central (foveal) vision. This is not the most serious ophthalmologic disease, but in comparison with others of significance it is the most prevalent and offers, with early intervention, the best prognosis. Improvement in this condition is unlikely if treatment is instituted after the sixth year of life, and is best if instituted in early infancy. Since the two most common causes of amblyopia ex anopsia are *strabismus* and *anisometropia* (an eye with a refractive error 1.5 diopters or more greater than its pair), it is important to be able to test accurately for muscle weakness and visual acuity.

Obstructive amblyopia is secondary to a *cataract, corneal opacity,* or severe *ptosis.*

To examine the eye in early and late childhood, use the methods described for adults in Chapter 7 for the position and alignment of the eyes, each of their externally visible parts (eyebrows, eyelids, lacrimal apparatus, conjuctivas, scleras, corneas, irises, and pupils), and the function of the extraocular muscles. These methods are equally applicable for examinations during early and late childhood.

Paralytic and *nonparalytic strabismus* (as shown in Table 7-8, Deviations of the Eyes, p. 218) are due to ocular muscle weaknesses and to unequal visual acuity in the two eyes (*anisometropia*). They are common during infancy and childhood and, when found, should be referred to an ophthalmologist as soon as possible.

Visual Acuity. Testing visual acuity in early childhood is not simple. The variables of the child, the examiner, the test environment, and the test itself all contribute significantly to the outcome and should be carefully considered if valid results are to be obtained. Unfortunately, there is no test that accurately measures visual acuity in children under the age of 3 years. Since each eye must be tested separately to detect amblyopia, one eye must be covered by an elastoplast bandage to ensure complete occlusion. Resistance to placement of the patch may be overcome by calling it a "pirate's patch." A child with amblyopia might accept the patch on the amblyopic eye but *not* on the good eye.

Opticokinetic testing is the most accurate method for determining visual acuity in this age group; however, this method requires too much technical equipment to use in most practice settings.

In children over the age of 3 years, the *Snellen E chart* (a form of direct visual testing) is very adequate. Most youngsters cooperate in indicating the direction of the E, either orally or by pointing. For those who initially have difficulty with this test, an E card can be sent home with the child for practice. Charts with pictures instead of Es are often used but have no special advantage, nor have any other testing methods generally available. The normal visual acuity at age 3 years is ±20/40, at 4 to 5 years, ±20/30, and at 6 to 7 years, 20/20. Any difference in visual acuity between the eyes (e.g., 20/20 on the left and 20/30 on the right) is abnormal, might lead to amblyopia, and should be referred to an ophthalmologist.

Visual Fields. The *visual* fields can be examined in infants and young children with the child sitting on the parent's lap. **Hold the head in the midline while bringing an object, such as a small toy, into the child's field of vision from behind the child, into the upper and lower temporal fields on both sides. Eyes deviating in its direction indicate that the child has seen the object.**

Late Childhood

Visual Acuity. The eye problems and methods of examining the eye for this age group have been covered in the adult section. In general, vision testing machines used for mass screening in schools tend to underrate visual acuity and produce over-referrals. Because visual acuity may change during the school year, vision testing during periodic well-child visits is recommended beginning at age 4 years, as shown in Recommendations for Preventive Pediatric Health Care on p. 623.

Distinguish a simple refractive error from organic causes of diminished vision by asking the child to look through a pinhole punched in a card.

Visual acuity improves by using the pinhole card when refractive errors are present, but not when organic ocular disease exists.

The Ear

Infancy

Inspection
Note the position of the ears in relation to the eyes. Normally the upper portion of the auricle (pinna) joins the scalp on or above the extension of a line drawn across the inner and outer canthi of the eye.

Small, deformed, or low-set auricles may indicate associated congenital defects, especially *renal agenesis* (*Potter's syndrome*), or anomalies.

Inspect the ear and surrounding skin.

Examination of the ear with an otoscope in the immediate neonatal period establishes only the patency of the ear canal, because the tympanic membranes are obscured by accumulated vernix caseosa for the first 2 or 3 days of life. In infancy the ear canal is directed downward from the outside; therefore, the auricle should be pulled gently downward for the best view of the ear drum. The light reflex on the tympanic membrane is diffuse and does not become cone-shaped for several months.

Acoustic Blink Reflex. **Test the infant's hearing by eliciting the acoustic blink reflex, which is positive when the infant can hear. Observe blinking eyes in response to a sudden sharp sound produced at a distance of about 12 inches from the ear by snapping the fingers, clapping the hands, or using a bell or other kind of mechanical noisemaking device. Be sure that in generating the sound you do not produce an airstream that could cause the baby to blink.**

The acoustic blink reflex is difficult to elicit during the first 2 or 3 days of life, and may disappear temporarily after it is elicited a few times. This test is crude at best, and the absence of blinking in response to sound is not diagnostic of deafness, nor does its presence assure normal hearing. At 2 weeks of age, the infant may jump in response to a sudden noise; at 10 weeks, the infant may cease body movements momentarily. Between 3 and 4 months of age, the eyes and head will turn toward the sound. Even before this, the respiratory rate may increase and the facial expression may change when familiar sounds, generating anticipation of forthcoming pleasures such as feeding, are heard.

Screening of infants for hearing loss is very costly and produces unacceptable levels of false-positive and false-negative results. Selective screening of newborn infants who are at high risk for hearing deficits by virtue of family history, physical findings, or perinatal difficulties should be performed using brainstem-evoked response audiometry.

Early Childhood

The Ear Canal and Drum
The examination of the ear becomes more difficult as children grow. They resist because their ear canals are sensitive and they cannot observe the procedure.

A small skin tab, cleft, or pit found just forward of the tragus represents a remnant of the first branchial cleft.

The parents' impression of the baby's auditory acuity is usually correct. When they believe that their baby cannot hear, it should be assumed that they are correct until proven otherwise.

Perinatal problems that increase the risk for hearing defects include birth weight <1,500 grams, anoxia, treatment with potentially ototoxic medications (e.g., aminoglycosides), exchange transfusion, congenital infection, hyperbilirubinemia >20 mg/dl, and meningitis.

Positioning the Child. Often it is helpful if you initially place the otoscopic speculum gently into the external auditory canal of one ear, remove it instantly, and repeat the procedure on the other. Then you can begin again, taking the necessary time in the actual examination, because the child's apprehensions have probably been allayed.

The ears can be examined successfully even in struggling children if you restrain them carefully and manipulate both ear and otoscope gently.

Place the patient supine and ask the parent or an assistant to hold the child's arms extended and close to the sides of the head, thus limiting movement from side to side. Approach from the child's right side and lean across the lower chest and upper abdomen to restrict movements of the trunk. A third person may be needed to hold the feet and legs if the child struggles unduly; however, this is rarely necessary.

This same restraining procedure may be used in examining the eyes, nose, and throat, as illustrated below.

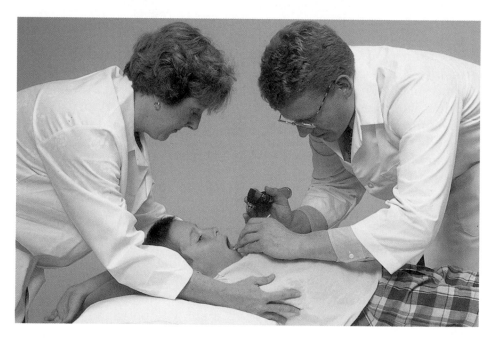

Using the Otoscope. **When examining the right ear, turn the child's head to the left and hold it firmly with the lateral aspect of your right hand and wrist. Hold the otoscope inverted in your right hand and manipulate the auricle with your left hand, the lateral aspect of which can be used to help keep the child's head still. In this age group, the external auditory canal is directed upward and backward from the outside, and the auricle must be pulled upward, outward, and backward to afford the best view. The thumb and forefinger of your right hand, which holds the otoscope, should be buffered from sudden movements of the child's head by your restraining right hand and your forearm, which rests firmly on the examining table. See the illustration on p. 669.**

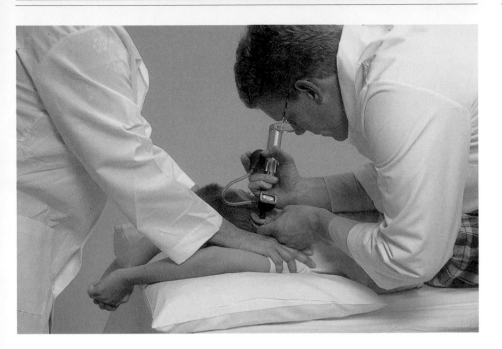

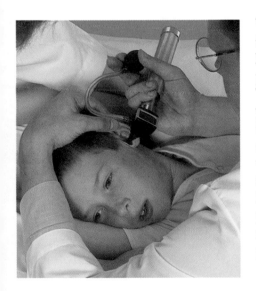

When examining the left ear, turn the patient's head to the right and hold it firmly with the lateral aspect of your left hand and wrist. The thumb and forefinger of your left hand should manipulate the auricle and your right hand should hold the otoscope inverted. The lateral aspect of the fifth finger of your right hand is held against the patient's head to provide a buffer against sudden movement by the patient. This procedure is illustrated at the left.

The speculum of the otoscope should be as large in diameter as will allow for comfortable ¼- to ½-inch penetration into the external auditory canal. This provides a maximum view of the canal and drum and a reasonable seal for observing the effects of pneumatic otoscopy (see below). Some examiners attach a rubber tip to the end of the speculum to gain a tighter, more comfortable seal.

The Tympanic Membrane. Accumulation of cerumen in the ear canal commonly obscures the view of the tympanic membrane. Often this accumulation is unilateral. There are several instruments and ear-washing techniques for removing ear wax comfortably. (These are described in Schuller DE, Schleuning AJ II: DeWeese and Saunders Otolaryngology—Head and Neck Surgery, 8th ed. St Louis, Mosby–Year Book, 1994.)

Pneumatic otoscopy. **Checking the movement of the tympanic membrane should be part of every otoscopic examination; it is accomplished by observing the tympanic membrane as the pressure in the external auditory canal is increased or decreased. You can do this by introducing and removing air from the canal—by applying positive and negative pressures with a rubber squeeze bulb, as shown in the figure here and the figures on p. 669.**

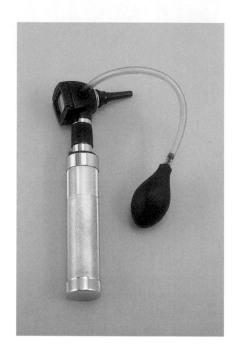

Acute *otitis media* in children is characterized by a tympanic membrane that is red, bulging, has a dull or absent light reflex, and shows diminished movement with pneumatic otoscopy. Purulent material may also be seen behind the intact tympanic membrane.

When air is introduced into the normal ear canal, the tympanic membrane and its light reflex move inward. When air is removed, the tympanic membrane moves outward, toward the examiner. This to-and-fro movement of the tympanic membrane has been likened to the luffing of a sail.

You may detect purulent material and debris in the ear canal both in otitis externa and in otitis media with a ruptured tympanic membrane. Avoid washing out the ear canal, in the first instance because of the pain created by the procedure and in the second instance because the cleansing fluid and canal debris are forced into the middle ear through the perforated tympanic membrane.

This movement is absent in chronic middle ear infection (*serous otitis media*), and diminished in some cases of *acute otitis media*.

Otitis media and *otitis externa* may be differentiated clinically by gently moving the pinna, which will cause exquisite pain in otitis externa but no discomfort in purulent otitis media. Acute *mastoiditis* in children is accompanied by a forward protrusion of the auricle of the affected ear, in addition to redness, swelling, and tenderness overlying the mastoid bone.

Screening for Hearing Deficits. Simple auditory screening in this age group can be accomplished by whispering at a distance of 8 feet.

Ask the child questions or give commands, taking care that lip reading is not possible. In addition, you can use a tuning fork to screen for hearing, using your own auditory acuity as the control.

If these screening methods reveal any diminution of hearing, full audiometric testing should be performed. Furthermore, all children should be given a full-scale acoustic screening test with an audiometer before beginning school, as should all children, regardless of age, with delayed speech development. Because of their complexity, audiometric screening devices used for older children are often unsatisfactory for use in early childhood; when speech is delayed or defective, direct referral to a hearing and speech center may be more appropriate.

Significant, temporary hearing loss for several months may follow an episode of acute otitis media, and may accompany serous otitis media.

Late Childhood

As the child grows, the ease and techniques of examining the ears and testing the hearing approach the levels and methods used for adults. There are no ear abnormalities or variations of normal unique to this age group. A possible exception is the "selective deafness" some children and adolescents demonstrate in hearing only what they choose when spoken to in either soft or loud voices by their parents and teachers.

The Nose and Throat

Infancy

Patency of the Nasal Passages. **Test the patency of the *nasal passages* by occluding each nostril alternately while holding the infant's mouth closed.** This will not cause stress in a normal baby, since most newborns are nasal breathers. On the other hand, occluding both nares simultaneously and allowing the mouth to open will cause considerable distress. Indeed, some infants (*obligate* nasal breathers) are unable to breathe through their mouths. **Confirm obstructed posterior nasal passages by attempting to pass a number-14 French catheter through each nostril into the posterior nasopharynx.**

The nasal passages in newborns may be obstructed in *choanal atresia* and by displacement of the nasal cartilage during delivery.

Inspecting the Mouth and Pharynx. **Inspect the mouth and pharynx with a tongue blade and flashlight, while the baby is lying supine.**

The newborn's *mouth* is edentulous. The gums are smooth with a raised, 1-mm, serrated fringe of tissue on the buccal margins. Occasionally, pearl-like retention cysts are seen along the ridges and are easily mistaken for teeth—they disappear spontaneously within a month or two.

Petechiae are commonly found on the soft palate after birth.

Rarely, *supernumerary teeth* are found. These are soft, have no enamel, and shed within a few days. They should be removed, however, to prevent their aspiration into the lower respiratory tract.

The frenulum of the upper lip may be quite thick and extend from the superior aspect of the inner lip to the posterior portion of the upper gum, creating a deep notch in the gum's midline. The frenulum of the tongue varies in consistency from a thin, filamentous membrane to a thick, fibrous cord. Its length varies, such that it may attach midway on the undersurface of the tongue or at its very tip. A heavy fibrous frenulum that extends to the tip of the tongue may interfere with its protrusion (*ankyloglossia* or *tongue tie*). No difficulties will be encountered with

Epstein's pearls, pinhead-sized, white or yellow, rounded elevations that are located along the midline of the hard palate near its posterior border, are caused by retained secretions and disappear within a few weeks or months.

nursing or speech, however, if the tongue can be extended as far forward as the anterior mandibular gum line, which is usually possible.

The *pharynx* can best be seen while the baby is crying. This is true throughout infancy and early childhood. A tongue blade produces strong reflex elevation of the base of the tongue and obstructs the view of the infant's pharynx. Tonsillar tissue is not seen in the newborn.

Oral candidiasis (*thrush*) is a common malady in infants, usually contracted from mothers with *Candida* vaginitis. In thrush, a lacy white material with an erythematous base is seen on the surface of the oral mucous membranes. Difficulty in removing it distinguishes it from milk curds, which wipe away. See pp. 237 and 242 for illustrations of oral candidiasis.

Little saliva is produced during the first 3 months of life. As infants begin to produce saliva, drooling occurs because there are no lower teeth to provide a dam for retention.

The presence of large amounts of saliva in the newborn may be a sign of *esophageal atresia*, since saliva cannot be swallowed.

The Infant's Cry. **Listen to the infant's breathing and the quality of the cry. Take care to note unusual shrillness, hoarseness, or audible breathing such as stridor.**

Infant Cries	
Type	**Possible Related Condition**
Shrill or high-pitched	Increased intracranial pressure. Such cries also occur in newborn infants born to narcotic-addicted mothers.
Hoarse	Hypocalcemic tetany or congenital hypothyroidism.
Continuous inspiratory and expiratory stridor	Caused by upper airway obstruction due to a variety of lesions (e.g., a polyp or hemangioma), a relatively small larynx (*infantile laryngeal stridor*) or a delay in the development of the cartilage in the tracheal rings (*tracheomalacia*).
Absence of cry	Suggests severe illness, vocal cord paralysis, or profound brain damage.

Early and Late Childhood

The Nose and the Sinuses
Look at the anterior portion of the *nose* by pushing up its tip. Use a large-bore speculum attached to the otoscope to look deeper into the nostrils. Inspect the nasal mucous membranes, noting their color and

Pale, boggy nasal mucous membranes with or without the presence of gelatinous, peeled-

condition. **Look for nasal septal deviation and the presence of polyps posteriorly.**

pink-grape–appearing polyps in the posterior nasal passages, which are found with chronic (perennial) allergic rhinitis

Palpate over the frontal and maxillary sinuses, applying pressure to elicit tenderness.

When sinusitis is suspected because tenderness is elicited, transillumination should be performed. This requires a completely dark room and a cooperative child.

- **Transilluminate the frontal sinuses. Firmly place the tip of the transilluminator light above each eye against the inner aspect of the supraorbital ridge of the frontal bone.**

Normally, one sees a faint glow of light transmitted through the bone outlining the frontal sinus on the same side. Frontal sinuses are not developed well enough for this procedure to be helpful until approximately age 10 years.

Transillumination is absent or diminished when sinusitis is present. While this finding is not sufficiently sensitive or specific in ruling the diagnosis of sinusitis in or out, it helps make the diagnosis when combined with supporting history and corresponding localized sinus tenderness.

- **Transilluminate the maxillary sinuses. Cover the neck and head of the transilluminator light with a sleeve made by cutting the finger off a plastic glove. Place the covered light in the patient's mouth and press the tip against first one side of the hard palate and then the other. Instruct the patient to seal both lips around the shaft of the transilluminator attachment while you look for the maxillary sinus glow on the corresponding side of the face. Discard the sleeve after use.**

The Mouth and Pharynx

This examination may present difficulties in early childhood, and restraints are usually needed (see figure on p. 668). The young child may be more comfortable sitting in the parent's lap, as shown below.

The presence of *Koplik's spots* on the buccal mucosa opposite the first and second molars in a child with fever, coryza, and cough is proof positive of prodromal measles (*rubeola*), and the appearance of a generalized maculopapular rash within 24 hours is confirmatory. Koplik's spots appear as grains of salt on individual erythematous bases. Their number varies according to when in the course of the illness they are observed. When three or more appear in a particular area they are recognized easily. See p. 238.

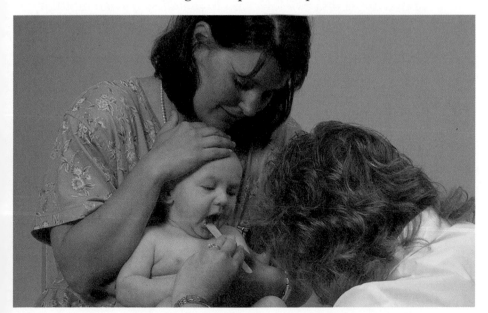

When children clamp their teeth and purse their lips, gently push the tongue blade through the lips along the buccal mucosa and between the gums behind the molars. This produces a gag reflex and, with it, a complete view of the pharynx.

A direct assault on the front teeth will only meet with failure and a splintered tongue blade. Most children, however, are not that resistant and can be enticed easily to open their mouths, especially if they do not see a throat stick in the examiner's hand. Children who can stick out their tongues and say "ahhh!" do not require further manipulation for a complete view of the pharynx. A good examiner can determine all that needs to be known with one quick look. Older children will permit placement of the tongue blade on one side of the base of the tongue and then the other. A transilluminator attached to the otoscope handle is more useful than a penlight or flashlight because it delivers concentrated light closer to the recesses of the oral cavity and the pharynx.

The Teeth

Examine the *teeth* for timing and sequence of eruption, number, character, condition, and position. Abnormalities of the enamel may reflect past or present, general or localized disease.

Dental caries, caused by bacterial activity, reflect frequent consumption of carbohydrates. Extensive decay of the primary teeth may be due to prolonged bottle feeding ("nursing-bottle caries"), especially in children who are given bottles at night and during naps.

The *primary teeth* erupt more predictably than do the permanent teeth. There is wide variation in age of eruption. African American children tend to have earlier eruption of permanent teeth than do Caucasian children. At age 10 months, most infants have two upper and two lower central incisors. From that point on, four teeth are added every 4 months, so that there are 8 at 14 months, 12 at 18 months, 16 at 22 months, and a full complement of 20 at 26 months. Normally, the shedding of primary teeth begins at about age 6 years; it precedes the eruption of corresponding *permanent teeth,* which begins at the onset of late childhood between 6 and 7 years of age and ends in early adulthood at age 17 to 22 years.

Irregular white specks or patches on tooth enamel are present with excess exposure to *fluorides*; grayish mottling of the enamel may result from giving tetracycline to infants and children under 8 years of age.

Look for malocclusion in late childhood. Most malocclusion and misalignment of teeth due to thumb sucking in early childhood is reversible if the habit is substantially arrested by age 6 or 7 years.

When examining for maxillary protrusion (*overbite*) or mandibular protrusion (*underbite*), do *not* ask the child to "show your teeth," because the upper and lower teeth are aligned reflexly when they are presented for inspection. Rather, ask the child to bite down as hard as

Malocclusion is most often due to hereditary predisposition, but may be due to premature loss of primary teeth. Maxillary overgrowth is associated with *chronic hemolytic anemia.* Mandibular overgrowth occurs rarely in the initial stages of *juvenile rheumatoid arthritis,* affect-

possible. **Part the lips and observe the *true* bite.** In normal children the lower teeth are contained within the arch formed by the upper teeth.

ing the temporomandibular joint; however, in chronic cases, a shortened mandible (*micrognathia*) eventually ensues.

The Tongue, Throat, and Tonsils

Inspect the dorsal and ventral surfaces of the tongue and its sides. Ask the patient to stick the tongue out and to move it from side to side.

The appearance of the *tongue* may indicate disease. The *coated* tongue is nonspecific, the *smooth* tongue is found in avitaminosis, and the *strawberry* and *raspberry* tongues are seen at specific stages of scarlet fever.

When the *throat* is examined, the size and appearance of the *tonsils* should be noted. In both early and late childhood the tonsils are relatively larger than in infancy and adolescence, as demonstrated by the abundance of lymphoid tissue at this time of life (see figure on p. 621). They appear even larger as they move out of their fossae toward the midline and forward when the gag reflex is elicited or when the tongue is voluntarily protruded and the traditional "ahhh!" is sounded. The tonsils usually have deep crypts on their surfaces, which often have white concretions or food particles protruding from their depths. This does not indicate disease, current or past.

A white exudate on the tonsils suggests *streptococcal tonsillitis*, particularly if accompanied by a beefy-red uvula and palatal petechiae; a thick gray, adherent exudate suggests *diphtheritic tonsillitis*; and necrosis (a grayish discoloration of the tonsillar tissue itself) suggests *infectious mononucleosis*. All three conditions produce a fetid odor. When one tonsil is red and protrudes forward and medially, a *peritonsillar abscess* is almost certainly present.

The *adenoids*, also called *pharyngeal tonsils*, consist of hyperplastic lymphoid tissue located on both sides of the nasopharynx, medial to the eustachian tube orifices. They are not ordinarily visible unless extremely enlarged or unless the soft palate is elevated with the tongue blade to expose them. Adenoidal size can be determined indirectly by noting the degree of posterior nasal obstruction present when the patient sniffs through each nostril, and the nasal quality they produce in the voice. Their size may also be determined directly by palpation. Adenoidal palpation should be carried out when a history of recurrent fever, headaches, and cough suggest *chronic adenoiditis* or *adenoidal abscess*.

Palpate the adenoids when these diagnoses are suggested. During this procedure, position and restrain the child as for examining the throat (see p. 668). Tape three tongue blades together and, with your left hand, place them between the molars and turn them on edge to ensure wide exposure. Place your plastic-gloved right index finger through the mouth into the nasopharynx behind the soft palate, and very rapidly and thoroughly massage the adenoidal and surrounding lymphoid tissue. The procedure is accomplished with three or four quick strokes of the finger from above downward, moving across the posterior nasopharynx.

In cases of chronic adenoiditis and adenoidal abscess, palpation reveals enlarged, boggy adenoidal tissue; massage produces copious amounts of bloody mucus and pus.

Children with markedly enlarged adenoids will mouth breathe and snore, and may have recurrent bouts of otitis media and sinusitis.

The child and parents should be warned that this procedure is uncomfortable and is likely to produce vomiting.

Use this same method to palpate (1) a peritonsillar abscess to determine the presence of fluctuation, and (2) the posterior pharyngeal wall to determine the presence of a retropharyngeal abscess.

Note absence or asymmetrical movement of the soft palate in response to gagging and phonation, which indicates paralysis or weakness.

Asymmetry and corresponding voice change are often observed for varying periods after tonsillectomy.

Do not examine the throat when acute epiglottitis is suspected. Inadvertently invoking the gag reflex during the examination could produce complete laryngeal obstruction and death. Therefore, the throat should be examined only by an otolaryngologist or other physician who is skilled in placing an endotracheal tube in the event of laryngeal obstruction. This is done best in an operating room where resuscitation can be effected if need be.

The child who has high fever, sore throat, croupy cough, hoarseness, drooling, and difficulty in swallowing may have acute *epiglottitis*. In such cases, the epiglottis is markedly swollen and cherry red.

Look for clues of a submucosal cleft palate, such as notching of the posterior margin of the hard palate or a bifid uvula. Because the mucosa is intact, the underlying defect is easily missed.

Children with *submucosal cleft palate* may have hypernasal speech, but many have no voice changes.

The Thorax, Breasts, and Lungs

Infancy

Chest Anatomy. The infant's *thorax* is rounded, with the anteroposterior diameter being equal to the transverse diameter. The *thoracic index,* which is the ratio of the transverse diameter to the anteroposterior diameter, is 1 at birth. At 1 year of age it is 1.25, and it reaches 1.35 at 6 years without much change thereafter.

The chest wall in infancy is thin with little musculature, and the bony and cartilaginous rib cage is very soft and pliant. The tip of the xiphoid process is often seen protruding anteriorly immediately beneath the skin at the apex of the costal angle.

Pectus excavatum may manifest in early infancy by marked midline sternal retractions with normal inspiration; however, it and other thoracic deformities, such as *pectus carinatum* ("chicken breast" deformity), do not ordinarily become evident until early childhood (see Table 8-2, Deformities of the Thorax, p. 270).

The *breasts* of the newborn in both male and female are often enlarged and engorged with a white liquid, sometimes colloquially called "witch's milk." This is due to maternal estrogen effect and usually lasts only a week or two. Supernumerary nipples occasionally are found on the thorax or the abdomen along a vertical line below the true nipple(s), as shown on p. 335. They appear as small, round, flat or slightly raised, pigmented lesions and are not clinically significant.

Assessing Respiration. The respiratory rate and patterns in infancy and early childhood are discussed on p. 640. Breathing is predominantly effected by movement of the diaphragm, with little assistance from the

When breathing is predominantly thoracic, suspect intra-abdominal or intrathoracic

thoracic muscles. This results in protrusion of the abdomen on inspiration and the reverse on expiration—so-called abdominal breathing.

Newborn infants, especially those born prematurely, exhibit irregular breathing characterized by periods of breathing at normal rates (30 to 40 per minute) alternating with "periodic breathing," during which the respiratory rate slows markedly and may even cease (*apnea*) three or more times for 3 seconds or longer. These alternating respiratory patterns have been observed in 30% to 95% of premature babies during sleep, but less often in full-term infants. The short apneic periods are not accompanied by bradycardia.

Feel for tactile fremitus in infants by placing your hand on the chest when the baby cries. Place your whole hand, palm and fingertips, over the anterior, lateral, or posterior thorax to detect gross changes in sound transmission through the chest. Percuss the infant's chest directly by tapping the thoracic wall with one finger, or indirectly by using the finger-on-finger method.

The percussion note is normally hyperresonant throughout. Any decrease in hyperresonance detected over the lung fields has the same significance as dullness in the adult.

Use the bell or small diaphragm of the stethoscope when auscultating the infant's chest to pinpoint findings.

The breath sounds are louder and harsher than in adults because the stethoscope is closer to the origin of the sounds. Breathing in newborns is usually intermittently slow and shallow, then rapid and deep. Breath sounds are often diminished on the side of the chest opposite the direction in which the head is turned. Fine crackles at the end of deep inspiration may be heard in normal newborns and older infants. Crying, fortunately, will produce all of the deep breaths one could want and actually enhances auscultation, except in the unusual baby who cries on inspiration as well as expiration.

In infants, it is difficult to distinguish transmitted upper airway sounds from sounds originating in the chest. Expiratory sounds usually originate below the vocal cords and inspiratory sounds from anywhere in the respiratory tract. Those from the upper airway are symmetrical and are louder closer to the head and on deep breathing.

Because of the smallness of the thoracic cage and the ease of sound transmission within it, breath sounds are rarely absent entirely. Even with atelectasis, effusion, empyema, and pneumothorax, breath sounds are diminished rather than absent. In infants, pure bronchial breathing is rarely heard, even when consolidation is present. Wheezes, which are

pathology that restricts the use of the diaphragm. An *increase* in abdominal breathing suggests pulmonary disease.

Periods of apnea lasting longer than 20 seconds and accompanied by bradycardia may indicate the presence of cardiopulmonary or central nervous system disease or a high risk for *sudden infant death syndrome (SIDS)*.

Dullness to percussion in infants may be due to consolidation of the lung, an intrathoracic mass, or pleural fluid.

Extension or other movement of the head with inspiration indicates use of accessory muscles of respiration, and usually accompanies severe respiratory disease.

palpable and audible, occur more frequently in infancy and early child-hood than in older children and adults because the small lumen of the tracheobronchial tree is easily narrowed by slight swelling of the mu-cous membranes or by small amounts of mucus. Often mucus and swollen nasal and pharyngeal mucous membranes cause loud, rhon-chorous inspiratory and expiratory sounds that are transmitted through-out the lung fields. Listening with the stethoscope placed over the cheeks and the lateral neck helps to localize the origin of these sounds—upper airway sounds being louder and lower airway sounds softer.

An inspiratory wheeze is called *stridor* and indicates nar-rowing high in the tracheo-bronchial tree; an expiratory wheeze suggests narrowing lower down.

Early and Late Childhood

Breast development for girls may begin normally as early as 8 years of age. Asymmetrical growth with resulting differences in breast size dur-ing preadolescence is common. Completion of growth through adoles-cence usually corrects these inequalities. It is often helpful to explain this to parents and the young person herself, even if neither mentions the subject.

As in infancy, the breath sounds on auscultation of the lungs are louder and harsher in early and late childhood than in adulthood because of the continued relative lack of musculature and subcutaneous tissue overlying the thorax. Respiratory patterns are more regular than in in-fancy, and cooperation in taking deep breaths and conducting other breathing maneuvers during auscultation of the lungs increases with age.

The stethoscope may be threatening to the very young child; therefore, your success in placing it on the chest will be enhanced if you say what it is and if you allow the child to manipulate it or even listen through it.

Generate tactile fremitus by feeling the chest wall while carrying on a conversation with the child. A surprising number say "99" or "1, 2, 3" when asked to. Gain the child's cooperation in deep breathing and breath holding by demonstrating each maneuver. If this is not suc-cessful, ask the child to blow out the light in your flashlight. This al-most always produces full inspiration.

The Heart

The examination of the heart in infants and children is, with few excep-tions, conducted like that in adults.

The Pulse. **Feel for the femoral pulse along the inguinal ligament midway between the iliac crest and the symphysis pubis as the ex-aminer is doing with her left hand in the figure on the next page.**

Diminution of the femoral pulses, as compared with the radial pulses, or their absence may be the only finding to suggest *coarctation of the aorta* in infancy and early childhood.

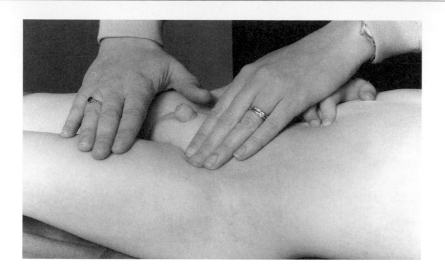

Because the respiratory rate may approximate the heart rate in infancy, breath sounds may be mistaken for murmurs. **Occlude the nares momentarily to interrupt the respirations long enough to clarify this issue.**

Apical Impulse, Heart Rhythm, and Heart Sounds. There are some distinct cardiac characteristics in normal infants and children that are not found in adults. The apical impulse or point of maximal impulse (PMI), which is often visible, is at the level of the 4th interspace until age 7 years, when it drops to the level of the 5th interspace. It is to the left of the midclavicular line until age 4 years, at the midclavicular line between ages 4 and 6, and to the right of it at age 7. On percussion the heart appears larger than it is because of its more horizontal position and the overlying thymus gland at its base. *Sinus arrhythmia* (heart rate faster on inspiration and slower on expiration) is almost always present, and *premature ventricular contractions* are quite common. The heart sounds are louder than those in adults because the chest wall is thinner, and they are of higher pitch and shorter duration. S_1 is louder than S_2 at the apex. Splitting of S_2 at the apex is found in 25% to 33% of infants and children, but is of no significance. S_2 is louder than S_1 in the pulmonic area.

Assessing Murmurs. During the first 48 hours of life, heart murmurs caused by the transition from intrauterine to extrauterine circulation are heard frequently. These are systolic in timing and less than grade 2 in intensity, and disappear spontaneously upon closure of the ductus arteriosus and the foramen ovale.

In the pediatric cardiac examination the *murmur* assumes great significance in differential diagnosis, because more than 50% of all children (indeed, some say all) develop an innocent murmur at some time during childhood and because significant heart disease in the pediatric age group is infrequent in the absence of a murmur. The examiner must therefore distinguish between the innocent and the organic murmur. The intensity of murmurs is graded on a scale of 1 to 6, as shown on p. 315.

The physical indications of severe heart disease include those not found with the stethoscope: poor weight gain, delayed development, tachypnea, tachycardia, a prominent, active, heaving or thrusting precordium, cyanosis, and clubbing of the fingers and toes. Heart failure is marked by poor feeding, tachycardia, tachypnea, venous engorgement, pulsus alternans, gallop rhythm, and hepatic enlargement. Pulmonary and peripheral edema appear late in the course of heart failure. (Peripheral edema, when it occurs in children, is more likely to be periorbital, and caused by renal failure.)

When S_2 is equal to or greater than S_1 at the apex, pulmonary hypertension should be suspected.

Innocent Murmurs and Venous Hum. The *innocent murmur* has received more than 120 labels, indicative of its benign or functional nature, its origin, or its auscultatory characteristics. It is systolic, is usually of short duration and of less than grade 3 in intensity, and has a low-pitched, vibratory, musical groaning quality. It is usually loudest along the left sternal border, either in the 2nd or 3rd intercostal spaces or in the 4th or 5th intercostal spaces medial to the apex. It is poorly transmitted, and is heard best with the bell of the stethoscope with the patient supine. Its intensity may vary with change in position, with the phase of respiration, with exercise, with the presence or absence of fever, and from day to day. The most important characteristic of the innocent murmur is that it is heard in the absence of any other demonstrable evidence of cardiovascular disease.

A *venous hum* (see Table 9-12, Cardiovascular Sounds With Both Systolic and Diastolic Components, p. 332) is heard commonly during childhood.

Hemic Murmurs. *Hemic murmurs* are caused by increased blood flow through the heart. This occurs when the body's tissues require more oxygen than usual (increased metabolism or muscular activity) or when hemoglobin-depleted red blood cells are not delivering ordinary amounts of oxygen to the tissues (anemia). These murmurs are located at the base of the heart, are soft (less than grade 3), occur during systole, and are accompanied by tachycardia. Two other common "innocent" murmurs heard in childhood are the *carotid bruit*, which is loudest in the neck and transmitted over the entire precordium, and *pulmonary branch stenosis*, which is heard best in the pulmonic area, radiates loudly to the axillae and back, and should disappear after the first few months of life as the branch pulmonary arteries enlarge.

Congenital and Acquired Murmurs. The noninnocent or *organic murmurs* are caused by congenital or acquired heart disease. *Acute rheumatic fever* is the major cause of acquired heart disease productive of murmurs of childhood. An organic murmur first appearing before 3 years of age is almost always caused by a congenital cardiac defect; one first appearing after that age is usually caused by rheumatic carditis.

The murmurs of congenital cardiac defects are caused either by abnormal communication between the arterial and venous circuits of the heart and great vessels or by valvular deformities. They are usually coarse in character, systolic in timing, and heard best at the base of the heart. The murmurs of *ventricular septal defect* and of *patent ductus arteriosus* have been described on pp. 330 and 332, respectively. Those of *aortic stenosis* and *pulmonic stenosis* are described on pp. 329 and 328.

The presence or absence of cyanosis may be helpful to the examiner in differentiating the various types of congenital heart disease that have similar murmurs (see Table 19-9, Cyanosis and Congenital Heart Disease, on p. 681).

Murmurs of grade 3 or higher usually indicate heart disease.

In *atrial septal defect*, a grade 1 to 3 coarse systolic murmur is heard at the 2nd and 3rd left interspaces. It is less coarse than the murmur of a ventricular septal defect, is rarely accompanied by a thrill, and is not widely distributed. The murmur of *coarctation of the aorta* (adult type) is heard in the same area, is louder, is transmitted to the back medial to the scapula, and may be accompanied by a visible pulsation and a palpable thrill at the suprasternal notch. It is also associated with decreased to absent femoral pulses and elevated blood pressure in

Usually the final diagnostic impression must await the results of electrocardiograms, chest x-rays, cardiac catheterization, echocardiograms, and more sophisticated studies.

The murmurs associated with acquired rheumatic heart disease include those of mitral stenosis (see p. 331), mitral regurgitation (see p. 330), aortic stenosis (see p. 329), and aortic regurgitation (see p. 331). Stenosis and regurgitation usually occur concomitantly when either the mitral or the aortic valve is affected from rheumatic carditis. Mitral valvular disease occurs in 90% of children who develop heart disease following acute rheumatic carditis, either alone or in combination with aortic valvular disease. Aortic valve involvement occurs in approximately 25% of cases. The tricuspid and pulmonic valves are rarely involved in the rheumatic process.

The examiner should be able to differentiate normal from abnormal findings. Final decisions regarding specific abnormalities, however, must often be left to the pediatric cardiologist, whose experience and access to special diagnostic tools will be more likely to produce accurate diagnoses and appropriate management. Therefore, the infant or child with evidence of congenital or acquired heart disease should be referred to a pediatric cardiologist early on.

the upper extremities. The murmurs associated with *tetralogy of Fallot, pure pulmonic stenosis, tricuspid atresia, transposition of the great vessels,* and *Eisenmenger's syndrome* are systolic and grades 3 to 5, may be heard best at the left 2nd and 3rd interspaces, are not well transmitted, may or may not be accompanied by a thrill, and have no distinguishing characteristics. These murmurs may be absent in infancy. In addition, palpable liver pulsations may be present with tricuspid atresia and pure pulmonic stenosis.

TABLE 19-9 *Cyanosis and Congenital Heart Disease*

No Cyanosis	Septal defects—small
	Patent ductus arteriosus
	Pure pulmonic stenosis—mild
	Coarctation of the aorta
	* Anomalous origin of left coronary artery
	* Subendocardial fibroelastosis
	* Glycogen storage disease
Early Cyanosis	Tetralogy of Fallot—severe
	Tricuspid atresia
	Transportation of the great vessels
	Two- and three-chambered hearts
	Severe pulmonic stenosis with intact ventricular septum
Late Cyanosis	Eisenmenger's complex
	Pure pulmonic stenosis—mild
	Tetralogy of Fallot
	Septal defects—large

* Presents with cardiac enlargement, tachycardia, and tachypnea, but without a heart murmur

The Abdomen

Infancy

Inspection. **Inspect the abdomen with the infant lying supine.** The abdomen in infants is protuberant, due to poorly developed abdominal musculature.

A newborn with a concave abdomen should immediately be investigated for *diaphragmatic hernia* with displacement of some of the abdominal organs into the thoracic cavity.

Check the umbilical cord at birth for the number of vessels present. Normally there are two thick-walled umbilical arteries and one thin-walled umbilical vein. The diameter of the arteries is smaller than that of the vein, and the vein is usually found at the 12 o'clock position at the level of the abdominal wall.

A high correlation exists between a variety of congenital anomalies and the presence of only a *single umbilical artery*.

The umbilicus in the newborn may have a relatively long cutaneous portion (*umbilicus cutis*), which is covered with skin, or a relatively long amniotic portion (*umbilicus amnioticus*), which is covered by a firm gelatinous substance. The amniotic portion dries up within 1 week and falls off within 2, while the cutaneous portion retracts to become flush with the abdominal wall.

The navel often fails to heal, and granulomatous tissue forms at its base.

Infants are prone to *umbilical hernias* (see p. 380), *ventral hernias,* and *diastasis recti.* However, these are not usually discernible until 2 or 3 weeks of age. All are easily detected with crying.

A diastasis recti may reflect a congenital weakness of the abdominal musculature (rare) or result from a chronically distended abdomen. Most, however, are normal variants and disappear in early childhood.

The defect in the abdominal wall at the umbilicus may be as large as 1½ inches in diameter, and the hernia itself may protrude 3 to 4 inches from the abdominal wall when intraabdominal pressure is increased. Many umbilical hernias disappear by 1 year of age, and almost all do by age 4 to 5 years.

A superficial abdominal venous pattern is observable until puberty. Abdominal reflexes are usually absent until after the first year of life.

Dilated veins may indicate portal vein obstruction. The direction of venous flow in *portal hypertension* is downward in veins below the umbilicus.

Auscultation and Percussion. **Auscultate the abdomen.** Metallic tinkling every 10 to 30 seconds is heard normally.

An increase in pitch or frequency of bowel sounds, or a marked diminution, indicates *intestinal obstruction* and *ileus,* respectively. A venous hum is a sign of *portal hypertension.*

Percuss the infant's abdomen as in the adult, but allow for a greater amount of air within the stomach and the intestinal lumen because infants frequently swallow air when feeding and crying.

Marked abdominal distention with tenderness may indicate an *acute surgical abdomen.*

Palpation. Palpation of the infant's abdomen is relatively easy. **Relax the infant by holding the legs flexed at the knees and hips with one hand; palpate with the other.**

The *liver edge* and *spleen tip* are more often palpable than not, and frequently both *kidneys* can be palpated by placing the fingers of one hand in front of and those of the other behind each kidney. The *bladder* is often felt and normally percussed to the level of the umbilicus. The *descending colon* is easily felt as a sausagelike mass in the left lower quadrant. Any abdominal masses of other origin are easily outlined.

In *Hirschsprung's disease* (congenital megacolon), a midline suprapubic mass representing a feces-filled rectosigmoid is often found.

Avoid the spasm and rigidity encountered in palpating the abdomen of a crying infant by giving a bottle or a pacifier.

Special Technique for Pyloric Stenosis
The abdominal examination technique is altered when *pyloric stenosis* is suspected.

Place the unclothed infant supine and stand at the foot of the table. Direct a bright light at table height across the abdomen from the patient's right side. Feed the infant a bottle of sugar water or milk and observe the abdomen closely. When pyloric stenosis is present, peristaltic waves are seen to go across the upper abdomen from left to right. These become increasingly large and frequent as the feeding progresses, as shown in the figure below. Inevitably, the baby will vomit with projectile force.

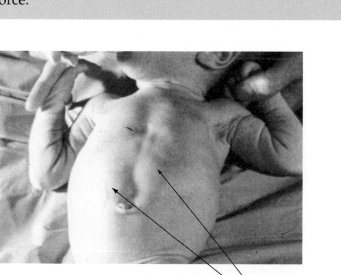

Peristaltic waves

At this point, palpate deeply in the right upper quadrant with your extended middle finger. This usually reveals the presence of a pyloric mass roughly 2 cm in diameter. Similar palpation with the baby prone may prove more successful.

Early and Late Childhood

A protuberant abdomen, apparent when the child is upright and disappearing when the child is supine, is typical in most children until adolescence.

Palpation. Children are almost universally ticklish when you first place your hand on their abdominal wall. This reaction disappears in most cases, particularly if you distract the child by conversation and place your whole hand flush on the surface for a few moments without probing with your fingers. **With children whose sensitivity persists, place the child's hand under yours, as shown in the illustrations below, to reduce apprehension and increase relaxation of the abdominal musculature.**

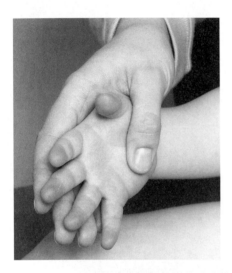

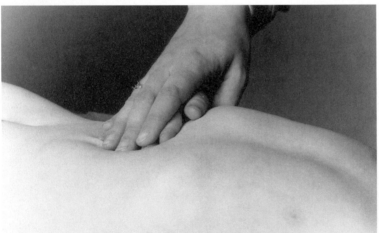

Flexing the knees and hips also relaxes the abdominal wall. Palpate lightly and then deeply in all quadrants. Examine last the area that the history suggests as the site of pathology.

Tenderness may be detected by the child's telling you, by a change in the child's facial expression, or in the pitch of the child's cry.

The Liver and Spleen. The *liver* is easily palpated in most children. The edge of the liver is normally felt 1 cm to 2 cm below the right costal margin. It is sharp and soft and moves easily when pushed from below upward during deep inspiration. The size of the liver is determined better by percussion than by palpation. The table below shows the expected liver span by percussion in the right midclavicular line for male and female patients by age.

A pathologically enlarged liver is usually palpable at more than 2 cm below the costal margin, and has a round, firm edge.

TABLE 19-10 *Expected Liver Span of Infants, Children, and Adolescents by Percussion*						
	Mean Estimated Liver Span (cm)				**Mean Estimated Liver Span (cm)**	
Age in Years	*Males*	*Females*	**Age in Years**		*Males*	*Females*
0.5 (6 mo)	2.4	2.8	8		5.6	5.1
1	2.8	3.1	10		6.1	5.4
2	3.5	3.6	12		6.5	5.6
3	4.0	4.0	14		6.8	5.8
4	4.4	4.3	16		7.1	6.0
5	4.8	4.5	18		7.4	6.1
6	5.1	4.8	20		7.7	6.3

The lower border of the liver can be determined with a *scratch test.* **Place the diaphragm of your stethoscope just above the right costal margin at the midclavicular line. With your fingernail, lightly scratch the skin of the abdomen along the midclavicular line, moving from below the umbilicus toward the costal margin.** When your scratching finger reaches the liver's edge, you will hear the scratching sound as it passes through the liver to your stethoscope.

As a rule the *spleen,* like the liver, is felt easily in most children. It too is soft with a sharp edge, and it projects downward like a tongue, from under the left costal margin.

You often can palpate the spleen between the thumb and forefinger of your right hand, and find it to be moveable.

The Aorta. Pulsations in the epigastrium caused by the aorta are seen normally.

Deeply palpate the abdomen to the left of the midline to feel the *aorta* and its pulsations.

Because the omentum is poorly developed in early childhood, localization of intraabdominal infection or other inflammatory reaction is less apt to occur than in late childhood and adolescence.

The pulsations of an enlarged right ventricle may be transmitted through the diaphragm and be visible in the epigastrium.

Tenderness and spasm of the abdominal musculature are usually diffuse whenever serious pathology occurs within the abdomen; *generalized peritonitis* should be suspected.

Ask the child to sit up from a supine position while you push down against the forehead with your hand.

This maneuver will elicit pain in the right lower quadrant in *acute appendicitis* when the appendix is lying anteriorly. When the appendix lies retrocecally over the psoas and obturator muscles, *psoas* and *obturator signs* are often present (see p. 353).

The Genitalia and Rectum

Infancy

The Male Genitalia. **Examine the *male genitalia* with the infant in the supine position.** The *foreskin* adheres to the *glans penis,* covers it completely, and has a tiny orifice at its distal end. Retraction of the foreskin over the glans in the uncircumcised male occurs months to years later, after regular gentle retraction. Circumcision exposes the glans penis to its base. The rate of circumcision has declined in recent years, but it is still a common practice.

Locate the *urethral orifice* and inspect the *shaft* of the penis.

Hypospadias is present when the urethral orifice appears at some point along the ventral surface of the glans or the shaft of the penis (see Table 12-1, Abnormalities of the Penis, p. 399). The foreskin in these instances is incompletely formed ventrally.

Palpate the contents of the scrotal sacs and the inguinal canal. Locate the testes, which are found normally in the scrotal sacs. If found in the inguinal canal, use steady, gentle pressure from above to push them down into the scrotum.

In approximately 3% of all male neonates, one or both testes cannot be felt in the scrotum or inguinal canal. (See Cryptorchidism, p. 394, and Table 12-2, Abnormalities of the Scrotum, pp. 400–401). By age 1 year, two thirds of these testes will have descended into the scrotum.

Bilateral *cryptorchidism* strongly suggests *adrenogenital syndrome* in which the infant's sex is female, and hyponatremia, dehydration, and shock may ensue within the first 2 weeks of life.

Generalized scrotal edema may be present for several days postdelivery due to the effects of maternal estrogens and of breech delivery, when bruising is also present.

Hydroceles overlying the testes and the spermatic cord are common in infancy and often associated with actual or potential *inguinal hernias.* Hydroceles may be differentiated easily from hernias in that the former transilluminate and are not reducible (see Table 12-2, Abnormalities of the Scrotum, pp. 400–401). Most hydroceles detected in infancy resorb by age 18 months.

The Female Genitalia. In the newborn female, the *mons pubis, labia majora,* and *labia minora* are prominent due to the effects of maternal estrogen; this prominence decreases within a month or two. Sometimes there is a bloody vaginal discharge during the first weeks of life, which may be replaced by a serosanguineous discharge for several more weeks.

Examine the female genitalia with the infant in the supine position. Separate the labia majora at their midpoint with the thumb of each hand, applying traction laterally and posteriorly. Inspect the *uretheral orifice* and the *vestibule,* defined by the labia minora laterally, the clitoris anteriorly, and the posterior fourchette. Look for the *hymen,* a thickened, avascular structure with a central orifice, covering the vaginal opening.

Enlargement of the clitoris and posterior fusion of the labia majora are signs of *ambiguous genitalia* due to inborn errors of testosterone biosynthesis, a chromosomal defect, teratogenic agents, or a simple developmental abnormality. When ambiguous genitalia are present, it is essential that the sex of the child be determined before sex assignment is made.

The absence of a central hymenal orifice (*imperforate hymen*) is rare and of no clinical significance in the neonate; should it persist, *hydrocolpos* may occur during childhood, and *hematocolpos* will occur following initial menstruation in the adolescent girl. Both conditions are rare.

The genitalia of female breech babies may be markedly edematous and bruised for several days following delivery.

The Rectal Examination. The rectal examination is not routinely performed during infancy, but should be done whenever intraabdominal, pelvic, or perirectal disease is suspected. It should be performed with the patient supine. This allows for deeper penetration of the examining finger and for combined abdominal and rectal examination.

Hold the feet together and flex the knees and hips on the abdomen with one of your hands while introducing the gloved and lubricated index finger of your other hand into the rectum. Then place your first hand on the abdomen to conduct a bimanual examination. The index finger is preferred for the rectal examination, even for infants, because of its greater length and tactile sensitivity. Regardless of the size of your examining finger, slight bleeding and protrusion of the rectal mucosa usually will occur upon its removal.

Early and Late Childhood

The Male Genitalia. The size of the penis in early childhood and pre-pubescence is of little significance unless it is very large. In obese boys the fat pad over the symphysis pubis may envelop the penis, obscuring it completely. The testes in young boys are quite retractile and are often found in the inguinal canal rather than in the scrotum.

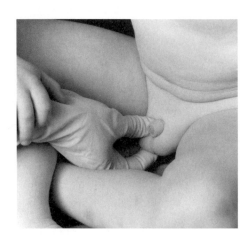

The testes should be well descended into the scrotum. They may be seen to move upward when the medial aspect of the ipsilateral thigh is scratched lightly (*cremasteric reflex*).

Warm your hands when attempting to locate undescended or retractile testes.

Overcome the cremasteric reflex by having the child sit cross-legged on the examining table, as illustrated here. Undescended testicle should not be diagnosed until you have palpated the inguinal canal and scrotum with the patient in this position.

The examination for *inguinal hernia* in this age group is similar to that performed on the adult and should be done with the patient standing (see p. 395).

The child's cough or attempts at performing a Valsalva maneuver may not be strong enough to demonstrate a reduced hernia. The hernia can sometimes be made evident if the child attempts to lift a heavy object, such as the end of the examining table or the chair in which you are sitting.

Tanner staging is used to track the sexual maturation of males during puberty, characterizing pubic hair distribution and penile and testicular size (see pp. 389–391).

The Female Genitalia. **Examine the female external genitalia while the patient is in the supine, frog-leg position on the examining table, or, for a young girl, while she is lying in the parent's lap.**

You can often make the examination of the female genitalia easier for yourself and more comfortable for the young child by using the child's

Enlargement of the penis to adolescent or adult size may occur in *precocious puberty*, due to an excess in circulating androgens of adrenal or testicular origin. This occurs with tumors of these organs or of the pituitary gland. Other signs of virilization—pubic and axillary hair, increased testicular size, increased somatic growth and muscle mass, hirsutism, and a deepening voice—usually accompany the penile enlargement.

Cryptorchidism, or undescended testicle, may persist unilaterally or bilaterally, with the testicle(s) remaining in the abdomen or within the inguinal canal.

Fusion of the labia minora is seen occasionally in girls under

own hands to distract and reassure her and to assist you, as shown in the figure below.

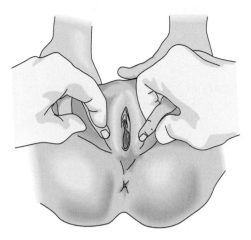

During the preschool years, the external genitalia are characterized by flattened labia majora, thin labia minora, and a small clitoris. The hymen, once thickened and avascular, becomes thin, with a well-defined edge and a lacy vascular pattern. The hymenal orifice is usually easily appreciated with lateral labial traction.

During the early school years, the external genitalia show signs of estrogen stimulation. The labia majora and minora become fuller, and the hymen becomes thicker. These changes progress as the child nears puberty and the genitalia assume adult characteristics. Tanner staging is also used to track the sexual maturation of pubertal females. This system includes a description of pubic hair and breast development (see pp. 407–408, and 335–337). Girls as young as 8 years may develop these secondary sexual characteristics.

Vaginoabdominal palpation as a method of examining the pelvic structures and direct inspection of the vagina and cervix are not considered part of the ordinary physical examination in childhood. When inspection of the vagina and cervix is indicated, it is done best with an otoscope equipped with a vaginal speculum, as shown below.

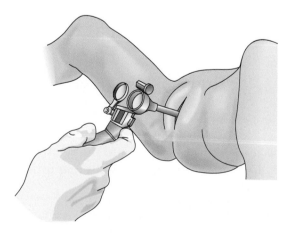

4 years of age. It may be partial, with only the posterior portion of the labia fused, or it may be complete. A thin membrane that joins the labial edges is easily lysed with a cotton swab or a probe. The labia will also separate if an estrogen-containing cream is applied to the labia once or twice daily for several days.

The appearance of pubic hair or breast enlargement before 8 years of age in girls may be due to *precocious puberty,* and must be thoroughly evaluated.

Foreign bodies are often inserted by the child into the vagina and cause irritation and infection, which lead to a purulent vaginal discharge.

Examination of the vagina and cervix is indicated when *sexual abuse* is suspected.

In the prepubertal and pubertal female, examination of the external genitalia is sufficient. The presence of vaginal bleeding in the prepubertal female is one of the few indications for a pelvic examination. These examinations are best left to an experienced practitioner. A speculum examination is indicated if the patient is sexually active, has nonmenstrual bleeding, or has a vaginal discharge.

While *physiologic leukorrhea* (a thin whitish vaginal discharge) is common in adolescents, a purulent vaginal discharge may be due to a foreign body, *irritant vulvovaginitis, bacterial infections,* and *sexually transmitted diseases.*

The Rectal Examination. The rectal examination is not part of the routine pediatric examination, but should be done whenever intraabdominal, pelvic, or perirectal disease is suspected.

Place the child in the supine position with the knees and hips flexed and the legs abducted. Drape from the waist down. Provide frequent reassurance during the course of the examination. Try to gain greater relaxation and cooperation by first demonstrating and then asking the child to breathe in and out through the mouth rapidly, "like a puppy dog." Spread the buttocks and observe the anus. Look for perianal skin tabs (frequently present but usually of no significance). Insert the lubricated index finger of your gloved hand slowly and gently through the anal sphincter, aiming it toward the umbilicus. Ask the child to "push down" to relax the sphincter. Proceed with a bimanual rectoabdominal examination. With the fingers of your other hand, palpate deeply in the lower abdomen, trying to feel the lower abdominal and pelvic structures between your two hands.

The prostate gland is not palpable in young boys.

Bimanual rectoabdominal palpation in females reveals a small midline mass, which is the *cervix.* Any other mass that is palpable on this examination should be considered abnormal, since none of the other anatomical structures are normally palpable until adolescence.

The Musculoskeletal System

Infancy

The range of motion at all joints is greatest in infancy, and gradually lessens throughout childhood to adult levels.

The Feet and Legs. At birth, the feet may appear deformed if they retain their intrauterine positioning. Such positional deformities can be distinguished by the ease with which the affected foot can be manipulated to neutral and overcorrected positions. Scratching or stroking along the outer edge of the positionally deformed foot will cause it to assume a normal position.

True deformities do not return to the neutral position even with manipulation.

Look for inversion of the feet (a turning inward so that the medial margin is elevated). Note the relationship of the forefoot to the hindfoot. Is the forefoot adducted at the metatarsal–tarsal line (a line across the junctions of the tarsal and metatarsal bones)?

Adduction of the forefoot distal to the metatarsal–tarsal line (*metatarsus adductus deformity*) is common; spontaneous correction occurs within the first 2 years of life.

During infancy there is a distinct *bowlegged growth pattern.* This begins to disappear at 18 months of age, when a transition from bowlegs to knock-knees occurs. The *knock-knee pattern* usually persists from age 2 years until age 6 to 10 years, when a balancing takes place and, for most, the legs straighten. Some babies exhibit a twisting or torsion of the tibia inwardly or outwardly on its longitudinal axis. This invariably corrects itself during the second year of life.

When the forefoot is twisted inward on its longitudinal axis (inverted) in addition to being adducted, *metatarsus varus* exists, as shown in the figure below.

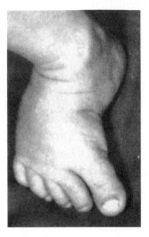

(Reprinted with permission from Tachdjian MO: Pediatric Orthopedics, 2nd ed. Philadelphia, WB Saunders, 1990)

Talipes varus is present when the forefoot is adducted and the entire foot is inverted.

Talipes equinovarus (clubfoot) is characterized by forefoot adduction and inversion and plantar flexion (equinus position) of the entire foot, as shown below.

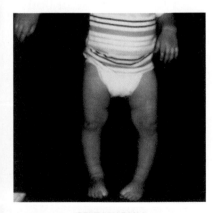

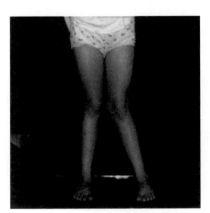

GENU VARUM (BOW LEGS)

GENU VALGUM (KNOCK-KNEES)

(Reproduced from a color photograph in Seidel HM et al. [Eds.], Mosby's Guide to Physical Examination, St. Louis, CV Mosby, 1987)

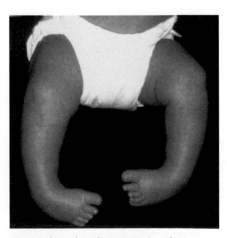

(Reproduced with permission from Prechtl HFR: The Neurological Examination of the Full-Term Newborn Infant, 2nd ed. Philadelphia, JB Lippincott, 1977)

When infants stand, their legs are set wide apart and the weight is borne on the inside of the feet. When they walk, a wide-based gait is used for the first year or two. This causes a certain degree of *pronation of the feet* and incurving of the Achilles tendons (viewed from behind).

The longitudinal arch in infancy is obscured by adipose tissue, giving the foot a flat appearance. This is accentuated by pronation of the foot, so the infant is often misdiagnosed as being flatfooted.

The Hips. The *hips* of all infants should be examined for signs of dislocation.

Place the baby supine with the legs pointing toward you. Flex the legs to right angles at the hips and knees, placing your index fingers over the greater trochanter of each femur and your thumbs over the lesser trochanters, as shown in the figures below. Abduct both hips simultaneously until the lateral aspect of each knee touches the examining table. This maneuver is known as the *Ortolani test*.

Spastic flat foot is very rare in childhood and nonexistent during infancy. It is characterized by pronation of the entire foot, eversion of the forefeet, and pain on walking.

When a *congenitally dislocated hip* is present, you will see and feel a "clunk," and sometimes hear a "click" as the femoral head, which in this condition lies posterior to the acetabulum, enters the acetabulum at some point in the 90° abduction arc. This finding is known as *Ortolani's sign*.

Beyond the newborn period, as the muscles surrounding the hip increase in strength, the clunk and click of the Ortolani sign is less obtainable; then decreased abduction of the flexed legs (at the hip on one or both sides) becomes the significant finding in detecting unilateral or bilateral congenital dislocation of the hip.

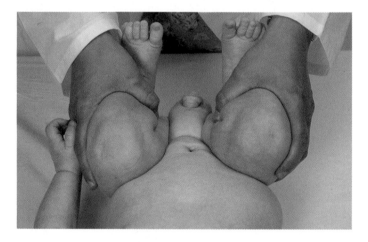

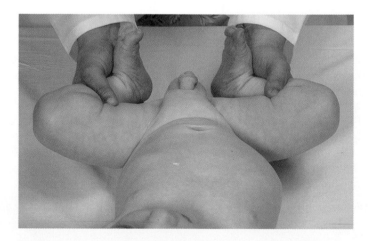

Detect an unstable (nondislocated but potentially dislocatable) hip by placing your thumbs medially over the lesser trochanters and your index fingers laterally over the greater trochanters, as shown in the figure below; press your thumb backward and outward. Feel for movement of the head of the femur laterally against some resistance as it slips out onto the posterior lip of the acetabulum. Normally no movement is felt. Then, with your index finger, press the greater trochanter forward and inward. Feel for a sudden movement of the femoral head inward as it returns to the hip socket. Again, movement is not normally felt. Movement in both directions constitutes *Barlow's sign.*

Barlow's sign is not diagnostic of a congenital dislocated hip, but it indicates the need to observe the baby very carefully for this possibility.

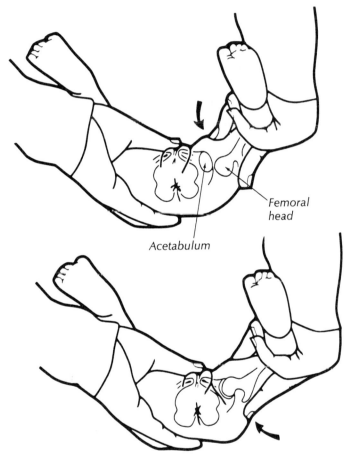

Femoral head

Acetabulum

(Reproduced with permission from Burnside JW: Physical Diagnosis: An Introduction to Clinical Medicine, 16th ed. Baltimore, Williams & Wilkins, 1981)

The Spine. Massive defects in the spine, such as meningomyelocele, are quite obvious at birth, but others that may lead to serious consequences present more subtly.

Palpate the spine carefully, particularly in the lumbosacral region, to determine if there are any deformities of the vertebrae or any abnormalities of the overlying skin, pigmented spots, hairy patches, or

Spina bifida occulta (a defect of the vertebral bodies) may be associated with defects of the underlying spinal cord (*diastematomyelia*) that can cause malfunctioning of the bladder and rectum and weakness or

deep pits that might overlie external openings of sinus tracts that extend to the spinal canal.

paralyses of the lower extremities. A sinus track provides potential entry to the spinal canal of organisms that can cause meningitis.

Early and Late Childhood

From both in front and behind, watch the child standing upright. Closely observe the child in various postures from the front and the rear (e.g., while the child is standing upright with the feet together, walking, stooping to obtain an object from the floor, rising from the supine position, and touching the toes or the shins while standing).

Various musculoskeletal difficulties can be detected using these observations.

In childhood, the thoracic convexity is decreased and the lumbar concavity increased. Lordosis is common and rarely causes symptoms.

Test for severe hip disease with its associated weakness of the gluteus medius muscle by observing the child from behind as the weight is shifted from one leg to the other. The pelvis remains level when the weight is borne on the unaffected side (*negative Trendelenburg sign*).

The pelvis tilts toward the unaffected hip when weight is borne on the affected side (*positive Trendelenburg sign*).

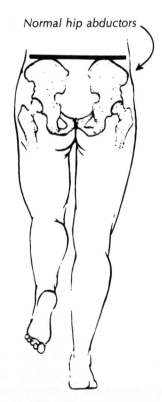
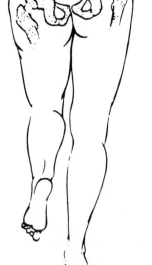
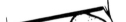

Normal hip abductors

Weak hip abductors

(Reproduced with permission from Chung SMR: Hip Disorders in Infants and Children. Philadelphia, Lea & Febiger, 1981)

Determine any *leg shortening* in hip disease by comparing the distance from the anterior superior spine of the ilium to the medial malleolus on each side (see p. 540).

When you suspect *scoliosis* (see p. 540), ask the child to bend forward. Mark the spinous processes with a felt-tip pen. From behind, watch for asymmetry of the scapulas, rib cage, and hips as the child slowly stands erect. Then look for a curve in the line of ink dots.

The Nervous System

Infancy

General Examination. Neurologic screening includes assessment of positioning, spontaneous and induced movements, cry, and knee and ankle jerk reflexes, and elicitation of the rooting, grasp, tonic neck, and Moro automatisms. It should be performed on all newborns. Babies showing abnormalities in these areas and those at risk for central nervous system disease should be completely assessed neurologically at frequent intervals.

The findings during the neurologic examination in infancy, especially in the newborn period, differ markedly from those present in children and adults.

The central nervous system at birth is underdeveloped, and cortical function cannot be tested entirely until early childhood. Findings of normal brainstem and spinal functioning do not ensure an intact cortical system, and abnormalities of the brainstem and spinal cord may exist without concomitant cortical abnormalities. A number of specific reflex activities (*infantile automatisms*) are found in the normal newborn that disappear in early infancy (see p. 697).

The absence of infantile automatisms in the neonate or the persistence of some beyond their expected time of disappearance may indicate severe central nervous system dysfunction.

Assess *mental status* by observing the ease of transition between states of alertness and drowsiness, ease of consolability, orientation to visual or auditory stimuli, and habituation to various stimuli.

The neurologic examination in infancy will enable the clinician to detect extensive disease of the central nervous system, but will be of little use in pinpointing minute lesions and specific functional deficits.

The general appearance, positioning, activity, cry, and alertness of the newborn baby should be noted, because these observations are important in the neurologic assessment of this age group.

Test for *motor function* by putting each major joint through its range of motion to determine whether normal muscle tone, spasticity, or flaccidity is present.

Postural indications of severe intracranial disease include persistent asymmetries, predominant extension of the extremities, and constant turning of the head to one side. Marked extension of the head, stiffness of the neck, and extension of the arms and legs (*opisthotonus*) indicate severe meningeal or brainstem irritation, seen in

Beyond the newborn period, throughout infancy, specific *gross and fine motor coordination testing* can be done using an age-appropriate protocol, such as the Denver Developmental Screening Test (see pp. 623–633). This is also a test of social and language development. Discrepancies in achievement in the motor and communication areas may suggest whether the deficit is in the motor, sensory, or intellectual sphere. Knowledge of when developmental landmarks are normally achieved is essential in assessing the function of the infant's nervous system.

The *sensory examination* for infants is rather limited in terms of defining neurologic disease. Thresholds of touch, pain, and temperature are higher in older children, and reactions to these stimuli are relatively slow.

Test for pain sensation by flicking the infant's palm or sole with your finger. Observe for withdrawal, arousal, and change in facial expression. Do not use a pin to test for pain sensation.

The *cranial nerves* are tested in infancy as in the adult. The difficulties encountered in assessing the function of the 2nd and 8th nerves have already been mentioned.

The 12th nerve is easily tested. Pinch the nostrils of the infant. This produces a reflex opening of the mouth and raising of the tip of the tongue.

Because the corticospinal pathways are not developed fully in infants, the *spinal reflex mechanisms* (deep tendon reflexes and plantar response) during infancy are variable. Their exaggerated presence, or their absence, has very little diagnostic significance unless this response is different from that in a previous testing.

The technique for eliciting these reflexes is similar to that used with adults, except that your semiflexed index or middle finger can substitute for the neurologic hammer, its tip acting as the striking point. Your thumbnail may be used to elicit the plantar response.

The *Babinski response* to plantar stimulation can be elicited in some normal infants, and sometimes until 2 years of age. However, a flexion response to plantar stimulation is elicited in more than 90% of normal newborns. The *triceps reflex* is usually not present until after 6 months of age. Rapid, rhythmic plantar flexion of the foot in response to eliciting of the ankle reflex (*ankle clonus*) is common in newborns; as many as eight to ten such contractions in response to one stimulus may occur normally (*unsustained ankle clonus*).

intracranial infection or hemorrhage (see figure below).

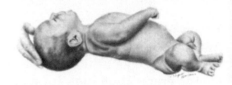

(Redrawn from Paine RS: *Neurological examination of infants and children.* Pediatr Clin North Am 7:477, 1960)

Absence of withdrawal when a painful stimulus is applied to an extremity indicates anesthesia or paralysis. If a facial expression or a cry changes in the absence of withdrawal, paralysis rather than anesthesia is indicated. With spinal cord lesions, the extremity withdraws reflexly in response to pain, but the baby's facial expression or cry will not change.

In *12th-nerve paresis,* the tongue tip deviates toward the affected side.

When the contractions are continuous (*sustained ankle clonus*), severe central nervous system disease should be suspected.

You also can elicit ankle clonus by pressing your thumb over the ball of the infant's foot and abruptly dorsiflexing the foot.

The *abdominal reflexes* are absent in the newborn but appear within the first 6 months of life. The *anal reflex*, however, is normally present in newborns, and is important to elicit when spinal cord lesions are present or suspected.

With the baby supine, straighten and raise the lower legs, stroke the perianal region with a paper clip, and observe the external anal sphincter contract.

An absent anal reflex strongly suggests loss of innervation of the external sphincter muscle due to a spinal cord lesion at the level of the lower sacral segments (or higher), such as a congenital anomaly (*spina bifida*), a tumor, or an injury.

Infantile Automatisms

The infantile automatisms are reflex phenomena present at birth or appearing shortly thereafter. Some remain only a few weeks while others persist well into the second year of life. Automatisms have prognostic value for central nervous system integrity. Eliciting any of them (except the rooting, grasp, tonic neck, and Moro responses) should be attempted only when central nervous system function is questionable. Each automatism is listed here with the method of elicitation and the prognostic significance of its presence or absence. All are present at birth unless otherwise indicated. The time of disappearance is also shown.

Blinking (Dazzle) Reflex. Disappears after first year. The eyelids close in response to bright light.

Absence may indicate blindness.

Acoustic Blink (Cochleopalpebral) Reflex. Disappearance time is variable. Both eyes blink in response to a sharp loud noise.

Absence may indicate decreased or absent hearing.

Palmar Grasp Reflex. Disappears at 3 or 4 months

With the baby's head positioned in the midline and the arms semi-flexed, place your index fingers from the ulnar side into the baby's hands and press against the palmar surfaces. The baby responds by flexing all of its fingers to grasp your fingers. This method allows for comparison of both hands. If the reflex is absent or weak, you can enhance it by offering the baby a bottle, since sucking facilitates grasping.

Persistence of the grasp reflex beyond 4 months suggests cerebral dysfunction. Note that babies normally clench their hands during the first month of life. Persistence of the clenched hand beyond 2 months also suggests central nervous system damage, particularly when the fingers overlap the thumb.

Rooting Reflex. Disappears at 3 or 4 months; may be present longer during sleep

Absence of this reflex indicates severe generalized or central nervous system disease.

With the baby's head positioned in the midline and the hands held against the anterior chest, stroke with your forefinger the perioral skin at the corners of the baby's mouth and at the midline of the upper and lower lips.

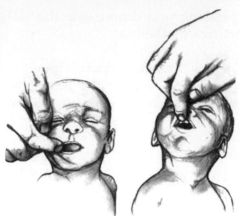

In response, the mouth will open and turn to the stimulated side. When the upper lip is stimulated, the head will extend; when the lower lip is stimulated, the jaw will drop. This response will also occur when the infant's cheek is stimulated at some distance from the corners of the mouth.

Trunk Incurvation (Galant's) Reflex. Disappears at 2 months

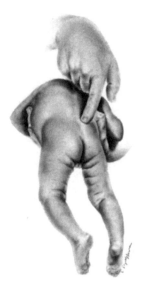

(Redrawn from Paine RS: Neurological examination of infants and children. Pediatr Clin North Am 7:490, 1960)

Hold the baby horizontally and prone in one of your hands. Using the index finger of your other hand, stimulate one side of the baby's back approximately 1 cm from the midline moving along a paravertebral line extending from the shoulder to the buttocks or vice versa. This produces a curving of the trunk toward the stimulated side, with shoulders and pelvis moving in that direction.

This reflex is absent in transverse spinal cord lesions or injuries.

Vertical Suspension Positioning. Disappears after 4 months

While you support the baby upright with your hands under the axillae, the head is normally maintained in the midline and the legs are flexed at the hips and knees.

Fixed extension and adduction of the legs (scissoring) indicates *spastic paraplegia* or *diplegia*, as shown in the figure on the next page.

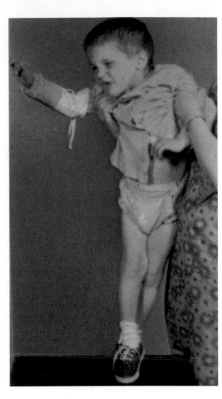

Placing Response. Best elicited after the first 4 days. Disappearance time is variable.

Hold the baby upright from behind by placing your hands under the baby's arms with your thumbs supporting the back of the head, and allow the dorsal surface of one foot to touch the undersurface of a table top. Take care not to plantar flex the foot.

(Reprinted from Atlas of Mental Retardation Syndromes, US Department of Health Education and Welfare, 1968.)

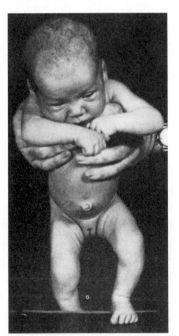 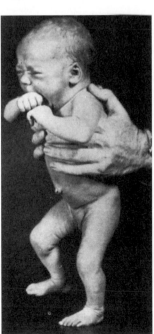

(Reprinted with permission from Paine RS: Neurologic examination of infants and children. In MA Perlstein [Ed]: Symposium on Neuropediatrics. Pediatr Clin North Am 7:471–510, 1960)

The baby responds by flexing the hip and knee and placing the stimulated foot on the table top. The opposite foot then steps forward and a series of alternate stepping movements occurs as you move the baby gently forward.

Rotation Test. Disappearance time is variable.

Hold the baby under the axillae, at arm's length facing you, and turn him or her in one direction and then the other. The head turns in the direction in which you turn the baby. If you restrain the head with your thumbs, the baby's eyes will turn in the direction in which you turned (see figure on p. 662).

Tonic Neck Reflex. May be present at birth, but usually appears at 2 months and disappears at 6 months

With the baby supine, as shown below, turn the head to one side, holding the jaw over the baby's shoulder. The arm and the leg on the side to which the head is turned extend, while the opposite arm and leg flex. This "fencing posture" response does not normally occur each time this maneuver is performed. Repeat the maneuver, turning the head to the opposite side.

Other Reflexes. Two mass reflexes occur in the presence of normal subcortical mechanisms that are not yet under significant inhibitory control from higher cerebral centers. They are present at birth and disappear by the third month.

Perez Reflex. **Suspend the baby prone in one of your hands. Place the thumb of your other hand on the baby's sacrum and move it firmly toward the head along the entire length of the spine. Extension of the head and spine, flexion of the knees on the abdomen, a cry, and emptying of the bladder are the usual responses.**

The last part of the response occurs with sufficient frequency to be useful in the collection of urine specimens from neonates.

These responses are absent when paresis is present and in babies born by breech delivery.

The head and eyes do not move in the presence of vestibular dysfunction. *Strabismus* may be detected early with this maneuver.

When this reflex is elicited every time it is evoked, it should be considered abnormal, at any age. It will persist beyond the time of expected disappearance with major cerebral damage.

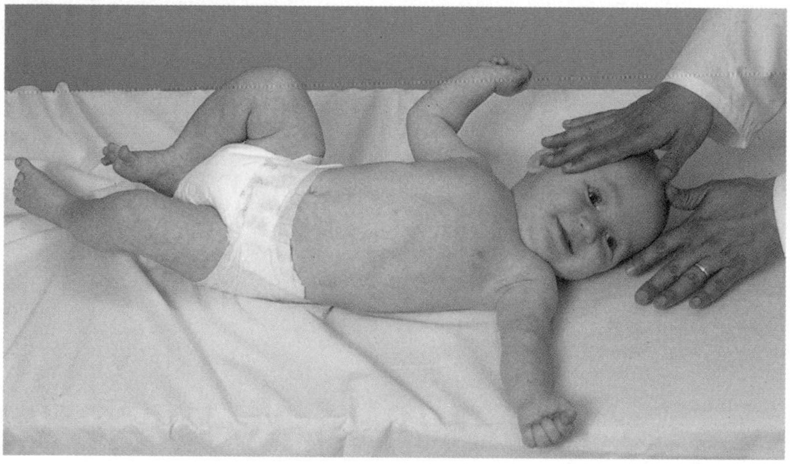

Bilateral cerebral injury produces hypotonia with normal or brisk deep tendon reflexes, delay in reaching motor milestones, and persistence of the tonic neck reflex.

Absence of either reflex during the first 3 months of life may indicate severe cerebral insult, injury to the upper cervical cord, advanced anterior horn cell disease, or severe myopathy.

Moro Response (Startle Reflex). You can produce the Moro response in several ways; the two most commonly used are described below.

- **Hold the baby in the supine position, supporting the head, back, and legs. Then suddenly lower the entire body about 2 feet and stop abruptly, as shown below.**

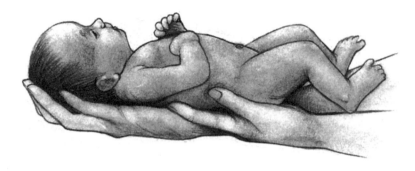

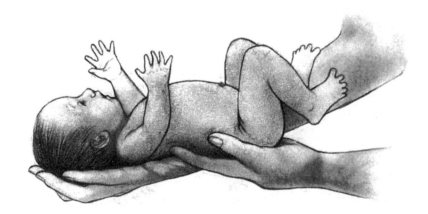

- **Produce a loud noise (e.g., strike the examining table with the palms of your hands on both sides of the baby's head).**

The response itself (elicited using either method) is one in which the arms briskly abduct and extend with the hands open and fingers extended, and the legs flex slightly and abduct (but less so than the arms). The arms then return forward over the body in a clasping maneuver and the baby cries simultaneously.

Persistence of the Moro response beyond 4 months may indicate neurologic disease; persistence beyond 6 months is almost conclusive evidence of such. An asymmetrical response in the upper extremities suggests hemiparesis, injury to the brachial plexus, or fracture of the clavicle or humerus. Low spinal injury and congenital dislocation of the hip may produce absence of the response in one or both legs.

Certain combinations of findings in infancy suggest specific diagnoses. In a baby with a history of hemolytic disease of the newborn and extreme neonatal jaundice, the presence of the setting sun sign, opisthotonos, and a disappearing or absent Moro response suggest *kernicterus*.

General Indicators of Central Nervous System Disease During Infancy

The following should suggest to the clinician the presence of central nervous system disease:

1. Abnormal localized neurologic findings
2. Asymmetry of movements of extremities
3. Failure to elicit expected infantile automatisms
4. Late persistence of infantile automatisms
5. Reemergence of vanished infantile automatisms
6. Delays in reaching developmental milestones (see Denver Developmental Screening Test, pp. 632–633)

In *congenital hemiplegia*, unilaterally absent or diminished movement of an extremity, along with abnormal posturing, is seen. Reflexes and muscle tone may be normal.

The *spastic diplegias* produce variable dystonic spasms, followed by hypotonia early in infancy and persistent clenched fists coupled with scissoring after the first few months.

Early and Late Childhood

Beyond infancy when the infantile automatisms have disappeared, the neurologic examination is conducted much like the adult examination. Samples of handwriting and figure drawing with both hands help to detect fine motor defects. Capacities for stereognosis, sensing vibration and position, two-point discrimination, number identification, and extinction are not usually testable in the child under 3 years of age and in many under 5 years. Hand preference is demonstrated by age 1 to 2 years and is firmly established by age 5.

The gait should be observed with the child both walking and running. Asymmetric arm movements in walking or running may indicate a hemiparesis, as may unequal wear of the soles and heels of the child's shoes. There are also localized neurologic and orthopedic conditions that may produce unequal shoe wear.

Observe the child rising from the floor from a supine position so that you can note the manner in which the muscles of the neck, trunk, arms, and legs are used to assume the standing position. Normally, the sitting position is first assumed; the legs are then flexed at the knees, while the arms are extended to the side of the body to push off from the floor, gaining an upright position in one smooth motion.

In certain forms of *muscular dystrophy* with pelvic girdle weaknesses, rising from a supine to a standing position is accomplished as shown on p. 703 (*Gower's sign*). Because of weakness of the hip extensor muscles, the child rolls over to a prone position and pushes off

Evidence of neurologic deficits, muscular weaknesses, and orthopedic defects may be detected here that would not otherwise be noted.

the floor with the arms, bringing the legs to a flexed position under the trunk; the legs are extended with the help of the hands and forearms, which push up on the thighs until the upright position is gained.

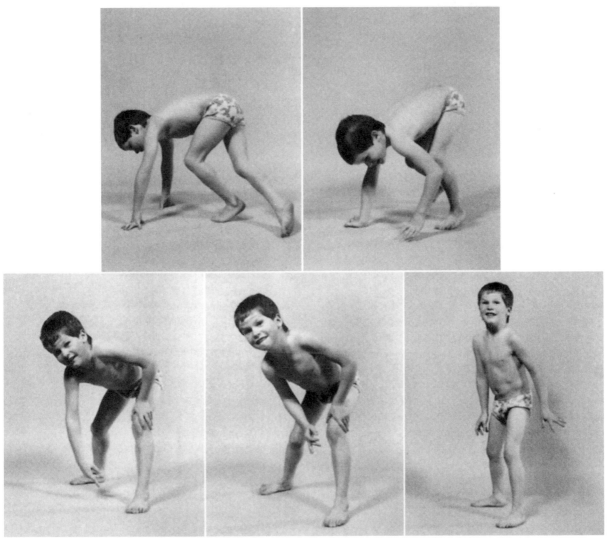

(Reprinted with permission from Swaiman KF: Pediatric Neurology: Principles and Practice. St. Louis, CV Mosby, 1989)

At All Ages

The neurologic examination in infancy and childhood includes elements from the general physical examination as well as the more specific techniques outlined in this section. Correlate all these observations to assess the integrity of the central and peripheral nervous systems. This principle also applies to evaluating adults.

Clinical Thinking: From Data to Plan

Like colors on an artist's palette, clinical data lack form and meaning. The clinician must not only gather data through interviewing and examination; he or she must also analyze them, identify the patient's problems, evaluate the patient's responses to the illness, and, together with the patient, formulate a plan to deal with the situation. This chapter describes this sequence of activities and focuses on the clinical thinking that underlies it.

From Data Base to Plan

Since the introduction of the problem-oriented system of recordkeeping, certain terms have gained wide acceptance. Information given by the patient, or possibly by family members or significant others, is called *subjective data. Objective data* include two kinds of information: physical findings and laboratory reports. Since both physical examination and laboratory work are human activities, they too involve subjective elements, and, as we shall see later, all kinds of data are subject to error. A comprehensive set of subjective and objective data, such as you might gather in evaluating a new patient, makes up a *data base* for that patient.

In recording the data base you should describe your findings as accurately as possible, whether they relate to what the patient tells you or to what you observe. Although inference and interpretation inevitably affect the organization of your materials, statements in the data base should describe, not interpret. Thus, "late inspiratory crackles at the bases of both lungs" is appropriate, while "signs of congestive heart failure" is not.

In the *assessment* process, however, you go beyond perception and description to analysis and interpretation. Here you select and cluster relevant pieces of data, think about their possible meanings, and try to explain them logically. For example, a patient's complaint of a "scratchy throat" and "stuffy nose," together with your observations of a swollen nasal mucosa and slight redness of the pharynx, give you the subjective and objective data on which to base a presumptive diagnosis of viral na-sopharyngitis.

Assessment also includes the patient's responses to the illness and to your diagnostic and therapeutic ideas. What are the patient's feelings, concerns, questions, and goals?

Once you have made these assessments, you are ready to work out a *plan* with the patient. In the problem-oriented record system, this plan has three parts: diagnostic, therapeutic, and educational. For example, you might decide on a throat culture, a decongestant for the patient's stuffy nose, cautionary advice against overfatigue, and a brief review of upper respiratory infections, their causes, and their modes of transmission.

Defining part of the plan as "educational" has one misleading connota-tion—that the process of communication is unidirectional. It should not be. The patient should participate in making the plan. Appropriate "ed-ucation" depends on what the patient already knows and wants to know. Give the patient an opportunity to tell you. Other parts of the plan may well be influenced by the patient's goals, economic means, and competing responsibilities, and the opinions of family or friends—to name just a few variables. Establishing a successful plan requires in-terviewing skills and interpersonal sensitivity, along with knowledge of diagnostic and therapeutic techniques.

The diagram below summarizes the sequence from data base to plan. The effects of the assessment process on the data base, as implied by the bidirectional arrows between them, are discussed later in the chapter.

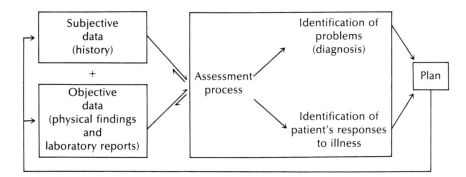

After a plan has been implemented, the process recycles. The clinician gathers more data, assesses the patient's progress, modifies the problem list if indicated, and adjusts the plan appropriately.

Assessment: The Process of Clinical Thinking

Because assessment takes place in the clinician's mind, its processes often seem inaccessible, even mysterious, to the beginning student. Ex-perienced clinicians, moreover, think so quickly, with little overt or con-scious effort, that they sometimes have difficulty in explaining their own logic. They also think in different ways, with different, individual-istic personal styles. Some general principles underlie this analytic process, however, and certain explicit steps may help you to think constructively and purposefully about your data. The thinking process starts at the beginning of your patient encounter, not at the end, but assume for the moment that you already have a data base to consider. You must answer the questions, "What is wrong with the patient? What are the problems?" To do so, try the following steps:

- *Identify the abnormal findings* in the patient's data base. Make a list of the *symptoms* noted by the patient, the *signs* that you observed on physical examination, and any *laboratory reports* that are available to you.

- *Localize these findings anatomically.* This step may be easy. The symptom of scratchy throat and the sign of a reddened pharynx, for example, clearly localize a problem in the pharynx. Other data, however, present greater difficulty. Chest pain, for example, might originate in the heart, the pleural surfaces, the esophagus, or the musculoskeletal system. If the pain consistently occurs with exercise and disappears with rest, either the heart or the musculoskeletal system is probably involved. If the patient notes pain only when carrying groceries with the left arm, the musculoskeletal system becomes the likely culprit. Be as explicit in your localization as your data allow, but no more so. You may have to settle for a body region (e.g., the chest) or a body system (e.g., the musculoskeletal system), or you may be able to define the exact structure involved (e.g., left pectoral muscle). Some symptoms and signs, such as fatigue or fever, have no localizing value but may be useful in the next step.

- *Interpret the findings in terms of the probable process.* A patient's problem may stem from a *pathological* process involving a body structure. There are a number of such processes, variably classified, including congenital, inflammatory, immunologic, neoplastic, metabolic, nutritional, degenerative, vascular, traumatic, and toxic. Other problems are *pathophysiological*, such as increased gastrointestinal motility or congestive heart failure, while others still are *psychopathological*, such as a disorder of mood or of thought processes. Redness and pain are two of the four classic signs of inflammation, and a red, painful throat, even without the other two signs—heat and swelling— strongly suggests an inflammatory process in the pharynx.

- *Make one or more hypotheses about the nature of the patient's problem.* Here you will have to draw on all the knowledge and experience you can muster, and it is here that reading will be most helpful in learning about abnormalities and diseases. Until your experience and knowledge broaden you may not be able to reach highly explicit hypotheses, but proceed as far as you can with the data and knowledge you have. The following steps should help:

  1. *Select the most specific and central findings* around which to construct your hypothesis. If a patient reports loss of appetite, nausea, vom-

iting, fatigue, and fever, for example, and if you find a tender, somewhat enlarged liver and mild jaundice, build your hypothesis around jaundice and hepatomegaly rather than fatigue and fever. Although the other symptoms are useful diagnostically, they are much less specific.

2. Using your inferences about the structures and processes involved, *match your findings against all the conditions you know that can produce them.* For example, you can match your patient's red throat with a list of inflammatory conditions affecting the pharynx; or you can compare the symptoms and signs of the jaundiced patient with the various inflammatory, toxic, and neoplastic conditions that might produce this kind of clinical picture.

3. *Eliminate the diagnostic possibilities that fail to explain the findings.* You might consider conjunctivitis as a cause of the patient's red eye, for example, but eliminate this possibility because it does not explain the dilated pupil or decreased visual acuity. Acute glaucoma would explain all these findings.

4. *Weigh the competing possibilities and select the most likely diagnosis* from among the conditions that might be responsible for the patient's findings. You are looking, of course, for a *close match* between the patient's clinical presentation and a typical case of a given condition. Other clues help in this selection too. The *statistical probability* of a given disease in a patient of this age, sex, ethnic group, habits, lifestyle, and locality should have major impact on your selection. You should consider the possibilities of osteoarthritis and metastatic prostatic cancer in a 70-year-old man with back pain, for example, but not in a 25-year-old woman with the same complaint. The *timing of the patient's illness* also makes a difference. Productive cough, purulent sputum, fever, and chest pain that develop acutely over 24 hours suggest quite a different problem than do identical symptoms that develop over 3 or 4 months. In making a tentative diagnosis, you can seldom reach certainty but must often settle for the most probable explanation. Such is the real world of applied science.

5. Finally, in considering possible explanations for a patient's problem, *give special attention to potentially life-threatening and treatable conditions* such as meningococcal meningitis, bacterial endocarditis, or subdural hematoma. Here you are trying to minimize the risk of missing conditions that may occur less frequently or be less probable but that, if present, would be particularly important.

- Once you have made a hypothesis about a patient's problem, you will usually want to *test that hypothesis.* You may need further history, additional maneuvers on physical examination, or laboratory studies to confirm or rule out your tentative diagnosis. When the diagnosis seems clear-cut—a simple upper respiratory infection, for example, or a case of hives—this step may not be necessary.

- You should then be ready to *establish a working definition of the problem.* Make this at the highest level of explicitness and certainty that the data allow. You may be limited here to a symptom, such as "pleuritic chest pain, cause unknown." At other times you can define a problem explicitly in terms of structure, process, and cause. Examples include "pneumococcal pneumonia, right lower lobe," and "hypertensive cardiovascular disease with left ventricular enlargement, congestive heart failure, and sinus tachycardia."

Difficulties and Variations

Limitations of the Medical Model. Although medical diagnosis is based primarily on identifying abnormal structures, disturbed processes, and specific causes, you will frequently see patients whose complaints do not fall neatly into these categories. Some symptoms defy analysis, and you may never be able to move beyond simple descriptive categories such as "fatigue" or "anorexia." Other problems relate to the patient's life rather than to the body. Events such as loss of a job or loved one threaten a person and may increase the risk of subsequent illness. Identifying such life events, evaluating a person's responses to them, and working out a plan to help the person cope with them are just as appropriate as dealing with the pharyngitis or duodenal ulcer. Health maintenance has become an increasingly important and legitimate item on problem lists for patients. Plans may include, for example, updating immunizations, advice on nutrition, exploring feelings about an important life event, and recommendations for seat belts or exercise.

Single Versus Multiple Problems. One of the greatest difficulties faced by the student is deciding whether to cluster the patient's symptoms and signs into one or into several problems. The patient's *age* may help, since young people are more likely to have single diseases while older people tend to have multiple ones. The *timing* of symptoms is often useful. An episode of pharyngitis 6 weeks ago is probably unrelated to fever, chills, chest pain, and cough today. To use timing effectively, you need to know the natural history of various diseases. A yellowish discharge from the penis followed in 3 weeks by a painless penile ulcer, for example, suggests two problems, gonorrhea and primary syphilis. A penile ulcer followed in 6 weeks by a maculopapular skin rash and generalized lymphadenopathy, on the other hand, suggests two stages of the same problem: primary and secondary syphilis.

Involvement of *different body systems* may help you to cluster the items of data. While symptoms and signs within a single system can often be explained by one disease, manifestations in different, apparently unrelated systems often require more than one explanation. Again, a knowledge of disease patterns is necessary. You might decide, for example, to group a patient's high blood pressure and sustained thrusting apical impulse together with the flame-shaped retinal hemorrhages, place them in the cardiovascular system, and label the constellation "hypertensive cardiovascular disease with hypertensive retinopathy." You will probably develop another explanation for the diarrhea and left lower quadrant tenderness.

Some diseases affect more than one body system. As you gain in knowledge and experience, you will become increasingly adept at recognizing such *multisystem conditions* and at building plausible explanations that link together their seemingly unrelated manifestations. In trying to explain the productive cough, hemoptysis, and weight loss reported by a 60-year-old man who has smoked cigarettes for 40 years, you probably even now would postulate lung cancer as a likely cause. You might even support this hypothesis by your observation of clubbed fingernails. With time you will also recognize that his other symptoms and signs can be linked to the same diagnosis. The dysphagia is caused by extension of the cancer to his esophagus; the pupillary inequality is a Horner's syndrome caused by pressure on the cervical sympathetic chain; and the jaundice results from metastases to the liver.

In another case of multisystem disease, a man's fever, weight loss, chronic diarrhea, dysphagia, white-coated tongue, generalized lymphadenopathy, and purplish skin nodules can all be explained by AIDS. The clinician who has not already explored the patient's risk factors for this disease should do so.

An Unmanageable Array of Data. In trying to understand a patient's problems, the clinician often is confronted with a relatively long list of symptoms and signs and an equally long list of potential explanations or labels. As already suggested, you can tease out separate clusters of observations and deal with them one cluster at a time.

You can also analyze a given group of observations by asking key questions, the answers to which steer your thinking in one direction and allow you to ignore others temporarily. For example, you may ask what produces and relieves a person's chest pain. If the answer is exercise and rest, respectively, you can concentrate on the cardiovascular system (and possibly the musculoskeletal system as well) and put aside the gastrointestinal tract. If the pain results from eating quickly and is relieved by regurgitating the food, you logically concentrate on the upper gastrointestinal tract. A series of such discriminating questions forms a branching logic tree or algorithm and is helpful in collecting data, analyzing them, and reaching conclusions that probably explain them.

Quality of the Data. Virtually all the information with which the clinician works is subject to error. Patients forget symptoms, misremember the sequence in which they occurred, hide important but embarrassing facts, and shape their stories toward what interviewers seem to want to hear. Clinicians misunderstand their patients, overlook some relevant information, fail to ask the one key question, jump to premature diagnostic conclusions, or forget to examine the genitals of a patient with asymptomatic testicular carcinoma. You can avoid some of these errors by being thorough, by keeping an open mind as you gather data, and by analyzing any mistakes that you might make. Clinical data, however, including laboratory work, are inherently imperfect. The quality of information may be judged by its reliability, validity, sensitivity, specificity, and predictive value.

- *Reliability* refers to how well an observation repeatedly gives the same result. This may be measured for one observer or for more than one. If on several occasions one clinician consistently percusses the same span of a patient's liver dullness, *intraobserver reliability* is good. If, on the other hand, several observers find quite different spans of liver dullness on the same patient, *interobserver reliability* is poor.

- *Validity* refers to a close agreement between an observation and the best possible measure of reality. The validity of blood pressures measured by a sphygmomanometer, for example, might be compared with levels obtained by intraarterial tracings.

- *Sensitivity* of an observation or test refers to the proportion of people with a disease (or other condition) who are positive for that disease on a given test (called "true positive"). When the observation or test is negative in a person who has the disease, the result is called "false negative." A highly sensitive test or observation reveals most of the people with a given condition (the true positives) and has few false negatives.

- *Specificity* of an observation or test refers to the proportion of people without a disease or condition who are negative on a given test (called "true negative"). A test that is 95% specific correctly identifies 95 out of 100 normal people. The other 5 are "false positives."

Heart murmurs provide good examples of sensitivity and specificity. The vast majority of patients with significant valvular aortic stenosis have systolic murmurs audible in the aortic area. A systolic murmur is, therefore, quite a sensitive criterion for valvular aortic stenosis. When auscultation for an aortic systolic murmur is used to detect this condition, it reveals most of the cases and misses only a few. The false negative rate is low. Such a murmur, however, sorely lacks specificity. Many other conditions, such as increased blood flow across a normal valve or the sclerotic changes associated with aging, may also produce this kind of murmur. If you were to use an aortic systolic murmur as your sole criterion for aortic stenosis, you would falsely label many patients as having it, thus producing many false positives. In contrast, the high-pitched decrescendo diastolic murmur heard best along the left sternal border is a murmur quite specific for aortic regurgitation. Normal people virtually never have such a murmur, and other conditions that might cause a similar sound are uncommon. The specificity of this murmur is very high.

- *Predictive value* is also a useful clinical tool. In a given population of individuals, a few may have a condition or disease and probably most do not. The clinician who has made an observation or obtained a test result—either positive or negative—wants to know how well this finding predicts the presence or absence of disease.

The *positive predictive value* of an observation or a test is the characteristic that is most relevant to the clinical setting. It refers to the proportion of "true" positive observations in a given population. In a group of women found to have suspicious breast nodules in a cancer screening program, for example, the proportion later determined to have breast cancer would constitute the positive predictive value of "suspicious nodules."

The *negative predictive value* of an observation or test refers to the proportion of "true" negative observations in a population. In a screening program for breast cancer, the proportion of women without suspicious nodules who really have no breast cancer constitutes the negative predictive value of the observation.

Predictive values depend heavily on the prevalence of the condition within the population. For any given sensitivity and specificity, the positive predictive value of an observation rises with increasing prevalence while the negative predictive value falls.

Calculating Sensitivity, Specificity, and Predictive Values. It is helpful to arrange data from an observation or test finding in a 2 × 2 table that shows the results of an observation, either positive or negative, in a group of people with and without the disease. Always using the exact format diagrammed below will allow you to avoid errors in calculating sensitivity and specificity. Note that presence or absence of disease implies use of a "gold standard" to establish whether the disease is truly present. This is usually the best test available, such as a coronary angiogram for coronary artery disease or tissue biopsy for malignancy.

Note that the numbers related to sensitivity and specificity are located in the left and right columns, respectively, and are indicated here by vertical red bars. Numbers related to positive and negative predictive values are found in the upper and lower rows, respectively, and are indicated by horizontal bars. The four boxes in the table are often identified by letters *a* through *d*, shown below in red.

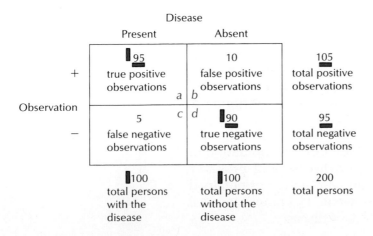

$$\textbf{Sensitivity} = \frac{a}{a+c} = \frac{\text{true positive observations (95)}}{\text{total persons with disease (95 + 5)}} \times 100 = 95\%$$

$$\textbf{Specificity} = \frac{d}{b+d} = \frac{\text{true negative observations (90)}}{\text{total persons without disease (90 + 10)}} \times 100 = 90$$

$$\textbf{Positive predictive value} = \frac{a}{a+b} = \frac{\text{true positive observations (95)}}{\text{total positive observations (95 + 10)}} \times 100 = 90.5\%$$

$$\textbf{Negative predictive value} = \frac{d}{c+d} = \frac{\text{true negative observations (90)}}{\text{total negative observations (90 + 5)}} \times 100 = 94.7\%$$

Two examples further illustrate these principles and show *how predictive values vary with prevalence.* Consider first (*Example 1*) an imaginary population *A* with 1000 people. The prevalence of disease X in this population is high—40%. You can quickly calculate that 400 of these people have X. You then set out to detect these cases with an observation that is 90% sensitive and 80% specific. Of the 400 people with X, the observation reveals .90 × 400, or 360 (the true positives). It misses the other 40 (400 − 360, the false negatives). Out of the 600 people without X, the observation proves negative in .80 × 600, or 480. These people are truly free of X, as the observation suggests (the true negatives). But the observation misleads you in the remaining 120 (600 − 480). These people are falsely labeled as having X when they are really free of it (the false positives). These figures are summarized below:

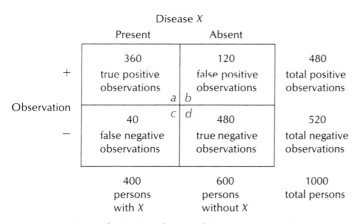

Example 1. Prevalence of Disease X = 40%

As a clinician who does not have perfect knowledge of who really does or does not have disease X, you are faced with a total of 480 people with positive observations. You must try to distinguish between the true and the false positives, and will undoubtedly use additional kinds of data to help you in this task. Given only the sensitivity and specificity of your observation, however, you can determine the probability that a positive observation is a true positive, and you may wish to explain it to the concerned patient. This probability is calculated as follows:

$$\text{Positive predictive value} = \frac{a}{a+b} = \frac{\text{true positives (360)}}{\text{total positives (360 + 120)}} \times 100 = 75\%$$

Thus 3 out of 4 of the persons with positive observations really have the disease, and 1 out of 4 does not.

By a similar calculation, you can determine the probability that a negative observation is a true negative. The results here are reasonably reassuring to the involved patient:

$$\text{Negative predictive value} = \frac{d}{c+d} = \frac{\text{true negatives (480)}}{\text{total negatives (480 + 40)}} \times 100 = 92\%$$

As *prevalence* of the disease in a population diminishes, however, the predictive value of a positive observation diminishes remarkably, while the predictive value of a negative observation rises further. In *Example 2*, in a second population, *B*, of 1000 people, only 1% have disease X. Now there are only 10 cases of X and 990 people without X. If this population is screened with the same observation, which has a 90% sensitivity and an 80% specificity, here are the results:

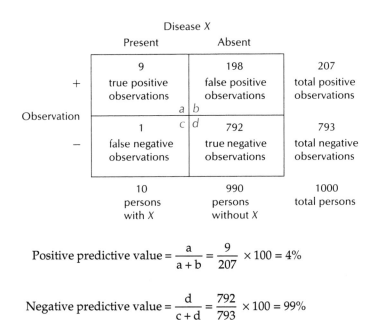

$$\text{Positive predictive value} = \frac{a}{a+b} = \frac{9}{207} \times 100 = 4\%$$

$$\text{Negative predictive value} = \frac{d}{c+d} = \frac{792}{793} \times 100 = 99\%$$

Example 2. Prevalence of Disease X = 1%

You are now confronted with possibly upsetting 207 people (all those with positive observations) in order to detect 9 out of the 10 real cases. The predictive value of a positive observation is only 4%. Improving the specificity of your observation without diminishing its sensitivity would be very helpful, if it were possible. For example, if you could increase the specificity of the observation from 80% to 98% (given the same prevalence of 1% and sensitivity of 90%), the positive predictive value of the observation would improve from 4% to 31%—scarcely ideal but certainly better. Good observations or tests have a sensitivity and specificity of 90%.

The Interplay of Assessment and Data Collection

The concepts of sensitivity and specificity help in both the collection and the analysis of data. They even underlie some of the basic strategies of interviewing. A question that is characterized by high sensitivity, if answered in the affirmative, may be particularly useful for screening and for gathering evidence to support a hypothesis. For example, "Have you had any discomfort or unpleasant feelings in your chest?" is a highly sensitive question for angina pectoris, and in patients with this condition would yield few false negative responses. It is a good first screening question, but because there are many other causes of chest discomfort it is not at all specific. With additional directed questions about location, quality, and duration of the discomfort, you can test further your hypothesis of angina pectoris. A pain that is retrosternal, pressing, and less than 10 minutes in duration—each a reasonably sensitive attribute of angina pectoris but not by itself specific—would add importantly to your growing evidence for the diagnosis. To confirm a hypothesis, a more specific question, if answered in the affirmative, is especially helpful. Precipitation of the pain by exercise and its prompt relief by rest are answers that serve this purpose.

Data with which to test a hypothesis come from the physical examination as well as from the history, and from both you can often screen, build your case, and clinch a diagnosis even before obtaining further diagnostic tests. Consider the following list of evidence: cough, fever, a shaking chill, left-sided chest pain that is aggravated by breathing, and dullness throughout the left lower posterior lung field with crackles, bronchial breathing, and increased voice sounds. Cough and fever are good screening items for pneumonia, the next items support the hypothesis, and bronchial breathing with increased voice sounds in this distribution is very specific for lobar pneumonia. A chest x-ray would confirm the diagnosis.

A negative response to a question or the absence of physical signs is also diagnostically useful, especially when the symptoms or signs are usually positive in a certain condition, i.e., when they have a high sensitivity. For example, if a patient with cough and left-sided pleuritic chest pain does not have fever, bacterial pneumonia becomes much less likely (except possibly in infancy and old age). Likewise, in a patient with severe dyspnea, the absence of orthopnea makes left ventricular failure a less probable explanation for the shortness of breath.

Skilled clinicians use this kind of logic in making assessments whether or not they are conscious of its statistical underpinnings. They often start to generate tentative hypotheses from the patient's identifying data and the chief complaint, and then build evidence for one or more of these hypotheses and discard others as they ask questions and look for physical signs. In developing a present illness they borrow items from other parts of the history, such as the family history, the past history, and the review of systems. If a middle-aged patient complains of chest pain, the skilled clinician does not stop after determining the attributes of the pain. If the pain suggests coronary artery disease, further questions probe the risk factors for this condition such as smoking, high blood pressure, diabetes mellitus, and a family history of the disease. In both history and physical examination, the clinician also focuses explicitly on other possible manifestations of coronary artery disease, such as congestive heart failure, and on evidence of atherosclerosis elsewhere in the body, such as intermittent claudication and diminished or absent pulses in the legs. By generating hypotheses early and by testing them sequentially, experienced clinicians improve their efficiency and enhance the relevance and value of the data they collect. They dig and collect less ore but they find more gold.

Because prevalence strongly affects the predictive value of an observation, prevalence too influences the assessment process. Because coronary artery disease is much more common in middle-aged men than in young women, you should pursue angina as a cause of chest pain more actively in the former group. The effect of prevalence on predictive value explains why your odds of making a correct assessment are better when you hypothesize a common condition rather than a rare one. The combination of fever, headache, myalgias, and cough probably has the same sensitivity and specificity for influenza throughout the year, but your chance of making this diagnosis correctly by using this cluster of symptoms is much greater during a winter flu epidemic than it is during a quiet August.

Prevalence varies importantly with clinical setting as well as with season. Chronic bronchitis is probably the most common cause of hemoptysis among patients seen in a general medical clinic. In the oncology clinic of a tertiary medical center, however, lung cancer might head the list, while in a group of postoperative patients on a general surgical service irritation from an endotracheal tube or pulmonary infarction might be most likely. In certain parts of Asia, in contrast, one should think first of a worm called a lung fluke. When you hear hoofbeats in the distance, according to the familiar saying, bet on horses, not on zebras, unless of course you're visiting the zoo.

While there is enormous value in structuring your data collection so as to test hypotheses, there are also risks. First, initial judgments are often wrong. They allow you to overlook important data and may prevent you from entertaining other, possibly sounder hypotheses. Second, premature formulation of hypotheses may lead you to the premature asking of direct questions, and thus you may miss important parts of the patient's story. Third, focusing in on a single problem may lead you to incomplete assessment. Not every patient needs a complete evaluation, of course, but some have hypertension, some are seriously depressed, and some have cervical cancer. You cannot detect these problems unless you make the proper observations; to do so you have to be reasonably complete.

Developing a Problem List and Plan

Turn now to the history and physical examination recorded for Mrs. N. in Chapter 21. Make a list of her symptoms and signs. Group these items together in a clinically rational way. Note that much of this clustering has already been done in constructing Mrs. N.'s present illness, since headache, nausea, vomiting, and psychological stress have all been placed together. You may or may not agree with this organization. Identify the problems to the degree that you can, and assess the patient's response to her illness.

Make a tentative problem list. In the problem-oriented record system, two parallel columns are used: active problems go on the left, inactive ones on the right. The problem list is placed at the front of the patient's clinical record, and all notes refer to these problems by name and number.

Date problem entered	No.	Active problems	Inactive problems
	1		

For each active problem, develop an initial plan insofar as you can. Some problems, of course, may need no immediate attention. Undoubtedly you will want more information in some areas. Make getting it part of your plan.

The Patient's Record

The clinical record documents the patient's history and physical findings. It shows how clinicians assess the patient, what plans they make on the patient's behalf, what actions they take, and how the patient responds to their efforts. An accurate, clear, well organized record reflects and facilitates sound clinical thinking. It leads to good communication among the many professionals who participate in caring for the patient, and helps to coordinate their activities. It also serves to document the patient's problems and health care for medicolegal purposes.

When creating a record, you do more than simply make a list of what the patient has told you and what you have found on examination. You must review your data, organize them, evaluate the importance and relevance of each item, and construct a clear, concise, yet comprehensive report. If you are a beginner, organizing the present illness will probably constitute one of the most difficult problems because considerable knowledge is needed to cluster related symptoms and physical signs. That muscular weakness, heat intolerance, excessive sweating, diarrhea, and weight loss all constitute a present illness, for example, may not be apparent to either the patient or the student who is unfamiliar with hyperthyroidism. Until your knowledge and judgment grow, the patient's story itself and the seven key attributes of symptoms listed on p. 9 are helpful guides.

Regardless of your experience, certain principles will help you to organize a good record. Order is imperative. Use it consistently and obviously so that future readers, including yourself, can easily find specific points of information. Keep items of history in the history, for example, and do not let them stray into the physical examination. Make your headings clear, use indentations and spacing to accentuate your organization, and asterisk or underline important points. Arrange the present illness in chronologic order, starting with the current episode and then filling in the relevant background information. If a patient with long-standing diabetes is hospitalized in coma, for example, start with the events leading up to the coma and then summarize the past history of the diabetes.

The amount of detail to record often poses a vexing problem. As a student, you may wish (or you may be required) to be quite detailed. This helps to build your descriptive skills, vocabulary, and speed—admittedly a painful, tedious process. Pressures of time, however, will ultimately force some compromises. The following guidelines may be useful in choosing what to record and what to omit:

- *Record all the data*—both positive and negative—*that contribute directly to your assessment.* No diagnosis should be made, no problem identified, unless you have clearly spelled out the data upon which your assessment is based.

- *Describe specifically any pertinent negative information* (i.e., the absence of a symptom or a sign) when other portions of the history or physical examination suggest that an abnormality might exist or develop in that area. For example, if the patient has large and unexplained bruises, you should specifically note the negative history for other kinds of bleeding, for injury and physical violence, for medications and nutritional deficits that might lead to bruising, and for familial bleeding disorders. If a patient feels depressed but not suicidal, state both facts. If the patient has no emotional problems, on the other hand, a comment on suicide is clearly unnecessary.

- *Data not recorded are data lost.* No matter how vividly you can recall a detail today, you will probably not remember it in a few months. The phrase "neurologic exam negative," even in your own handwriting, may leave you wondering a few months hence: "Did I really do a sensory exam?"

- On the other hand, information can be buried in a mass of excessive detail, to be discovered by only the most persistent reader. *Omit most of your negative findings* unless they relate directly to the patient's complaints or to specific exclusions in your diagnostic assessment. Do not try to list all the abnormalities that you did *not* observe. Instead, concentrate on a few major ones (such as "no heart murmurs") and try to describe structures in a concise, positive way. "Cervix pink and smooth" indicates that you saw no redness, ulcers, nodules, masses, cysts, or other suspicious lesions, but the description is shorter and much more readable. You can even omit certain body structures despite the fact that you examined them. You may thus leave out normal eyebrows and eyelashes even though you looked at them.

- Save valuable time and space by omitting superfluous words. *Avoid redundancies* such as those in parentheses in the following examples: pink (in color), resonant (by percussion), tender (to palpation), both (right and left) ears, (audible) murmur, and (bilaterally) symmetrical thorax. Repetitive introductory phrases such as "The patient reports no . . ." are also redundant and may be omitted. Unless you have indicated otherwise, readers will assume that the patient gave you the history. *Use short words* instead of long and probably fancier ones when they mean the same thing: "felt" for "palpated" and "heard" for "auscultated." Try to *describe what you observed, not what you did.*

"Optic discs seen" may mark an exciting moment in your career when you first glimpsed them, and it may be all you can claim during your first few tries at an ophthalmoscopic examination. "Disc margins sharp," however, adds important information with only two additional letters.

- *Be objective.* Hostility, moralizing comments, and disapproval have no place in the patient's record, whether conveyed in words, penmanship, or punctuation. Notes such as "PATIENT DRUNK AND LATE TO CLINIC AGAIN!!" tell more about the writer than about the patient and, furthermore, might prove embarrassing in court.

Because records are scientific and legal documents, they should be understandable. Employ abbreviations and symbols only if they are commonly used and understood. Some clinicians may wish to develop an elegant style, and should certainly be encouraged to do so. Time is usually scarce, however, and style may be sacrificed in favor of concise completeness. It is common to use words and brief phrases instead of whole sentences. Legibility is essential. Otherwise, all that you have done is worthless to potential readers.

Diagrams add greatly to the clarity of the record. Two examples follow:

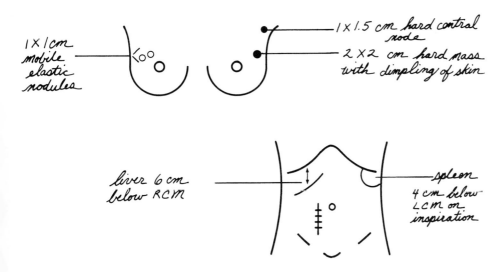

Make measurements in centimeters, not in fruits, vegetables, or nuts. "Pea-sized" and "walnut-sized" lesions preclude accurate evaluations and future comparisons. How big were the peas? Did the walnut have a shell?

You should write the record as soon as possible, before the data fade from your memory. In your initial attempts at interviewing, you will probably prefer just to take notes when talking with a patient. As you gain experience, however, work toward recording in final form the past medical history, family history, and review of systems during the interview. Leave spaces for filling in later the present illness, the psychosocial history, and any other complex areas. During a physical examination it is wise to record immediately specific measurements such as the blood pressures in three positions. Recording a large number of items and descriptions interrupts the flow of the examination, however, and you will soon learn to remember your findings and record them after you have finished.

Recording the history and physical examination is simplified by printed forms. If your institution or agency provides them, you may be expected to use them. You should also, however, be able to create your own record. The example that follows offers one moderately complete guide. Although it is longer than most you may see in patients' charts, it still does not reflect every question and technique that you have learned to use.

Note the difference in the statements that introduce the history and the physical examination. The basic identifying data start the history, while a descriptive paragraph that summarizes your general survey begins the physical examination.

Unless forms are used and carefully followed, records are not exactly alike in detail. Detail varies appropriately with the patient's symptoms and signs and with the clinician's diagnostic thoughts about them. In this record, additional pertinent negatives are sometimes listed when an abnormality is described. Because of the edema and varicose veins, for example, the clinician also reported "No stasis pigmentation or ulcers." If there had been neither edema nor varicose veins, these comments would not have been necessary.

Mrs. Audrey N., 1463 Maple Blvd., Capital City
11/13/97
Mrs. N. is a 54-year-old, widowed, white saleswoman, born in the U.S.

Referral. None

Source. Self, seems reliable

Chief Complaint. Headaches

Present Illness. For about 3 mo Mrs. N. has been increasingly troubled by headaches: bifrontal, usually aching, occasionally throbbing, mild to moderately severe. She has missed work only once because of headaches, when she felt nauseated and vomited several times. Otherwise, nausea is rare. Headaches now average once a wk, usually are present on waking and last all day. They are relieved by lying down and using a cold wet towel on head. Little relief from aspirin. No other related symptoms, no local weakness, no numbness or visual symptoms

"Sick headaches" with nausea and vomiting began at age 15, recurred through her mid-20s, then diminished to one every 2 or 3 mo and almost disappeared.

Has recently had increased pressure at work from a new and demanding boss, and is also worried about her daughter (see personal and social history). Thinks her headaches may be like those in the past, but wants to be sure because her mother died of a stroke. Concerned that they make her irritable with her family. Regular meals. Drinks three cups of coffer per day, cola at night.

Medications. Aspirin for headaches, multivitamins. "Water pill" at times for ankle swelling, none recently. *Allergies.* Ampicillin causes rash.

Past History

General Health. Good

Childhood Illnesses. Only measles and chickenpox

Adult Illnesses. Medical: Acute kidney infection 1982 with fever and right flank pain; treated with ampicillin. Generalized rash with itching developed several days later. Kidney x-rays said to be normal; infection has not recurred. Surgical: Tonsillectomy, age 6, appendectomy, age 13. ObGyn: G2, P2, 3 living children. Menarche age 12. Last menses 6 months ago. No concerns about HIV infection. Psychiatric: None

Accidents and Injuries. Stepped on glass at beach, 1991, laceration sutured, healed

Transfusions. None

Current Health Status. Tobacco. About 1 pack cigs per day from age 18 (36 pack yr)[†]. *Alcohol/Drugs.* Rare drink (wine) only. No drugs.

Exercise/Leisure. "No time." *Diet.* Low in calcium with little milk or cheese. Mid-morning and evening snacks. *Sleep.* Generally good, average 7 hr, sometimes has trouble falling asleep, is awakened by alarm.

Immunizations. Oral polio vaccine, yr uncertain; tetanus shots × 2 1991, followed with booster 1 yr later; flu vaccine 11/93, no reaction.

Screening Tests. Last pap smear 1991, normal. No mammograms.

---

*Asterisk or underline important points.
[†](Age 54 yr − 18 yr) × (1 pack) = 36 pack yr

Safety Measures. Uses seat belt regularly. Uses sunblock. *Hazards.* Medications kept in unlocked medicine cabinet. Cleaning solutions, furniture polish, and Drano in unlocked cabinet below sink. Mr. N's shotgun, with box of shells, in upstairs closet.

Family History
(There are two methods of recording the family history. The diagrammatic format is more helpful than the narrative in tracing genetic disorders. The negative family information follows either format.)

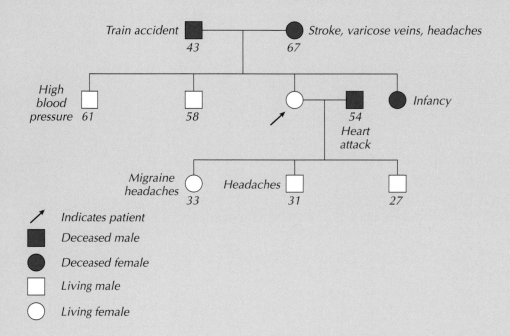

Indicates patient

◼ Deceased male

● Deceased female

☐ Living male

○ Living female

Outline

Father died, 43, train accident
Mother died, 67, stroke; had varicose veins, headaches
One brother, 61, has high blood pressure, otherwise well
One brother, 58, apparently well except for mild arthritis
One sister, died in infancy, ?cause
Husband died, 54, heart attack
Daughter, 33, "migraine headaches," otherwise well
Son, 31, headaches
Son, 27, well

No family history of diabetes, tuberculosis, heart or kidney disease, cancer, anemia, epilepsy, or mental illness

Personal and Social History. Born and raised in Lake City, finished high school, married at age 19. Worked as a clerk in store for 2 yr, then moved with husband to Capital City, had 3 children. Mr. N. had a fairly steady factory job, but to help with the family income Mrs. N. went back to work 15 yr ago. Children all married. 4 yr ago Mr. N. died suddenly of a heart attack, leaving little savings and no insurance. Finances now tight. Has moved to small apartment to be near daughter, Dorothy. Dorothy's husband, Arthur, has a drinking problem and is verbally though not physically abusive. Mrs. N.'s apartment serves as a haven for Dorothy and her 2 children, Kevin, 6 yr, and Linda, 3 yr. Mrs. N. feels responsible for helping them, is tense and nervous, but denies depression. She has a few good friends but doesn't like to bother them with her family's trouble. "I'd rather keep it to myself. I don't like gossip." No church or other organizational support

Typically up at 7:00 a.m., works 9:00 to 5:30, eats dinner alone. Dorothy or the children visit most evenings and weekends. Moderate number of squabbles and considerable strain

Review of Systems

General. Has <u>gained</u> about <u>10 lb</u> in the past 4 yr

Skin. No rashes or other changes

Head. See present illness. No head injury

Eyes. Reading glasses for 5 yr, last checked 1 yr ago. No symptoms

Ears. Hearing good. No tinnitus, vertigo, infections

Nose, Sinuses. Occasional mild cold. No hay fever, sinus trouble

Mouth and Throat. Some <u>bleeding of gums</u> recently. Last to dentist 2 yr ago. Occasional canker sore, has had one for 4 days

Neck. No lumps, goiter, pain

Breasts. No lumps, pain, discharge. Does breast self-exams sporadically

Respiratory. No cough, wheezing, pneumonia, tuberculosis. Last chest x-ray 1986, St. Mary's Hospital, normal

Cardiac. No known heart disease or high blood pressure; last blood pressure taken in 1992. No dyspnea, orthopnea, chest pain, palpitations. No ECG

GI. Appetite good; no nausea, vomiting, indigestion. Bowel movement about once daily though sometimes has <u>hard stools for 2–3 d when especially tense</u>; no diarrhea or bleeding. No pain, jaundice, gallbladder or liver trouble

Urinary. No frequency, dysuria, hematuria or recent flank pain; nocturia × 1, large volume. <u>Occasionally loses some urine</u> when coughs hard

Genital. No vaginal or pelvic infections. No dyspareunia. Little interest in sex now. Not sexually active.

Musculoskeletal. Mild <u>aching low back pain</u> often after a long day's work; no radiation down legs; used to do back exercises, but not now. No other joint pain

Peripheral Vascular. <u>Varicose veins</u> appeared in both legs during first pregnancy. Has had swollen ankles after prolonged standing for 10 yr; wears light elastic pantyhose; tried "water pill" 5 mo ago but it didn't help much; no history of phlebitis or leg pain

Neurologic. No faints, seizures, motor or sensory loss. Memory good

Hematologic. Except for bleeding gums, no easy bleeding. No anemia

Endocrine. No known thyroid trouble, temperature intolerance. Sweating average. No symptoms or history of diabetes

Psychiatric. See present illness and personal and social history

Physical Examination

Mrs. N. is a short, moderately obese, middle-aged woman who walks and moves easily and responds quickly to questions. She wears no makeup but her hair is fixed neatly and her clothes are immaculate. Although her ankles are swollen, her color is good and she lies flat without discomfort. She talks freely but is somewhat tense, with moist, cold hands.

    P 94, regular R 18 Temp 37.1°C (oral)
    BP 164/98 right arm, lying
        160/96 left arm lying
        152/88 right arm, lying (wide cuff)
    Ht (without shoes) 157 cm (5'2")
    Wt (dressed) 65 kg (143 lb)

Skin. Palms cold and moist, but color good. Scattered cherry angiomas over the upper trunk

Head. Hair of average texture. Scalp without lesions, skull intact

Eyes. Vision 20/30 in each eye. Visual fields full by confrontation. Conjunctiva pink. Sclera white. Pupils round, regular, equal, react to light.

Extraocular movements intact. Disc margins sharp. No arterial narrowing, A–V nicking

Ears. Wax partially obscures right drum. Left canal clear and drum negative. Acuity good (to whispered voice). Weber midline. AC > BC

Nose. Mucosa pink, septum midline. No sinus tenderness

Mouth. Mucosa pink. Several interdental papillae red and slightly swollen. Teeth in good repair. Tongue midline, with a (3 x 4 mm) shallow, white ulcer on a red base, located on the undersurface near the tip; it is slightly tender but not indurated. Tonsils absent. Pharynx negative

Neck. Trachea midline. Thyroid isthmus barely palpable, lobes not felt

Lymph Nodes. Small (< 1 cm), soft, nontender, and mobile tonsillar and posterior cervical nodes bilaterally. No axillary or epitrochlear nodes. Several small inguinal nodes bilaterally—soft and nontender

Thorax and Lungs. Thorax symmetrical. Good expansion. Lungs resonant. Breath sounds vesicular with no added sounds

Cardiovascular. Jugular venous pressure 1 cm above the sternal angle, with head of bed raised to 30°. Carotid upstrokes brisk, without bruits, and symmetrical. Apical impulse discrete and tapping, barely palpable in the 5th left interspace 8 cm from the midsternal line. Physiologic split of S_2. No S_3 or S_4. A 2/6 medium-pitched midsystolic murmur at the 2nd right interspace; does not radiate to the neck. Diastole clear

Breasts. Large, pendulous, symmetrical. No masses. Nipples erect and without discharge

Abdomen. Obese, but symmetrical. Well healed right lower quadrant scar. Bowel sounds normal. Sigmoid colon slightly tender, no other masses or tenderness. Liver span 7 cm in right midclavicular line; edge smooth and palpable 1 cm below right costal margin. Splenic percussion sign negative. Spleen and kidneys not felt. No CVA tenderness

Genitalia. Vulva normal. Mild cystocele on straining. Vaginal mucosa pink. Cervix parous, pink, without discharge. Uterus anterior, midline, smooth, not enlarged. Adnexa difficult to feel because of obesity and poor relaxation. No cervical or adnexal tenderness. Pap smears taken. Recto-vaginal exam unremarkable

Rectal. No masses. Brown stool, negative for occult blood

Peripheral Vascular. 2+ edema of feet and ankles with 1+ edema extending up to just below knees. Moderate varicosities of saphenous veins bilaterally from mid-thigh to ankles, with spider veins on both lower legs. No stasis pigmentation or ulcers. No calf tenderness

Pulses:

	Radial	Femoral	Popliteal	Dorsalis Pedis	Posterior Tibial
RT	N	N	N	↓	N
LT	N	N	N	0	N

Musculoskeletal. No joint deformities. Good range of motion in hands, wrists, elbows, shoulders, spine, hips, knees, ankles

Neurologic

Mental Status. Tense but alert and cooperative. Thought coherent. Oriented. Cognitive testing not done in detail

Cranial Nerves. See head and neck. Also—

I—Not tested
V—Sensation intact, strength good
VII—Facial movement good
XI—Sternomastoids and trapezii strong

Motor. Normal muscle bulk and tone. Strength 5/5 throughout. Rapid alternating movements and point-to-point movements intact. Gait normal. No pronator drift

Sensory. Romberg negative. Pinprick, light touch, position, vibration, and stereognosis intact

Reflexes. (Two methods of recording may be used, depending upon personal preference: a tabular form or a stick figure diagram, as shown below and at right.)

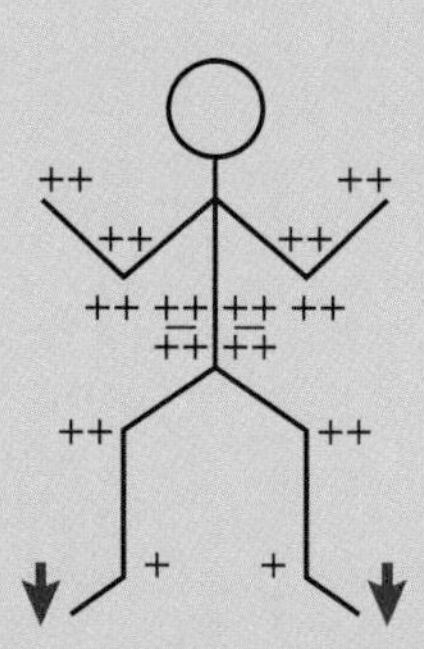

	Biceps	Triceps	Sup	Abd	Knee	Ankle	Pl
RT	2+	2+	2+	2+/2+	2+	1+	↓
LT	2+	2+	2+	2+/2+	2+	1+	↓

Before reading farther, assess Mrs. N.'s symptoms and physical findings. Then construct your own problem list for Mrs. N., as suggested in Chapter 20.

One way to organize Mrs. N.'s problem list is shown below. The clinician constructed the following problem list for Mrs. N. and placed it at the front of the chart. When a new assessment indicates changing the name of a problem, the original name is crossed out and a new name is given to the old number.

Date Problem Entered	No.	Active Problems	Inactive Problems
11/13/97	1	Migraine headaches	
11/13/97	2		Acute kidney infection
11/13/97	3	Allergy to ampicillin	
11/13/97	4	Tensions secondary to family situation, finances, and stress at work	
11/13/97	5	Gingivitis	
11/13/97	6	Low back pain	
11/13/97	7	Varicose veins with venous insufficiency	
11/13/97	8	Cystocele with occasional stress incontinence	
11/13/97	9	Possible high blood pressure	
11/13/97	10	Diet high in calories, fat, and carbohydrates, low in calcium	
11/13/97	11	Home hazards: kitchen supplies, medicines, gun	

Different clinicians often organize somewhat different problem lists for the same patient, and yours probably does not agree exactly with this one. Good lists vary in their emphases, length, and detail according to many factors, including clinicians' philosophies, specialties, and perceptions of their role in the care of the patient. The list illustrated here includes problems that need some attention now (such as the headaches) or may need further observation or possible future attention (such as the blood pressure and cystocele). The allergy is listed as an active problem to warn against inadvertent future prescriptions of penicillins.

A few items noted in the history and physical examination, such as canker sores and hard stools, do not appear in this problem list because they are relatively common phenomena that do not seem to demand attention. Such judgments may be wrong. Problem lists that are cluttered with relatively insignificant items, however, diminish in value. Some clinicians would undoubtedly judge this list too long; others would bring greater explicitness to problems such as "tensions," "diet," and "gingivitis."

The patient's record included notes on two of Mrs. N.'s problems:

1. Migraine headaches

   Assessment. Supporting this diagnosis are "sick headaches" in earlier life, recurrent course of headaches, their duration, their relief by cold and quiet, associated nausea and vomiting (once at least), and positive family history. Further, no related neurologic symptoms or signs. Headaches may be somewhat more frequent than typical migraine headaches, pain is usually aching rather than throbbing, and there are obvious tensions at work and at home. Tension headaches should also be considered, therefore, but the headaches fit this pattern less well.

   Plan
   Diagnostic. Observation only. Mrs. N. to look for possible precipitating factors.
   Therapeutic. Continue aspirin as needed.
   Education. Nature of migraine discussed. Patient pleased and relieved

9. Possible high blood pressure

   Assessment. Some of apparent elevation clearly related to obese arms, and some may be related to anxiety of a first visit. No evidence of target organ damage

   Plan
   Diagnostic. Repeat BP in one month. Use wide cuff. Urinalysis
   Therapeutic. None now. Consider diet change on next visit.
   Education. Need for BP checks explained

A month later Mrs. N. returned for a second visit. Part of the progress notes read as follows:

1. Migraine headaches

   Subjective (S). Has had only 2 headaches, both mild, without associated symptoms. No longer worried about them. Cannot detect any precipitating factors
   Objective (O). Not reexamined
   Assessment (A). Improved
   Plan (P). Return as needed.

4. Tensions

S. Dorothy is now attending Al-Anon meetings and tensions at home seem somewhat better.
O. Mrs. N. is more relaxed today.
A. Somewhat improved.
P. Encouraged to discuss situation with me as needed

9. Possible high blood pressure

S. None
O. BP 146/84 right arm, lying (wide cuff). Urinalysis normal
A. If systolic pressure is high next time, it will indicate isolated systolic hypertension.
P. Repeat BP in 6 months.

Although you have insufficient information about most of Mrs. N.'s other problems, including her own priorities, try to develop an approach to them. What further data do you need?

What information do you need and how do you obtain it? These questions appear implicitly in Chapter 1 and continue throughout the book—and long afterward. The process of learning about a patient continues far beyond the first encounter, and understanding grows in depth, complexity, and fascination. Although your knowledge of Mrs. N. is incomplete, you know a great deal about her and have the tools with which to expand your knowledge further. Needed now is repetitive practice, with supervision, in polishing your newly acquired skills.

Bibliography

General References

Anatomy and Physiology

Agur, AMR: Grant's Atlas of Anatomy, 9th ed. Baltimore, Williams & Wilkins, 1991.

Berne RM, Levy MN (eds): Physiology, 3rd ed. St. Louis, Mosby–Year Book, 1993.

Guyton AC: Textbook of Medical Physiology, 9th ed. Philadelphia, WB Saunders, 1996.

Moore KL: Clinically Oriented Anatomy, 3rd ed. Baltimore, Williams & Wilkins, 1992.

Netter FH: Atlas of Human Anatomy. New Jersey, Ciba-Geigy Corp, 1989.

Williams PL: Gray's Anatomy, 38th ed. New York, Churchill Livingstone, 1995.

Medicine, Surgery, and Physical Examination

Barker LR, Burton, JR, Zieve PD: Principles of Ambulatory Medicine, 4th ed. Baltimore, Williams & Wilkins, 1995.

Clain A (ed): Hamilton Bailey's Demonstration of Physical Signs in Clinical Surgery, 17th ed. Bristol, England, John Wright, 1986.

Fauci AS, Braunwald E, Isselbacher KJ, et al (eds): Harrison's Principles of Internal Medicine, 14th ed. New York, McGraw-Hill, 1998.

Judge RD, Zuidema GD, Fitzgerald FT (eds): Clinical Diagnosis: A Physiologic Approach, 5th ed. Boston, Little, Brown & Co, 1989.

Kelley WN (ed): Textbook of Internal Medicine, 3rd ed. Philadelphia, Lippincott-Raven, 1997.

Mandell GL, Mildran D (eds): AIDS (Vol I) in Atlas of Infectious Diseases New York, Churchill Livingstone, 1997.

Noble J, Greene HL, Levinson W, Modest GA, Young MJ (eds): Primary Care Medicine, 2nd ed. St. Louis, Mosby, 1996.

Sabiston DC Jr (ed): Textbook of Surgery: The Biological Basis of Modern Surgical Practice, 15th ed. Philadelphia, WB Saunders, 1997.

Sapira JD: The Art and Science of Bedside Diagnosis. Baltimore, Urban & Schwarzenberg, 1990.

Schwartz SI (ed): Principles of Surgery, 6th ed. New York, McGraw-Hill, 1994.

Walker HK, Hall WD, Hurst JW: Clinical Methods: The History, Physical, and Laboratory Examinations, 3rd ed. Boston, Butterworths, 1990.

Wyngaarden JB, Smith LH Jr, Bennett JC (eds): Cecil Textbook of Medicine, 20th ed. Philadelphia, WB Saunders, 1996.

Youngkin EQ, Davis MS: Women's Health: A Primary Care Clinical Guide. Norwalk, CT, Appleton and Lange, 1994.

Changes with Age

Adolescents

Freidman SB, Fisher M, Schonberg SK, Alderman EM (eds): Comprehensive Adolescent Health Care, 2nd ed. St. Louis, Mosby, 1998.

McAnarney ER, Kriepe RE, Orr DP, Comerci GD (eds): Textbook of Adolescent Medicine. Philadelphia, WB Saunders, 1992.

Older Persons

Hazzard WR, Bierman EL, Blass JP, et al: Principles of Geriatric Medicine and Gerontology, 3rd ed. New York, McGraw-Hill, 1994.

Kane RL, Ouslander JG, Abrass IB: Essentials of Clinical Geriatrics, 3rd ed. New York, McGraw-Hill, 1994.

Lachs MS, Feinstein AR, Cooney LM Jr, et al: A simple procedure for general screening for functional disability in elderly patients. Ann Intern Med 112:699, 1990.

Schectel SM, Fleming KC, Chulka DS, Evans JM: Geriatric Health Maintenance. Mayo Clin Proc 71:289, 1996.

Health Promotion and Counseling

American Nurses Association: Clinician's Handbook on Preventive Services: Put Prevention into Practice. Waldorf, MD, American Nurses Publishing, 1994.

Gardner P, Eickhoff T, Poland GA et al: Adult Immunizations. Ann Intern Med 12:35, 1996.

Henrahan JP, Sherman CB, Bresnets EA, et al: Cigarette smoking and health. Official statement of American Thoracic Society. Am J Respir Crit Care 153:861, 1996.

U.S. Preventive Services Task Force: Guide to Clinical Preventive Services, 2nd ed. Baltimore, Williams & Wilkins, 1996.

Woolf SH, Jonas S, Lawrence RS: Health Promotion and Disease Prevention in Clinical Practice. Baltimore, Williams & Wilkins, 1996.

Chapter 1. Interviewing and the Health History

Angelou M: I Know Why the Caged Bird Sings. New York, Bantam Books, 1971:21–27. [*Memories of a woman*]

Beckman HB, Frankel RM: The effect of physician behavior on the collection of data. Ann Intern Med 101:693, 1984.

Billings JA, Stoeckle JD: The Clinical Encounter: A Guide to the Medical Interview and Case Presentation. Chicago, Year Book Medical Publishers, 1989.

Bird J, Cohen-Cole SA: The three-function model of the medical interview. Adv Psychosom Med. 65:20, 1990.

Conant EB: Addressing patients by their first names. N Engl J Med 308:226, 1983. [*A patient's view*]

Delbanco TL: Enriching the doctor–patient relationship by inviting the patient's perspective. Ann Intern Med 116:414, 1992.

Engel GL, Morgan WL Jr: Interviewing the Patient. Philadelphia, WB Saunders, 1973.

Heller ME: Addressing patients by their first names. N Engl J Med 308:1107, 1987. [*Short report of a survey of obstetrical outpatients*]

The Skills of Quality Interviewing

Branch WT, Malik TK: Using 'windows of opportunities' in brief interviews to understand patients' concerns. JAMA 269:1667, 1993.

Brown JB, Weston WW, Stewart AM: Patient-centred interviewing, Part I: Understanding patients' experiences. Can Fam Physician 147:35, 1989.

Brown JB, Weston WW, Stewart AM: Patient-centred interviewing, Part II: Finding common ground. Can Fam Physician 153:35, 1989.

Smith RC: The Patient's Story, Integrated Patient–Doctor Interviewing. Boston, Little, Brown Co, 1996.

Waitzkin H: Doctor–patient communication: Clinical implications of social scientific research. JAMA 252:2441, 1984.

Challenges to the Clinician

American Academy of Addiction Psychiatry: Supplement to the American Journal on Addictions: Identification and Treatment of Substance Abuse in Primary Care Settings. Vol 5(4), 1996.

Council on Ethical and Judicial Affairs, AMA: Sexual misconduct in the practice of medicine. JAMA 266:2741, 1991.

Council on Scientific Affairs, AMA: Health care needs of gay men and lesbians in the U.S. JAMA 275:1354, 1996.

Cyr MG, Wartman SA: The effectiveness of routine screening questions in the detection of alcoholism. JAMA 259:51, 1988.

Drugs that cause sexual dysfunction: An update. Med Lett Drugs Ther 34:73, 1992.

Ewing JA: Detecting alcoholism: The CAGE Questionnaire. JAMA 252:1905, 1984.

Fleming MF, Barry KL: Practical Guide for the Treatment of Substance Abuse. St. Louis, Mosby–Year Book, 1992.

Freeman MG: The sexual history. In Walker HK, Hall WD, Hurst JW: Clinical Methods: The History, Physical, and Laboratory Examinations, 3rd ed. Boston, Butterworths, 1990.

Gabbard GO, Nadelson C: Professional boundaries in the physician–patient relationship. JAMA 273:1445, 1995.

Harrison AE: Primary care of lesbian and gay patients: Educating ourselves and our students. Family Medicine 28:10, 1996.

Helman CG: Culture Health and Illness, 3rd ed. Oxford, England, Butterworth & Heinemann, 1994.

Kleinman A, Eisenberg L, Good B: Culture, illness, and care: Clinical lessons from anthropologic and cross-cultural research. Ann Intern Med 88:251, 1978.

Mayfield D, McLeod G, Hall P: The CAGE Questionnaire: Validation of a new alcoholism screening instrument. Am J Psychiatry 131:1121, 1974.

Spitzer RL, Williams JB, Kroenke K, et al: Utility of a new procedure for diagnosing mental disorders in primary care. JAMA 272:1749, 1994.

Zimmerman M: Diagnosing DSM-IV Psychiatric Disorders in Primary Care Settings: An Interview Guide for the Nonpsychiatrist Physician. Rhode Island, Psych Products Press, 1994.

Patients at Different Ages

Kubler-Ross E: On Death and Dying. New York, Macmillan, 1997.

McDaniel SH, Campbell TL, Seaburn DB: Family Oriented Primary Care: A Manual for Medical Providers. New York, Springer-Verlag, 1990.

Nuland SB: How We Die: Reflections on Life's Final Chapter. New York, Alfred A. Knopf, 1994.

Situations That Call for Specific Responses

Davis TC, Long SW, Jackson RH, et al: Rapid estimate of adult literacy in medicine: A shortened screening instrument. Family Medicine 25:391, 1993.

Goldoft M: A piece of mind: Another language. JAMA 268:23, 1992.

Mayeaux EJ, Murphy PW, Arnold C, et al: Improving patient education for patients with low literacy skills. Amer Fam Phys 53:205, 1996.

Putsch RW: Cross-cultural communication: The special case of interpreters in health care: JAMA 254:3344, 1985.

Chapter 2. An Approach to Symptoms

For most symptoms in this chapter, refer also to the relevant references in later chapters and the textbooks of general medicine and surgery.

Alpert JS: The patient with angina: The importance of careful listening. J Am Coll Cardiol 11:27, 1988.

Calkins H, Shyr Y, Frumin H, et al: The value of the clinical history in the differentiation of syncope due to ventricular tachycardia, atrioventricular block and neurocardiogenic syncope. Am J Med 98:365, 1995.

Deyo RA, Rainville J, Kent DL: What can the history and physical examination tell us about low back pain? JAMA 268:760, 1992.

Douglas PS, Ginsburg GS: The evaluation of chest pain in women. N Engl J Med 334:1311, 1996.

Kost RG, Straus SE: Posttherapeutic neuralgia—pathogenesis, treatment, and prevention. N Engl J Med 335:32, 1996.

Kroenke K, Lucas CA, Rosenberg ML, et al: Causes of persistent dizziness: A prospective study of 100 patients in ambulatory care. Ann Intern Med 117:898, 1992.

Kupfer DJ, Reynolds CF: Management of insomnia. N Engl J Med 336:341, 1997.

Moore, AA, Siu AI: Screening for common problems in ambulatory elderly: Clinical confirmation of a screening instrument. Am J Med 100:438, 1996.

Nathan DM: Long-term complications of diabetes mellitus. N Engl J Med 328:1676, 1993.

Sager MA, Franke T, Inouye S et al: Functional outcomes of acute medical illness and hospitalization in older persons. Arch Intern Med 156:645, 1996.

Solomon S: Diagnosis of primary headache disorders. Neuro Clinics 15: 15, 1997.

Talbot, Land-Curtis L: The challenges of assessing skin indicators in people of color. Home Healthcare Nurse 14:167, 1996.

Chapter 3. Mental Status

American Psychiatric Association: Diagnostic and Statistical Manual of Mental Disorders, 4th ed. Washington DC, American Psychiatric Association, 1994.

Beck AT, Ward CH, Mendelson M, Mock T, Erbaugh T: An Inventory for Measuring Depression. Arch Gen Psychiatry 4:561, 1961.

Carpenter WT Jr, Buchanan RW: Schizophrenia. N Engl J Med 330:681, 1994.

Cummings JL, Coffey E: Textbook of Geriatric Neuropsychiatry. Washington DC, The American Psychiatric Press, 1994.

Damasio AR: Aphasia. N Engl J Med 326:531, 1992.

Fleming KC, Adams AC, Petersen RC: Dementia: Diagnosis and evaluation. Mayo Clin Proc 70:1093, 1995.

Fogel BS, Schiffer RB (eds): Neuropsychiatry. Baltimore, Williams & Wilkins, 1996.

Folstein M, Folstein SE, McHugh PR: Mini-mental state. J Psych Res 12:189, 1975.

Geldmacher DS, Whitehouse PJ: Evaluation of dementia. N Engl J Med 335:330, 1996.

Hales RE, Hilty DA, Hise MG: A treatment algorithm for the management of anxiety. J Clin Psychiatry 58 (Suppl 3):76, 1997.

Hales RE, Yudofsky SC, Talbott JA: The American Psychiatric Press Textbook of Psychiatry, 2nd ed. Washington, DC, The American Psychiatric Press, 1994.

Kaplan HI, Sadock BJ, Grebb JA: Kaplan and Sadock's Synopsis of Psychiatry, 7th ed. Baltimore, Williams & Wilkins, 1994.

Kroenke K, Spitzer RL, Willans JBW, et al: Physical symptoms in primary care: Predictors of psychiatric disorders and functional impairment. Arch Fam Med 3:774, 1993.

Lipowski ZJ: Delirium in the elderly patient. N Engl J Med 320:578, 1989.

Some drugs that cause psychiatric symptoms. Med Lett Drugs Ther 40:21, 1998.

Spitzer RL, Williams JBW, Kroenke K, et al: Utility of a new procedure for diagnosing mental disorders in primary care: The PRIME-MD 1,000 study. JAMA 272:1749, 1994.

Waldinger RJ: Psychiatry for Medical Students, 3rd ed. Washington DC, American Psychiatric Press, 1996.

Chapter 4. Physical Examination: Approach and Overview

Oboler SK, LaForce FM: The periodic physical examination in asymptomatic adults. Ann Intern Med 110:214, 1989.

Sackett DL: A primer on the precision and accuracy of the clinical examination. JAMA 267:2638, 1992.

Schneiderman H, Peixoto AJ: Bedside Diagnosis, 3rd ed. Philadelphia, American College of Physicians, 1997.

Sox HC Jr: Preventive Services Task Force: Guide to Clinical Preventive Services: An Assessment of the Effectiveness of 169 Interventions. Baltimore, Williams & Wilkins, 1989.

Chapter 5. The General Survey

Andres R, Muller DC, Sorkin JD: Long-term effects of change in body weight on all-cause mortality: A review. Ann Intern Med 119:737, 1993.

Blair SN, Shaten J, Brownell K, et al: Body weight change, all-cause mortality, and cause-specific mortality in the Multiple Risk Factor Intervention Trial. Ann Intern Med 119:749, 1993.

Pamuk ER, Williamson DF, Serdula MK, et al: Weight loss and subsequent death in a cohort of U.S. adults. Ann Intern Med 119:744, 1993.

Rosenbaum M, Leibel RL, Hirsch J: Obesity. N Engl J Med 337:396, 1997.

Sawaya ME: Clinical updates in hair. Derm Clinics 15:37, 1997.

Tanner JM: Growing up. Sci Am 229:34, 1973.

Chapter 6. The Skin

Bisno AL, Stevens DL: Streptococcal infections of the skin and soft tissues. N Engl J Med 334:240, 1996.

Drake LA, Dinehart SM, Farmer ER, et al: Guidelines of care for superficial mycotic skin infections of the skin: Onychomycosis. J Am Acad Dermatol 34:116, 1996.

Fine JD: Management of acquired bullous skin diseases. N Engl J Med 333:1475, 1995.

Fitzpatrick TB: Dermatology in General Medicine, 4th ed. New York, McGraw-Hill, 1993.

Fitzpatrick TB: Color Atlas and Synopsis of Clinical Dermatology: Common and Serious Diseases, 3rd ed. New York, McGraw-Hill, 1997.

Goldsmith LA, Lazarus GS, Thorp MD: Adult and Pediatric Dermatology: A Color Guide to Diagnosis and Treatment. Philadelphia, FA Davis, 1997.

Greaves MW, Weinstein GD: Treatment of psoriasis. N Engl J Med 332:581, 1995.

Hacker SM: Common disorders of pigmentation. Postgrad Med 99:177, 1996.

Habif TP: Clinical Dermatology: A Color Guide to Diagnosis and Therapy, 3rd ed. St. Louis: CV Mosby, 1996.

Jeghers H, Edelstein LM: Skin color in health and disease. In Blacklow RS: MacBryde's Signs and Symptoms: Applied Pathologic Physiology and Clinical Interpretation, 6th ed. Philadelphia, JB Lippincott, 1983.

Kalve E, Klein JE: Evaluation of women with hirsutism. Am Fam Physician 54:117, 1996.

Moschella SL, Hurley HJ: Dermatology, 3rd ed. Philadelphia, WB Saunders, 1992.

Noronha PA, Zubkov B: Nails and nail disorders in children and adults. Am Fam Med 55:2129, 1997.

Sauer GC: Manual of Skin Diseases, 7th ed. Philadelphia, Lippincott-Raven 1996.

Tucker MA, Halpern A, Holly EA, et al: Clinically recognized dysplastic nevi: A central risk factor for cutaneous melanoma. JAMA 277:1439, 1997.

Young EM Jr, Newcomer VD, Kligman AM: Geriatric Dermatology: Color Atlas and Practitioner's Guide. Philadelphia, Lea & Febiger, 1993.

Chapter 7. Head and Neck

Eyes

Albert DM: Principles and Practice of Ophthalmology. Philadelphia, WB Saunders, 1994.

Anglade E, Whitcup SM: The diagnosis and management of uveitis. Drugs 49:213, 1995.

Bankes JLK: Clinical Opthalmology: A Text and Colour Atlas. Edinburgh, Churchill Livingstone, 1994.

D'Amico DJ: Diseases of the retina. N Engl J Med 331:95, 1994.

Gaston H: Ophthalmology for Nurses. London, Croom Helar, 1986.

Gold DH: Eye in Systemic Disease. Philadelphia, JB Lippincott, 1990.

Kritzinger EE, Beaumont HM: A Colour Atlas of Optic Disc Abnormalities. London, Wolfe Medical Publications, 1987.

Newell FW: Ophthalmology: Principles and Concepts, 8th ed. St. Louis, Mosby–Year Book, 1996.

O'Neill D: Perkin's & Hansell's Atlas of Diseases of the Eye, 4th ed. Edinburgh, Churchill Livingstone, 1994.

Quigley HA: Open-angle glaucoma. N Engl J Med 328:1097, 1993.

Singer DE, Nathan DM, Fogel HA, Schachat AP: Screening for diabetic retinopathy. Ann Intern Med 116:660, 1992.

Sommers A, Tielsch JM, Katz J, Quigley HA, et al: Racial differences in the cause-specific prevalence of blindness in East Baltimore. N Engl J Med 325:1412, 1991.

Spalton DJ: Atlas of Clinical Ophthalmology. Philadelphia, JB Lippincott, 1984.

Tasman W, Jaeger EA: Duane's Clinical Ophthalmology, 16th ed. Philadelphia, JB Lippincott, 1992.

Walsh TJ (ed): Neuro-ophthalmology: Clinical Signs and Symptoms, 4th ed. Baltimore, Williams & Wilkins, 1997.

Yanoff M: Ocular Pathology: A Text and Atlas, 2nd ed. Philadelphia, Harper and Row, 1992.

Ears, Nose, and Throat

Bain J, Carter P, Morton R: Colour Atlas of Mouth, Throat and Ear Disorders in Children. San Diego, CA, College-Hill Press, 1985.

Bull TR: A Colour Atlas of E.N.T. Diagnosis, rev 2nd ed. London, Wolfe Medical Publications, 1987.

Hawke M, Bruce B: A Color Atlas of Otorhinolaryngology. Philadelphia, JB Lippincott, 1995.

Nadol JB Jr: Hearing loss. N Engl J Med 329:1092, 1993.

O'Donoghue GM, Bates GJ, Narula AA: Clinical ENT: An Illustrated Textbook. Oxford, Oxford University Press, 1992.

Russell J: Ear screening. Comm Nurse 1:14, 1995.

Schuller DE, Schleuning AJ II: DeWeese and Saunders' Otolaryngology: Head and Neck Surgery, 8th ed. St. Louis, Mosby–Year Book, 1994.

Williams JW, Simel DL, Roberts L, Sampsa GP: Clinical evaluation for sinusitis: Making the diagnosis by history and physical examination. Ann Intern Med 117:705, 1992.

Mouth

Beaven DW, Brooks SE: Color Atlas of the Tongue in Clinical Diagnosis. Chicago, Year Book Medical Publishers, 1988.

Carranza FA Jr (ed): Glickman's Clinical Periodontology, 7th ed. Philadelphia, WB Saunders, 1990.

Cawson RA, Eveson JW: Oral Pathology and Diagnosis: Colour Atlas with Integrated Text. London, Gower Medical Publishing, 1987.

Genco RJ, Goldman HM, Cohen DW (eds): Contemporary Periodontics. St. Louis, CV Mosby, 1990.

Langlais RP, Miller CS: Color Atlas of Common Oral Diseases, 2nd ed. Baltimore, Williams & Wilkins, 1998.

Neville BW, Damm DD, White DK, et al: Color Atlas of Clinical Oral Pathology. Philadelphia, Lea & Febiger, 1991.

Regezi JA, Sciubba JJ: Oral Pathology: Clinical–Pathologic Correlations, 2nd ed. Philadelphia, WB Saunders, 1993.

Robinson HBG, Miller AS: Colby, Kerr, and Robinson's Atlas of Oral Pathology, 5th ed. Philadelphia, JB Lippincott, 1990.

Rogers RS: Common lesions of the oral mucosa. Postgrad Med 91:141, 1992.

Tyldesley WR: Color Atlas of Orofacial Diseases, 2nd ed. St. Louis, Mosby–Year Book, 1991.

Neck

Brook I: The swollen neck. Infect Dis Clin North Am 2:221, 1988.

Franklyn JA: The management of hyperthyroidism. N Engl J Med 330:1731, 1994.

Jeghers H, Clark SL Jr, Templeton AC: Lymphadenopathy and disorders of the lymphatics. In Blacklow RS: MacBryde's Signs and Symptoms: Applied Pathologic Physiology and Clinical Interpretations, 6th ed. Philadelphia, JB Lippincott, 1983.

Mazzaferri EL: Management of a solitary thyroid nodule. N Engl J Med 328:553, 1993.

Trivalle C, Doucet J, Chassagne P, et al: Differences in the signs and symptoms of hyperthyroidism in older and younger patients. J Am Ger Soc 44:50, 1996.

Chapter 8. The Thorax and Lungs

Abenhaim L, Moride Y, Brenot F, et al: Appetite-suppressant drugs and the risk for primary pulmonary hypertension. N Engl J Med 335:609, 1996.

American Thoracic Society: Standards for the diagnosis and care of patients with chronic obstructive pulmonary disease (COPD). Am J Respir Crit Care Med 152:S78, 1995.

American Thoracic Society: Treatment of tuberculosis and tuberculosis infection in adults and children. Am J Respir Crit Care Med 149:1359, 1994.

Badgett RG, et al: Can moderate obstructive pulmonary disease be diagnosed by historical and physical findings alone? Am J Med 94:188, 1993.

Bartlett JG, Mundy LM: Community-acquired pneumonia. N Engl J Med 333:1618, 1995.

Baum GL, Wolinsky E (eds): Textbook of Pulmonary Diseases, 5th ed. Boston, Little, Brown & Co, 1994.

Bettancourt PE, DelBono EA, Speigelman D, Hertzmark E, Murphy RL: Clinical utility of chest auscultation in common pulmonary disease. Am J Resp Crit Care Med 150:1921, 1994.

Cugell DW: Lung sound nomenclature. Am Rev Respir Dis 136:1016, 1987.

Epler GR, Carrington CB, Gaensler EA: Crackles (rales) in the interstitial pulmonary diseases. Chest 73:333, 1978.

Koster MEY, Baughmann RP, Loudon RG: Continuous adventitious lung sounds. J Asthma 27:237, 1990.

Kraman SS: Lung sounds for the clinician. Arch Intern Med 146:1411, 1986.

Lehrer S: Understanding Lung Sounds, 2nd ed. Philadelphia, WB Saunders, 1993. (With audiocassette)

Loudon RG: The lung exam. Clin Chest Med 8:265, 1987.

Nath AR, Carpel LH: Inspiratory crackles—early and late. Thorax 29:223, 1974.

Nath AR, Carpel LH: Lung crackles in bronchiectasis. Thorax 35:694, 1980.

Patrick H, Patrick F: Chronic cough. Med Clin North Am 79:361, 1995.

Pioped Investigators: Value of the ventilation/perfusion scan in acute pulmonary embolism: Results of the prospective investigation of pulmonary embolism diagnosis (PIOPED). JAMA 263:2753, 1990.

Schapira RM, et al: The value of the forced expiratory time in the physical diagnosis of obstructive airways disease. JAMA 270:731, 1993.

Stead WW, To T: The significance of the tuberculin skin test in elderly persons. Ann Intern Med 107:837, 1987.

Swensen SJ, Silverstein MD, Ilstrup DM, et al: The probability of malignancy in solitary pulmonary nodules. Arch Intern Med 157:849, 1997.

Weinberger SE: Principles of Pulmonary Medicine, 3rd ed. Philadelphia, WB Saunders, 1998.

Chapter 9. The Cardiovascular System

Cardiovascular Assessment

American College of Physicians: Clincal Guideline, Part 1: Guidelines for using serum cholesterol, high density lipoprotein cholesterol, and triglycerides levels as screening tests for preventing coronary heart disease in adults. Ann Intern Med 124:515, 1996.

Braunwald E (ed): Heart Disease. A Textbook of Cardiovascular Medicine, 5th ed. Philadelphia, WB Saunders, 1997.

Butman SM, Ewy GA, et al: Bedside cardiovascular examination in patients with severe chronic heart failure: Importance of rest or inducible jugular venous distension. J Am Coll Card 22:968, 1993.

Califf RM, Bengtson JR: Cardiogenic shock. N Engl J Med 330:1724, 1994.

Carabello BA, Crawford FA: Valvular heart disease. N Engl J Med 337:32, 1997.

Cohn JN: The management of chronic heart failure. N Engl J Med

Dajani AS, Taubert KA, Wilson W, et al: Prevention of bacterial endocarditis. Recommendations by the American Heart Association. JAMA 277:1794, 1997.

Don Michael TA: Auscultation of the Heart: A Cardiophonetic Approach. New York, McGraw-Hill, 1998.

Folland ED, Kriegel BJ, Henderson WG, et al: Implications of third heart sounds in patients with valvular heart disease. N Engl J Med 327:458, 1992.

Garber AM, Browner WS, Hulley SB: Clinical guideline, Part 2: Cholesterol screening in asymptomatic adults, revisited. Ann Intern Med 124:518, 1996.

Grodstein F, Stampfer MJ, Manson JE, et al. Postmenopausal estrogen and progestin use and the risk of cardiovascular disease. N Engl J Med 335:453, 1996.

Grossman E, Messerli FH: Diabetic and hypertensive heart disease. Ann Intern Med 125:304, 1996.

Harvey WP, Canfield DC: Clinical auscultation of the cardiovascular system. Newton. Laennec Publishing, 1996.

Kupari M, Koskinen P, Virolainen J et al: Prevalence and predictors of audible physiological third heart sound in a population sample aged 36 to 37 years. Circulation 89:1189, 1994.

Lembo NJ, Dell' Italia LJ, Crawford MH, et al: Bedside Diagnosis of Systolic Murmurs. N Engl J Med 318:1572, 1988.

Muller JE, Mittelman MA, Maclure M, et al: Triggering myocardial infarction by sexual activity. JAMA 275:1405, 1996.

Novey DW, Pencak M, Stang JM: The Guide to Heart Sounds: Normal and Abnormal. Boca Raton, FL, CRC Press, 1988. (*Audiocassette with pamphlet*)

Perloff JK: Physical Examination of the Heart and Circulation, 2nd ed. Philadelphia, WB Saunders, 1990.

Sandok BA, Whisnant JP, Furlan AJ, et al: Carotid artery bruits: Prevalence survey and differential diagnosis. Mayo Clin Proc 57:227, 1982.

Schlant RC, Alexander RW, O'Rourke KA, et al (eds): Hurst's The Heart, Arteries, and Veins, 8th ed. New York, McGraw-Hill, 1994.

Weibers PO, Whisnant JP, Sandok BA, O'Fallin WM: Prospective comparison of a cohort of asymptomatic carotid bruit and a population-based cohort without carotid bruit. Stroke 21:984, 1990.

Blood Pressure

Appel LJ, Moore TJ, et al: A clinical trial of the effects of dietary patterns on blood pressure. N Engl J Med 336:1117, 1997.

Cavallini MC, Roman MJ, Blank SG, Pini R, Pickering TG, Devereux RB: Association of the ausculatory gap with vascular disease in hypertensive patients. Ann Intern Med 124:877, 1996.

Joint National Commission on Prevention, Detection, Evaluation, and Treatment of High Blood Pressure and the National High Blood Pressure Education Program Coordinating Committee: The Sixth Report on Prevention, Detection, Evaluation, and Treatment of High Blood Pressure. Arch Intern Med 157:2413, 1997.

Kaplan NM: Clinical Hypertension, 6th ed. Baltimore, Williams & Wilkins, 1994.

Lipsitz LA: Orthostatic hypotension in the elderly. N Engl J Med 321:952, 1989.

Reeves RA: Does this patient have hypertension? JAMA 273:1211, 1995.

Sague A, Larson MG, Levy D: The natural history of borderline isolated systolic hypertension. N Engl J Med 329:1912, 1993.

Schmeider RE, Martus P, Klingbeil A: Reversal of left ventricular hypertrophy in essential hypertension. JAMA 275:1507, 1996.

SHEP Cooperative Research Group: Prevention of stroke by anti-hypertensive drug treatment in older persons with isolated systolic hypertension. JAMA 265:3255, 1991.

Chapter 10. The Breasts and Axillae

Pubertal Changes

Harlan WR, Harlan EA, Grillo GP: Secondary sex characteristics of girls 12 to 17 years of age. The U.S. Health Examination Survey. J Pediatr 96:1074, 1980.

Marshall WA, Tanner JM: Variations in pattern of pubertal changes in girls. Arch Dis Child 44:291, 1969.

Tanner JM: Growth at Adolescence, 2nd ed. Oxford, Blackwell Scientific Publications, 1962.

General Assessment

Baines CJ: The Canadian National Breast Screening Study: A perspective on criticisms. Ann Intern Med 120:326, 1994.

Bartow SA, Pathak DR, Mettler FA, et al: Breast mammographic pattern: A concatenation of confounding and breast cancer risk factors. Am J Epidemiol 142:813, 1995.

Bland KJ, Copeland EM: Breast Chapter. In Schwartz S (ed): Principles of Surgery, 6th ed. New York, McGraw-Hill, 1994.

Braunstein GD: Gynecomastia. N Engl J Med 328:490, 1993.

Feig SA: Mammographic screening of women aged 40 to 50 years. Obstet Gynecol Clin North Am 21:587, 1994.

Harris JR: Disease of the Breast. Philadelphia: Lippincott-Raven, 1996.

Harris JR, Morrow M, Bonadonna G: Cancer of the Breast. In DeVita VT, Hellman S, Rosenberg SA (eds): Cancer Principles & Practice of Oncology, 5th ed. Philadelphia, Lippincott-Raven, 1997.

Kaufman Z, Garstin WH, Hayes R, et al: The mammographic parenchymal patterns of women on hormonal replacement therapy. Clinical Radiology 43:389, 1991.

Love SM: Dr. Susan Love's Breast Book, 2nd ed. Reading, MA, Addison-Wesley Publishing, 1995. (*Although this book is written for general readers, professionals can learn much from it.*)

Schultz MZ, Ward BA, Reiss M: Chapter 149. Breast Diseases. In Noble J, Greene HL, Levinson W, Modest GA, Young MJ (eds): Primary Care Medicine, 2nd ed. St. Louis, Mosby, 1996.

Breast Conditions and Diseases

Breast Mass

Cancer Committee of the College of American Pathologists: Is fibrocystic disease of the breast precancerous? Arch Pathol Lab Med 110:171, 1986.

Deckers PJ, Ricci A: Pain and lumps in the female breast. Hosp Practice 67, 1992.

Donegan WL: Evaluation of the palpable breast mass. N Engl J Med 327:937, 1992.

Dupont WD, Page DL: Risk factors for breast cancer in women with proliferative breast disease. N Engl J Med 312:146, 1985.

Dupont WD, Page DL, Parl FF: Long-term risk of breast cancer in women with fibroadenoma. N Engl J Med 331:10, 1994.

Breast Malignancy

Bilmoria MM, Morrow M: The woman at increased risk for breast cancer. Evaluation and management strategies. Cancer 45:263, 1995.

Harris JR, Lippman ME, Veronesi U, et al: Breast cancer. N Engl J Med 327:319, 1992.

Jaiyesimi IA, Buzday AU, Sahin AA, et al: Carcinoma of the male breast. Ann Intern Med 117:771, 1992.

Long E: Breast cancer in African-American women. Cancer Nursing 16:1, 1993.

Marchant DJ: Risk factors in contemporary management of breast disease, II: Breast cancer. Obstet Gynecol Clin North Am: 561, 1994.

Marcus JN, Watson P, Page DL, et al: Pathology and heredity of breast cancer in younger women. Mongr Natl Cancer Inst 16:23, 1994.

Miller AB, Baines CJ, To T, et al: Canadian National Breast Screening Study: 1. Breast cancer detection and death rates among women aged 40 to 49 years; 2. Breast cancer detection and death rates among women aged 50 to 59 years. Can Med Assoc J 147:1459, 1477, 1992.

Velentgas P, Daline JR: Risk factors for breast cancer in younger women. Monogr Natl Cancer Inst 16:15, 1994.

Chapter 11. The Abdomen

Arnell TD, DeVirgilio C, Doneyre C, Grant E, Baker JD: Abdominal aortic aneurysm in elderly males with atherosclerosis: The value of physical exam. Am Surgeon 62:661, 1996.

Sherlock SD, Summerfield JA: Color Atlas of Liver Disease, 2nd ed. St. Louis Mosby–Year Book, 1991.

Silen, W: Cope's Early Diagnosis of the Acute Abdomen, 19th ed. New York, Oxford University Press, 1996.

Sleisenger MH, Fordtran JS (eds): Gastrointestinal Disease: Pathophysiology, Diagnosis, Management, 5th ed. Philadelphia, WB Saunders, 1993.

Williams JW Jr, Simel DL: Does this patient have ascites? How to divine fluid in the abdomen. JAMA 267:2645, 1992.

Evaluation of the Liver

Meidl EJ, Ende J: Evaluation of liver size by physical examination. J Gen Intern Med 8:835, 1993.

Naylor CD: Physical examination of the liver. JAMA 271:1859, 1994.

Zoli M, Magliotti D, Grimaldi M, Gueli C, Marchesini G, Pisi E: Physical examination of the liver: Is it still worth it? Am J Gastroenterol 90:1428, 1995.

Evaluation of the Spleen

Barkun AN, Camus M, Green L, et al: The bedside assessment of splenic enlargement. Am J Med 91:512, 1991.

Grover SA, Barkum AN, Sackett DL: Does this patient have splenomegaly? JAMA 270:2218, 1993.

Sullivan S, Wiliams R: Reliability of clinical techniques for detecting splenic enlargement. Br Med J 2:1043, 1976.

Tamayo SG, Rickman LS, Matthews WC, Fullerton SC et al: Examiner dependence on physical diagnostic tests of splenomegaly: A prospective study with multiple observers. J Gen Intern Med 8:69, 1993.

Chapter 12. Male Genitalia and Hernias

Pubertal Changes

Harlan WR, Grillo GP, Comoni-Huntley J, et al: Secondary sex characteristics of boys 12 to 17 years of age. The U.S. Health Examination Survey. J Pediatr 95:293, 1979.

Marshall WA, Tanner JM: Variations in the pattern of pubertal changes in boys. Arch Dis Child 45:13, 1970.

McAnamey ER, Kreipe RE, Orr DP, et al: Textbook of Adolescent Medicine. Philadelphia, WB Saunders, 1992.

Tanner JM: Growth at Adolescence, 2nd ed. Oxford, Blackwell Scientific Publications, 1962.

Urology

Gillenwater TY, Grayhack JT, Howards SS, et al: Adult and Pediatric Urology, 3rd ed. St Louis, Mosby, 1996.

Sande MA, Volberding PA: The Medical Management of AIDS, 4th ed. Philadelphia, WB Saunders, 1995.

Tanagho EA, McAninch JW: Smith's General Urology, 14th ed. Norwalk, CT, Appleton and Lange, 1995.

Walsh PC, Retik AB, Staney TA, et al (eds): Campbell's Urology, 6th ed. Philadelphia, WB Saunders, 1992.

Hernias

Eubanks S: Hernias. In Sabiston DC Jr (ed): Textbook of Surgery: The Biological Basis of Modern Surgical Practice, 15th ed. Philadelphia, WB Saunders, 1997.

Wantz GE: Abdominal wall hernias. In Schwartz SI (ed): Principles of Surgery, 6th ed. New York, McGraw-Hill, 1994.

Genito-Urinary Conditions

Davis-Joseph B, Tiefer L, Melman A: Accuracy of the initial history and physical examination to establish the etiology of erectile dysfunction. Urology 40:498, 1995.

Handsfield HH: Color Atlas and Synopsis of Sexually Transmitted Diseases. New York, McGraw-Hill, 1992.

Holmes KK, Mardh PA, Sparling PF (eds): Sexually Transmitted Diseases, 2nd ed. New York, McGraw-Hill, 1990.

Howards SS: Treatment of male infertility. N Engl J Med 332:312, 1995.

McDowell BJ, Burgie KL, Dombrowski MD, et al: An interdisciplinary approach to the assessment and behavioral treatment of urinary incontinence in geriatric outpatients. J Am Geriatr Soc 40:370, 1992.

Smith DS, Catalona WJ, Herschman JD: Longitudinal screening for prostate cancer with prostate specific antigen. JAMA 276:1309, 1996.

Wisdom A: Colour Atlas of Sexually Transmitted Diseases, 2nd ed. London, Year Book Medical Publishers, 1989.

Chapter 13. The Female Genitalia

Pubertal Changes

See references in Chapter 10.

Gynecology

Berek JS, Adasti EY, Hillard PA: Novak's Gynecology, 12th ed. Baltimore, Williams & Wilkins, 1996.

Greydanus DE, Shearin RB, Langdon D: Adolescent Sexuality and Gynecology. Philadelphia, Lea & Febiger, 1990.

Herbst AL, Mishell DR Jr, Stenchever MA, et al: Comprehensive Gynecology, 3rd ed. St Louis, Mosby, 1997.

Scott JR, DiSaia PJ, Hammond CB, et al (eds): Danforth's Obstetrics and Gynecology, 7th ed. Philadelphia, JB Lippincott, 1994.

The Pelvic Examination

Blake J: Gynecologic examination of the teenager and young child. Obstet Gynecol Clin North Am 19:27, 1992.

Brink CA, Sampselle CM, Wells TJ, et al: A digital test for pelvic muscle strength in older women with urinary incontinence. Nurs Res 38:196, 1989.

Pearce KF, et al: Cytopathological findings on vaginal papanicolau smears after hysterectomy for benign gynecologic disease. N Engl J Med 335:1559, 1996.

Primrose RB: Taking the tension out of a pelvic exam. Am J Nurs 84:72, 1984.

Rimsza ME: An illustrated guide to adolescent gynecology. Pediatr Clin North Am 36:639, 1989.

Wilcox LS, Mosher WD: Factors associated with obtaining health screening among women of reproductive age. Public Health Rep 108:76, 1993.

Willard MA, Heaberg GL, Pack JB: The educational pelvic examination: women's responses to a new approach. J. Obstet Gynecol Neonatal Nurs 15:135, 1986.

Vaginal and Pelvic Conditions

Bickley LS: Acute vaginitis. In Black ER, Panzer RJ, Bordley DR, Tape TG (eds): Diagnostic Strategies for Common Medical Problems, 2nd ed. Philadelphia, American College of Physicians, in press.

Ho GYF, Bierman R, Beardsley L, et al: Natural history of cervicovaginal papillomavirus infection in young women. N Engl J Med 338:423, 1998.

McCormack WM: Pelvic inflammatory disease. N Engl J Med 330:115, 1994.

Rose PG: Endometrial carcinoma. N Engl J Med 335:640, 1996.

Scholes D, et al: Prevention of pelvic inflammatory disease by screening for cervical chlamydial infection. N Engl J Med 334:1362, 1996.

Spiroff L, Rowan J, Symons J, Genant H, Wilborn W: The comparative effect on bone density, endometrium, and lipids of continuous hormones as replacement therapy (CHART study). JAMA 276:1397, 1996.

Genito-Urinary Conditions

See references listed on this topic in Chapter 12.

Brown JS, Steely DG, Fong J, et al: Urinary incontinence in older women: Who is at risk? Obstet Gynecol 87:715, 1996.

Chapter 14. The Pregnant Woman

General

Baron TH, Ramirez B, Richter JE: Gastrointestinal motility disorders during pregnancy. Ann Intern Med 118:366, 1993.

Beebe JE, Duperret M (consultants): Programmed instruction: Examination of the female pelvis, Part I. Am J Nurs 78:10, 1978.

Cunningham FG, MacDonald PC, Gant NF: Williams Obstetrics, 20th ed. Norwalk, CT, Appleton & Lange, 1997.

Merkatz IR, Thompson JE (eds): New Perspectives on Prenatal Care. New York, Elsevier, 1990.

Myles M: Textbook for Midwives, 12th ed. London, E & S Livingstone, 1993.

Thompson JE: Primary health care nursing for women. In Mezey MD, McGivern DO: Nurses, Nurse Practitioners. New York, Springer, 1993.

U.S. Public Health Service, Department of Health and Human Services: Caring for Our Future: The Content of Prenatal Care. Washington, DC, U.S. Government Printing Office, 1989.

Vaney H: J Nurse Midwifery, 3rd ed. Boston, Jones & Bartlett, 1997.

Nutrition

Enkin M, Keirse MJNC, Renfrew M, Neilson J: A Guide to Effective Care in Pregnancy and Childbirth, 2nd ed. New York, Oxford, 1995.

Food and Nutrition Board; Recommended Dietary Allowances, 10th ed. National Research Council, National Academy of Sciences, Washington, DC, 1989.

Institute of Medicine: Nutrition During Pregnancy. Part I, Weight Gain; Part II, Nutrient Supplements. Committee on Nutritional Status During Pregnancy and Lactation, Food and Nutrition Board, National Academy Press, Washington, DC, 1990.

Institute of Medicine: Nutrition During Pregnancy and Lactation: An Implementation Guide. Subcommittee for a Clinical Application Guide, Committee on Nutritional Status During Pregnancy and Lactation, Food and Nutrition Board, National Academy Press, Washington, DC, 1992.

Worthington-Roberts B: Nutrition. In Fogel CI, Woods NF (eds): Women's Health Care: A Comprehensive Handbook. California: Sage Publications, 1995.

Worthington-Roberts B, Klerman L: Maternal nutrition. In Merkatz IR, Thompson JE (eds): New Perspectives on Prenatal Care. New York, Elsevier, 1990.

Exercise

ACOG, Technical Bulletin No. 189, February 1994.

Bell R, O'Neill M: Exercise and pregnancy: A review. Birth 2:85, 1994.

Yeo S: Exercise guidelines for pregnant women. Image 26:265, 1994.

Violence

Adler C: Unheard and unseen: Rural women and domestic violence. J Nurs Midwifery: 41:463, 1996.

Bohn DK, Holz KA: Sequelae of abuse: Health effects of childhood sexual abuse, domestic battering, and rape. J Nurse Midwifery: 41:442, 1996.

Center for Disease Control and Prevention. MMWR 43:132, 1994.

King MC, Ryan J: Woman abuse: The role of nurse-midwives in assessment. J Nurs Midwifery 41:436, 1996.

Paluzzi PA, Houde-Quimby C: Domestic violence: Implications for the American College of Nurse-Midwives and Its Members. J Nurse Midwifery: 41:430, 1996.

Chapter 15. The Anus, Rectum, and Prostate

American College of Physicians: Suggested technique for fecal occult blood testing and interpretation of colorectal cancer screenings. Ann Intern Med 126:808, 1997.

Donowitz M, Kokke FT, Saidi R: Evaluation of patients with chronic diarrhea. N Engl J Med 332:725, 1995.

Hanauer SB: Inflammatory bowel disease. N Engl J Med 334:841, 1996.

Madoff RD, William JG, Caushaj PF: Fecal incontinence. N Engl J Med 326:1002, 1992.

Schrock TR: Examination of anorectum and diseases of anorectum. In Sleisinger MH, Fordtran JS (eds): Gastrointestinal Disease: Pathophysiology, Diagnosis, Management, 5th ed. Philadelphia, WB Saunders, 1993.

Chapter 16. The Peripheral Vascular System

Baraff LJ: Capillary refill: Is it a useful sign? Pediatrics 92:723, 1993.

Caputo GM, Cavanaugh PR, Ulbrecht JS, et al: Assessment and management of foot disease in patients with diabetes. N Engl J Med 331:854, 1994.

Cantwell-Gaw K: Identifying chronic peripheral arterial disease. Am J Nurs 96:43, 1996.

Coleman RW, Hirsh J, Marder VJ, Salzman EW: Hemostasis and Thrombosis: Basic Principles and Clinical Practice, 3rd ed. Philadelphia, JB Lippincott, 1994.

Harris AH, Brown-Etris M, Troyer-Caudle J: Managing vascular leg ulcers. Part I. Am J Nurs 96:38, 1996.

Loscalzo J, Creager MA, Dzau VJ (eds): Vascular Medicine: A Textbook of Vascular Biology and Diseases. Boston, Little, Brown & Co. 1992.

Tibbs DJ: Varicose Veins and Related Disorders. Boston, Butterworth-Heinemann, 1992.

Verstraite M: The diagnosis and treatment of deep-vein thrombosis. N Engl J Med 329:1418, 1993.

Chapter 17. The Musculoskeletal System

Alexander NB: Gait disorders in older adults. J Am Geriatr Soc 44:434, 1996.

American Orthopedic Association: Manual of Orthopedic Surgery, 1985.

Baker DG, Schumacher HR Jr: Acute monoarthritis. N Engl J Med 329:1013, 1993.

Bland JH: Disorders of the shoulder, Ch. 71. In Noble J (ed): Primary Care Medicine, 2nd ed. St. Louis, Mosby, 1996.

Doherty M, Doherty J: Clinical Examination in Rheumatology. London, Wolfe Publishing, 1992.

Emerson BT: The management of gout. N Engl J Med 334:445, 1996.

Hoppenfeld S: Physical Examination of the Spine and Extremities. Norwalk, CT, Appleton-Century-Crofts, 1976.

Katz WA: Diagnosis and Management of Rheumatic Diseases, 2nd ed. Philadelphia, JB Lippincott, 1988.

Kelley WN: Textbook of Rheumatology, 5th ed. Philadelphia, WB Saunders, 1997.

Koopman WJ: Arthritis and Allied Conditions: A Textbook of Rheumatology, 13th ed. Baltimore, Williams & Wilkins, 1997.

Polley HF, Hunder GG: Rheumatologic Interviewing and Physical Examination of the Joints, 2nd ed. Philadelphia, WB Saunders, 1978.

Schumacher HR, Klippel JH, Koopman WJ: Primer on the Rheumatic Diseases, 10th ed. Atlanta, Arthritis Foundation, 1993.

Snider RK (ed): Essentials of Musculoskeletal Care. Rosemont; IL, American Academy of Orthopedic Surgeons, 1997.

Chapter 18. The Nervous System

Anatomy and Physiology

DeGroot J, Chusid JG: Correlative Neuroanatomy, 21st ed. Norwalk, CT, Appleton & Lange, 1991.

Gilman SG, Newman SW: Manter and Gatz's Essential of Clinical Neuroanatomy and Neurophysiology, 9th ed. Philadelphia, FA Davis, 1996.

Neurology

Adams RD, Victor M, Ropper AH: Principles of Neurology, 6th ed. New York, McGraw-Hill, 1997.

Bennett DA, et al: Prevalence of parkinsonian signs and associated mortality in a community population of older people. N Engl J Med 334:71, 1996.

Drachman DB: Myasthenia gravis. N Engl J Med 330:1797, 1994.

Joynt RJ, Griggs RC: Clinical Neurology. Philadelphia, Lippincott-Raven, 1996.

Kankam CG, Sallis R: Guillain-Barré syndrome. Postgrad Med 101:279, 1997.

Kapoor WN: Evaluation and management of the patient with syncope. JAMA 268:2553, 1992.

Rowland LP (ed): Merritt's Textbook of Neurology, 9th ed. Baltimore, Williams & Wilkins, 1995.

The Neurologic Examination

Aids to the Examination of the Peripheral Nervous System: Medical Research Council Memorandum No. 45. London, Her Majesty's Stationery Office, 1976.

Dawson DM: Entrapment neuropathies of the upper extremities. N Engl J Med 329:2013, 1993.

DeMyer WE: Technique of the Neurologic Examination, A Programmed Text, 4th ed. New York, McGraw-Hill, 1994.

Haerer AF: DeJong's The Neurologic Examination, 5th ed. Philadelphia, JB Lippincott, 1992.

Mancall EL: Alpers and Mancall's Essentials of the Neurologic Examination, 2nd ed. Philadelphia, FA Davis, 1981.

Coma

Edwards RH, Simon RP: Coma. Vol 2 (19). In Joynt RJ, Griggs RC (eds): Clinical Neurology. Philadelphia, Lippincott-Raven, 1996.

Lipowski ZJ: Delirium (acute confusional states). JAMA 258:1789, 1987.

Plum F, Posner JB: The Diagnosis of Stupor and Coma, 3rd ed. Philadelphia, FA Davis, 1980.

Chapter 19. The Physical Examination of Infants and Children

Emmanouilides GC, et al (eds): Heart Disease of Infants, Children and Adolescents, including the Fetus and Young Adult, 5th ed. Baltimore, Williams & Wilkins, 1994.

Fanaroff AA, Martin RJ: Neonatal–Perinatal Medicine, 6th ed. St. Louis, Mosby–Year Book, 1997.

Hoekelman RA, et al (eds): Primary Pediatric Care, 3rd ed. St. Louis, Mosby–Year Book, 1997.

Lowrey GH: Growth and Development of Children, 8th ed. Chicago, Year Book Medical Publishers, 1986.

Newell FW: Ophthalmology: Principles and Concepts, 8th ed. St. Louis, Mosby–Year Book, 1996.

Rodnitzky RL: Van Allen's Pictorial Manual of Neurologic Tests, 3rd ed. Chicago, Year Book Medical Publishers, 1988.

Swaiman KF: Pediatric Neurology: Principles and Practice, 2nd ed, (2 vols). St. Louis, Mosby–Year Book, 1994.

Tachdjian MO: Pediatric Orthopedics, 2nd ed, (4 vols). Philadelphia, WB Saunders, 1990.

Chapter 20. Clinical Thinking: From Data to Plan

Alfaro-Lefevre R: Critical Thinking in Nursing: A Practical Approach. Philadelphia, WB Saunders, 1995.

Black ER, Panzer RJ, Bordley DR, Tape TG, (eds): Diagnostic Strategies for Common Medical Problems, 2nd ed. Philadelphia, American College of Physicians, in press.

Carpenito LJ: Nursing Diagnosis: Application to Clinical Practice, 7th ed. Philadelphia, Lippincott-Raven, 1997.

Cutler P: Problem Solving in Clinical Medicine; From Data to Diagnosis, 3rd ed. Baltimore, Williams & Wilkins, 1997.

Diamond GA, Forrester JS: Analysis of probability as an aid in the clinical diagnosis of coronary artery disease. N Engl J Med 300:1350, 1979.

Fletcher RH: Clinical Epidemiology: The Essentials, 3rd ed. Baltimore, Williams & Wilkins, 1996.

Hunt DL, McKibbon KA: Locating and appraising systemic reviews. Ann Intern Med 126:531, 1997.

Nettina SM: The Lippincott Manual of Nursing Practice, 6th ed. Philadelphia, Lippincott-Raven, 1996.

Orem DE, Taylor SG, Renpenning KM: Nursing Concepts of Practice, 5th ed. St. Louis, Mosby, 1995.

Rubenfield MG, Scheffer BK: Critical Thinking in Nursing: An Interactive Approach. Philadelphia, JB Lippincott, 1995.

Sackett DL: A primer on the precision and accuracy of the clinical examination. JAMA 267:2638, 1992.

Sackett DL, Haynes RB, Tugwell P: Clinical Epidemiology: A Basic Science for Clinical Medicine, 2nd ed. Boston, Little, Brown & Co, 1991.

Chapter 21. The Patient's Record

Hurst JW, Walker HK (eds): The Problem-Oriented System. New York, Medcom, 1972.

Subject Index

NOTE: A t following a page number indicates tabular material.

A

A₂, 283, 312, 312t, 325t

Abdomen, 134, 355–386
  acute, in infants, 682
  age-related changes in, 358
  anatomy and physiology of, 355–358
  back pain referred from, 100t
  in children, 684–686
  contour of, 360–361
  examination of, 134, 359–378
    auscultation in, 361–362, 441–442, 682
    in children, 684–686
    general approach to, 359
    in infants, 682–683
    inspection in, 360–361, 440
    palpation in, 363–364, 440–441
      in children, 684–686
      in infants, 683
    percussion in, 362
      in infants, 682
    in pregnant patient, 437, 440–442
      modified Leopold's maneuvers in, 444–446
    special techniques in, 374–377
      in infants, 683
  health promotion and counseling and, 378–379
  in infants, 682–683
  masses in
    abdominal wall masses differentiated from, 377
    palpation in assessment of, 363–364
  protuberant, 381t
    in children, 684
    in infants, 682
    in pregnancy, 381t, 432–433
  quadrants/sections of, 356
  sounds in, 382t
    in infants, 682
Abdominal aorta, pulsations of, 356
  in children, 685
Abdominal bloating, 55
Abdominal breathing, in infants, 677
Abdominal cavity, 357. See also Abdomen
Abdominal fullness, 55
Abdominal pain/tenderness, 55–57, 86–87t, 383–384t
  in appendicitis, 56, 86–87t, 376–377
  assessment of, 363–364, 376–377
  in children, 684, 685–686
  in cholecystitis, 86–87t, 377
  joint pain and, 69
Abdominal reflexes, 561, 593
  in aging patient, 568
  in infants, 697

Abdominal striae, 358
  in pregnant patient, 440
Abdominal wall. See also Abdomen
  anatomy of, 355
  bulges in, 380t. See also Hernia
  masses in, masses in abdominal wall differentiated from, 377
  tenderness originating in, 383t
Abducens nerve (cranial nerve VI), 558
  examination of, 570
  functions of, 559t, 569
  paralysis of, 190
    strabismus in, 218t
Abduction, assessing
  at fingers and thumb, 518, 578
  at hip, 528, 580
Abduction stress test, 535t
Abductor muscles, of hip, 499–500
Abscesses
  adenoidal, 675
  lung, cough and hemoptysis associated with, 84t
  peritonsillar, 675, 676
Absence seizures, 105t
Abstract thinking, in higher cognitive functioning, 108
  assessment of, 118
Abuse
  alcohol. See Alcohol use/abuse
  child
    clues to in interview, 634
    facies in, 659t
    sexual, examination of vagina and cervix and, 689
  in pregnancy, health promotion and counseling and, 448
  substance. See Drugs; Substance use/abuse
Acanthosis nigricans, 345
Accessory muscles of breathing, use of, 253
Accidents, information about
  in child health history, 40
  recording, 723
Accommodation, 169
  aging affecting (presbyopia), 47, 182
Acetabulum, 498
Achalasia, dysphagia associated with, 85t
Achilles tendon, 505
  examination of, 537
Aching neck, 101t. See also Neck, pain/stiffness in
ACL. See Anterior cruciate ligament
Acne, 150, 181
  comedones in, 154t

Acoustic blink reflex, 667, 697
Acoustic nerve (cranial nerve VIII), 558
  examination of, 573
  functions of, 559t, 569
  tumor impinging on, vertigo caused by, 79t
Acoustic neuroma, findings in, 614t
Acquired immunodeficiency syndrome. See HIV infection/AIDS
Acrocyanosis, in infants, 650
Acromegaly, facies in, 211t
Acromioclavicular arthritis, 545t
Acromioclavicular joint, 488, 510
  examination of, 511
Acromion, 487, 489–490, 509–510
Actinic cheilitis, 234t
Actinic keratosis, 147, 157t
Actinic lentigines ("liver spots"), 147, 160t
Actinic purpura, 147
Activities of daily living, 28t
  assessment of in aging patient, 28–29
  musculoskeletal assessment and, 507–508
Acuity
  auditory. See also Hearing
    testing, 197, 233t
  visual. See also Vision
    age-related changes in, 182
    testing, 184–185
Acute necrotizing ulcerative gingivitis, 239t
Acute stress disorder, 125t
Acute surgical abdomen, in infants, 682
Addison's disease, 72
Adduction, assessing
  at fingers and thumb, 518
  at hip, 529, 579
Adduction stress test, 535t
Adductor muscles, of hip, 499–500
Adductor tubercle, 501
  examination of, 531
Adenitis, cervical, in children, 657
Adenoidal abscess, 675
Adenoiditis, chronic, 675
Adenoids (pharyngeal tonsils), examination of, 675
Adhesive capsulitis (frozen shoulder), 545t
Adie's (tonic) pupil, 189, 217t
Adipose tissue (fat)
  abdominal, aging affecting, 358
  of breast, 334
ADLs. See Activities of daily living
Adnexa, ovarian, 407
  examination of, 418
    in pregnant patient, 443
  masses of, 430t

Cutaneous hyperesthesia, in appendicitis, 377
Cuticle, 145–146
Cutis marmorata, 650
CVAs. *See* Cerebrovascular accidents
Cyanosis, 146–147, 149, 155*t*, 253
  in congenital heart disease, 680, 681*t*
Cyclothymic disorder, 124*t*
Cystitis, painful urination and, 60
Cystocele, 424*t*
  in pregnant patient, 442
  uterine prolapse and, 428*t*
Cystourethrocele, 424*t*
Cysts
  behind ear, 228*t*
  breast, 349*t*, 353*t*
  epidermoid
    behind ear, 228*t*
    scrotal, 400*t*
    vulvar, 423*t*
  of epididymis, 400*t*
  ovarian, 430*t*
  pilonidal, 457*t*
  popliteal ("baker's"), 533
  porencephalic, transillumination in identification of, 655
  thyroglossal duct, 655

D

Dacryocystitis, 214*t*
Daily life, information about in health history, 37
Data
  arranging, 710
  collection of, assessment and, 715
  in health history
    identifying, 2
      in adult, 35
      in child, 39
    recording, 720–722
    source of, 2–3, 35
      family and friends as, 34, 35
      reliability of, 2, 35
  objective, 705
  planning and, 705–706
  quality of, 710–714
  recording, 719–731
  subjective, 705
  unmanageable array of, 710
Data base, 705. *See also* Data
Date, in health history, 2, 35
Date of confinement, expected, 436
Dazzle reflex. *See also* Blink reflex
  in infants, 697
DDST. *See* Denver Developmental Screening Test
Deafness. *See also* Hearing loss
  interviewing techniques and, 33
Decerebrate rigidity, 602, 620*t*
Decorticate rigidity, 602, 620*t*
Decreased intracranial pressure, in infants and children, 653
Decrescendo murmur, 314
Deep breathing, apnea alternating with (Cheyne–Stokes breathing), 269*t*
  in coma, 618*t*
Deep retinal hemorrhage, 222*t*

Deep tendon reflexes (spinal reflexes), 560–561, 590–596. *See also specific type*
  in central nervous system disorders, 614*t*
  eliciting, 561, 590
    reinforcement and, 590, 591
  in infants, 696–697
  in pregnant patient, 444
Deep veins, of leg, 462
Deep venous insufficiency (post-phlebitic/postthrombotic) syndrome, edema in, 482*t*
Deep venous thrombosis, 96–97*t*, 472–473
Defecation reflex, constipation associated with inadequate time or setting for, 89*t*
Degenerative joint disease (osteoarthritis), 98–99*t*. *See also* Arthritis
  hands affected in, 514, 547*t*
Déjà vu, in complex partial seizures, 104*t*
Delayed puberty
  in females, 412
  in males, 392
Delirium, 109, 127*t*
Deltoid ligament, 505
Deltoid muscle, 488
Delusional disorder, 126*t*
Delusions, 115*t*
Dementia, 109, 121–122, 127*t*
  detection of, 604
Dental caries, 240*t*
  in children, 674
  prevention of, 209–210
Dentate (pectinate) line (anorectal junction), 449–450
Dentures, care of, counseling about, 210
Denture sore mouth, 200
Denver Developmental Screening Test, 631, 632–633
Deoxyhemoglobin, 146
Dependent edema, 52–53, 474
Depersonalization, feelings of, 115*t*
Depression (depressive disorder), 124*t*
  in aging patient, 109
  assessment of, 113–114, 121, 124*t*
  constipation associated with, 89*t*
DeQuervain's tenosynovitis, 516
Derailment (loosening of associations), 114*t*
Dermatitis, atopic, 161*t*
Dermatomes, 566–567
  back pain radiation along (sciatica), 100*t*
  neck pain radiation along, 101*t*
Dermis, 145
DES. *See* Diethylstilbestrol
Descending colon, 356
  in infants, 683
Developmental milestones, 622, 631
  assessing, 621–622, 631, 631–632
  in child health history, 41
Deviated nasal septum, 198, 199
Dextrocardia, 304
Diabetes insipidus, 92*t*
Diabetes mellitus, 72
  peripheral vascular disease and, 477
  polyneuropathy of, findings in, 615*t*
Diabetic retinopathy

  fundus changes in, 222*t*, 224*t*, 227*t*
  nonproliferative, 227*t*
  proliferative, 222*t*, 224*t*, 227*t*
Diagnoses, generating and testing hypotheses about, 9, 707–708
Diaphragm, 251
  liver displaced by, 385*t*
Diaphragmatic dullness, 260
Diaphragmatic excursion, estimation of, 260
Diaphragmatic hernia, in infant, 682
Diarrhea, 58, 90–91*t*
  joint pain and, 69
Diastasis recti, 380*t*
  in infants, 682
  in pregnancy, 433
Diastematomyelia, 693–694
Diastole, 280
  events during, 280–282
  extra sounds in, 312*t*, 327*t*
  relationship of to electrocardiogram, 286
Diastolic hypertension, 298
Diastolic murmurs, 312*t*, 313, 331*t*
Diastolic pressure, 287, 288
  aging and, 291
  classification of, 298, 298*t*
  in infants and children, 641, 643*t*, 644*t*
Diencephalon, 555
Diet, information about in health history, 36
  recording, 723
Dietary intake, rapid screen for, 318
Diethylstilbestrol, fetal exposure to, 426*t*
Diffuse esophageal spasm
  chest pain associated with, 80–81*t*
  dysphagia associated with, 85*t*
Diffuse interstitial lung disease, dyspnea associated with, 82–83*t*
Digital rectal examination. *See* Rectal examination
Digit span, for testing attention, 117
Dimpling, of breast, 341–342, 344, 352*t*
Diphtheria, 236*t*
Diphtheritic tonsillitis, 675
Diplegia, spastic, 576
  scissoring in, 698, 699
Diplopia (double vision), 47
  amblyopia and, 665
DIPs. *See* Distal interphalangeal joints
Direct questions, in health history interview, 8
Direct reaction to light, 168–169, 188
"Disc diameters," 195
Discipline, in child health history, 41
Discriminative sensations, testing, 588–589
Discs
  intervertebral, 484, 494, 496
    age-related changes in, 506
    herniated, 521–522
      findings in, 615*t*
Disease
  illness differentiated from, 10
  psychotic disorder associated with, 126*t*
Disorientation, 116. *See also* Orientation
  in delirium and dementia, 127*t*

overview/bony structures/joints of, 490–491

swollen/tender, 513–514, 546*t*

Elderly. *See* Aging patient

Electrocardiogram, 285–286

relationship of to cardiac cycle, 286

Embolism, pulmonary

cough and hemoptysis associated with, 84*t*

dyspnea associated with, 82–83*t*

syncope associated with, 102–103*t*

Empathic responses, in interviewing, 13

Emphysema

dyspnea associated with, 82–83*t*

physical signs in, 275*t*

Encephalopathy, lead, Macewen's sign in, 654

Endemic goiter, 244*t*

Endocervical swab, for cervical cytology, 416

Endocrine system/glands

in review of systems, 39

symptoms related to, 72–73

Enteritis, regional (Crohn's disease), diarrhea associated with, 90–91*t*

Entropion, 213*t*

in aging patient, 182, 213*t*

Environment (setting), for health history interview, 5–6, 7

Epicanthus, 213*t*

Epicondyles, of humerus, 490

examination of, 514

Epicondylitis, 514, 546*t*

lateral (tennis elbow), 514, 546*t*

medial (pitcher's/golfer's/Little League elbow), 514, 546*t*

Epidermis, 145

Epidermoid cyst

behind ear, 228*t*

scrotal, 400*t*

vulvar, 423*t*

Epididymis, 387, 388

cyst of, 400*t*

palpation of, 394

Epididymitis

acute, 401*t*

tuberculous, 400*t*

Epigastric (subxiphoid) area, 304, 356

inspection and palpation of, 308–309

Epigastric hernia, 380*t*

Epigastric pain, 55

Epiglottitis, acute, 676

Episcleritis, 214*t*

Episiotomy, 442

Epistaxis, 49, 199

Epitrochlear lymph nodes, 133, 464, 465, 468

Epstein's pearls, in infants, 671

Epulis (pregnancy tumor/pyogenic granuloma), 240*t*

Equilibrium, 172

Erb's palsy, 509

Erectile dysfunction, 66

Erosion, skin, 153*t*, 161*t*

Erythema

multiforme, 160*t*

nodosum, 96–97*t*

toxicum, 651

Erythroplakia, 243*t*

Esophageal atresia, 629, 672

Esophageal cancer, dysphagia associated with, 85*t*

Esophageal dysphagia, 54, 85*t*

Esophageal rings, dysphagia associated with, 85*t*

Esophageal spasm, diffuse

chest pain associated with, 80–81*t*

dysphagia associated with, 85*t*

Esophageal stricture, dysphagia associated with, 85*t*

Esophageal webs, dysphagia associated with, 85*t*

Esophagitis, reflux. *See also* Gastroesophageal reflux

chest pain associated with, 80–81*t*

Esotropia, 218*t*

Estrogen replacement therapy, 422

health promotion and counseling and, 543

Ethical considerations, 23–24

Ethmoid sinuses, 174

E-to-A change (egophony), 263, 271*t*

Eustachian tube, 170

Eversion, assessing, at ankles and feet, 538

Excoriation, 154*t*, 161*t*

Exercise

cardiovascular health and, 319

information about in health history, 36

recording, 723

musculoskeletal health and, 542–543

during pregnancy, health promotion and counseling and, 447–448

work of breathing affected by, 252

Exophthalmometer, 206

Exophthalmos, 206, 213*t*

Exostoses, 196

Exotropia, 218*t*

Expected date of confinement, 436

Expected weeks of gestation by dates, 436

Expiration, 251

assessment of, 253, 267

Expression (facial), assessment of, 143, 184

cranial nerve function and, 572

mental status and, 112

Extension, assessing

at elbow, 577

at hip, 528, 580

at knee, 580

at neck, 522

at spine, 524

at wrist and hand, 517–518, 577

Extensor muscles, of hip, 499

External anal sphincter, 449, 450

External ear, 170–171

External genitals. *See* Female genitals; Male genitals

External inguinal ring, 389, 395, 402*t*

External jugular vein, 179

pressure/pulsation assessment in, 288, 299, 301

External (cervical) os, 406, 407

examination of, 415

in pregnant patient, 442

variations in shapes of, 425*t*

Extinction, 589

visual, 570

Extrahepatic bile ducts, jaundice in obstruction of, 59

Extraocular movements, 169–170

assessment of, 189–190, 191, 570

in coma/stupor, 600

in infants, 662–663

Extraocular muscles

assessment of functions of, 189–190, 191, 570

in strabismus, 218*t*

Extremities. *See also* Arms; Legs

examination of, in pregnant patient, 443–444

Exudates

hard, 223*t*

soft (cotton wool patches), 195, 223*t*

Eyeball, 165

Eyebrows, 186

Eyelids, 164

age-related changes in, 182

eversion of, in conjunctival examination, 207

examination of, 186–187

herniated fat in, 213*t*

periorbital edema and, 213*t*

retracted, 213*t*

variations and abnormalities of, 213*t*

Eyes. *See also under* Visual *and* Vision

age-related changes in, 182–183

anatomy and physiology of, 163–170

autonomic nerve supply to, 169

in children, 665–666

deviations of, 189, 218*t*. *See also* Strabismus

disorders of, headache associated with, 74–75*t*

dry, 187

in aging patient, 182

examination of, 132, 184–195

in children, 665–666

in infants, 662–665

in pregnant patient, 439

special techniques in, 206–208

health promotion and counseling and, 209

in infants, 662–665

lumps and swellings in and around, 214*t*

measurements within, 195

movements of, 169–170

evaluation of, 189–190, 191, 570

in infants, 662–663

position and alignment of, 186

protrusion of (prominent), 206, 213*t*

pupillary reactions and, 168–169

red, 47, 187, 215*t*

in review of systems, 38

structures of, 163–166

symptoms related to, 46–47

visual fields of, 166–167

visual pathways of, 167–168

F

Face. *See also* Facial expression

examination of, 184, 211*t*, 572

in infants, assessment of shape and symmetry and, 653–654

in pregnant patient, 439

Fluid exchange, 465–466
Fluid wave, in ascites assessment, 375
Flush technique, for blood pressure measurement in infants and children, 641
Flutter, atrial, 320*t*, 321*t*
FOBT. *See* Fecal occult blood test
Fontanelles, 653
Foot. *See* Feet
Forced expiratory time, 267
Fordyce spots/granules, 238*t*
Foreign bodies, in vagina, in children, 689
Foreskin (prepuce), 387, 388
    examination of, 392
    in infants, 686
Forgetfulness, "benign," 109
Fornix, 406
Fourth heart sound, 282, 327*t*
    age and, 290
    assessment of, 310, 311, 312*t*
        inspection and palpation in, 303, 307
        relationship of to electrocardiogram, 286
Fovea, 166
    examination of, 194
Fractured rib, identification of, 267
Frank breech presentation, position of infants born in, 630
Fremitus, tactile, 255, 264, 271*t*
    in children, 678
    in infants, 677
    locations for identification of, 256, 265
    in selected chest disorders, 274–275*t*
Frenulum
    labial, 175
        in infants, 671–672
    lingual, 177
        in infants, 671–672
Frequency, urinary, 61, 92*t*, 93*t*
    in pregnancy, 434*t*
Friction rub
    abdominal, 362, 382*t*
    pericardial, 314, 332*t*
    pleural, 272*t*
Friends, as information source for health history interview, 34, 35
Frontal lobe, 555
Frontal sinuses, 174
    examination of, 200, 208
    transillumination of, 208
    in children, 673
Functional incontinence, 62, 94–95*t*
Functional scoliosis, 551*t*
Fundal height, measurement of, 440–441
Fundus
    ocular, 166, 225–227*t*, 570
        in aging patient, 182, 226*t*
        in diabetic retinopathy, 222*t*, 224*t*, 227*t*
        in hypertensive retinopathy, 226*t*, 227*t*
        in infants, 664–665
        light-colored spots in, 223–224*t*
        normal
            in dark-skinned person, 225*t*
            in fair skinned person, 225*t*
            in older person, 226*t*
        red spots and streaks in, 222*t*
    of uterus, 406
Funnel chest (pectus excavatum), 270*t*, 676

G

Gag reflex
    in aging patient, 568
    assessing, 573
Gait, 142
    abnormalities of, 616–617*t*
    assessing, 584–585
        in hip evaluation, 525
        in knee evaluation, 530
    in children, 702
    in infants, 692
    of old age, 617*t*
Galactorrhea, 50
    nonpuerperal, 346
Galant's (trunk incurvation) reflex, 698
Gallbladder, 357
Gallbladder disease, jaundice in, 60
Ganglion, 548*t*
Gangrene, in arterial insufficiency, 478*t*, 479*t*
Gas
    excessive, 55
    protuberant abdomen caused by, 381*t*
Gases, irritating, cough and hemoptysis associated with, 84*t*
Gastric cancer, abdominal pain/tenderness associated with, 86–87*t*
Gastroesophageal reflux, cough and hemoptysis associated with, 84*t*
Gastrointestinal system. *See also specific organ or structure and* Abdomen
    in review of systems, 38
    symptoms related to, 54–60, 85–91*t*
Gaze, cardinal directions of, 169–170
Gaze preference, in coma/stupor, 600
Gegenhalten, 612*t*
Gelling, 68
Generalized anxiety disorder, 125*t*
Generalized seizures, 105*t*
General survey, 132, 137–144
    anatomy and physiology relevant to, 137–140
    in infants and children, 638–649
    technique for, 141–144
Genital herpes
    in female, 423*t*
    in male, 399*t*
Genitals. *See also* Female genitals; Male genitals
    ambiguous, in infants, 687
    in review of systems, 38–39
Genu valgum (knock-knees), 530, 691
Genu varum (bowlegs), 530, 691
Geographic tongue, 242*t*
Gestation, expected weeks of, by dates, 436
Gestational age
    assessment of, 625, 626, 627*t*
    newborn classification by, 625, 626, 628
Giant cell arteritis, headache associated with, 76–77*t*
Gibbus, 551*t*
Gingiva (gums), 174–175
    abnormalities of, 239–241*t*
    bleeding from, 49
    examination of, 201
        in pregnant patient, 439
    hyperplasia of, 239*t*

    in infants, 671
    infection of, in infants and children, submaxillary lymphadenopathy in, 660*t*
    pregnancy tumor (epulis/pyogenic granuloma) of, 240*t*
    recession of, 241*t*
Gingival hyperplasia, 239*t*
Gingival margin, 174, 175
    examination of, 201
Gingival sulcus, 175
Gingivitis, 201
    acute necrotizing ulcerative, 239*t*
    chronic, 239*t*
    marginal, 239*t*
    prevention of, 209–210
Glandular tissue, of breast, 334
Glans penis, 387, 388
    examination of, 393
    in infants, 686
Glaucoma
    headache associated with, 74–75*t*
    iris changes and, 188
    red eye in, 215*t*
    surveillance for, 209
Glaucomatous cupping, 220*t*
Glenohumeral joint, 488
    examination of, 512
Glossitis, atrophic (smooth tongue), 242*t*
    in children, 675
Glossopharyngeal nerve (cranial nerve IX), 558
    examination of, 573
    functions of, 559*t*, 569
Gluteus maximus muscle, 499
Gluteus medius muscle, 499–500
Gluteus minimus muscle, 500
Goiter, 50, 204, 244*t*
    in children, 659*t*
Golfer's elbow (medial epicondylitis), 514, 546*t*
Goniometers, for describing limited range of motion, 541
Gonococcal arthritis, wrist affected in, 515
Gonococcal tenosynovitis, 515
Gonococcal urethritis, 393
Gout, 98–99*t*
    acute, 98–99*t*
        great toe affected in, 552*t*
    chronic tophaceous, 98–99*t*
        ear involvement and, 229*t*
        hand involvement and, 548*t*
Gouty arthritis, joint pain in, 98–99*t*
Gower's sign, 702–703
Grandiose delusions, 115*t*
Grand mal seizures, 105*t*
Granuloma, pyogenic, of gums (pregnancy tumor/epulis), 240*t*
Granulomatous colitis (Crohn's disease), diarrhea associated with, 90–91*t*
Graphesthesia (number identification), 588, 589
Grasp reflex, 697
Graves' disease (hyperthyroidism), 73, 244*t*
    bruits in, 206
    diffuse thyroid enlargement in, 244*t*
    in infants and children, facies in, 659*t*
    lid lag of, 190

Hip *(continued)*
  in children, 694–695
  congenitally dislocated, 692–693
  examination of, 525–530
    in children, 694–695
    in infants, 692–693
    inspection in, 525–526
    palpation in, 526
    range of motion and maneuvers in,
      527–530
  flexion deformity of, 527–528
  in infants, 692–693
  muscle groups of, 499–500
    assessing strength of, 579–580
  overview of, 497
  unstable, in infants, 693
Hirschsprung's disease (congenital mega-
    colon), in infants, 683
His bundle, 285
History, 1–2. *See also* Interview
  comprehensive, 2–4, 35–42
    adult patient, 35–39
    child patient, 39–42
  confusion about, mental disorders and,
    31–32
  family, 3
    in adult, 3
    recording, 724–725
  feeding, 40
  past, 3
    in adult, 36
    in child, 40–41
    recording, 723
  personal and social, 3
    recording, 725
  pregnancy, 435–436
  recording data from, 722–725
  sensitive issues and, 14–23
  source of, 2–3, 35
    families and friends as, 34, 35
  structure and purposes of, 2–4
Hives, joint pain and, 69
HIV infection/AIDS, 65, 66
  health promotion and counseling and
    in females, 421–422
    in males, 398
  Kaposi's sarcoma in, 157*t*
    of gums, 240*t*
    of palate, 237*t*
  testing for, 64, 66
Hoarseness, 50, 573
Hobbies, information about in health his-
    tory, 37
Hodgkin's disease, cervical lym-
    phadenopathy in, 660*t*
Holosystolic (pansystolic) murmurs, 313,
    330*t*
Home situation, information about in
    health history, 37
Homonymous hemianopsia, 185, 186, 212*t*
"Hooking technique," for liver palpation
    in obese patient, 368
Hopping in place, in gait assessment, 584
Hordeolum, acute (sty), 214*t*
Horizontal diplopia, 47
Horizontal (minor) fissure, 249
Horizontal nystagmus, 606*t*
Horizontal visual field defect, 212*t*

Horner's syndrome, 217*t*
  ptosis in, 213*t*, 217*t*
Hostility, interviewing techniques and, 30
Hot flushes/flashes, 64, 422
"Housemaid's knee" (prepatellar bursitis),
    530, 533
Houston, valves of, 449, 450
HSV infection. *See* Herpes simplex infec-
    tion
Human immunodeficiency virus infection.
    See HIV infection/AIDS
Humeroulnar joint, 491
Humerus, 487, 490
  greater tubercle of, 488, 490
Huntington's disease, 611*t*
Hutchinson's teeth, in congenital syphilis,
    241*t*, 658*t*
Hydrocele, 394, 400*t*
  in infants, 686–687
  transillumination of, 394, 400*t*, 686–687
Hydrocephalus, in infants and children,
    head circumference measurement
    and, 646
Hydrocephaly, 654, 656*t*
  craniotabes in, 654
Hydrocolpos, 687
Hydrostatic pressure, 465
Hygiene, personal, assessment of, 142
  mental status and, 111–112
Hymen, 405
  in children, 689
  imperforate, 419, 687
  in infants, 687
Hyoid bone, 179
Hypalgesia, 587
Hyperactive reflexes, 590
Hyperalgesia, 587
Hyperemesis, in pregnancy, 438
Hyperesthesia, 587
Hyperkinetic impulse, 323*t*
Hyperopia (farsightedness), 47
  headache associated with, 74–75*t*
Hyperplasia, gingival, 239*t*
Hyperpnea, 269*t*
Hyperpyrexia, 143
Hyperresonance, 259*t*
  in chest, 259, 265
    in selected disorders, 275*t*
Hypertension
  aging and, 291
  in children, 642
  control of, in stroke prevention, 604
  definition of, 297–298, 298*t*
  portal, in infants, 682
  pregnancy-induced, 438
  retinal arteries in, 221*t*
  systolic, 291
Hypertensive retinopathy, fundus changes
    in, 226*t*
  macular star and, 227*t*
Hyperthyroidism, 73, 244*t*
  bruits in, 206
  in infants and children, facies in, 659*t*
  lid lag of, 190
Hypertonia, 612*t*
Hypertrophic cardiomyopathy
  assessment of, 317*t*
  murmur associated with, 329*t*

syncope associated with, 102–103*t*
Hypertrophic scar, 154*t*
Hypertrophy, muscle, 575
Hyperventilation, 269*t*
  anxiety causing, dyspnea associated
    with, 82–83*t*
  hypocapnia caused by, 102–103*t*
  tetany caused by, Chvostek's sign in,
    655
Hypesthesia, 587
Hypoalbuminemia, edema in, 480*t*
Hypocalcemic tetany
  Chvostek's sign in, 654
  in infants, hoarse cry and, 672
Hypocapnia, hyperventilation causing,
    102–103*t*
Hypogastric (suprapubic) region, 356
Hypoglossal nerve (cranial nerve XII),
    558
  examination of, 574
    in infants, 696
  functions of, 559*t*, 569
  tongue affected in lesions of, 201, 574,
    696
Hypoglycemia, syncope mimicked by,
    102–103*t*
Hypomanic episode, 124*t*
Hypospadias, 393, 399*t*, 686
Hypotension
  postural (orthostatic), 102–103*t*, 297
    in aging patient, 291, 297
  supine, in pregnant patient, 437
Hypothalamus, 556
Hypothenar eminence
  atrophy of, 515, 575
  examination of, 515
Hypothermia, 143
Hypothyroidism, 73, 244*t*
  congenital (cretinism), 658*t*
    facies in, 658*t*
    posterior fontanelle in, 653
    skin appearance in, 650
Hypotonia, 576, 612*t*
Hysterical fainting, conversion reaction
    causing, 102–103*t*

I

IADLs. *See* Instrumental activities of daily
    living
Icterus. *See* Jaundice
Icthyosis, congenital, 650
Identifying data, in health history, 2
  in adult, 35
  in child, 39
Idiopathic pulmonary fibrosis, dyspnea
    associated with, 82–83*t*
Ileopectineal (iliopsoas) bursa, 500
  examination of, 526
Ileus, in infants, 682
Iliac arteries, pulsations of, 356
Iliac crests, 355, 494, 498
  unequal heights of, 520
Iliac spine
  anterior superior, 355, 388, 389, 395, 498
  posterior superior, 494, 499
Iliac tubercle, 498
Iliofemoral thrombosis, 473

Lumbricals, 492
Lumps/masses, breast, 50, 349t, 353t. See also Breast cancer; Breast cysts; Breast nodules
in pregnant patient, 440
Lung abscess, cough and hemoptysis associated with, 84t
Lung cancer, cough and hemoptysis associated with, 84t
Lung fields, 250
Lungs, 133
age-related changes in, 252
anatomy of, 249–250
auscultation of, 260–263, 266–267. See also Lung (breath) sounds
locations for
on anterior chest, 265
on posterior chest, 259
bases of, 250
in children, 678
examination of, 133, 253–267
general approach to, 253
in infants, 676–677
in pregnant patient, 439
special techniques in, 267
fissures and lobes of, 249–250
health promotion and counseling and, 268
in infants, 676–677
Lung (breath) sounds, 261–263, 267
abnormal, 262–263, 262t, 267, 272t, 274–275t
adventitious (added), 262–263, 262t, 267, 272t, 274–275t
altered, 271t
bronchial, 261, 261t, 271t, 274–275t
bronchovesicular, 261, 261t, 267, 271t, 274t
characteristics of, 261t
in children, 678
location of, quality affected by, 250
normal, 261–262, 261t, 267, 271t, 274t
in selected chest disorders, 274–275t
tracheal, 261, 261t
vesicular, 261, 261t, 271t, 274t
Lunula, 145
Lymphadenitis, acute posterior cervical, 660t
Lymphadenopathy, 468
in head and neck, 50, 203–204
in infants and children, 655, 657–661, 660t
Lymphangitis, acute, 96–97t
Lymphatics (lymphatic system), 464–465. See also Lymph nodes
breast drained by, 338–339
in children, 657
genitals drained by
in females, 407
in males, 388
Lymphatic stasis. See Lymphedema
Lymphedema, 473, 481t, 482t
of hand and arm, 467
in venous insufficiency, 473
Lymph nodes, 464–465. See also Lymphatics (lymphatic system)
age-related changes in, 466

axillary, 338–339, 464, 465
palpation of, 345–346
cervical, 180–181
age-related changes in, 181
deep, 180, 203
enlarged, 50, 203–204
in infants and children, 655, 657–661, 660t
examination of, 203–204
posterior, 180, 203
superficial, 180–181, 203
tender, 203–204
epitrochlear, 133, 464, 465, 468
of head and neck, 180–181. See also Lymph nodes, cervical
in infants and children, 655, 657–661, 660t
infraclavicular, 464
inguinal, 464, 465
palpation of, 468
occipital, 180, 203
pectoral, 338
palpation of, 346
posterior auricular, 180, 203
preauricular, 180, 203, 464
submandibular, 180–181, 203
submental, 180, 181, 203
subscapular, 338
palpation of, 346
supraclavicular, 180–181, 203
enlargement of, 203
tonsillar, 180–181, 203
Lymphoma, cervical lymphadenopathy in, 660t

M

Macewen's sign, 654
McMurray test, 536t
Macula, 166
examination of, 194
Macular degeneration of aging, 194
Macular star, in hypertensive retinopathy, 226t
Macule, 153t, 160t
Major depressive episode, 124t. See also Depression
Major (oblique) fissure, 249
Malabsorption syndromes, diarrhea associated with, 90–91t
Male breast, 335
in adolescent, 338
examination of, 345
in newborn, 676
Male genitals, 134, 387–403
in adolescent, 389–391, 392
age-related changes in, 389–391, 392
in aging patient, 391
anatomy and physiology of, 387–391
in children, 688
development of, 389–391, 392
examination of, 134, 392–398
in children, 688
general approach to, 392
in infants, 686–687
special techniques in, 397
health promotion and counseling and, 398

in infants, 686–687
lymphatics draining, 388
in review of systems, 38
symptoms related to, 65–67
Males, growth in, 137, 138, 648
Malignant melanoma, 152, 157t
Malleolus
lateral, 504
medial, 504
Malleus, 170
examination of, 197
Malocclusion, in children, 674
Mammary duct ectasia, 343
Mammary souffle (pregnancy-related heart murmur), 290, 439
Mammography, for breast cancer screening, 351
Mandible, 485, 486
Mandibular protrusion (underbite), 674–675
Manic episode, 124t
Manner, assessment of, mental status and, 112
Manubrium, 487
Marginal gingivitis, 239t
Masseter muscle, 486
assessing strength of, 570, 571
Mass reflexes, in infants, 700
Mastectomy, examination of patient after, 347
Mastoiditis, in children, 670
acute posterior cervical lymphadenitis in, 660t
Mastoid process, 170, 171
Maxillary protrusion (overbite), 674
Maxillary sinuses, 174
examination of, 200, 208
in children, 673
transillumination in, 208, 673
MCL. See Medial collateral ligament
MCPs. See Metacarpophalangeal joints
Measles (rubeola), Koplik's spots in, 238t, 673
Medial collateral ligament, 503
examination of, 532, 535t
Medial condyle
tibial, 502
femoral, 531
Medial epicondyle
femoral, 531
humeral, 513, 514
tibial, 501
Medial epicondylitis (pitcher's/golfer's elbow), 514, 546t
Medial malleolus, 504
Medial meniscus, 503
examination of, 532, 536t
Median nerve, 491, 493
compression of in carpal tunnel, 515
assessment of, 539
testing function of, 518
Mediastinal crunch (Hamman's sign), 272t
Medical model diagnosis, limitations of, 709
Medical records, 719–731
reviewing before interview, 4
Medications

allergies to, identification of in health history, 36, 723
constipation associated with, 89*t*
current, in health history, 36
   recording, 723
diarrhea caused by, 90–91*t*
fever and, 46
incontinence caused by, 94–95*t*
nasal stuffiness caused by, 49
psychotic disorder associated with, 126*t*
vertigo caused by, 79*t*
Medulla, 556
Medullated nerve fibers, 219*t*
Mees' lines, 159*t*
Megacephaly, 654
Megacolon, congenital (Hirschsprung's disease), in infants, 683
Meibomian glands, 164
Melanin, 146
   changes in, 155*t*
Melanoma, 152, 157*t*
Melena, 57, 88*t*
Memory, 107
   in delirium and dementia, 127*t*
   impairments in with aging, 109
Menarche, 63, 408
   relationship of to breast development, 337
Meniere's disease, vertigo associated with, 79*t*
Meningeal signs, testing for, 597–598
Meningitis
   headache associated with, 76–77*t*
   in infants and children, neck mobility affected in, 661–662
Menisci
   of knee, 503
     examination of, 532, 536*t*
Menopause, 64
   health promotion and counseling and, 422
Menorrhagia, 63
Menstrual age, 436
Menstrual history, 63
   breast cancer risk and, 350, 351*t*
Menstruation, cessation of, in pregnancy, 434*t*
Mental status, 107–127
   aging affecting, 108–109
   assessment of, 110–120, 135
     Mini-Mental State Examination for, 120
     screening for, 73
   components of mental function and, 107–109
   confusing behavior/history and, 31–32
   in delirium and dementia, 127*t*
   health promotion and counseling and, 121–122
   in infants, 695
   physical disorders affecting, 108
Mesenteric ischemia, abdominal pain/tenderness associated with, 86–87*t*
Metabolic disorders, constipation associated with, 89*t*
Metabolic–toxic coma, 618*t*
Metacarpals, 491
   examination of, 515

Metacarpophalangeal joints, 492
   examination of, 516
Metastatic disease, cervical lymphadenopathy in, 660*t*
Metatarsalgia, 537
Metatarsals
   examination of, 537
   heads of, 505
Metatarsophalangeal joint, 505
   examination of, 537, 538
   of great toe, in acute gouty arthritis, 552*t*
Metatarsus adductus, 691
Metatarsus varus, 691
Metopic suture, 653
Metrorrhagia, 63
Microaneurysms, retinal, 222*t*
Microcephaly, 646, 654
Micrognathia, 654, 675
Micturition syncope, 102–103*t*
Midaxillary line, 248
Midbrain, 555, 556
Midclavicular line, 248
Middiastolic murmurs, 313, 331*t*
Middle ear, 171
Midposition fixed pupils, in coma, 618*t*, 619*t*
Midsternal line, 248
Midsystolic murmurs, 313, 328–329*t*
Migraine headaches, 74–75*t*
Milia, 651
Miliaria rubra, 651
"Milking" urethra
   in female, 413
   in male, 393
"Milk line," supernumerary breasts along, 335
Mindset, clinician's, health history interview and, 5
Mini-Mental State Examination (MMSE), 120
Minor (horizontal) fissure, 249
Miosis, 188
Mitgehen, 612*t*
Mitral regurgitation, 681
   murmur associated with, 330*t*
   systolic murmur of, 291
Mitral sound, 283
Mitral stenosis, 681
   cough and hemoptysis associated with, 84*t*
   dyspnea associated with, 82–83*t*
   murmurs associated with, 331*t*
Mitral valve, 279
   age-related changes in, 291
   auscultation of sounds and murmurs originating in, 284, 310
     diastolic murmurs, 331*t*
     pansystolic (holosystolic) murmurs, 330*t*
   rheumatic heart disease affecting, 681
Mitral valve prolapse, assessment of, 317*t*
Mixed episode, 124*t*
Mixed hearing loss, 232*t*
MMSE. *See* Mini-Mental State Examination
Mobility
   eardrum (tympanic membrane), 197
     pneumatic otoscopy for assessment of in children, 670

neck, assessing, 597
   in infants and children, 661–662
skin, 150
Modified Leopold's maneuvers, 444–446
Molding, 653
Mole (nevus), 154*t*
Mongolian spots, 650
Monilia, 427*t*
Monocular vision, 167
Mononeuropathy, findings in, 615*t*
Mononucleosis, infectious, cervical lymphadenopathy in, 660*t*
Mons pubis, 405
   in infants, 687
Montgomery's glands, in pregnancy, 431–432, 439
Mood, 108
   assessment of, 113–114, 124*t*
   in delirium and dementia, 127*t*
   disorders of, 124*t*
Moro response, 701
Motility disorders, esophageal, dysphagia associated with, 85*t*
Motion, limitation of, joint pain and, 68
Motor (efferent) fibers, 560
Motor neurons
   lower, 561, 562
     damage to, 563
       flaccidity caused by, 612*t*
   upper, 561
     damage to
       facial paralysis caused by, 608–609*t*
       spasticity caused by, 612*t*
Motor pathways, 561–563. *See also* Motor system
   lesions of, 562–563
Motor system (motor activity/function), 135, 142
   assessment of, 135, 142, 574–585
     in infants, 695–696
     mental status and, 111
   in central nervous system disorders, 614*t*
   changes in in aging patient, 568
   disorders of, 562–563
     in infants, 695–696
Mouth, 133. *See also* Oral mucosa
   age-related changes in, 183
   anatomy of, 174–178
   cancer of, 243*t*
   in children, 673–674
   examination of, 133, 200–202
     in children, 673–674
     in infants, 671–672
     in pregnant patient, 439
   health promotion and counseling and, 209–210
   in infants, 671–672
   in review of systems, 38
   symptoms related to, 49–50
Movements, involuntary, 71
Mucocutaneous lymph node syndrome (Kawasaki's disease), 660*t*
Mucoid sputum, 53
Mucopurulent cervicitis, 426*t*
Mucopurulent sputum, 53
Mucous patch of syphilis, 243*t*
Mucous plug, 434

in infants, 695–702
peripheral, anatomy and physiology of, 558–560
in review of systems, 39
symptoms related to, 70–71, 102–105t
Neuralgia, trigeminal, headache associated with, 76–77t
Neurofibromatosis, 520
skin manifestations in, 161t, 520
Neurologic disorders. *See* Nervous system, disorders of
Neurologic examination, 134, 134–135, 569–603
in children, 702–703
in coma/stupor, 600–603
general approach to, 569
in infants, 695–702
special techniques in, 596–603
symmetry of findings and, 568
Neuroma, acoustic, findings in, 614t
Neuromuscular junction, 561
lesions of, 615t
Neuromuscular maturity, assessment of, in gestational age assessment, 626, 627t
Neuronitis, vestibular (acute labyrinthitis), vertigo associated with, 79t
Neurons (nerve cells), 556
Neuropathic ulcer, 479t
of foot, 553t
Nevus, 154t
flammeus, 651
telangiectatic, 651
vasculosus, 651
Newborn. *See also* Infants
classification of, 625–628, 629
examination of
approach to, 624–630
auscultation and palpation in, 630
inspection in, 630
normal full-term, 630
skin in, 650–652
New learning ability, assessment of, 118
Nicotine replacement therapy, 268
Night sweats, 45
Nipples, 333, 335
discharge from, 50
assessment of, 346, 347
in pregnant patient, 440
examination of
inspection in, 340, 341
in male, 345
palpation in, 344
in pregnant patient, 439, 440
inverted, 341, 439
Paget's disease of, 352t
during pregnancy, 431, 439, 440
retraction of, 341, 352t
supernumerary, 335, 676
Nits, 184. *See also* Lice
Nocturia, 61, 93t
Nocturnal emissions, 391
Nodal (supraventricular) premature contractions, 320t, 321t
Nodules
breast, 343, 344, 353t
physiologic, 337
rheumatoid

ear involvement and, 229t
at elbow, 546t
skin, 153t, 160t, 161t
thyroid, 244t
Non-Hodgkin's lymphoma, cervical lymphadenopathy in, 660t
Noninflammatory infectious diarrhea, 90–91t
Nonmaleficence, 23
Nonparalytic strabismus, 218t
in children, 665
Nonproliferative diabetic retinopathy, 227t
Nonpuerperal galactorrhea, 346
Nonverbal communication, 11–12
Normal sinus rhythm, 320t
Nose, 133. *See also under Nasal*
anatomy of, 172–173
in children, 672–673
examination of, 133, 198–200
in children, 672–673
in infants, 671
in pregnant patient, 439
in infants, 671
in review of systems, 38
symptoms related to, 49
Nosebleed (epistaxis), 49, 199
Nostrils (nares), 173
Notching, of teeth, 241t
Note taking, during health history interview, 5
Nuchal rigidity, in infants and children, 661–662
Nuclear cataract, 216t
Nucleus pulposus, 484
Number calculation, in higher cognitive functioning, 108
assessment of, 118
Number identification (graphesthesia), 588, 589
Numbness, 71
"Nursing bottle caries," 674
Nutrition
musculoskeletal health and, 542
in pregnancy, health promotion and counseling and, 447
recording information about, 723
Nystagmus, 189, 573, 606–607t
in infants, 663

O

Obesity (overweight), 44
blood pressure cuff selection and, 294, 298
prevention of, cardiovascular health and, 318–319
Objective data, 705
Oblique (major) fissure, 249
Oblique muscles of eye, 169, 170
Obsessions, 115t, 125t
Obsessive–compulsive disorder, 125t
Obstipation, 58
Obstreperous patient, interviewing, 30–31
Obstructive breathing, 269t
Obtundation, 111
level of consciousness assessment and, 600t

Obturator sign, in appendicitis, 377
in children, 686
Occipital lobe, 168, 555
Occipital lymph nodes, 180
enlarged (occipital lymphadenopathy), in infants and children, 660t
examination of, 203
Ocular fundus, 166, 225–227t, 570
in aging patient, 182, 226t
in diabetic retinopathy, 222t, 224t, 227t
in hypertensive retinopathy, 226t, 227t
in infants, 664–665
light-colored spots in, 223–224t
normal
in dark-skinned person, 225t
in fair skinned person, 225t
in older person, 226t
red spots and streaks in, 222t
Ocular movements. *See* Extraocular movements
Oculocephalic reflex (doll's-eye movements), in coma/stupor, 601
Oculomotor nerve (cranial nerve III), 164, 558
examination of, 570
functions of, 559t, 569
paralysis of
pupillary abnormalities in, 217t
strabismus in, 218t
Oculovestibular reflex, with caloric stimulation, in coma/stupor, 601
Odynophagia, 54
Olecranon bursa, 491
Olecranon bursitis, 485, 513, 546t
Olecranon process, 490, 491
examination of, 513
Olfactory nerve (cranial nerve I), 558
examination of, 570
functions of, 559t, 569
Oligomenorrhea, 63
Onycholysis, 158t
Open-angle glaucoma, 188
Open-ended questions, in health history interview, 7–8
Opening snap, 282, 312t, 327t
Ophthalmia neonatorum, prophylaxis in newborn and, 663
Ophthalmoscope, technique for use of, 191–192
Ophthalmoscopic examination, 166, 191–195
in aging patient, 182–183
in glaucoma surveillance, 209
in infants, 664–665
Opisthotonus, 695–696
Opposition, thumb, assessing, 518, 579
Optical blink reflex, in newborn, 664
Optic atrophy, 220t
Optic chiasm, 168, 212t
visual field defects caused by lesions of, 212t
Optic disc, 166, 192–193
abnormalities of, 220t
finding, 192–193
inspecting, 193
normal variations of, 219t
in papilledema, 195, 220t
Optic fundus. *See* Ocular fundus

Optic nerve (cranial nerve II), 166, 168, 212*t*, 558
  examination of, 570
  functions of, 559*t*, 569
  visual field defects caused by lesions of, 212*t*
Opticokinetic testing, in children, 666
Optic radiation, 168, 212*t*
  visual field defects caused by lesions of, 212*t*
Optic tract, 168, 212*t*
  visual field defects caused by lesions of, 212*t*
Oral candidiasis (thrush)
  in infants, 672
  palate affected in, 237*t*
  tongue affected in, 242*t*
Oral cavity (mouth), 133
  age-related changes in, 183
  anatomy of, 174–178
  cancer of, 243*t*
  in children, 673–674
  examination of, 133, 200–202
    in children, 673–674
    in infants, 671–672
    in pregnant patient, 439
  health promotion and counseling and, 209–210
  in infants, 671–672
  in review of systems, 38
  symptoms related to, 49–50
Oral–facial dyskinesias, 610*t*
Oral health, health promotion and counseling and, 209–210
Oral leukoplakia, 238*t*, 243*t*
  hairy, 242*t*
Oral mucosa
  abnormalities of, 236–238*t*
  examination of, 200–201
Oral temperature, 143
  normal, 144
Orchitis, acute, 401*t*
Organic murmurs, 680
Orientation, 107
  assessment of, mental status and, 112, 116–117
  in delirium and dementia, 127*t*
Orthopnea, 52
Orthostatic edema, 481*t*, 482*t*
Orthostatic (postural) hypotension, 102–103*t*, 297
  in aging patient, 291, 297
Ortolani's sign, 692
Ortolani test, 692
OS. *See* Opening snap
Osmotic diarrhea, 90–91*t*
Osmotic pressure, colloid
  interstitial, 465
  of plasma proteins, 465–466
Ossicles, auditory, 170, 171
Osteoarthritis (degenerative joint disease), 98–99*t*. *See also* Arthritis
  hands affected in, 514, 547*t*
Osteoporosis
  estrogen replacement therapy and, 422
  health promotion and counseling and, 543
  height loss and, 506

Otitic barotrauma, 231*t*
Otitis externa, 195, 196, 231*t*, 670
  acute posterior cervical lymphadenitis in, 660*t*
  otitis media differentiated from, 195, 231*t*, 670
Otitis media, 195, 197, 231*t*, 670
  acute, 670
  otitis externa differentiated from, 195, 231*t*, 670
  with purulent effusion, 231*t*
  with serous effusion, 231*t*, 670
Otoscope
  for examination of ear canal and drum, 195–196
    in children, 667–670
    in infants, 667
  for examination of nose, 199
  pneumatic, 670
Ova, 407
Ovarian adnexa, 407
  examination of, 418
    in pregnant patient, 443
  masses of, 430*t*
Ovaries, 406, 407
  age-related changes in, 409, 417–418
  cysts and tumors of, 430*t*
  palpation of, 417–418
  in pregnant patient, 435, 443
Overbite (maxillary protrusion), 674
Overflow incontinence, 62, 94–95*t*
Overtalkative patients, interviewing, 29–30
Overweight (obesity), 44
  blood pressure cuff selection and, 294, 298
  prevention of, cardiovascular health and, 318–319
Oxyhemoglobin, 146, 149

P
P$_2$, 283, 312, 312*t*, 325*t*
Paget's disease of nipple, 352*t*
Pain
  abdominal, 55–57, 86–87*t*, 383–384*t*
    in appendicitis, 56, 86–87*t*, 376–377
    assessment of, 363–364, 376–377
    in children, 684, 685–686
    in cholecystitis, 86–87*t*, 377
    joint pain and, 69
  anal lesions causing, constipation associated with, 89*t*
  in arms and legs, in peripheral vascular disorders, 67, 478*t*
  back (backache), 69, 100*t*, 521–522
    in pregnancy, 434*t*
    prevention of, 542
    with radiation to leg, 100*t*
    assessment of, 540
  chest, 50–51, 80–81*t*
  chest wall, 80–81*t*
  in/around ears, 48–49
    in otitis externa and media, 195, 231*t*, 670
  in/around eyes, 47
  facial, 571
  headache, 46, 74–77*t*

  with intercourse (dyspareunia), 65
  joint, 67–68, 98–99*t*, 508
    symptoms associated with, 68–69
  kidney, 60, 373
  knee, 531–532
  neck, 70, 101*t*, 519, 522
  neurologic, 71
  in peripheral vascular disorders, 67, 96–97*t*, 478*t*
  pleural, 80–81*t*
  referred
    to abdomen, 56
    to back, 100*t*
  rest, in arteriosclerosis obliterans, 96–97*t*
  sensation of
    fibers conducting, 564
    testing, 587
      on face, 571
      in infants, 696
  shoulder, 510, 511–513, 544–545*t*
  on swallowing (odynophagia), 54
  in urinary tract disorders, 60–61
  on urination, 60–61
Palate
  abnormalities of, 236–238*t*
  in children, 676
  cleft, submucosal, 676
  hard, 178
  soft, 177, 178
    in children, 676
    in cranial nerve X (vagus nerve) paralysis, 202, 573
    examination of, 202, 573
      in children, 676
      in infants, 671
      in newborn, 671
  thrush (candidiasis) affecting, 237*t*
Pallor, 149
  in infants, 650
Palmar aponeurosis, thickening of in Dupuytren's contractures, 515, 549*t*
Palmar grasp reflex, 697
Palmar interossei muscles, 492
Palmar space infections, 548*t*
Palpation. *See also specific system or structure*
  blood pressure measurement by, 299
  in infants and children, 641
Palpebral conjunctiva, 164
  examination of, 187, 207
Palpebral fissure, 163
Palpitations, 51–52
Pancreas, 357
Pancreatic cancer, abdominal pain/tenderness associated with, 86–87*t*
Pancreatitis
  acute, 86–87*t*, 384*t*
  chronic, 86–87*t*
Panic attack, 125*t*
Panic disorder, 125*t*
Pansystolic (holosystolic) murmurs, 313, 330*t*
Papanicolaou smears
  health promotion and counseling and, 421
  obtaining specimens for, 415–416
    in pregnant patient, 438, 442

Papillae
  interdental, 174
    examination of, 201
  of tongue, 176–177
Papilledema, 195, 220t
  in infants, 664–665
Papilloma, benign intraductal, 347
Papule, 153t, 160t
Paradoxical pulse, 317, 322t
Paralanguage, 12
Paralysis (plegia), 70–71, 576
  abducens nerve (cranial nerve VI), 190
    strabismus in, 218t
  cranial nerve III (oculomotor nerve)
    pupillary abnormalities in, 217t
    strabismus in, 218t
  cranial nerve IV (trochlear nerve), stra-
    bismus in, 218t
  cranial nerve VI (abducens nerve), 190
    strabismus in, 218t
  cranial nerve X (vagus nerve), pharyn-
    geal findings in, 202, 573
  facial, 608–609t
  flaccid, in response to painful stimulus,
    602
  hemiplegia, 576
    early, 620t
    in infants, 702
    muscle tone assessment in, 602–603
  paraplegia, 576
  quadriplegia, 576
Paralytic strabismus, 218t
  in children, 665
Paranasal sinuses, 133. See also Sinusitis
  anatomy of, 174
    in children, 672–673
  examination of, 133, 200, 208
    in children, 672–673
  in review of systems, 38
  symptoms related to, 49
  transillumination of, 200, 208
    in children, 673
Paraphasias, 112
Paraphimosis, 392
Paraplegia, 576
  scissoring in, 698, 699
Parasternal muscles, 251
Parasympathetic nervous system, eye sup-
  plied by, 169
Paratonia, 612t
Paraurethral (Skene's) glands, 405
  in pregnant patient, 442
Paravertebral muscles, 494
  examination of, 521
Parent–infant interaction, assessment of, 631
Paresis, 576
Paresthesias, 71
Parietal bone, percussion of in infants, 654
Parietal lobe, 555
Parietal pain, 56
Parietal pleura, 251
Parkinsonian gait, 617t
Parkinsonism
  facies in, 211t
  findings in, 614t
    gait abnormalities, 617t
  resting tremor of, 610t
  rigidity in, 612t

Paronychia, 158t
Parotid (Stensen's) ducts, 177
  examination of, in infants, 657
Parotid gland, 163
  enlargement of, facies in, 211t
  examination of, in children, 657
Paroxysmal nocturnal dyspnea, 52
Pars flaccida, 171, 196
Pars tensa, 171, 196
Partial seizures, 104t
Past history, 3
  in adult, 36
  in child, 40–41
  recording, 723
Past pointing, 583
Patch, skin, 153t, 161t
Patella femoral grinding test, 532
Patella (knee cap), 501, 502
  examination of, 531–532
  swelling over, 530
Patellar clonus, 596
Patellar tendon, 502
  examination of, 531
  tear of, 531
Patellofemoral compartment, examination
  of, 531
Patellofemoral joint, 502
Patent ductus arteriosus, murmurs associ-
  ated with, 332t
Patient autonomy, 23
Patient-centered questions, 10–11, 10t
Patient–clinician relationship
  building partnership and, 17
  establishing rapport for health history
    interview and, 6–7, 7
    with children, 24
  sexuality in, 23
Patient comfort, during health history in-
  terview, 7
Patient education. See also Health promo-
  tion and counseling
  planning and, 706
Patient problems, single vs. multiple,
  709–710
Patient record (clinical record), 719–731
  reviewing before interview, 4
PCL. See Posterior cruciate ligament
Pectinate (dentate) line (anorectal junction), 449–450
Pectoralis major muscle, 333, 489
  examination of, 513
Pectoralis minor muscle, 489
Pectoral lymph nodes, 338
  palpation of, 346
Pectoriloquy, whispered, 263, 271t
Pectus carinatum (pigeon chest/chicken
  breast deformity), 270t, 676
Pectus excavatum (funnel chest), 270t, 676
Pedersen speculum, 411, 419
Pedicle, vertebral, 495
Pediculosis capitis (head lice), in children,
  acute posterior cervical lymph-
  adenitis and, 660t
Pediculosis pubis (crab lice)
  in females, 412
  in males, 393
Pelvic disease, abdominal pain/tender-
  ness caused by, 383t

Pelvic examination, 410–420
  in children, 689–690
  equipment for, 411–412
    pregnant patient and, 438
  external, 412–413
  general approach to, 410–412
  internal, 413–419
  lubricants for, contamination of, 419
  patient position for, 412
    for pregnant patient, 437
  in pregnant patient, 437, 442–443
Pelvic inflammatory disease, 430t
Pelvic muscles, assessment of strength of,
    418
  in pregnant patient, 443
Pelvic tilt, 520
Pelvis
  back pain referred from, 100t
  changes in during pregnancy, 433–435
Pemphigus, 160t
Pendular nystagmus, 606t
Penis, 387, 388
  abnormalities of, 66, 399t
  age-related changes in, 389, 390, 391, 392
  carcinoma of, 399t
  in children, 688
  corona of, 388
  discharge from, 66, 393
  examination of, 392–393
  lymphatics draining, 388
  shaft of, 387, 388
  in infants, 686
Peptic ulcer disease, abdominal pain/ten-
  derness associated with, 86–87t
Perceptions, 107
  assessment of, 116, 116t
  in delirium and dementia, 127t
Percussion. See also Percussion notes
  in abdominal examination, 362
    ascites assessment and, 374–375
    of infants, 682
    liver assessment and, 365–366
    spleen assessment and, 369, 370
  in cardiac examination, 309
  in chest examination
    anterior, 265–266
      locations for, 265
    posterior, 256–260
      locations for, 259
    in selected disorders, 274–275t
  technique for, 257–259, 265–266
Percussion notes, 259, 259t. See also specific
  type and Percussion
  in infants, 677
Perez reflex, 700
Perforating (communicating) veins, 463
Perforation of eardrum, 230t, 670
  healed, 230t
Perianal area
  abnormalities of, 457–458t
  examination of, 452
Perianal skin tabs, in children, 690
Pericardial friction rub, 314, 332t
Pericarditis, chest pain associated with,
    80–81t
Perimetry, in glaucoma surveillance, 209
Perineum, 405, 406
Periodic breathing, in newborn, 677

Periodontal disease, 239*t*
  in aging patient, 183
  prevention of, 209–210
Periodontitis, 239*t*
Periorbital edema, 213*t*
Peripheral cataract, 216*t*
Peripheral cyanosis, 147, 149
Peripheral nerves, 560
  lesions of, 615*t*
Peripheral nervous system, 555. *See also*
  Nervous system
  anatomy and physiology of, 558–560
  disorders of, 615*t*
Peripheral vascular disease, prevention of,
  477
Peripheral vascular system, 134, 461–482
  age-related changes in, 466
  anatomy and physiology of, 461–466
  arteries in, 461–462
  capillary bed in, 465–466
  examination of, 134, 467–476
    in bedfast patient, 474
    special techniques in, 473–476
  fluid exchange and, 465–466
  health promotion and counseling and,
    477
  lymphatics in, 464–465
  lymph nodes and, 464–465
  painful disorders of, 67, 96–97*t*, 478*t*
    disorders mimicking, 67, 96–97*t*
  in review of systems, 39
  symptoms related to, 67, 96–97*t*
  veins in, 462–463
Peristalsis, assessment of, 361
Peritoneal inflammation, assessing, 363, 364
Peritoneal reflection, 449
Peritonitis, generalized, in children, 686
Peritonsillar abscess, 675, 676
Periumbilical pain, 55
Permanent teeth, 674
Perpendicular lighting, 135, 136
Persecution, delusions of, 115*t*
Perseveration, 114*t*
Persistent posterior lenticular fiobrovascu-
  lar sheath, in infants, 664
Person, orientation to, 112, 117
Personal history, 3, 37
  recording, 725
Personal hygiene, assessment of, 142
  mental status and, 111–112
Personality, in child health history, 41
Pes anserine bursitis, 530, 533
Petechiae, 72, 156*t*
  in buccal mucosa, 238*t*
Petit mal absences, 105*t*
Peutz-Jeghers syndrome, lips affected in,
  235*t*
Peyronie's disease, 399*t*
Phalanges, 491
  examination of, 515
Phalen's test, 539
Pharyngeal tonsils (adenoids), examina-
  tion of, 675
Pharyngitis (sore throat), 49, 236*t*
  cervical lymphadenopathy in, 660*t*
  joint pain and, 69
Pharynx (throat), 133, 178
  abnormalities of, 236–238*t*

anatomy of, 174–178
  in children, 673–674, 675–676
  in cranial nerve X (vagus nerve) paraly-
    sis, 202, 573
  examination of, 133, 202
    in children, 673–674, 675–676
    in infants, 672
  in infants, 672
  in review of systems, 38
  sore (pharyngitis), 49, 236*t*
    cervical lymphadenopathy in, 660*t*
    joint pain and, 69
  symptoms related to, 49–50
Phenothiazines
  dystonia caused by, 611*t*
  tics caused by, 611*t*
Phimosis, 392
Phobias, 115*t*, 125*t*
Physical abuse, in pregnancy, health promotion and counseling and, 448
Physical activities of daily living, 28*t*
  assessment of in aging patient, 28–29
Physical examination, 129–136
  completeness of, 131
  examiner's position for, 132
  general approach to, 129–132
    in infants and children, 624–649
  in infants and children, 621–703
    approach to patient for, 624–638
    general survey in, 638–649
  lighting for, 130, 135–136
  overview of, 132–136
  with patient standing, 134
  with patient supine, 138
  recording data from, 726–728
  relating findings to patient and, 130
  right- vs. left-handed approach for, 132
  sequence of, 131
Physical growth, 137, 138, 642–646
  age affecting, 137, 138
  in child health history, 41
  norms for, 622, 642, 647, 648
Physiologic cupping, 193, 219*t*
Physiologic jaundice, of newborn, 651
Physiologic murmurs, 328–329*t*
PID. *See* Pelvic inflammatory disease
Pigeon chest (pectus carinatum), 270*t*, 676
Pigmentation changes, 149. *See also* Skin,
  color of
  in infants, 650
  in melanin, 155*t*
PIH. *See* Pregnancy-induced hypertension
Pilar (trichilemmal) cyst, behind ear, 228*t*
Pill-rolling tremor of parkinsonism, 610*t*
Pilonidal cyst and sinus, 457*t*
Pinguecula, 214*t*
Pinna. *See* Auricle
Pinpoint pupils, in coma, 618*t*, 619*t*
PIPs. *See* Proximal interphalangeal joints
Pitcher's elbow (medial epicondylitis),
  514, 546*t*
Pitting edema, 471–472, 482*t*
Place, orientation to, 117
Placing response, 699–700
Plagiocephaly, 653–654
Plan, 706
  development of, 717
    data base in, 705–706

Plantar fasciitis, 537
Plantar flexion, 505, 581
Plantar reflex, 561, 595–596
Plantar wart, 553*t*
Plaque
  dental, in gingivitis, 239*t*
  skin, 153*t*, 161*t*
Plasma proteins, colloid osmotic pressure
  of, 465–466
Plateau murmur, 314
Platelet disorders, bleeding in, 72
Plegia. *See* Paralysis
Pleura, anatomy of, 251
Pleural effusion, physical signs in, 275*t*
Pleural pain, 80–81*t*
Pleural rub, 272*t*
Pleural space, 251
Pleurisy, abdominal pain/tenderness
  caused by, 383*t*
PMI. *See* Point of maximal impulse
PMS (premenstrual syndrome), 64
Pneumatic otoscopy, in children, 670
Pneumonia
  cough and hemoptysis associated with,
    84*t*
  dyspnea associated with, 82–83*t*
Pneumothorax
  physical signs in, 275*t*
  spontaneous, dyspnea associated with,
    82–83*t*
Point localization, 589
Point of maximal impulse (apical impulse), 278
  age-related changes in, 290
  amplitude of, 306
  assessment of, 303–307
  diameter of, 306
  duration of, 307
  in infants and children, 679
  location of, 306
  in pregnant patient, 439
Point-to-point movements, assessing, 583
Polio, findings in, 615*t*
Polydipsia, 61
  in diabetes mellitus, 72
  polyuria caused by, 92*t*
Polymenorrhea, 63
Polymyalgia rheumatica, 98–99*t*
Polyneuropathy
  distal hip muscles affected in, 580
  findings in, 615*t*
  sensory loss in, 586, 587
Polyphagia, in diabetes mellitus, 72
Polyps
  cervical, 426*t*
  nasal, 199
  rectal, 458*t*
Polyuria, 61, 92*t*
  in diabetes insipidus, 92*t*
  in diabetes mellitus, 72
Pons, 555, 556
Popliteal angle, in newborn, 626, 627*t*
Popliteal artery, 462
Popliteal ("baker's") cyst, 533
Popliteal pulse, 462
  assessment of, 469–470
Porencephalic cysts, transillumination in
  identification of, 655

Pubertal gynecomastia, 338
Puberty. *See also* Adolescents
  breast development in
    in females, 335–337
    in males, 338
    delayed, in males, 392
  genital development in
    in females, 407–409, 412
    in males, 389–391, 392
  precocious, 688
Pubic hair, development of
  in females, 336, 337
  in males, 389, 390, 391, 392
Pubic tubercle, 355, 388, 389, 498
Pulmonary artery, 277, 278, 279
  inspection and palpation of area over-
    lying, 309
Pulmonary branch stenosis, heart murmur
    in, 680
Pulmonary disease
  abdominal pain/tenderness caused by,
    383t
  chronic obstructive, anteroposterior di-
    ameter of chest in, 254
  diffuse interstitial, dyspnea associated
    with, 82–83t
Pulmonary embolism
  cough and hemoptysis associated with,
    84t
  dyspnea associated with, 82–83t
  syncope associated with, 102–103t
Pulmonary fibrosis, idiopathic, dyspnea
    associated with, 82–83t
Pulmonary function, clinical assessment
    of, 267
Pulmonary vein, 279
Pulmonic ejection sound, 326t
Pulmonic regurgitation, murmur associ-
    ated with, 328t
Pulmonic stenosis, murmur associated
    with, 328t, 681
Pulmonic valve, 279
  auscultation of sounds and murmurs
    originating in, 284, 310, 328t
Pulse amplitude, assessment of, 292–294
Pulse contour, assessment of, 292–294
Pulse pressure, 287
  in infants and children, 639–640
  widened, 291
Pulses
  arterial, 287–288, 461–462
    abnormalities of, 322t
    age-related changes in, 466
    alternating amplitudes of (pulsus al-
      ternans), 316, 322t
    in aneurysm identification, 467, 469
    in arm, 292, 293–294, 461, 467–468
    assessment of, 292–294, 467–468,
      468–471
      tips on, 471
    diminished/absent, 469, 478t
    in infants and children, 678–679
    large and bounding, 322t
    in leg, 298, 462, 468–471
    normal, 322t
    paradoxical, 317, 322t
    small and weak, 322t
  venous, jugular, 289, 299–230, 301

carotid pulsations differentiated from,
    300t
Pulsus alternans, 316, 322t
Puncta (lacrimal), 165
Pupillary reactions, 168–169
  autonomic supply to eye and, 169
  in coma/stupor, 600, 618t
  in infants, 663, 663–664
  testing, 188–189, 570
Pupils
  abnormalities of, 217t
  age-related changes in, 182
  Argyll Robertson, 189, 217t
  in coma/stupor, 600, 618t, 619t
  dilation of for ophthalmoscopic exami-
    nation, 191
    contraindications to, 191, 664
    in infants, 664
  equal, one blind eye and, 217t
  examination of, 188–189
    in coma/stupor, 600
    in infant, 663
  Marcus Gunn, 208
  small and irregular, 189, 217t
  tonic (Adie's), 189, 217t
  unequal (anisocoria), 188, 217t
Purgatives, osmotic, diarrhea caused by
    abuse of, 90–91t
Purpura, 156t
  actinic, 147
Purulent sputum, 53
Pustule, 153t, 160t, 161t
P wave, of electrocardiogram, 285, 286
Pyloric stenosis, abdominal examination
    and, 683
Pyogenic granuloma, of gums (pregnancy
    tumor/epulis), 240t
Pyramidal (corticospinal) tract, 562, 563
  damage to, 562
Pyrexia, 143. *See also* Fever

Q
QRS complex, of electrocardiogram, 285,
    286
Quadrantic visual field defects, 185, 212t
Quadriceps femoris muscle, 502, 503
Quadriplegia, 576
Quadruple rhythm, 327t
Q wave, of electrocardiogram, 285

R
Radial artery, 461
  testing patency of, 475
Radial deviation, assessment of, 517
Radial nerve, testing function of, 518
Radial pulse, 461, 467
  for heart rate assessment, 292
Radicular pain, assessment of, 540
Radiocarpal (wrist) joint, 492
Radiohumeral joint, 491
Radioulnar joint, 491
  distal, 492
Radius, 490
  distal, 491
    examination of, 515
Range of motion

assessing, 507
  at ankles and feet, 538
  at elbow, 514
  at feet and ankles, 538
  at hip, 527–530
  at knee, 534–536
  at neck, in infant, 657
  at shoulder, 510
  at spine, 522–524
  at temporomandibular joint, 509
  at wrist and hand, 517–518
  in infants, 690
  limited, describing, 541
Rape, 410
Rapid alternating movements, assessing,
    582–583
Rapport with patient, health history inter-
    view and, 6–7, 7
  with children, 24
Rash, joint pain and, 69
Raspberry tongue, 675
Raynaud's disease/phenomenon, 96–97t,
    467
Reading ability, assessment of in inter-
    view, 32
Reassurance, in interviewing, 13
Rebound tenderness, peritoneal inflamma-
    tion/appendicitis and, 364, 376
  referred, 377
Recent (short-term) memory, 107. *See also*
    Memory
  assessment of, 117–118
Recession of gums, 241t
Rectal examination, 451–454
  for cancer screening, 379, 453, 456
  in children, 690
  in females, 134, 418–419, 454
    lubricants for, contamination of, 419
    in pregnant patient, 442–443
  in infants, 687–688
  in males, 134, 451–454
  in prostate cancer screening, 455
Rectal shelf, 454, 458t
Rectal temperature, 143
  in infants and children, 639
  normal, 143
  in stupor/coma, 599
Rectocele, 424t
  in pregnant patient, 442
  uterine prolapse and, 428t
Rectosigmoid cancer. *See also* Rectum, can-
    cer of
  sigmoidoscopy in identification of, 451
Rectouterine pouch (pouch of Douglas),
    406, 407
Rectovaginal examination, 418–419
  lubricants for, contamination of, 419
  in pregnant patient, 443
Rectum, 449–459. *See also under* Rectal
  abnormalities of, 457–458t
  anatomy and physiology of, 449, 450
  cancer of, 453, 458t
    constipation associated with, 89t
    screening for, 379, 453, 456
  examination of
    for cancer screening, 379, 453, 456
    in females, 134, 418–419, 454
      lubricants for, contamination of, 419

in pregnant patient, 442–443
in males, 134, 451–453
polyps of, 458t
prolapse of, 458t
Rectus abdominis muscle, 355
Rectus muscles of eye, 169, 170
Red eyes, 47, 187, 215t
Redness
joint, 69, 508
in peripheral vascular disease, 67
Red reflex, 192
in infants, 664
Red spots/streaks, in ocular fundus, 222t
Reference, delusions of, 115t
Referral source, in health history, 2, 35
recording, 722
Referred pain
abdominal, 56
to back, 100t
Reflection, in interviewing, 12
Reflexes. *See also specific type*
abdominal, 561, 593
in aging patient, 568
cutaneous, 561
deep tendon/spinal, 560–561, 590–596
in central nervous system disorders,
614t
eliciting, 561, 590
reinforcement for, 590, 591
in infants, 696–697
in pregnant patient, 444
in infants, 695, 697–701
oculocephalic (doll's-eye movements),
in coma/stupor, 601
oculovestibular, in coma/stupor, 601
plantar, 561
in pregnant patient, 444
Reflex hammer, 590
Reflux, gastroesophageal, cough and hemoptysis associated with, 84t
Reflux esophagitis, chest pain associated
with, 80–81t
Refractive errors, headache associated
with, 74–75t
Regional enteritis (Crohn's disease), diarrhea associated with, 90–91t
Regurgitation, 57
Reinforcement, in testing reflexes, 590, 591
Relationship to person and things. *See* Ori-
entation
Reliability
of data, 711
of data source in health history, 2, 35
Religious affiliations/beliefs, information
about in health history, 37
Remote (long-term) memory, 107. *See also*
Memory
assessment of, 117
Renal agenesis (Potter's syndrome), auri-
cle abnormalities in, 666
Renal colic, 60
Renal disease, edema in, 480t
Reproductive physiology, 431–435, 434t
Resonance, 259t
in selected chest disorders, 274t
Respiration (breathing), 251–252. *See also
under Respiratory*
abnormalities in, 269t

age-related changes in, 252
assessment of, 253–254
in children, 678
in infants, 672, 676–678
in children, 678
deep, apnea alternating with
(Cheyne–Stokes breathing), 269t
in coma, 618t
in infants, 672, 676–678
muscles of, 251
accessory, 251
use of, 253
age-related changes in, 252
rate and rhythm of
abnormalities of, 269t
assessment of, 253
in coma/stupor, 600, 618t
in infants and children, 640, 677, 678
normal, 269t
in stupor/coma, 599, 600, 618t
Respiratory expansion, assessment of, 255,
264
Respiratory irritants, cough and hemoptysis associated with, 84t
Respiratory muscles, 251
accessory, 251
use of, 253
age-related changes in, 252
Respiratory rate and rhythm
abnormalities in, 269t
assessment of, 253
in infants and children, 640, 677, 678
normal, 269t
Respiratory system
physical signs in selected disorders of,
274–275t
in review of systems, 38
upper, viral infection of, cervical lymphadenopathy in, 660t
Resting (static) tremor, 610t
Restless legs syndrome, 71
Rest pain, in arteriosclerosis obliterans,
96–97t
Retching, 57
Retention cysts
cervical (nabothian), 425t
oral, in infants, 671
Reticular activating (arousal) system, 556
Retina
coloboma of, 224t
examination of, 193–194
lesions of, 194
ophthalmoscopic visualization of, 166
in visual pathway, 167
Retinal arteries, 193–194, 193t
arteriovenous crossing and, 221t
in hypertension, 221t
normal, 221t
Retinal detachment, in infants, 664
Retinal hemorrhages
deep, 222t
in infants, 664–665
superficial, 222t
Retinal veins, 193–194, 193t
Retinoblastoma, in infants, 664
Retinopathy
diabetic
fundus changes in, 222t, 224t, 227t

nonproliferative, 227t
proliferative, 222t, 224t, 227t
hypertensive
fundus changes in, 226t
macular star and, 227t
of prematurity, 664
Retracted drum, 230t
Retracted lid, 213t
Retracted nipple, 341
Retroflexion, of uterus, 429t
Retrograde filling (Trendelenburg) test,
474
Retroversion, of uterus, 417
rectovaginal palpation in assessment of,
419
Review of systems, 3, 3–4
in adult, 37–39
patient with multiple symptoms and, 30
recording data from, 725–726
Rhagades, in congenital syphilis, 658t
Rheumatic fever, acute, heart murmurs
caused by, 680
Rheumatoid arthritis, 98–99t
juvenile, mandibular overgrowth in,
674–675
wrists and hands in, 515, 547t
Rheumatoid nodules
of ear, 229t
of elbow, 513, 546t
of hand, 547t
Rhinitis, 49
perennial allergic, 672–673
facies in, 659t
Rhinorrhea, 49
Rhomboid muscles, 488
Rhonchi, 262, 262t, 263, 272t
Ribs, 245
counting, 246–247
fractured, identification of, 267
Rickets, craniotabes in, 654
Riedel's lobe, 385t
Right atrium, 278, 279
Right-handed approach, for physical examination, 132
Right second interspace, 304
auscultation at, 310
inspection and palpation of, 309
Right-sided congestive heart failure,
edema in, 480t
Right ventricle, 277, 278, 279
variations and abnormalities of im-
pulses of, 323t
Right ventricular area (left sternal border),
304
inspection and palpation of, 307
Rigidity, 612t
decerebrate, 602, 620t
decorticate, 602, 620t
Rings
esophageal, dysphagia associated with,
85t
in optic disc, 219t
Rinne test, 133, 198, 233t
Romberg test, 585
Roof of mouth, examination of, 201
Rooting reflex, 697–698
Roseola infantum, occipital lymphadenopathy in, 660t

Rotary nystagmus, 606t
Rotation, assessing
  at hip, 530
  at neck, 522
  at spine, 524
Rotation test, 700
Rotator cuff, 488
  examination of, 511–512
  tears of, 511–512, 544t
Rotator cuff tendinitis, 544t
Rovsing's sign, in appendicitis assessment, 377
Rubella, occipital lymphadenopathy in, 660t
Rubeola (measles), Koplik's spots in, 238t, 673
Rubor, in arterial insufficiency, 476, 478t
R wave, of electrocardiogram, 285

S

S₁ (first heart sound), 281, 324t
  assessment of, 302–303, 310, 312t
  in infants and children, 679
  relationship of to electrocardiogram, 286
  splitting of, 283, 312t, 324t
  variations in, 324t
S₂ (second heart sound), 281
  assessment of, 302–303, 310, 312t
  in infants and children, 679
  relationship of to electrocardiogram, 286
  splitting of, 283, 312, 312t, 325t
    age-related changes in, 290
    in infants and children, 679
  variations in, 325t
S₃ (third heart sound), 282, 327t
  age and, 290
  assessment of, 310, 311, 312t
    inspection and palpation in, 303, 307
  physiologic, 327
S₄ (fourth heart sound), 282, 327t
  age and, 290
  assessment of, 310, 311, 312t
    inspection and palpation in, 303, 307
  relationship of to electrocardiogram, 286
Saber shins, in congenital syphilis, 658t
Sacral edema, 474
Sacral pain, 55
Sacral promontory, 356
Sacrococcygeal area, examination of, 452
Sacroiliac joint, 499
  examination of, 521
Saddle nose, in congenital syphilis, 658t
Safety awareness/precautions, information about in health history
    in adult, 37
    in child, 41–42
    recording, 724
Sagittal suture, 653
Saliva, in newborn, 672
Salpingitis
  acute, abdominal pain/tenderness caused by, 383t
  in pelvic inflammatory disease, 430t
Salpingo-oophoritis, in pelvic inflammatory disease, 430t
Salt retention, renal, edema in, 480t
Saphenous veins, 463
  varicose, 473

Sarcoidosis, dyspnea associated with, 82–83t
Sarcoma, Kaposi's, in HIV infection/AIDS, 157t
  of gums, 240t
  of palate, 237t
Scabies, burrow of, 154t
Scale, 153t
Scalene muscles, 251, 252
Scalp, examination of, 184
Scalp infections, in infants and children
  acute posterior cervical lymphadenitis in, 660t
  occipital lymphadenopathy in, 660t
  preauricular lymphadenopathy in, 660t
Scalp veins, assessment of in infant, 653
Scapula, 487, 494
  coracoid process of, 488, 510
  Sprengel's deformity of, 520
  winging of, 520, 597
Scapular line, 249
Scapulohumeral muscles, 488
Scapulothoracic articulation, 487
Scar, 154t
Scarf sign, 616, 627t
Scheuermann's disease, kyphosis in, 550t
Schizoaffective disorder, 126t
Schizophrenia, 126t
Schizophreniform disorder, 126t
Schooling, in child health history, 41
Sciatica, 100t
Sciatic nerve, 500
  examination of, 521–522
Scissoring, 698, 699
Scissors gait, 616t
Sclera, 164
  examination of, 187
  in infant, 663
Scleroderma, dysphagia associated with, 85t
Scoliosis, 520, 551t, 695
  shoulder asymmetry in, 509
Scotomas, 47
Scratch test, 685
Screening tests
  for breast cancer, 351
  Denver Developmental, 631, 632–633
  information about in health history
    in adult, 37
    in child, 41
    recording, 723
  in mental status assessment, 73
  visual field, 185
Scrotal edema, 401t
  in infants, 686
Scrotal hernia, 396, 400t
Scrotal swelling, 394
Scrotal (fissured) tongue, 242t
Scrotum, 387, 388
  abnormalities of, 66, 400–401t
  age-related changes in, 389, 390
  examination of, 393–394, 686–687
  in infants, 686–687
Sebaceous glands, 145, 146
Seborrheic keratosis, 147, 157t
Secondary amenorrhea, 63
Second-degree atrioventricular block, 320t
Second heart sound, 281

assessment of, 302–303, 310, 312, 312t
  in infants and children, 679
  relationship of to electrocardiogram, 286
  splitting of, 283, 312, 312t, 325t
    age-related changes in, 290
    in infants and children, 679
  variations in, 325t
Secretory diarrhea, 90–91t
Seizure disorders, 70, 104–105t
Self-awareness, 16
Self-examination
  breast, 347–348
  testicular, 397
Semen, 388
Semilunar valves, 279
Semimembranosus bursa, 504
Seminal vesicle, 388
Senile ptosis, 182
Sensation. *See also specific type*
  assessment of, 135, 586–589
    in infants, 696–697
    patterns of testing for, 586–587
  in central nervous system disorders, 614t
  in infants, 696–697
  lost or altered, 71, 564–565
    mapping boundaries of, 586, 587
    symmetry and, 586
Sensitivity, 711
  calculating, 712–714
  in data collection and assessment, 715–716
Sensorineural hearing loss, 47–48, 172, 197–198, 232–233t
Sensorineural phase of hearing, 172
Sensory ataxia, 617t
Sensory cortex, 564, 565
Sensory (afferent) fibers, 560
Sensory mapping, 586, 587
Sensory pathways, 564–567
  lesions of, 564–565
Sensory receptors, 564
Sensory system. *See also Sensation*
  examination of, 135, 586–589
    patterns of testing in, 586–587
  symptoms related to, 71
Sentinel tag, 457t
Septum, nasal, 133
  deviated, 198, 199
  examination of, 199
Serial 7's, for testing attention, 117
Serous effusion, 231t
Serous otitis media, 231t, 670
Serratus anterior muscle, 333, 488
Sex maturity ratings
  in females, 137–139, 336, 406–409, 412, 689
    breast development and, 336, 341, 409
    pubic hair development and, 336, 337, 408, 409, 412
  in males, 390, 391, 392, 688
Sexual abuse, of child, examination of vagina and cervix and, 689
Sexual development, 137–139, 141
  assessment of
    in females, 336, 337, 341, 407–409, 412, 689
    in males, 389–391, 392, 688

Tympanosclerosis, 230t
Tympany, 259t
in abdomen, 362
in ascites assessment, 374, 375
in selected chest disorders, 275t

U

Ulcerative colitis, diarrhea associated
with, 90–91t
Ulcers
aphthous (canker sores), 200–201, 243t
nasal, 199
neuropathic, 479t
of foot, 553t
peptic, abdominal pain/tenderness associated with, 86–87t
skin, 153t, 160t
in arterial insufficiency, 478t, 479t
in venous insufficiency, 473, 478t, 479t
of tongue, 201
Ulna, 490
distal, 491
examination of, 515
Ulnar artery, 461
testing patency of, 475
Ulnar deviation, assessment of, 517
Ulnar nerve, 491
testing function of, 518
Ulnar nerve compression, 515
Ulnar pulse, 461
assessment of, 475
Umbilical artery, single, 682
Umbilical cord, examination of at birth,
682
Umbilical hernia, 380t
in infants, 682
Umbilical region, 356
Umbilicus, 355
amnioticus, 682
cutis, 682
examination of, 358
in newborn, 682
Umbo, 171, 196
Underbite (mandibular protrusion),
674–675
Undescended testicle (cryptorchidism),
394, 401t, 686, 688
Unreality, feelings of, 115t
Upper motor neurons, 561
damage to
facial paralysis caused by, 608–609t
spasticity caused by, 612t
Upper respiratory tract infections, viral,
cervical lymphadenopathy in,
660t
Ureteral pain/colic, 60
Urethra
in females, 406
bulges and swelling of, 424t
in males, 387, 388
Urethral caruncle, 424t
Urethral meatus/orifice
in females, 405
examination of, 412
in infants, 687
in males, 387, 388
discharge from, 66, 393

in infants, 686
position of, 393, 686
Urethral mucosa, prolapse of, 424t
Urethral stricture, 393
Urethritis
in females, 413
gonococcal, 393, 413
joint pain and, 69
in males, 393
painful urination and, 60
Urge incontinence, 61, 94–95t
Urinary bladder. See Bladder
Urinary frequency, 61, 92t, 93t
in pregnancy, 434t
Urinary hesitancy, 61, 62
Urinary incontinence, 61–62, 94–95t
Urinary stream, changes in, 61, 62
Urinary system. See also specific structure or
organ
in review of systems, 38
symptoms related to, 60–62, 92–95t
Urinary urgency, 61, 94–95t
Urination
nonpainful symptoms associated with,
61–62
painful, 60–61
Urine, color of, 62
in jaundiced patient, 59
Urticaria, 161t
Uterine contractions, during abdominal
palpation, 440
Uterus, 406
abnormalities of, 428t
bicornuate, 443
myomas (fibroids) of, 428t
in pregnant patient, 443
palpation of, 417
positions of, 428–429t
pregnant, 433–434, 443
location of, 356, 432, 433
size of, 436
prolapse of, 428t
retroflexion of, 429t
retroversion of, 417, 429t
rectovaginal palpation in assessment
of, 419
Uvula, 177, 178
examination of, 202

V

Vagina, 405, 406
age-related changes in, 409
bulges and swelling of, 424t
carcinoma of, DES exposure and, 426t
examination of, 416, 687
in infants, 687
in pregnant patient, 433, 442
Vaginal adenosis, DES exposure and, 426t
Vaginal bleeding, in prepubertal female,
690
Vaginal discharge, 64
in adolescents, 690
in infants, 687
in pregnancy, 434t, 442
Vaginal speculum, 411–412
for examination of pregnant patient,
438, 442

insertion of, 413–414
Vaginal vestibule, 405
in infants, 687
Vaginal walls
assessing support of, 413
in pregnant patient, 442
inspection of, in pregnant patient, 442
Vaginismus, 65
Vaginitis, 427t
during pregnancy, 433
Vaginosis, bacterial, 427t
Vagus nerve (cranial nerve X), 558
examination of, 573
functions of, 559t, 569
pharyngeal findings in paralysis of, 202,
573
Valgus stress, 535t
Validation, in interviewing, 13
Validity, of data, 711
Valsalva maneuver, systolic murmurs affected by, 316, 317t
Values, 16
Valves
cardiac, 279
in cardiac cycle, 280–282
of Houston, 449, 450
venous, 463
evaluating competency of, 474
Varicocele, 394, 400t
Varicose veins
hemorrhoidal
external, 458t
internal, 458t
in pregnant patient, 442
in leg, 444, 473
mapping, 473
in pregnant patient, 444
around tongue (caviar lesions), 243t
Varus stress, 535t
Vascular disease, prevention of, 477
Vascular headaches
migraine, 74–75t
toxic, 74–75t
Vascular skin lesions, 156t
in infants, 651
Vascular system, peripheral, 134, 461–482
age-related changes in, 466
anatomy and physiology of, 461–466
arteries in, 461–462
capillary bed in, 465–466
examination of, 134, 467–476
in bedfast patient, 474
special techniques in, 473–476
fluid exchange and, 465–466
health promotion and counseling and,
477
lymphatics in, 464–465
lymph nodes and, 464–465
painful disorders of, 67, 96–97t, 478t
disorders mimicking, 67, 96–97t
in review of systems, 39
symptoms related to, 67, 96–97t
veins in, 462–463
Vas deferens, 387, 388
Vasodepressor syncope (fainting/common
faint), 70, 102–103t
Veins, 462–463. See also specific named vein
age-related changes in, 291, 466